NURSING,
PHYSICIAN CONTROL,
AND THE MEDICAL
MONOPOLY

NURSING, PHYSICIAN CONTROL, AND THE MEDICAL MONOPOLY

Historical Perspectives on Gendered Inequality in Roles, Rights, and Range of Practice

THETIS M. GROUP
JOAN I. ROBERTS

Indiana University Press
Bloomington and Indianapolis

This book is a publication of

Indiana University Press
601 North Morton Street
Bloomington, IN 47404-3797 USA

http://www.indiana.edu/~iupress

Telephone orders   800-842-6796
Fax orders   812-855-7931
Orders by e-mail   iuporder@indiana.edu

The paper used in this publication meets the
minimum requirements of American National
Standard for Information Sciences—Permanence
of Paper for Printed Library Materials, ANSI
Z39.48-1984.

Manufactured in the United States of America

Library of Congress Cataloging-in-Publication Data

Group, Thetis M.
   Nursing, physician control, and the medical monopoly : historical perspectives on
gendered inequality in roles, rights, range of practice / Thetis M. Group, Joan I.
Roberts.
      p.   cm.
   Includes bibliographical references and index.
   ISBN 0-253-33926-X (cl : alk. paper)
      1. Nurse and physician—History. 2. Sexism in medicine—History.
   3. Feminism—History. 4. Nursing—History. 5. Nursing—Social aspects—History.
   6. Discrimination against women—History.   I. Roberts, Joan I.   II. Title.
      [DNLM: 1. Physician-Nurse Relations. 2. Nursing—Trends. 3. Prejudice.
   4. Women's Rights. WY 87 G882n 2001]
   RT86.4 .G76 2001
   610.73′09—dc21
                                                                      00-069714

1   2   3   4   5   06   05   04   03   02   01

In loving memory

My mother
Thetis Miller Group
1899–1992

My father
Dr. Edward F. Group, Sr.
1897–1995

My brother
Dr. Edward F. Group, Jr.
1935–1990

CONTENTS

ACKNOWLEDGMENTS

Funding assistance for manuscript preparation has been provided by the Omicron Chapter of Sigma Theta Tau (Syracuse University College of Nursing), the Syracuse University Senate Research Committee, the Syracuse University Small Grants Program, and Syracuse University Office of Research. Special thanks are extended to Ben Ware, Vice President of the Office of Research, who believed in our project and provided financial support throughout the manuscript revisions. We also extend our thanks for the library support and professional assistance provided by Dr. Linda K. Amos, Associate Vice President for Health Sciences, University of Utah, and Dr. Imogene Rigdon, Associate Dean, University of Utah College of Nursing.

We especially appreciate Irene Quinlan, who is not only a superb typist and formatter, but a contextual editor as well. She spent many hours helping prepare the manuscript for submission, always giving us invaluable assistance in critiquing meaning and consistency. We are fortunate indeed to have had her expertise in preparing this book for publication.

Thetis M. Group
Joan I. Roberts
Scottsdale, Arizona, 2001

Acknowledgments for the Use of Quoted Material

Quotes from G. I. Alfano, K. Kowalski, L. R. Levin, and G. B. McFadden (1976, Fall), "Prerequisite for Nurse-Physician Collaboration: Nursing Autonomy," *Nursing Administration Quarterly, 1,* 1, pp. 45–63, reprinted with the permission of Aspen Publishers, Inc.

Quotes from D.C. Celentano (1982), "The Optimum Utilization and Appropriate Responsibilities of Allied Health Professionals," *Social Science and Medicine, 16,* pp. 687–698, reprinted with the permission of Elsevier Science.

Quotes from D. Diers and S. Molde (1979), "Some Conceptual and Methodological Issues in Nurse Practitioner Research," *Research in Nursing and Health, 2,* pp. 73–84, reprinted with the permission of [Jossey-Bass, Inc./Wiley-Liss, Inc., a subsidiary of] John Wiley and Sons, Inc.

Quotes from A. K. Dolan (1980, Winter), "Antitrust Law and Physician Dominance of Other Health Practitioners," *Journal of Health Politics, Policy and Law, 4* (4), pp. 675–691, reprinted with the permission of Duke University Press.

Quotes from R. Froh (1988, Sept./Oct.), "An Interview with AMA's James Sammons: Responding to Critics of the RCT Proposal," *Nursing Economic$, 6*

(5), pp. 221–230, reprinted with permission of the publisher, Jannetti Publications, Inc.

Quotes from M. Godfrey (1978), "Job Satisfaction—Or Should That Be Dissatisfaction?" *Nursing '78, 8* (4), pp. 89–102, reprinted with the permission of Springhouse Corporation.

Quotes from M. J. Hughes (1968), *Women Healers in Medieval Life and Literature,* reprinted with the permission of Ayer Company Publishers.

Quotes from T. Ingles (1976, Spring), "The Physicians' View of the Evolving Nursing Profession: 1873–1913," *Nursing Forum, 15* (2), pp. 123–164, reprinted with the permission of NurseCom, Inc.

Quotes from B. J. Kalisch and P. A. Kalisch (1984, May), "The Dionne Quintuplets Legacy: Establishing the 'Good Doctor and His Loyal Nurse' Image in American Culture," *Nursing and Health Care, 5* (5), pp. 242–250, reprinted with the permission of Technomic Publishing Co., Inc.

Quotes from B. Keddy, M. J. Gillis, P. Jacobs, H. Burton, and M. Rogers (1986), "The Doctor-Nurse Relationship: A Historical Perspective," *Journal of Advanced Nursing, 11* (6), pp. 745–753, reprinted with the permission of Blackwell Science Ltd., U.K.

Quotes from N. Krantzler (1986), "Media Images of Physicians and Nurses in the United States," *Social Science and Medicine, 22* (9), pp. 933–952, reprinted with the permission of Elsevier Science.

Quotes from D. Mechanic and L. Aiken (1982, September), "A Cooperative Agenda for Medicine and Nursing," *New England Journal of Medicine, 307* (12), pp. 747–750, reprinted with the permission of Massachusetts Medical Society. All rights reserved.

Quotes from B. Melosh (1983), "Doctors, Patients, and 'Big Nurse': Work and Gender in the Postwar Hospital," in *Nursing History: New Perspectives, New Possibilities,* ed. E. C. Lagemann, pp. 157–179, reprinted with the permission of Teachers College Press, Teachers College, Columbia University. All rights reserved.

Quotes from L. Newton (1981, June), "In Defense of the Traditional Nurse," *Nursing Outlook, 29* (6), pp. 348–354, reprinted with the permission of Mosby, Inc.

Quotes from "Responses to 'Traditional Nurse,'" *Nursing Outlook, 29* (9), pp. 500–503, reprinted with the permission of Mosby, Inc.

Quotes from S. M. Reverby (1987), *Ordered to Care: The Dilemma of American Nursing, 1850–1945*, reprinted with the permission of Cambridge University Press.

Quotes from S. Rothman (1978), *Woman's Proper Place*, reprinted with the permission of Perseus Books Group.

Quotes from B. Safriet (1992, Summer), "Health-care Dollars and Regulatory Sense: The Role of Advanced Practice Nursing," *Yale Journal on Regulation, 9* (2), pp. 417–488, reprinted with the permission of *Yale Journal on Regulation*.

Quotes from M. C. Versluysen (1980), "Old Wives' Tales? Women Healers in English History," in *Rewriting Nursing History*, ed. C. Davis, pp. 175–199, reprinted with the permission of Barnes and Noble Books–Imports. World rights granted by Routledge Ltd., London.

Quotes from K. Williams (1980), "From Sarah Gamp to Florence Nightingale: A Critical Study of Hospital Nursing Systems from 1840–1897," in *Rewriting Nursing History*, ed. C. Davis, pp. 41–75, reprinted with the permission of Barnes and Noble Books–Imports. World rights granted by Routledge Ltd., London.

Quotes from A. Yankauer and J. Sullivan (1982), "The New Health Professionals: Three Examples," *Annual Review of Public Health, 3*, pp. 249–276, reprinted with the permission of Annual Reviews.

GENERAL INTRODUCTION*

Over the past three decades, significant changes have occurred in the nursing profession and in the conventional societal definitions of women and their roles. As the women's movement reemerged in the late 1960s and many women refused to uphold the traditional roles allocated to them, a parallel trend in nursing centered on the development of "expanded" roles for nurses: the "independent" practitioner, nurse clinician, and nurse practitioner. As these professional and societal trends gained momentum in the 1970s, the conflicts inherent in integrating professional and gender roles became overt and critically important. In nursing it became obvious that it would be improbable, if not impossible, to prepare assertive, independent nurse practitioners if they were socialized to be dependent females. Similarly, it is improbable, if not impossible, for female nurses to implement expanded roles if they are unaware of or unwilling to recognize the social constraints imposed on them because they are women. Indeed, the successes or failures of the nursing profession in its struggle to grow in stature and gain autonomy during its long history cannot be fully understood unless they are integrally linked to the relationship between gender and professional roles as these have changed over time.

Women in nursing have not consistently or systematically documented these interrelationships; thus, the analysis of nurses' perceptions of themselves as both women and nurses has only recently emerged. Ironically, nursing, one of the few occupations available to women in the industrial period, has seldom and only recently been the subject of women's studies scholars. The absence of an extended dialogue between women scholars in the broader academic community and women in nursing has led to difficulties in understanding nursing as a predominantly woman's profession. On one hand, some feminists have advised women to enter medicine, believing nursing to be subservient—a model of professional domesticity. On the other hand, some women in nursing have seen the women's movement as peripheral to their long fight for independent professional status. Both inside and outside of nursing, women have too often neglected or misperceived each other because of a fundamental misunderstanding of the historical relationship of the nursing profession to the general societal subordination of women.

Documenting a Lineage of Concern

In the summer of 1975 a preliminary bibliography developed by the authors for a course on nursing and women's studies produced scanty and sparse

---

*Readers who have read our previous book(s) in this series may wish to skim this section and proceed to the overview to this volume.

published materials on gender and professional roles of nurses; at that time, no centralized and comprehensive bibliographic sources related to this issue could be located. This contrasted sharply with more extensive bibliographic sources on women as physicians, women as health-care consumers, and the politics of sexism in the health-care system, all areas of considerable long-term interest to feminists. Indeed, the *Cumulative Index of Nursing and Allied Health Literature* (*CINAHL*) did not include the topics "sexism" (sex discrimination) and "women's rights" (feminism) until 1983, and it was not until 1984 that *CINAHL* was computerized. Thus, a painstaking review of all topics in the nursing literature was required, making our research task more complex.

Feminist scholars have documented the politics of sexism in medicine and health care in the nineteenth century and again in the twentieth century with the reemergence of feminism. For example, Barbara Ehrenreich and Deirdre English in *Complaints and Disorders: The Sexual Politics of Sickness* (1973), Ellen Frankfort in *Vaginal Politics* (1972), Germaine Greer in *The Female Eunuch* (1971), and Barbara Seaman in *Free and Female* (1972) brought issues of discriminatory medical practices against women to the public's notice. From these earlier exposés, books documenting sexist practices in women's health care emerged. In the later 1970s, for example, typical sources included Belita Cowan's *Women's Health Care* (1977); Sheryl B. Ruzek's *The Women's Health Movement: Feminist Alternatives to Medical Control* (1978); Diane K. Kjervik and Ida M. Martinson's *Women in Stress* (1979) and later their work on *Women in Health and Illness* (1986). Continuing the lineage of concern in the 1980s were, for example, Helen I. Marieskind's *Women in the Health Delivery System: Patients, Providers, and Programs* (1980); Margarete Sandelowski's *Women, Health, and Choice* (1980); Elizabeth Fee's *Women and Health: The Politics of Sex in Medicine* (1983); Gena Corea's *The Hidden Malpractice: How American Medicine Mistreats Women* (1985); Ellen Lewin's *Women, Health, and Healing* (1985); Sue Fisher's *In the Patient's Best Interest* (1986); and Alexandra D. Todd's *Intimate Adversaries: Cultural Conflict between Doctors and Women Patients* (1989). In the 1990s, the lineage continued with, for example, Clarice Feinman's *The Criminalization of a Woman's Body* (1992); Helen Roberts's *Women's Health Matters* (1992); Beverly McElmurry, Kathleen Norr, and Randy Parker's *Women's Health and Development: A Global Challenge* (1993); Leslie Doyal's *What Makes Women Sick: Gender and the Political Economy of Health* (1995); Marcia Bayne-Smith's *Race, Gender, and Health* (1996); Judith A. Lewis and Judith Bernstein's *Women's Health: A Relational Perspective across the Life Cycle* (1996); Barbara Laslett, Sally Kohlstedt, Helen Longino, and Evelynn Hammonds's *Gender and Scientific Authority* (1996); and Sheryl B. Ruzek, Virginia I. Oleson, and Adele E. Clarke's *Women's Health: Complexities and Differences* (1997). To his credit, Robert S. Mendelsohn, one of the few male physicians to write on sexism and medicine, made a scathing indictment of medical practices in *Malepractice: How Doctors Manipulate Women* (1982). Equally damning was the exposé by Charles Inlander, Lowell Levin, and Ed Weiner in their book, *Medicine on Trial* (1988).

Much more has been written about sexism and women in medicine than about sexism and women in nursing. Some books of several published over the past four decades analyze the major problems: Carol Lopate's *Women in Medicine* (1968); Margaret Campbell's *Why Should a Girl Go into Medicine?* (1974); Mary Walsh's *Doctors Wanted: No Women Need Apply: Sexual Barriers in the Medical Profession, 1835–1975* (1977); Judith Lorber's *Women Physicians: Careers, Status, and Power* (1984); and Delese Wear's *Women in Medical Education: An Anthology of Experience* (1996).

Even with the reemergence of feminism, fewer works appeared on sexism and nursing, but probably the earliest is *Witches, Midwives, and Nurses* (Ehrenreich and English, 1972). This was followed by the historical study of American nursing by Jo Ann Ashley in *Hospitals, Paternalism, and the Role of the Nurse* (1976), and the more sociological analysis, *WomanPower and Health Care,* by Marlene Grissum and Carol Spengler (1976). A later anthology by Janet Muff, *Socialization, Sexism, and Stereotyping* (1982), focused on women's issues in nursing. Although only somewhat concerned with gender and sexism, some later histories on nursing have some relevance, such as *Ordered to Care: The Dilemma of American Nursing, 1850–1945,* by Susan Reverby (1987). In a variety of articles and books, Vern and Bonnie Bullough (e.g., 1978; 1984) and Beatrice and Phillip Kalisch (1977; 1983; 1984a; 1984b) have contributed most consistently to issues of sexism and gender in nursing from historical perspectives. Two more recent histories of nursing specifically focused on sexism and nursing are our own book, Joan I. Roberts and Thetis M. Group, *Feminism and Nursing: An Historical Perspective on Power, Status, and Political Activism in the Nursing Profession* (1995), and Sandra Lewenson's *Taking Charge: Nursing, Suffrage, and Feminism in America, 1873–1920* (1993). In addition, with the founding of the International History of Nursing Society in 1980 (renamed the American Association for the History of Nursing in 1983), the *Nursing History Review,* inaugurated by the association in 1993, has included some relevant articles on sexism and nursing and is a welcome resource for contemporary nursing history research scholars.

Nevertheless, the general paucity of sources focused specifically on gender and nursing forced a historical search of materials published by women in nursing and by scholars from other disciplines. From these sources, hundreds of articles and books were analyzed for possible relevance to this key area of concern. The organization and analysis of these sources confirmed the compellingly important influence of gender stratification and sex discrimination within the health occupations, in which about 70 percent of the workers are female. Discrimination, as documented in all social systems, adversely affects the individual nurse as well as her or his profession. Sexism is particularly important in understanding the development of the nursing profession, since it is almost totally female (95 percent).

Our primary focus has been to analyze the voices of nurses themselves, and of some non-nurses who have been concerned with gender issues in nursing. We have tried to stay as close to the words of the authors as possible, providing synthesis with other sources and critical analyses as appropriate. Our perspective is clearly directed toward women and their problems. Using sources only from English-speaking countries, we found that some of the writings are very sophisticated and some less so; thus, our syntheses and analyses are subject to both the quality and the quantity of published works. Since these are differentially distributed in varied cultures, the extent to which crossnational integration is possible also changes with the topics considered. For example, the interconnections between gender and expanded roles are more likely to be considered, even if only indirectly, in American sources. In comparison, British sources have been very concerned with the impact of men in nursing. Thus, the crosscultural emphasis varies according to the sources available. Similarly, subcultural linkages among gender, race, and class are also limited to what is available in the literature. These linkages are infrequently made by many authors; thus, the interconnections among different forms of discrimination have yet to be fully explored.

Ironically, in analyzing the published literature, it has been difficult to find writings from some historical periods that systematically express the interrelation of gender and nursing as a woman's profession. Nevertheless, we can establish and demonstrate a lineage of concern about women's roles, sex discrimination, health care, and nursing that extends over a century. In the writings of nurses themselves, there is great diversity in awareness of sex discrimination as a phenomenon to which all women are subjected. Thus, it is common to find in the earlier sources an underlying assumption that a gender-stratification system exists, for example, in economics and nursing, but no explication of that fact in the analyses presented. Also, it is common to find articles that do explicate facets of gender, such as in writings on nurses as mother surrogates, but do not within the body of the work implicate *systematic* sexism. In contrast, some women, even in the earlier periods, were acutely aware of the gender-stratification system and clearly espoused feminist principles in their writings. Though we have chosen to focus on those sources that exhibit some understanding of the effects of sex discrimination and gender on the nursing profession, some nurses even now seem to be caught in the traditional subordination of women and exhibit little understanding of their own subjugation. The variations in current tactics and strategies for change still reflect the diversity of opinion on what a woman should be and what a "woman's" profession should be; thus, achieving political consensus in nursing has been extremely difficult.

Historically, there is a lack of a consistent theoretical position related to gender and a woman's profession; thus, it is difficult to analyze the historical materials from a coherent theoretical perspective. It was not until the 1980s that nurses themselves attempted to connect feminist theory to fundamental issues in nursing. Perhaps the best initial work comes from Peggy L. Chinn and Charlene Eldridge Wheeler (1985), who were among the first nurses to elaborate on four philosophic approaches in feminist theory as they applied to nurses and nursing. Liberal feminism, stemming from a civil libertarian emphasis on equal rights, stresses equal opportunity for women relative to men. Marxist feminist theory originates in social structural thinking in which women and children are regarded as property within each social class. Socialist feminist theory goes beyond traditional class analysis to focus on the integral relation between the private sphere of person, family, and reproduction and the public sphere of production and labor. Radical feminism arises from a woman-centered worldview and postulates that women's oppression is a fundamental universal experience. Chinn and Wheeler emphasize that feminism is not to be equated with lesbian ideologies; rather, "it is committed to ending the isolation and divisiveness that exist among women in male-defined systems, advocating that women value themselves and other women" (p. 75).

What are the commonalities between feminist and nursing theory? Chinn and Wheeler propose that some concepts are essentially harmonious, such as the integral unity of human existence and environment, the interactive processes of caring and nurturing that are devalued by patriarchal systems, and reverence for life, for environment, and for individual uniqueness. Feminism adds the systematic analysis of oppression and power that, when applied to nursing, helps explain the devaluation of nursing, the low affiliation with others who are seen as "powerless" in professional associations, and the frequent emulation of the powerful, as reflected in the medical model. But the analysis of power is not necessarily the enactment of power. It is a very common finding over the past three centuries that women who have written powerfully in behalf of women, or activists who have moved politically against discrimination, have taken the brunt of societal condemnation by men and even some women. In general, women can be activists as long as they agitate in behalf of others—children, sanitation, health, morality, and so on—but not for themselves. The most frequent accusation against activist women is that they are "unwomanly"; sometimes accusations of insanity and immorality have been directed toward women leaders. Perhaps the most distressing stereotypes have been "mannishness," common in the nineteenth century, and "queer" or lesbian, common in the twentieth century. These stereotypes are intended to demean and trivialize feminists as well as weaken the unity among them. It is clear that feminism cannot be for only some women; it must be for all women of whatever race, creed, religion, or lifestyle. Without this unity, the masculist game of divide and conquer can be played out indefinitely.

Although it would have been ideal, it has not been possible to incorporate all of the feminist theories and research in our books; limitations on manuscript length have precluded this. Of the major feminist theoretical positions, however, the one that has been most consistently apparent in the sources analyzed on gender and nursing is liberal feminism, derived from the liberal or humanistic perspective, originating in the human rights tradition associated with the European or, more particularly, the British philosophical approach emerging in the nineteenth century. This was most eloquently expressed by John Stuart Mill in his book *The Subjection of Women* (1869) and in Harriet Taylor Mill's essay "Enfranchisement of Women" (1851). Thus, most of the sources assume a position based on an equality of rights. Exceptions to this trend can be found earlier, for example, in the work of Lavinia L. Dock (1907; 1909b), who espoused in some of her thinking a more socialist-feminist position and sometimes even a radical-cultural feminism. These perspectives are best represented today by various writers who have been particularly concerned about the economic status of women as nurses, or who have been influenced by radical feminism, sometimes associated with feminist philosopher Mary Daly (1968, 1978), and observed in the thinking and writing of some nurses (e.g., Ashley, 1976, 1980; Campbell, 1981).

Newer perspectives from critical theory, especially feminist deconstructionism, have not predominated in the research and writing about nurses and nursing, although some are evident in recent critiques of nursing education: Allen's 1986 analysis of familialism in nursing textbooks, Hagell's 1989 concern with nursing's overreliance on scientific knowledge and quantitative research to define its knowledge base, and Doering's 1992 feminist poststructuralist viewpoint on the relationship of knowledge to power in nursing. More recently, at the tenth annual International Critical and Feminist Perspectives in Nursing Conference in October 1999, several presentations focused on, for example, deconstructing gender, poststructural analysis of domestic violence, paradigms of epistemology and ontology, and paradigm methodology and transformation. At the eleventh annual conference in October 2000, there was, for example, a critical discourse analysis of stories of "bad nursing" and explorations of the implications for nursing of the poststructural framework. Numerous theories specific to the fields of anthropology, psychology, and sociology clearly have influenced scholars writing about nursing: for example, feminist organizational theory, the role of women in complex organizations, psychological effects of war on nurses, and effects of employment on women and their children. Many of these theories, however, have not been used in a consistent manner to produce cumulative research-based bodies of knowledge.

Until relatively recently, research on gender and nursing has been somewhat limited. Few studies are available from the earlier periods, probably because nursing was yet to be established in university structures in which research was legitimized and expected. As more nurses have achieved advanced degrees, an increasing number of research studies on gender and nursing have appeared, and as more women's studies scholars attend to nursing, more analyses should be expected. Nevertheless, a large number of sources deal with personal expressions of dismay among nurses, and offer only short analyses of specific issues, often derived from the social sciences and, more recently, from feminist writers. These give us a sense of women's perceptions over time of nurses and nursing from a gender perspective.

It is apparent that a strong women's movement has directly affected the nursing profession. For example, at the turn of the century, when even non-feminist women were organizing to achieve the vote and the rhetoric of feminism was widely heard, the movement to strengthen the nursing profession was significant. This same relationship can be observed in the past three decades with the reemergence of feminism. For example, feminist issues such as pay equity are now widely espoused by nurses. Given this trend, however, it is clear that many nurses have followed the lead of women outside the profession, exhibiting a concern for gender issues somewhat later than that expressed by women external to nursing. Yet, a countervailing trend is also apparent: nurses have retained their concern for feminist issues, such as working conditions for women and greater equity between male and female workers, even during periods of extreme gender conservatism. Although an overt feminist analysis is not often apparent in some of their writing, still such efforts could be classified as attempts to achieve greater autonomy and power—both important goals of feminism.

These trends represent only a few of those observable in the history of gender and nursing. All these trends influence the current situation in nursing, and unless gender issues are resolved through the historical analysis of their impact in previous decades, nurses will be unable to make forward progress because they will have little clarity on the essential issues.

Creating New Perspectives for Understanding Nursing History

From the large number of sources collected and analyzed to clarify the effects of gender stratification on nurses and the health-care system, it became clear that one volume alone could not do justice to the complex relationship between the most fundamental social roles, defined by sex in gendered patterns, and the professional roles of nurses, whose lives, work, education, and practice represent in microcosm the realities of and restrictions on women in the general society. Thus, this book is the second of an interrelated set of texts that examine neglected areas in previous writing and research and provide a comprehensive perspective on gender and nursing. Drawing on sources from the United States, Great Britain, Canada, and, to a lesser extent, other predominantly English-speaking countries, the research on which these books is based interrelates historical sources to create new perspectives and to establish a basis for women's studies in nursing, a field until recently overlooked by most scholars.

The attitudes, beliefs, and behaviors that are directed toward women influence all segments of the practice and education of nurses. In the first published text, *Feminism and Nursing: An Historical Perspective on Power, Status, and Political Activism in the Nursing Profession* (Roberts and Group, 1995), the status of women is historically linked to the status of nursing and to nurses' awareness of feminist issues. The second volume in the series is *Nursing, Physician Control, and the Medical Monopoly: Historical Perspectives on Gendered Inequality in Roles, Rights, and Range of Practice*, which analyzes time-ordered resources that exemplify the writing of social scientists, nurses, and, to a lesser extent, physicians, on their gendered interrelationships from very early periods to the 1990s. A closely related companion text, currently being prepared for publication, is *Gender and the Nurse-Physician Game: The Impact of Changing Interrelationships on Autonomy and Range of Practice in Health Care. Nursing, Physician Control, and the Medical Monopoly* should be read first since it begins with earlier historical periods and provides more general analyses of gender and interprofessional relations. *Gender and the Nurse-Physician Game* begins with the 1960s and focuses on recent role changes involving nurses and their interactions with physicians. A special subset of nurse-physician relations, and the one most heavily contested, is related to childbirth, midwifery, and obstetrics. Although we have collected resources on midwives, nurses, and male control, a variety of competent histories have already been published that focus on this one area of health care, the one women have been most reluctant to allow men to control. As such, obstetrics, midwifery, and nursing, considered historically, represent most clearly the conflictual relations between gender and professional authority.

A fourth text, *Sexism and Nursing: Historical Perspectives on the Struggle to Overcome Educational and Economic Inequities,* focuses on the historical interrelation between nursing and the discriminatory patterns inherent in patriarchal educational and economic systems. Another text, *Nurses as Caregivers at Work and at Home: The Impact of Triple Duty, Inadequate Support, and Changing Gender Expectations on Their Families and the Nursing Profession,* analyzes major published sources, again historically organized, on the problems that nurses as women experience in juggling personal and professional roles in societies structured on male work patterns. Another text, *Men in Nursing: Historical Perspectives on Prejudice and Privilege,* is devoted to the problems of male nurses, whose gender role is often perceived as incongruent with the professional nursing role. Although the history of men in nursing is actually quite lengthy, we are most concerned with writings produced in this century, and, more particularly, during the past four decades, when publications on male nurses increased substantially.

To understand the interplay between gender and professional subordination, we have attended to the voices of all nurses, both female and male. Nevertheless, female terminology is used to refer to members of the nursing profession since the emphasis is on the status of women in the general society in relation to that of women in nursing. Almost all writings of nurses refer to physicians as male; pictures in nursing journals invariably depict male physicians; and until recently, even research did not usually distinguish between men and women physicians. In the not too distant past, when female physicians were studied, they were often dropped from analysis because of their small numbers. Ideally, a variegated analysis of the relations of male physicians and male nurses and of female physicians and female nurses should be compared with those of female physicians and male nurses and all these should be differentiated from the more common cross-gender interrelations of male physicians and female nurses. Given limited data, this is only partially possible at this time. Therefore, we follow the practice of nurses themselves, referring to physicians as male, except when there are differentiations made by specific researchers or authors. To the voices of nurses are added those of non-nurses, usually female, but sometimes male, social scientists or activists who were concerned about nursing. The medical point of view on nursing is, of course, represented, but the history of medicine is widely known; thus, we have selected only the sources pertaining to gender and nurses.

The complementary interconnections among the texts allow readers to obtain a comprehensive understanding of the processes of gender stratification and sex discrimination that influence nursing and health-care systems. Thus, it is possible to grasp the extent to which nurses have been aware of and have written about nursing issues from the perspective of their subjugation as women; to focus on nurses' conceptions of marriage and family roles as these influence the profession; to understand how societal institutions—economic, political, and educational—affect nursing and health care; to perceive the relationship between the "public" and "private" spheres of life; to connect these to interprofessional relations between men as physicians and women as nurses; to understand the search for autonomy in expanded roles in relation to gendered interactional patterns between professions; to see how women's biological functions in childbirth have been central to the gendered struggle for control; and to learn what happens to men who choose to enter nursing, a traditionally female field.

The selection and analysis of sources in the texts should accomplish several objectives. First, they further clarify the gendered historical development of the profession so it can be reconsidered from a broader perspective and more accurately understood. Second, they significantly modify existing and traditional conceptions of the nursing profession. To use standard definitions of the nature of a profession without reference to the gender roles of the members of that profession is a continuing exercise in futility; thus, in the sociology of professions, scholars may be able to rectify the muddled state of affairs on the meaning of professional identity. A third objective is to provide nursing, medicine, and the social sciences with resources organized both historically and substantively as a foundation for further research. A fourth objective is to uncover and define new areas of knowledge which may help refine existing concepts in nursing and provide directions for new research. A fifth objective is to influence curricular directions in nursing education by changing analyses of the nursing profession and its history, which, as currently presented to students and understood by most nurse educators, are inadequately interconnected to gender, race, and class. A sixth goal is to provide women, both nurses and non-nurses, with a more accurate and precise understanding of gender and professional role identities and to establish these as a component of women's studies. A seventh objective is to provide men, both those in and out of nursing and medicine, with a clearer understanding of the historical and current discriminatory practices so they can be sensitive to change and help create different, more equal institutional and societal arrangements for women and men in the health-care system. Finally, from these new, more equal arrangements, consumers can hopefully obtain health care that is more holistic, less expensive, and more directly available to them in their homes and communities.

Purpose and Organization of the First Published Text: *Feminism and Nursing*

We include this description of the first volume for readers who want to relate the contents to subsequent volumes. In *Feminism and Nursing*, cross-era, comparative sources are analyzed to better understand the relation between women's roles in society and the effect these have had on the nursing profession as it has evolved over time. Chapter 1 focuses on Florence Nightingale as the recognized founder of nursing. We examine her writings on and for women, particularly her philosophy of women's status, her feminist thinking, and her mystical perceptions of life and work. Included are others' perceptions of Nightingale's feminism and the changing images or moral iconography in publications over the past century of her as a woman speaking about women and nursing. In a sense, the debate on Nightingale as feminist or nonfeminist is a symbolic debate on nursing itself. In another sense, this issue revolves around her role as an early critic of family and of religion and in her creation of one woman's early system of "objective" spirituality.

Other voices from the past, other nursing leaders, have also spoken about women's roles and lives. In chapter 2 we meet Clara Barton, Margaret Sanger, Lillian D. Wald, Adelaide Nutting, Lavinia Lloyd Dock, and, more recently, Wilma Scott Heide, all of whom wrote on women's lives and experiences. Those choosing a feminist path external to nursing often have their early work in nursing discredited or overlooked. Those doing their major work on feminism within nursing often remain unknown to both scholars and the general public.

Paralleling the emergence of the women's movement are the continuing series of men's wars, which impacted very heavily on women in nursing. In chapter 3 we analyze nurses as healers in the military establishment over time. Devoted to healing and caring, nursing as a woman's profession has experienced both gains and losses as a result of male violence in the Crimean and U.S. Civil Wars and later in World War I, World War II, and the Korean, Vietnam, and Iraq wars. Certainly, there was considerable debate among nurses about the First World War and much distress about subsequent wars. During the Second World War, women were urged into public work, but following the war, in the late 1940s and throughout the 1950s, they were urged to return home. These contradictory directives were particularly problematic for nurses, who wrote extensively on nurses and the military during and following the war, but much less on broader women's issues. In general, the treatment of women and men nurses in the military has been discriminatory, causing substantial damage to individuals and forcing nurse leaders to struggle for decent treatment throughout this century.

In chapter 4 we examine the feminist actions of those early nursing leaders who aligned themselves with non-nurse feminists in fighting for women's suffrage. The lively debate among nurses on suffrage during the first two decades of this century and subsequently on the "Lucretia Mott Amendment," or the Equal Rights Amendment, exemplifies the commitment of a few nurse leaders to women's equality, as well as illustrating the divisions in the ranks of professional nursing.

Chapter 5 makes it clear that, from the late 1950s through the 1960s, the sounds of transition could be detected in the few voices speaking about women's issues in nursing publications. They expressed their concerns about their status in the sense that every report or commission on nurses described a largely female group trying to sustain their public professional roles during a time of severe conservatism about women's roles in general. In chapter 6 we see how the early 1970s were a turning point that gave rise to the much more decisive ring of feminism in nursing in the latter part of the decade. In chapter 7, the dilemma of women leaders in nursing is analyzed. While power in nursing was being openly discussed, so was the fragmented diversity of nurses. Clearly, gender and professional role expectations were differently configured for women, both in and outside of nursing. The critical need for politically astute leaders and administrators was proclaimed with nurses presumably entering a confrontation-negotiation era. As we see in chapter 8, this continued into the 1980s, although the conservative Reagan era had a significant effect in deflecting attention from feminist goals and activism.

Finally, chapter 9 considers current relationships among gender, power, and leadership. Personal power gradually came to be associated with political action, which many nurses had previously seen as "unprofessional, unworthy, and unwomanly." Obviously, feminism had influenced nurses sufficiently that they begin to reject such assertions. Indeed, many authors asserted that the most significant change in the profession was a newly found sense of women's competencies and worth associated with a determination to act. The newer thinking connected women's and nurses' rights with overt calls for action. Resocialization in consciousness-raising groups was connected to a call for cohesive, strong participation in political action to counteract male domination and authoritarianism. The struggles both inside and outside nursing's body politic again called for assertive action. Nursing history was presented more frequently to gain a new perspective on the preparation of leaders. Organizational analyses of nursing, medicine, and hospital administration led to recommendations for different coalitions. By the 1980s women in nursing were writing on the politics of medical deception, challenging the trajectory of medical history. By the early 1990s an analysis of structured misogyny had emerged, detailing implications for the politics of care.

Articles on barriers to women in top-level management and structural similarities between the corporate worlds of hospitals and business appeared simultaneously with those discussing nurses in feminist organizations, such as the National Organization for Women, and others that considered new power strategies for women in management. Canadian and British nurses joined American nurses in analyzing power and legitimizing political action, connecting both to the provision of adequate patient care. Stories of inbreeding and infighting among American nurses in practical politics appear alongside British accounts of surgical sisters' successes and failures in retaining power in surgical theaters. Assertiveness training is advocated, and nurses are urged to speak out for their patients and the profession. More restrained but still useful analyses of gender and leadership are connected to nursing in some sociological work in women's studies. The need for women mentors for women (as detailed in earlier women's studies organizational analyses) is reconsidered in fine-tuned analyses of gender and sponsorship. Projections on power and gender are viewed from a futuristic perspective. Finally, recent successful efforts to wrest the control of home care and other areas of practice from physicians is documented, marking an increased sophistication in political actions by nurse leaders.

Nursing's Feminist Future

In the first and second published texts, and in all subsequent volumes, we obviously stress the importance of gender. Is this emphasis justified? Contrary to popular opinion, many feminists argue that women's status has not substantially improved during the past few decades. Indeed, Susan Faludi (1991) asserts that women have been convinced that their dissatisfaction and distress are caused by *too much* feminism; however, any minimal progress has actually been undermined. According to Faludi, virtually all outlets of popular culture have spread the backlash against women's rights. Promoting questionable studies on issues such as the "shortage" of men or the "epidemic" of infertility, the media have been joined by political actions that have reduced women's employment and reproductive rights. Indeed, the image of a "New Traditional Woman" covers up the actual losses in the struggle for equality. The rise of violence against women in films, television, homes, and jobs and on the streets tells women that if they question their subordination beyond a certain level they will suffer the consequences. Indeed, Faludi claims that there is much left to be achieved and contends that feminism is *not* women's worst enemy but their only hope for real change.

Nursing professor Phyllis B. Kritek (1991) analyzes Faludi's work, praising it for its thorough documentation, but is appalled with the disturbing trends so obvious in Faludi's critique. Kritek agrees that there is a backlash and that women have lost ground over the past ten years. As a female-dominant discipline, nursing reflects the status of women in any culture; thus, Kritek wonders how the backlash of the 1980s has affected nurses. She urges nurses to return to Lavina Lloyd Dock, who a century ago perceived the intimate linkages among the status of women, women's health, nurses, and nursing. In environments not conducive to the collective hopes and visions of the future, Kritek warns that "the full development and worth of women is a troublesome and threatening agenda. . . . Sometimes the opposition will be substantial and deeply destructive" (p. 4).

Equally impressed with Faludi's work, attorney Sondra Henry (1992) interviewed her because of the Pulitzer Prize–winning journalist's persuasive documentation (eighty pages of endnotes). Faludi's major contention is that women have become convinced that their dissatisfaction and stress come from too much independence and feminism rather than minimal economic and political progress. Faludi claims that society, not feminists, has downgraded women's work. The women's movement calls attention to the systematic condescension and degradation of women's roles, for example, in the imbalances, status, and pay of nurses compared to physicians: "The goals of feminism were, and remain, to . . . honor in real ways the work that women do" (p. 40).

In Faludi's view, there was historically a conscious campaign to chase women out of the healing profession, which was originally theirs. The situation for nurses today reflects that takeover. Indeed, it is a wonder to her that so many nurses, conscious of the power differentials, can remain in the profession while often being underpaid, overworked, and disrespected. According to Faludi, the key problem is the glorification of physicians in the medical structure, which must change if authority is to return to women. In mental health, women are now the majority of psychologists, competing effectively by being more affordable and offering solutions that are less invasive and drastic and more short-term than those of higher-priced psychiatrists. Could not nurses use this as a model for entrepreneurial "medicine"?

Can nurses simultaneously sustain their own values while also changing inequities? Faludi warns that women's values cannot be fully expressed unless women have real authority in decision making. Both efforts, then, must be undertaken simultaneously, and, if possible, in coalition with women physicians. But how, asks Henry, can nurses change the stereotypes of them as self-sacrificing caretakers, intellectually inferior to physicians and unable to make informed clinical judgments? These myths, says Faludi, are perpetuated for a reason. If physicians continue to espouse publicly the handmaiden image of nurses, this will justify lower pay and diminished authority. Nurses need to engage in publicity blitzes, lawsuits, and strikes, but they are often discouraged from banding together on a massive scale and from recognizing their allied interests.

In the interview Henry pointed out that leaders of the backlash will often use the fear of change as a threat *before* the major changes can happen. Faludi agreed that there had been the veneer of change; thus, physicians pay lip service to the contributions of nurses instead of accepting even their relative independence and authority. Henry said that despite changes, nurses are still patronized by physicians, who advise them to be happy so everyone can be happier. To this Faludi replied, "Nurses are not rocking the boat enough! No one was happy with the old arrangements. Fear kept our mouths closed. No one enjoys being devalued, looked upon as a glorified bed-pan changer" (p. 45). But when nurses challenge physicians, the medical profession tries to import nurses from other countries or even creates new categories of workers, such as registered care technologists. To this, Faludi said, "Backlash is felt more keenly when women challenge a profession that is seen as 'male'" (p. 45).

Despite these difficult problems for nurses, the most significant gain in the past few decades, said Faludi, is a change in women's own heads. Sexism was not even a word until the late 1960s. Women, even if not feminists, now say they expect equal treatment. Although women now have a different vision of themselves, only a small minority of men support *real* change; the majority in surveys still perceive the "ideal" woman as the one who puts family before work and defers to a man. Certainly men in power have not reshaped societal institutions to accommodate women's new vision. The enormous resurgence in women's anger is the most promising sign, and this, with strength of numbers, can create change. The key tool in the backlash has been "to load down the word feminist with every epithet imaginable" (p. 134), forcing women to back off from the term but not the tenets of feminism. Women must get over the fear of public identification with feminism—to obtain the fruits of a political movement, women must participate in it.

Even without identification, have women around the world incorporated any feminist ideas? Have there been any changes in their own heads? At the end of the twentieth century, the latest of *The Economist*'s world polls was conducted by the Angus Reid Organization, interviewing about three thousand women in eleven, mostly developed, countries. The belief that women's lot had improved over the past two generations was supported by 93 percent, who thought they were better off than their grandmothers (although Mexican and South African women were less likely to agree). However, only 8 percent of the sample thought that women had all the same rights as men; 31 percent said most of the rights and 37 percent only some. Perhaps Faludi was right when she said that the most important feminist change is in women's heads, since 58 percent said they should have "all" the rights men enjoy and 24 percent said "almost all." However, in Japan only 21 percent wanted such equality, and in Switzerland the figure was only 39 percent. Clearly, much remains to be done.

"The Most Neglected Tragedy of Our Times": Global Subjugation of Women; the Need for a Better Model of Health Care and Nursing

The United Nations Fourth World Conference on Women in 1995 brought together some 50,000 women from 185 countries and from 2,500 national and international nongovernment organizations. From 1945, when the U. N. Commission on the Status of Women was created, to 1975 and the International Women's Year Tribune in Mexico City, to the 1980 Second Conference on Women in Copenhagen, and to the 1985 Third Conference on Women in Nairobi, the subordinate condition of women and girls has been well established: inadequate health care; persistent and increasing poverty; unequal access to education and economic decision making; unequal power sharing in politics and government. To these, add violence against women, the extremely negative effects of armed conflict on them, little governmental commitment to women's rights, lack of media attention, and little recognition of women's problems and achievements.

The sixth annual *U.N. Human Development Report* in 1995 asserted that in *no* society do women enjoy the same opportunities as men. Among the world's 900 million illiterates, females outnumber males 2 to 1. Of the 130 million children without access to primary school, 60 percent are girls. Of the 1.3 billion people in poverty, 70 percent are female. In 55 countries the average female wage is 75 percent of that of men. In Sweden, the top-ranked country, women earned 83.4 percent and in Bahrain, the lowest-ranked country, 20.9 percent of men's earnings. In the United States in 1995, women working full-time made 71 cents to a man's dollar. African American women earned 63 cents and Latinas 57 cents. This is exacerbated by the lack of compensation for work done at home. About 61 percent of American women still work in female-dominated workplaces and 60 percent of them make less than $25,000 a year. Only childless women's income approaches equity. Obviously, women with children should not be penalized. Quality child care is still lacking, as is child support for children of divorced mothers: Some 30 million children are owed

$50 billion in support and in only 23 percent of all cases is money being col-
lected. At work, women are still blocked from assuming upper-level jobs; by
2000 only 10 percent of senior managers in the top 500 companies were female. Indeed, some researchers said that "women were not blocked by a glass
ceiling," but by the *whole structure,* the entire edifice of organizations. Furthermore, research in the late 1990s found that women political candidates not
only had more difficulty raising funds, but were treated differently by the
media, which focused on them as personalities, not leaders. Thus, it is not
surprising that globally women occupy only 10 percent of parliamentary and
6 percent of government cabinet positions.

Women do more and men less of the world's work. Unpaid child care,
housework, and farm labor totaled $16 trillion; of this, $11 trillion was attributed to women, shattering the myth that men are the main breadwinners. Nevertheless, the number of women in poverty grew during the past 20 years by
50 percent compared to 30 percent for men. In a 1998 AFL-CIO survey in the
United States, 37 percent of working women said that making a living had
become harder over the past five years and 32 percent said that they did not
receive equal pay for equal work, although there was 99 percent agreement
that such equality is important.

In September 2000, the next Conference on Women met at the United
Nations in New York City to review progress on the 150-page platform for
action in achieving equality for women that was adopted at the 1995 Beijing
conference. Although more girls are going to school and more women are
working and receiving some health care, women around the world remain
underpaid, underrepresented in government, and threatened with physical
and sexual abuse. Of the world's poorest people, 75 percent are still women
and children. In the United States, an advocacy group, U.S. Women Connect,
published a report card in 2000, *Making the Grade on Health,* in which the U.S.
government's attempts to reduce the number of women in poverty received an
"F." This failing grade was caused in large part by the 1996 Welfare Reform
Act, which has actually driven the poorest deeper into poverty and only slightly
raised the incomes of those better off. Although the overall rate of poverty in
the United States has decreased over the past five years, that of women and
children has increased.

The mass rape and torture of women is a widespread weapon of war, but
instances are seldom prosecuted as war crimes. Indeed, most human rights
casualties of war are, according to Amnesty International, women and children. Child trafficking and sexual slavery are still common, particularly in
South Asia, where about nine thousand girls a year are transported across national borders. Laws are still unequal and, where equality is legislated, they
often go unenforced. The United States is no paragon, as is made very clear in
Lorraine Dusky's book *Still Unequal: The Shameful Truth about Women and
Justice in America* (1997). Despite laws outlawing sexual slavery, by the end of

the 1990s, the United Nations reported that some two million people, overwhelmingly female, are forced into the international sex trade each year. The U.S. State Department estimates that 50,000 are brought into this country annually. Although varied proposals have been debated in Congress, none is sufficient to deal with this outrage.

Probably the most damning evidence is enunciated in the UNICEF Annual Progress of Nations report in 1996 that said complications during pregnancy and childbirth kill 1,600 women every day and 585,000 women each year and create health problems for about a quarter of women worldwide. More than 140,000 women die each year from hemorrhaging; another 75,000 from trying to abort in the absence of adequate birth control techniques. Another 100,000 die of sepsis and 40,000 die from obstructed labor. More than three million women suffer chronic weakness and related symptoms from Sheehan's syndrome. A stunning silence surrounds the "most neglected tragedy of our times." In addition, some two million girls a year continue to suffer genital mutilation that is not required by any religion.

In September 2000, the United Nations Population Fund produced the *State of the World Population Report 2000,* compiled from U.N. agencies, the World Health Organization, the World Bank, and national governments and surveys. At the turn of a new century and millennium, the report noted that there are still 80 million unwanted or mistimed pregnancies, representing one-third of all pregnancies worldwide. Only 53 percent of births in developing countries are attended by professionals. This means that 52.4 million women are subject to neglect annually. Indeed, nearly 38 million women, or about 30 percent, who give birth in developing countries receive no care after giving birth. Each year there are an estimated 50 million abortions, 20 million of which are unsafe and result in the deaths of 78,000 women and the suffering of millions more.

In agreement with other reports, the *State of World Population Report 2000* said that at least one in three women have been beaten, coerced into sex, or otherwise abused in some way. Indeed, one in four women are abused *during pregnancy.* Violence against girls and women has increased, and the U.N. Conference on Women in 2000 has called for tougher measures against sex trafficking and domestic violence. Ironically, the hardest and most strongly contested issue at both the 1995 and 2000 conferences was women's right to decide freely all matters related to their sexuality and childbearing. Indeed, sexual and reproductive health care is still far from universally available. At the 2000 U.N. Conference on Women, the Vatican, India, and some Islamic countries—Algeria, Iran, Libya, and Pakistan—continued to reject women's right to control their own sexuality and childbearing. Yet girls and women continue to be subjected to violence, incest, rape, and dowry burnings, which are all on the increase globally. In addition, female circumcisions, forced prostitution, forced pregnancies, and forced marriages all continue.

Probably the worst situation for girls and women is in Afghanistan, where the Taliban has forced women to wear a garment covering them from head to toe; fired them en masse from their jobs, except for a few hospital workers; excluded them from schools or universities; prohibited them from leaving their homes except in the company of a close male relative; ordered households with adult women to paint their windows opaque; and even decreed that women's shoes must not make noise when they walk. According to the *Feminist Majority* in 1998, any violations of these rules have led to beatings, torture, or even killings. In late 1999, a human rights investigator from the United Nations, after two weeks of observations and interviews, reported on the Taliban's widespread, systematic, and officially sanctioned abuse of women and accused the Ministry of Vice and Virtue of being the most misogynist department in the whole world. Ministry employees, armed with rifles, patrol the streets in pickup trucks looking for women who violate the men's edicts. More than 120 American national and regional women's groups, including the American Nurses' Association (ANA), have taken a stand against this treatment of girls and women. As Eleanor Smeal said, "*If this were happening to any other class of people around the world, there would be a tremendous outcry.* We must make sure these same standards are applied when it is women and girls who are brutally treated" (Smeal, 1998, p. 4).

Women cannot demand the same standards if they reject identification with feminism and if they do not know their own history so they can learn from the successes of the past, not repeat its failures. For feminist and activist Naomi Wolf, women are again at a turning point, an "open moment" at the beginning of a new century when the level of historical awareness will determine the movement toward or away from equality. For Wolf, women's cultural and historical awareness is blocked by the media, which, according to Women, Men and Media, a national watchdog project, features women in only 15 percent of front-page news items, and then usually as victims or perpetrators of crime or misconduct. Women's history is omitted from women's culture in a variety of publications for women that presumably, as Wolf says, do little to suggest that women's destiny is determined by women themselves, as agents of historical change. Indeed, there is a recurrent ideological theme that says that if women take themselves seriously, they will lose their femininity and social status. And, finally, there is a simple lack of education that can cause a cultural forgetfulness of women's real history and, as Wolf notes, even shock them when women discover they do have a history!

Although the values of feminism have entered the lives of women, only 33 percent of American women and 16 percent of female college students call themselves feminists. Ironically, women in developed countries are often living feminist lives without admitting to feminism. Wolf warns that indifference to the history that led to these changed lives comes at the risk of losing it all. She believes that ignorance of women's history leaves women powerless to build toward greater equality and to learn lessons from women's strategies in the past.

We agree with Wolf. Women are at a turning point, an "open moment." We also agree that women's history is fundamental to determining the direction of change. In our first published volume on nursing and feminism, and in this second volume on nursing and the medical monopoly, and the other texts in process, we believe that the historical perspective provided may offer a real hope for substantial change in nursing and the health-care system, helping to free women health-care workers to provide the care and cure people really need, and to reconceptualize health care in a more humane way, creating a model of human health and equality that is worthy of adoption throughout the world—a world that is still marked by discrimination against women and girls and that very much needs feminism and women healers.

NURSING, PHYSICIAN CONTROL, AND THE MEDICAL MONOPOLY:
An Overview

Organized nursing and medicine are currently on a collision course, with the American Nurses' Association (ANA) often taking positions on nurses' roles, rights, and range of practice in opposition to those espoused by the American Medical Association (AMA). The strained relations in the last few decades have a very long history, but one that is largely unknown and incomplete. This history is also a chronology of gendered relations between predominantly male medical and predominantly female nursing groups. In this volume we examine sources on gendered nurse-physician relations over time to trace the centuries-old efforts of physicians to dominate and to achieve a monopoly over health care and the continuous efforts of women healers and nurses to sustain at least some of their medical-nursing functions, which were originally associated with their female roles in families and communities. Because medical histories have come to dominate both the scholarly and the public imagination, we must first consider the extent to which women healers actually existed in previous centuries, compare their contributions to those of physicians, and then assess how physicians reacted to women healers. From this longer historical perspective, nurse-physician relations in the nineteenth and twentieth centuries can be placed in a different and more inclusive context.

Medical histories usually exclude women healers and nurses, and nursing histories have often provided only limited information on women healers prior to the mid nineteenth century, when "modern" nursing emerged. Because of unknown sources, scholars studying nursing have had to rely too often on predominantly male medical sources for accounts of healing activities in earlier periods. Obviously, this creates potential and often very real gender and occupational biases. Although the negative impact of gender on nursing is clearly apparent in earlier sources, few provide an explicit gendered perspective or analysis. However, there are some feminist publications, such as Jeanne Achterberg's *Woman as Healer* (1991) and Elisabeth Brooke's *Women Healers through History* (1993), that survey women's healing activities from prehistoric times to the present. Unfortunately, such sources often do not focus specifically on nurses, probably because both medical and nursing functions were part of women's healing activities.

Despite the limitations of available data, it is our contention that the current perceptions of power relations between nurses and physicians are significantly altered by, first, taking a longer view of history; second, by including data on all kinds of women's healing activities; and, third, by placing these in the context of sex-stratified institutions and patriarchal societies. Indeed, the often spurious and even deleterious division between curing and caring in current health-care systems, which is assumed to rest on functional differences, is more likely a result of imposed gender distinctions. The blurred lines between the present functions of nurses and physicians today are, in part, a result of the exclusion of women from their previous healing functions—an exclusion that happened long before the emergence of a fully scientific approach in medicine. The present overlap of many functions of nursing and medicine exists because of the increasing medicalization of all healing tasks and the renaming of all health domains as belonging to physicians, most of whom are male. Whether this medical monopoly is good for the health of people is highly questionable.

Rendering the Invisible Visible

The historical approach provides a long-range perspective on gendered nurse-physician relations that best illuminates the current situation. To reconstruct nursing history is to rewrite the biased ideology that has infused medical history, which is a chronology that not only informs but also legitimizes physicians' power and justifies their economic advantage. Since nurses, as women, were largely excluded in previous centuries from both formal education and publication, the creation of new stories and the retelling of old medical tales is difficult, but within the context of women's history these will be very differently constructed. In historian Linda Gordon's (1986) words, we have "to render the invisible visible, the silent noisy, the motionless active (p. 21) . . . to proclaim a truth heretofore denied, disguised, distorted, defamed and thereby to expose the meretricious lies" (p. 22). From these efforts, the new stories of nurse-physician relations will gain a greater historical accuracy and may over time empower nurses today.

Early British nursing leader Ethel Gordon Fenwick claimed that "'the Nurse question is the Woman question, pure and simple'" (Nutting and Dock, 1912, vol. 3, p. 33). If this is so, no history of nursing in relation to medicine can be separated from the history of women, since, as Fenwick said, nurses too have had to deal with a past riddled with gender subordination, and thus have had to run "the gauntlet of those historic rotten eggs" (p. 33). Close to a century later, Judith Moore (1988) could still call the history of nursing the "unknown history." Indeed, Marion Ferguson (1979) asserted that the field of nursing history was "fragmented [and] lacking a central focus" (p. 121). More optimistically, Ellen Condliffe Lagemann (1983) stated that the growing interest in women's history has fostered a broader audience for nursing history, which is moving out of its obscurity to a wider relevance. This, coupled with different approaches to the history of professions and unions, and to the organization of women's work itself, leads Lagemann to a more hopeful view.

Questions derived from and informed by women's history are generating new inquiries and a deeper critique of the medical profession as "monopoly-seeking and monopoly-maintaining" (Lagemann, 1983, p. 4). From this new perspective, labeling nursing a "minor profession" (p. 5) is misleading and represents a value-laden perspective that is now superseded by a new understanding of women's organizations and the values placed on different kinds of work.

A major contradiction in research on women's history, claims Linda Gordon, is whether to "document oppression . . . specify the agents and authors of domination . . . [or] document our struggles and identify successes" (Gordon, 1986, p. 23). Do we stress women healers' and nurses' capability or their fragility? A second contradiction centers on the attribution of causation: structural and systemic versus individual. In nurse-physician relations, it is particularly difficult to deal with domination and resistance simultaneously, but as Gordon states, "To be less powerful is not to be power-less, or even to lose all the time" (p. 24).

Still another contradiction exists between the political history of power and powerlessness and the social or cultural history of everyday lives. If we pay tribute to a nurse working a sixteen-hour day in a hospital training school and applaud her stamina and see value in her work, are we romanticizing her oppression by medical and hospital authorities? Alternatively, if we examine published history, will we see only the recent "queens," the nursing leaders of the last 125 years? Or the physicians and hospital administrators, who directly or indirectly gained control of women healers and nurses? From a feminist perspective, the key question is power: how do nurses incorporate political activity and power in their professional relationships, their practice, and their daily lives? As Gordon says, the problem is to transcend the victim/heroine dualism by incorporating the complexity of power and weakness in women's lives. This may create very different histories of nursing and medicine and of the relationships between these disciplines.

What of differences among nurses as women? This issue is critical because people outside the health-care delivery system may see nursing in this century as simply an inferior form of medicine—women as merely the subsumed. But nurses do espouse a value system, which may be lost in a "neutral asymmetry," an espousal of "teamwork," that avoids the issue of professional domination. Nurses particularly are caught in the dichotomy between the uniquely female versus the common humanity of all women and men. Are nurses as women similar to men in medicine or are they superior in their claim to nurturing the whole person, not simply "curing" the pathological parts? A duality of this kind persists continuously as women attempt to work out both their female uniqueness and their commonality with men.

Institutionalized heterosexuality, says Gordon, also creates gender ideals that negate women's actual identities. In nursing, "femininity," as adherence to heterosexual norms, constrains identities and limits forthright action. Women nurses are not just different, they are also often in opposition—even if muted—to physicians and administrators. This opposition is experienced differently, according to the degree of acceptance or rejection of traditional women's identity. How do nurses unify women who perceive their gender roles differently? What exactly constitutes the traditions of women's culture and female consciousness that are not feminist? In nursing, the differences between female and feminist consciousness are at the heart of problems in achieving political unity. How can nurses, who are often viewed as the quintessence of the "feminine," simultaneously stand against medical domination, violation, and subordination of women as nurses? In Gordon's terms, how can women celebrate the female but reject the traditional subjugation of the female?

A chronology of nurse-physician relations that does not incorporate both female and feminist history is stranded—as Gordon would say, an island outside the stream. If isolated, nurses have to rely on medical history for definition, rather than on their own or women's studies scholars, who can make nursing history visible in the center of women's lives. This overreliance on medical history can only serve to legitimize medical and male domination. The challenge is to create a body of knowledge and a new and powerful mythos. Unless this is achieved, the historic "rotten eggs" will continue to stink. And the current fight for greater autonomy from physician control and a broader mandate for nurses' range of practice will rest on very shaky historical grounds. Fortunately, a few articles from the *History of Nursing Review* over the past few years have focused more specifically on gender and the medical monopoly, providing a more solid historical foundation for nurses. By understanding historical antecedents, current conflicts can be reconfigured, making possible quite different interpretations of the present struggle over nurses' relative autonomy from physicians.

Questioning the "Naturalness" of the Medical Monopoly

The effort of physicians to obtain a monopoly over all matters pertaining to health is not new. It has a long history, but medical men's success in these endeavors is relatively recent, although the monopoly is now considered by many to be "natural" and in the best interests of the patient. While this truism has some merit, it lacks validity when applied to the restriction on nurses and other health-care workers, who are now questioning their subordination. The medical monopoly is also increasingly questioned by consumers, who have turned to alternative therapies and herbal remedies to avoid total control by traditional medicine, which is too much based on illness, not health; drugs, not lifestyles; and surgery instead of prevention. Certainly, medicine can be congratulated for many achievements, particularly in the application of research findings from related fields; however, a growing number of consumers ask whether monopolistic control is for the good of physicians' economic status, rather than the good of patients.

These questions apply most directly to restrictions on nurses, physicians' closest and practically only direct competitors, who are also in a position to evaluate the efficacy of MDs' treatment of patients. Over time, some male-dominated health-care fields, such as dentistry, have carved out separate domains. Others, such as psychology and chiropractic, are in the process of defining their boundaries. But a female-dominated field, such as nursing, is still assumed to be a subordinate group of workers with little independence. Historically, gender has been overtly used as a rationale for nurses' subordination. In addition, medicine has been assumed to precede and therefore to have the right to define all health matters as within their scope. Thus, any overlap in functions between nurses and physicians is presumed to be automatically a *medical* matter. With the emergence of nurse practitioners, nurse clinicians, and nurse anesthetists and the reemergence of nurse midwives, all of the assumptions underpinning the medical monopoly are questionable. In addition, given the rise of the feminist movement, the use of gender as a rationale for nurses' subordination is flatly unacceptable.

Organization of the Text

In this book, we trace the development of the continual efforts by physicians to achieve a medical monopoly by subordinating their only genuine competitors: nurses. In part I, chapter 1, we analyze evidence of early women healers prior to the nineteenth century, focusing primarily on early Mediterranean and European societies, tracing the erosion of women healers' independence and influence, and their increasing subordination to physician control and authority.

We examine the evidence, first, for the prevalence of women healers in previous centuries and their usual healing activities and then consider the early efforts of medical men to exclude them, certainly from the 1300s, with the founding of major universities. Although the evidence will eventually grow, all we can do now is provide the groundwork for subsequent researchers. However, what is clear from the earliest period onward is the large overlap of functions between healers of whatever title. Indeed, the term "empiric" has been used by some researchers to describe women healers precisely because neither "nurse" nor "physician" fits the work since both nursing and medical functions were involved. It is also very apparent that male physicians over time constantly expanded their functions, medicalizing more and more aspects of human life, claiming them as the province of medicine. Eventually, the layperson came to believe that these functions had always been the province of physicians. Thus, it is necessary to ask in chapter 1 who preceded whom—physicians or women healers? Who were the most widespread healers? Whose clinical theories were better? What differences in treatments existed? Who supervised women healers—physicians or the women themselves? Was there any real separation between nursing and medicine? To what extent did male physicians purposely use gender as a means to obtain a monopoly?

Although more research is needed, our answers to these questions strongly suggest that women healers preceded or at least paralleled medical men; that they were the most widely used healers in families and communities; that they were in many situations quite independent of direct supervision by medical men; that the herbal treatments used by the women were often better and certainly no worse than the leeching and purging used by medical men; that both groups used charms, amulets, and other superstitions in their practice; that medical theories taught in universities were not superior to those of herbalists; and that medical men directly and unambiguously used gender as a means to get rid of women competitors. From this perspective, the current medical monopoly, in contrast to the usual great-men-of-medicine approach to history, provides little support for the primacy of medicine until late in the nineteenth century. Indeed, nurses who want greater autonomy have good historical reasons to believe they have a right to it. This does not justify the primitive treatment of patients in previous centuries, but it does suggest that both women and men were limited in their theories and health care. Given these inadequacies, the attempts by medical men to exclude women *because* they were women is a misogynous approach, unethically used for centuries and one that still echoes in the minds of many today, even though overt expression of gender discrimination is more muted.

In the second chapter in part I, we focus on nurses and women healers in Great Britain from the 1800s to early 1900s to determine the trajectory toward medical control and nursing subservience that subsequently influenced American health care. With increasing male monopolistic control, did the conditions and the quality of women's nursing in hospitals and other institutions improve? Was the scientific model adopted by most physicians and, if not, what was the basis for their claims for superior treatment and the rationale for their monopoly? What were the pre-Nightingale nurses or attendants really like? What did medical men do to help or to block Nightingale and her nurses? To what extent was sex discrimination and gender stereotyping used to prop up the medical monopoly? What differences are there in the historical accounts of the emergence of Nightingale nurses by women nurses and medical men? To what extent was the legally subordinate position of women in families used to justify the subservience of nurses? To what extent did physicians try to control emerging nurses' organizations? The answers to these questions suggest a pattern of repeated efforts by medical men to control women healers and later to subordinate women attendants and nurses using gender stereotypes and exclusionary practices, even *before* the widespread adoption of a scientific basis of care by the majority of physicians and *before* the standardization of medical training and licensure. Although some claim that medical men represented scientific and the nurse healers religious orientations, the evidence is clear that the majority of men practicing medicine did not fully agree on a scientific approach until well into the nineteenth century.

With the efforts of Florence Nightingale, the reemergence of educated nurses, previously and largely eliminated with the destruction of women's religious orders in England and their subordination by medical men on the European continent, was a threatening development to an occupation trying to achieve professional status and to create a monopoly over health care. The relations between Nightingale-type nurses and physicians in the nineteenth century were not marked with any great conviviality, and it is clear that Nightingale herself had no great respect for many medical practitioners. One of her most important reforms was to place nursing in the hands of women. Given a period in which women lacked legal, political, and social rights, this was no small achievement, particularly since women had no place in the public world of men. The early nurse reformers were made of stern stuff, but even they had to compromise to reenter a public world from which they had been excluded.

The evidence shows that the male monopoly of institutions often did not produce good care or even decent conditions in hospitals, almshouses, and other places presumably established for the humane care of human beings. These conditions were not in the best interest of patients or of nurses. It is difficult to grasp the often terrible working conditions for nurses. Given these circumstances it is not surprising that most nursing and medical functions were still carried out in homes and usually directed by women themselves.

Although the long history of women healers and the experiences of European, particularly British, nurses influenced American nurses, most research in the United States has focused on nursing from the mid to late nineteenth century and on nurses in a women's world; thus, the impact of the gendered medical monopoly is not fully explicated. In the third chapter of part I, we focus on different conceptualizations of American nursing history by historians who have studied different groups of women, some in religious orders, others in domestic medicine, in nursing during wartime, in women's hospitals, in health-reform activities, in early hospital nursing schools, and in public health nursing. From the history of religious orders, it is clear that nuns did not simply follow medical men's orders but founded a vast network of their own hospitals, orphanages, and infirmaries. Nor did early American nurses slavishly follow the European model of Nightingale, but started nursing from their own domestic roots, despite physicians' efforts to get the women under control. Such efforts are particularly obvious during the Civil War, when many physicians actively worked to eliminate or restrict women nurses, who nevertheless entered war zones to care for the wounded and dying and forced politicians to deal with the horrific conditions the men suffered (see Roberts and Group, 1995).

Women continued their health crusades following the war, and it is in this context that "modern" nursing arose. As in Great Britain, "modern" nurses were not always welcomed by physicians, who also strenuously objected to women physicians. The latter established with nurses hospitals for women, and the issue of the primacy of gender versus occupation in interprofessional relations became a key issue. Although the "modern" nurses in hospitals set up their own women's structure run by nurses, by the late nineteenth century the predominantly male physicians were increasingly successful in controlling what the women could do. Clearly, the men feared competition from educated females and used stereotyped military and family models to ensure obedience, which, to some historians, came to be internalized by the nurses themselves, whose own interior colonization led to nursing school and hospital structures that reinforced subordination. In contrast, other historians emphasize the strong feminism of early nursing leaders, who clearly understood medical men's opposition to women nurses' independence and grasped the implications of the growing medical monopoly for health-care givers and their patients.

In part II, we consider in chapter 4 nurse-physician relations just before and after the turn of the century, a time when the medical monopoly had gained strength from the standardization of medical education and from the increasing importance of medical organizations and their efforts to affect political decision making in favor of physicians. Gender continued to be used as a rationale for keeping women out of medical schools and limiting the education of women in nursing. As hospitals grew at a tremendous pace, physicians reinforced their monopoly by controlling patient admissions and hospital staff privileges. Hospital nursing schools were grossly underfunded; instruction was inadequate, and the free use of student nurses as unpaid employees working ten- to twelve-hour days was the norm. Efforts by nursing leaders to rectify this situation and to achieve greater autonomy were blocked by hospital administrators and organized medicine. Whether the medical monopoly was in the patients' best interest is questionable, given evidence of the development of the medical profession as a business. The AMA, for example, won its first major political battle against national health insurance following World War I and even opposed compulsory diphtheria inoculations and smallpox vaccinations, mandatory reporting of tuberculosis cases, and a variety of other public health measures that were clearly in the public's best interest, but not necessarily in the physicians' economic interest. Even the AMA Code of Ethics adopted in 1847 established MD ownership of patients and encouraged dependence. Information was withheld not only from patients but from nurses, who were sometimes forbidden to read patient histories; given medicine bottles with numbers, not names; and denied use of thermometers and other instruments. The sexist domination of nursing by medicine was not haphazard or accidental but structured and institutionalized.

Indeed, no nursing domain was free of attempted medical control, and this negatively affected women nurses' efforts to enact their own values; their relation to the state in licensure and practice laws; their access to and practice with patients; their level and types of education; and their access to and use of scientific knowledge and instrumentation. Physicians also tried to control nurses' functions, activities, standards, and ethics; their involvement in governing and ruling boards of governmental and institutional bodies; their nursing leaders and the degree of their authority; their recruitment, employment, salaries, and shortages; and even their character, demeanor, and interaction styles.

In part II, chapter 5, we consider the consolidation of the medical monopoly in the 1920s and 1930s, and, with the waning of feminism by the 1930s, the concretization of gendered stereotyped roles and of the two occupational groups. Nurses, however, joined with women health activists to create a national network and program to improve women's and children's health. Unfortunately, organized medicine opposed and eliminated this public health venture. Nurses continued to document and change the unsatisfactory state of nurses' licensure, education, and practice. These efforts were too often opposed by many physicians, making it much more difficult for the women nurses to achieve their goals. The AMA established committees on nursing and tightened controls by the 1930s. With the rise of radio and movies in the 1930s, the stereotyped images of the nurturing, obedient woman nurse and the sacrificing, scientific male doctor were widely disseminated. Women nurses who showed creativity and initiative were often sharply put down by physicians.

In chapter 6, part II, the growing unease in nurse-physician relations from the 1940s to the 1960s is evident. With expanding scientific knowledge, improvement in technological capacities, and widespread use of sulfa, penicillin, and antibiotic drugs, the basis for the medical monopoly was solidified. Shifting from private duty to hospitals, nurses were expected to coordinate without sufficient authority an ever increasing array of new technologists and auxiliary personnel. With a postwar shift to very conservative back-to-the-home gender roles for women, nurses' efforts to gain more autonomy—for example, in their efforts to move from hospital to university-based education—were made even more difficult. As nurses' dissatisfaction increased, the ANA demanded joint national conferences with the AMA, which culminated in the National Joint Practice Commission. Unionization, both in and outside of the ANA, was sharply constrained by the continued governmental restrictions on strike actions by nurses. Such strikes would not be fully allowed until the 1970s.

The tremendous growth of the health-care industry, the greater complexity of health care, and the increase in physicians' specialization all created heavier demands on nurses, who were more frequently specializing in, for example, intensive and coronary care units. By the mid-1960s, medical organizations unilaterally decided to create physician's assistants, enraging many nurses who were tired of being told what to do and with taking on the leftovers—the tasks MDs no longer wanted to do.

In part II, chapter 7, we consider the conflict between organized nursing and medicine, which entered a public and open phase of contention in the 1970s. Nurses countered the creation of the physician's assistant position with that of the nurse clinician or nurse practitioner, who could take on advanced functions while retaining a nursing identity. The issue of nursing autonomy was directly related to the rise of feminism, which made women's subordination a central issue and thus brought into question the nurse's stereotype as the loyal "right arm" of the physician. This meshed with the increasing unhappiness of consumers with the inadequate, fragmented, and costly "system" of health care. The nurses stepped up their efforts to move to university education, to obtain more federal education funds, to train more nurses with MA and PhD degrees, to achieve more equality in military ranks, to obtain more equitable salaries and better working conditions through more organized professional and union actions, and to change federal restrictions on union strikes and other labor initiatives. Despite these actions, medical sociologists at the start of the 1970s considered the medical monopoly to be unparalleled in the degree of its control over other occupations. Nevertheless, nurses worked to obtain legal diagnostic authority, to resocialize themselves in assertiveness training, and to gain more rights for nurse practitioners. Research on physicians' acceptance or rejection of nurse practitioners indicated a preference for physician's assistants, underutilization of the nurses, and a reluctance to delegate authority or to hire nurse practitioners. Increasing numbers of research studies proved nurse practitioners' competence equaled or exceeded that of physicians in primary care. By the end of the 1970s, some sociologists were recommending that nurses become the primary caregivers and physicians become specialized consultants. Organized medicine obviously rejected such recommendations.

In part III, we consider in chapter 8 whether gender stereotypes remained central to nurse-physician relations in the 1980s and into the early 1990s, a period marked by a backlash to feminism and a more conservative political agenda. The traditional stereotype of the nurse as a mother surrogate was resurrected to reduce the dissatisfaction with the impersonal health-care industry. Although more cooperation was advocated by medical sociologists, there was still continued devaluation of nurses and their work, rigid ritualization and standardization of procedures, and explicit and often unnecessary orders for every action. The AMA insisted on their supervision of nurse practitioners, yet were dismayed to learn physicians were a major cause of nurses' dissatisfaction! This dismay did not stop the AMA from withdrawing from the National Joint Practice Commission, causing its collapse.

Nurses from other countries, for example Great Britain, were also in conflict with physicians over nurses' autonomy. Women physicians and men nurses had different perspectives, as did lawyers and medical ethicists. The evidence for continued gender stereotyping in the 1980s and into the 1990s is strongly substantiated in research investigations that found physicians' negative portrayal of nurses in fiction written by MDs; stereotyping of nurses in television advertisements and programming and in medical journals, and even in cartoons in a major medical publication; and the devaluation of nurses as authoritative sources in the media. Indeed, research on the role of gender in the health-care hierarchy proved, despite increases in female MDs, to be substantially intact even by the late 1990s.

In chapter 9, we consider nurses' frontal attack on the medical monopoly, which only became possible after the Federal Trade Commission ruling that antitrust laws also applied to professionals, including physicians, who were engaging in monopolistic practices, such as group boycott, tying, and bottleneck agreements. To challenge these practices legally, nurses would have to prove that their quality of primary care was equal to or better than that of physicians. Research continued to support the argument that nurses offered not only equal but superior primary care and, more importantly, that there were differences in the clinical approaches of nurses and physicians. Economic competition became an open and public issue; the cost-effectiveness of nurse practitioners was researched and proof was provided of their potential to reduce the spiraling costs of health care.

Given the refusal of many physicians to hire them, nurse practitioners were, by the early 1980s, in a difficult situation. Indeed, some medical men claimed that a stalemate had been reached and accused nurses of engaging in "gender politics" rather than in actions related to patient care. Previous research on the continued gendering of the health-care hierarchy was sustained, for example, in the practice characteristics of physician's assistants and physicians, although there was a greater tendency toward androgyny in their self-characterizations. Despite excessive controls, nurses continued to open nurse-managed health-care centers across the nation and to conduct research on their own efficacy; the latter was strongly supported by the positive findings in the 1986 report of the U.S. Office of Technology Assessment. Nevertheless, the AMA passed resolutions to restrict federal nursing funds and limit the autonomy of nurse practitioners, and, in addition, proposed a new category of health-care provider, the registered care technologist, responsible to physicians. Thus, medicine engaged in a squeeze play, controlling and subordinating nurse practitioners at the top and replacing registered nurses at the bottom. Nevertheless, nurses continued to chip away at monopolistic practices, demanding legislative changes in diagnostic and prescriptive authority; direct reimbursement of services; and inclusion in hospital patient admission rights and staff privileges. By the beginning of the 1990s, the ANA produced the nurses' own agenda for health-care reform, insisting on nurses' autonomy and a national system of primary and preventive health care.

In chapter 10, we focus on the results of the medical monopoly, consider nurses' and consumers' critiques of the health-care "system," continue to document nurses' efforts to reform the "system," and the counterefforts by organized medicine to constrain nurses' practice and to overturn the antimonopolistic rulings of the Federal Trade Commission. In a period of multiple mergers of hospitals and other health-care institutions and the conversion of these from nonprofit to profit-making businesses, nurses have not fared very well. Nor have consumers. With the collapse of the Clintons' national health plan, health maintenance organizations (HMOs) rapidly enrolled millions of Americans, whose basic rights have been jeopardized, causing legislative consideration of a variety of ethical issues. The number of Americans without health insurance has not been substantially reduced by these organizational changes. Cost cutting has led to the reduction and elimination of thousands of registered nurses, who are often replaced with "unlicensed assistive personnel." In addition, a 1994 Supreme Court ruling, only recently reversed, classified vast numbers of nurses as supervisory, thus eliminating their participation in labor actions by unions and professional associations.

With the increasing number of female physicians, gender, though still important, is decreasingly stressed, although the blurring of gendered occupational lines has not substantially changed the male dominance in upper-echelon power positions. Nor have there been fundamental shifts in the subordination of women in the general population of working women. Thus, despite thirty years of research, which continued through the 1990s to prove the competence and cost-effectiveness of nurse practitioners, the nurses' push for a national system of preventive and primary care, and the widespread use of nurses as gatekeepers are still not widely adopted in the mergers and profit-making institutions and health organizations that have mushroomed. Unfortunately, true cost savings and better health care are often replaced by threats to patient safety as fewer nurses try to take care of more patients with more severe conditions. Despite these threats to patients, physicians continue to oppose more autonomy for nurses, while in large part sustaining their own economic status and while shifting to group practices, then investing their own profits in stocks of the organizations that assume power. Although complaining of a loss of control, the medical monopoly remains substantially intact. Nurses have made some changes in their legal rights, but these are offset by losses in their numbers that jeopardize patient care and safety and by the amount of time required by nurses to prove the lowering of standards of care.

With the support of some charitable foundations, nurses, sometimes with physicians, have developed community-based programs, but whether these will serve as nationwide models remains open to question. A fundamental restructuring of the health-care hierarchy and an overhaul of the entire system are needed, but again the AMA in a series of resolutions have opposed nurses' autonomy, thus limiting the extent to which health care could be refocused, causing staffing problems, and resulting in a "regulatory, and policy quagmire." Although the medical monopoly is still widely assumed to be in the best interest of patients, it is now possible to see that the exclusion of women healers and their subsequent subordination as nurses created severe imbalances in health care that are still not rectified, thus, negatively affecting the health of people. Although monopolistic control has provided some benefits, the cost to consumers is higher than they want to or should pay, both literally and figuratively.

Whenever a monopoly of any service exists, the exclusion of alternative modes of care restricts the potential for creativity and productivity and limits both caregivers and consumers. More particularly, when gender is the historical basis for such a monopoly, the full capacities and capabilities of the female half of the human race are stunted and the full possibilities for humane care of human beings are limited because of the exclusion of women. Although some would argue that the success of feminist demands to open all professions and occupations to women has substantially impacted the health-care system, we would argue that no system in the true sense of the word has been achieved and that monopolistic control of thousands of female health-care workers has made the development of such a system difficult if not impossible. Indeed, the small, though increasing, number of women in medicine can hardly solve the problems of large bureaucracies and the fragmentation of services, overpriced and undercoordinated in large part because of the domination by a small, predominantly male elite of physicians. Thus, an outdated, burdensome model of monopolistic control originating in a gender-stereotyped division of labor from previous centuries is still lumbering along and is likely to be sustained well into the twenty-first century. Anticipated changes in the future scientific and technological bases of medicine are evidently not going to be paralleled by a comparable advance in institutional arrangements or professional interrelations unless nurses themselves can force the health-care "system" to become a reality for all the world's people in the new millennium.

PART I | *"Exposing the Meretricious Lies":*
Early Women Healers and Nurses and
the Mythology of Medicine's "Natural"
Supremacy over Healing

1 | "The Mere Trivia of History?"
The Legacy of Early Women Healers and Physicians' Efforts to Exclude or Control Them

In this chapter, sources on gender and nursing are brought together to make visible a centuries-old lineage of women healers and nurses and to document its relationship to that of physicians. Taking a longer view of women healers over several centuries helps us to understand whether nurses indeed usurped medical rights and functions when they created "modern" nursing in the nineteenth century, or whether they were reclaiming only a portion of what women originally did. Perhaps nurses' current striving for greater autonomy is based not on a desire to "practice medicine" but rather on a need to retrieve and take back a part of the functions and authority women previously held.

There is substantial evidence that in previous centuries women were the majority of healers, providing most of the care for the health problems of most people. Whether women healers paralleled or preceded the emergence of medical men is still open to question; however, it is clear that women healers not only provided informally most of the domestic nursing and medical care in families, neighborhoods, and communities, but also created hospitals and other formal institutions of healing in which they provided both medical and nursing treatment.

To what degree were early women healers and caregivers, in both their communities and institutions, actually independent of physicians? Preliminary evidence suggests that these women enjoyed substantial independence from medical authority, and many, in fact, probably had considerable distrust of physicians and their treatments. Indeed, it is likely that some physicians at times depended on the women healers' knowledge, particularly of herbal concoctions. Were women healers' treatments and theories markedly different from or inferior to those of physicians? Were most earlier physicians giving superior treatment based on proven theories of disease and health? Certainly, prior to the later nineteenth century, the state of medical theory and practice was insufficiently advanced to give physicians any superior record over experienced women healers. The vast majority of physicians did not adopt any genuine scientific approach to medicine until well into the nineteenth century.

The emergence of universities from the thirteenth century onward eventually gave physicians their base for authority, which they used to justify excluding women healers from practice. Women's exclusion from colleges and universities prohibited them from receiving formal credentials and eventually, in the nineteenth century, from obtaining scientific training, a critical factor in the eventual subordination of most women healers by the twentieth century. There is further evidence that a number of physicians, even some involved in teaching nurses in the twentieth century, were opposed to theoretical and scientific training for nurses. Clearly, physicians *intentionally* used gender as a way to exclude women healers from obtaining formal credentials and, later, full scientific knowledge. They also *intentionally* colluded with male-dominated legal and religious authorities to eliminate or control women healers; this is most markedly obvious during the European witch hunts, particularly from the fifteenth to the seventeenth centuries.

Perhaps the best way to exclude women healers is to deny or denigrate their existence. Medical historians have eliminated or trivialized women healers, despite the fact that nursing and medicine have a very long history of overlapping tasks and functions. Indeed, it is inappropriate to take the current division of labor and extrapolate backwards to justify it. Throughout the historical stages of nursing and medicine, the professions were so closely interwoven that it is often impossible to distinguish one from the other. Written evidence of nursing appears as early as 4000 B.C., later in the Code of Hammurabi in Babylonia, and still later in religious sources from India. In Greece, records show that women provided health care for their families that involved the skills of both medicine and nursing. By 460 B.C., Hippocrates, the "father" of medicine, wrote notes on nursing for medical students, who carried out what would today be considered traditional nursing practice (Abdullah, 1972). Clearly, nursing and medicine have been so intermeshed that distinctions are difficult to determine or sustain. Despite functional overlap, accusations against women of black magic or, more generally, malpractice were made in the earliest era and have continued to the most recent; for example, Elizabeth Kenny, a twentieth-century nurse, faced such allegations for her pioneering work with victims of poliomyelitis.

Regardless of functional similarities, men have written and maintained the medical version, which, given women's previous exclusion from formal education and publishing, has prevailed over time. Indeed, even the daily lives of women over the centuries, which demonstrate nursing and domestic medicine as central to their work, have also been excluded from the record. Even when attempting to apply medical history to nursing, scholars, some well-intentioned, have failed to connect women's and nurses' histories; thus, any chronology of nurse-physician relations is fundamentally lacking. For example, in Richard H. Shryock's history of nursing (1959), the reader learns nothing of women healers in primitive medicine and nursing and little about them in ancient civilizations, even though in some cultures women had relatively high status. Shryock admitted, however, that in patriarchal Greek culture, women were not allowed to study medicine because of their subordinate status. Midwives were described as merely "folk practitioners." Unfortunately, such gender discrimination seems almost taken for granted. With scarcely any indication of incongruency or illogicality, Shryock maintained that Hellenic medical ideals were on a high level, establishing the foundations of medical ethics, even though medical knowledge could be legally passed only to sons or male students. It is ironic that medical men who excluded 50 percent of humanity from formal learning should be exalted for the formation of ethics. Shryock dealt briefly with Roman antecedents and credited women of the new Christian faith as most actively expressing the tenets of the Church by taking on the care of the sick and the poor; he speculated, "Perhaps they were more inclined to compassion than were the majority of men" (Shryock, 1959, p. 77).

After A.D. 300, women, claimed Shryock, entered nursing because of the improved position of Roman women, the Christian teaching of equality, and the appeal to heed those in distress. Feminist research calls into question such assertions. Indeed, Christian dogma became increasingly negative about women and, over time, reinforced their subordinate status. Shryock made another short reference to women healers of the Middle Ages, but only to female physicians, not nurses, although the development of women's religious orders is described. One secular order, the Beguines of Flanders, founded in 1184, unlike regular orders, permitted women to come and go in public as needed. The Catholic Church later required more restrictive rules for women's orders; however, the Beguines maintained lay status. Said Shryock: "A sort of feminist note is to be observed in the desire of Beguines to be free of male control through bishops or monastic connections ... [which] anticipated modern tendencies" (p. 107). With this one offhand sentence, women's struggle for autonomy in healing is noted.

Relying heavily on traditional medical histories, Shryock presented considerable information on medicine during the Renaissance and Reformation periods, but little on nursing and none on women healers. Secular trends in hospitals and nursing following the Reformation are discussed, but the reader finds only one short statement acknowledging women's subordinate status: during the French Revolution, the issue of women's subjugation was raised, but few changes in their status were subsequently allowed. However, noted Shryock, a conscious feminist campaign, one of many social reforms of the time, did emerge. After this brief acknowledgment, Shryock continued to focus on male-dominated science, medicine groping for the light, and the dark age of hospitals and nursing, before we again see mention of women in the mid nineteenth century when organized feminism is reported. But to Shryock, feminist actions in the nineteenth century seem more important to women physicians than to nurses, who, in his view, benefited only indirectly since they did not have to fight to nurse. These assertions are directly contested in this book. So is the statement that feminism was a reformist, not a radical movement. Many feminists then and now would take issue with this interpretation. Clearly, current nurse-physician relations cannot be accurately analyzed from a perspective that largely eliminates the development of a gendered medical monopoly. Even nursing texts and histories have often emphasized recent history, relied too much on medical perspectives, failed to connect nursing with women's history, and lacked a systematic analysis of the gendered division of labor. Often written as general texts for undergraduate students, some of these have gone through several editions over many decades, and thus these deficiencies have had a cumulative impact (for example, Dolan, 1958, 1963, 1968, 1973; Goodnow, 1916, 1919, 1923, 1928, 1933, 1938, 1942, 1949, 1953; Jensen, 1943, 1950, 1955, 1959, 1965).

Overcoming the Loss in Inspiration by Recovering a "Cherished Tradition"

One of the best histories of early women healers and nursing is found in the four-volume *History of Nursing* by Mary Adelaide Nutting and Lavinia Lloyd Dock (1907; 1912). Given the period in which they wrote, the authors' efforts to analyze the interconnections between gender and nursing prior to the nineteenth century and to stress the importance of feminism to nursing are remarkable. Before the turn of the century, feminists, such as Matilda Joslyn Gage in *Woman, Church and State* (1893), presented extensive research using overlooked historical sources to establish the variety, importance, and subordination of women in earlier periods of Western history. Paralleling this work, Nutting and Dock, in their first volume, traced nursing to the earliest periods of known history. Acknowledging the paucity of sources, they nevertheless hoped that their history would overcome the loss in the "inspiration which arises from cherished tradition," and provide each nurse with the "perspective which shows the relation of one progressive movement to others. Only in the light of history can she clearly see how closely her own calling is linked with the general conditions of education and of liberty that obtain—as they [women] rise, she rises, and as they sink, she falls" (Nutting and Dock, 1907, vol. 1, p. v).

Nutting and Dock believed that from the early beginnings of humanity women must have developed elementary health principles for the care of their children, and grandmothers must have gathered herbs for medicinal teas, as they still did in the early twentieth century: "Who, that knows the old women of remote mountain regions, can but be certain that the grandmothers were the first doctors and nurses thousands of years ago?" (p. 12). Nutting and Dock attempted to establish the honorable and lengthy history of nurses by tracing, for example, their origins to the early Greek god Asklepios and the goddess Hygieia, presumably the prototypic physician and nurse. They contrasted the sanity of early nurse-physicians with the later emergence of theories of demoniacal possession: "In ancient Greece and Egypt the treatment of the epileptic and insane was not only humane, but was largely remedial, and the general feeling toward 'witches' was one of veneration and awe, not of detestation.

This was also true of the ancient Teutons, who revered their 'wise women'" (p. 17).

In contrast, the later Christian medieval period was "one of the most tragic chapters in the whole course of human misery" (p. 18) and represented a period of incredible cruelty based on the idea of demonic possession, which was used to justify the persecution of witches. Nutting and Dock noted that a number of witches were older women who knew medicinal and dental secrets. These wise women served as the prototypes of later "witches," who in the episodes of witch hunting were cruelly tortured and then drowned or killed by burning. Nutting and Dock provide considerable evidence of the destruction of women, many of them healers. Of numerous records, one list of victims, for example, documents the slaying of between three and four thousand women in only one area of many. Such atrocities in Europe were continued to a lesser degree in colonial New England; indeed, the authors noted that even in the closing years of the nineteenth century "a demand for a trial for witchcraft was recently made in Pennsylvania" (p. 20).

Nutting and Dock paid a price for their efforts to produce a nursing history that connected gender and feminism to nursing's development. This is most obvious in the negative book reviews written by members of the medical profession. For example, volumes 3 and 4, covering the international development of nursing in the late nineteenth and early twentieth centuries, were criticized in the British journal *Hospital* (1913, March 8), forcing Nutting to send a letter to the editor (1913, May 7) and a copy to the *American Journal of Nursing* (1913, July). The review, said Nutting, was "written in a deeply hostile spirit and solely for the purpose of discrediting the '*History*'" (Nutting, 1913, p. 743). The reviewer charged that the history was written by a "small clique" engaged in "mutual laudation" and provided "a farrago of prejudice masquerading as history . . . [containing] misrepresentations·of fact . . . sufficient to condemn it" (p. 743). To these charges Nutting replied:

> Doubtless unpalatable truths are presented. It would be difficult to write any true history of nursing during the past quarter of a century, at least, which would form pleasant reading for those, who, in hospitals or out of them, have been concerned with that enterprise which one can only truthfully call the exploitation of nurses. The historian of the future who will have access to the facts will probably have to present a still less pleasant picture. (p. 743)

Nutting and Dock understood that any history of nursing, including midwifery, must be extended to embrace all women healers, even the beneficent or "white witch." This realization seems lost to some subsequent historians, but in a widely distributed and critically contested monograph, *Witches, Midwives, and Nurses*, feminists Barbara Ehrenreich and Deirdre English (1972) resurrected the idea that women have historically been the predominant healers, the unlicensed doctors, anatomists, abortionists, nurses, counselors, pharmacists, and midwives. Whether its practitioners were called wise women by the people, or witches or charlatans by the authorities, medicine is "part of our heritage as women, our history, our birthright" (p. 1). To these authors, the current mythology that male science replaced female superstition or "old wives' tales" belies history: "it was the male professionals who clung to untested doctrines and ritualistic practices" (p. 2). The women healers were the herbalists and empiricists.

Given current knowledge, the value of some of the women healer's remedies can certainly be questioned. Nevertheless, it is impossible to deny that misogyny, the hatred of women, was central to the mass murder of 500,000 to nine million people (estimates vary widely), of whom at least 85 percent were women or children. Ironically, said Ehrenreich and English, the most terrible and strongest evidence of witchcraft was that the women had "magical" powers that could either harm or heal others. In contrast, church-sanctioned incantations and charms for healing were evidently not magic because these were approved by male priests. Excluded from such legitimization, women were automatically a suspect class because of their gender. However, their herbal painkillers, digestive aids, and anti-inflammatory agents were all empirically tested, not based simply on faith: "So great was the witches' knowledge that in 1527, Paracelsus, considered the 'father of modern medicine,' burned his text on pharmaceuticals, confessing that he 'had learned from the Sorceress all he knew'" (p. 17).

Ehrenreich and English claimed that an active takeover by medical men occurred *before* science and technology became solidly established. The reason? To obtain a total and lucrative monopoly over all healing and the power to determine who would live or die, who was fertile or sterile, who was mad or sane. These authors, in agreement with Nutting and Dock, assert that the status of women healers has risen and fallen as women's status has improved or declined. Healers were attacked as women, and they have fought back in relation to other women. In short, the authors turn nursing history upside down: medicine was *part of nursing* and emerged from the age-old traditional, community-based wise women, who practiced *both* nursing and medicine.

From the thirteenth and fourteenth centuries on, European medicine as a profession actively eliminated female healers from universities and imposed strict controls within the limits set by the Catholic authorities; thus, they disengaged medicine from the "soul" while remaining within existing religious strictures. Ironically, the physicians' university training was distinctly not clinical but philosophical, sharply differentiated from that of barber-surgeons, who dealt directly with people. Bleeding, leeching, incantations, and rituals were commonly used by physicians.

Literate women healers, said Ehrenreich and English, were attacked first because they were more likely to have wealthy patients and thus were an economic threat. That they cared for patients was the issue; their presumption to treat at all was the problem. That they did so without formal, institutionalized "training" was the charge. Because they were excluded as women from such "training" made the conclusion automatic. By the fourteenth century, the emerging medical monopoly was extended to judging witches. Physicians over the next three centuries were consulted to make "scientific" judgments on whether or not women were witches. For women, healing came to equal heresy, torture, and even death.

Clearly, Nutting and Dock and, later, Ehrenreich and English were trying not only to establish the ancient, sacred origins of women healers, but to go beyond medical histories written by men. By the 1970s renewed feminist research on the early historical origins of women, when combined with feminist reconceptualizations of religions and the resurrection of the female sacred in the study of early goddesses, laid the foundation for a reconsideration of the sacred in nurses' early history. The influence of women's rethinking of early history is apparent in nurse Marie-Thérèse Connell's (1983) article on female consciousness in historical perspective. Connell, writing in the last decades of the twentieth century, seems unaware that Nutting and Dock had written on the same topic in the century's first decades. By the 1980s, however, Connell is able, because of subsequent research, to do what her foremothers could not: she too challenged the male versions of history but also found that women healers in sacred symbols may have *preceded* and later been usurped by physicians. Connell does not look to Hippocrates, the "father of medicine," or even to Fabiola, the "first nurse" (who in the fourth century founded the first free public hospital under Christian auspices), but to early Greek mythology, in which the goddess Hygieia is postulated as the source of nursing. Some historical sources refer to her as the daughter of the mythological first physician, Asklepios, thus, having no identity separate from him. However, Connell suggests a different story: Hygieia was a goddess "in her own right" at least as early as 600 B.C., one hundred years *before* the rise of Asklepios and two hundred years *before* she became his daughter. Greek patriarchy devalued the female and, as portrayed in votive tablets, the original prominent image of Hygieia gives way to Asklepios in the foreground, who, when absorbed into Roman culture, finally stands alone, "the solitary, benevolent image of healing and a prototype of the modern physician" (p. 7). To Connell, this imagery is false: a woman symbolized the earliest founder of nursing *and* medicine; only later was she usurped in male medical imagery.

Changing Images of Early Women Healers

Are there other images in later historical periods that suggest at least some prominence and independence of women healers? Little research has been conducted specifically on nurses, but art historian Natalie Boymel Kampen (1988) studied paintings and sculpture to provide a history of nursing before

Florence Nightingale's emergence and prominence in the mid nineteenth century. To Kampen, "nurses have a complicated history, invisible in many periods, hard to recognize in others, and only in this century assuming the look we take for granted" (p. 6). Kampen's research is a pioneering effort to uncover women healers in Greek and Roman art from the fifth century B.C. to the fourth century A.D. and then to compare these images with those from the late medieval and Renaissance periods, more particularly the fifteenth and sixteenth centuries. Given the extremely secluded lives of Greek women and the underrepresentation of women as artists, Kampen's search is valiant, difficult, and, of necessity, overly dependent on male perceptions and productions.

Kampen tracks iconography, the study of images as symbols or signs of ideas, as metaphors and analogies of the world of women healers. She finds that artists pictured the public and rarely the private worlds of women. On the few occasions in which women are portrayed, they are depicted in pleasant actions: "We are never permitted to see the sick slaves being nursed by women in the villa infirmaries described by Roman writers; nowhere do we find any illustration of the passages in Roman history that tell of women nursing men wounded in battle" (p. 8). Except for women preparing dead bodies for burial, the artistic imagery does not show what men's written records describe. Women midwives were, however, portrayed in rare childbirth scenes, and nurses were shown bathing newborn infants. Midwives did more than deliver babies, even though the images do not portray their pre- and postnatal care, nor their treatment of sick babies, nor their care of women's gynecological problems. The baby nurse was not, said Kampen, as highly valued as the midwife; however, both of these images lived through the Middle Ages and into the seventeenth century. The baby nurse was commonly represented in nativity scenes and at the birth of the Virgin Mary.

From the later Middle Ages, the iconography shifts to include individual women performing acts of mercy—for example, St. Elizabeth nursing the sick—and to groups of nursing sisters in hospitals. These pictures of women healing *outside* the family and home represent to Kampen a clear and distinct change in nursing iconography, which is even more pronounced in hospital scenes where the women are *never* pictured as subordinated to patients or doctors. In fact, pictures of nursing sisters at the Hôtel-Dieu in Paris show them gathered before the sick in the hospital ward, where they are not represented as assistants to physicians. Of one painting, Kampen notes, "Although the priest is present, there are no male physicians, nor is there evidence of anyone giving orders to the sisters" (p. 25). Northern European images differ from those of Italy, where women are not depicted at all or, for example, stand in the background as a physician visits a plague victim. Nevertheless, Kampen concludes that, in general, in comparison to later images, the nurses "seem remarkably independent of male physicians" (p. 29). She sees a synthesis of nurse as kin and nurse as public worker in the Christian version of sisters caring for others in hospices, hostels, and homes.

Over time, Kampen notes, there was, in some areas, increasing concern about women as nurses and as witches, whether they had good or evil intentions. At the same time, the physician, particularly the man conducting cesarean sections, grew more popular in the images than midwives or nurses. The tensions between Catholic and Protestant, scientific and spiritual, and male and female practitioners are all apparent in the male imagery. But what the women's artistic images were or would have been remains unclear; however, even without certainty on this issue, it is clear that the iconography does not support the view of a direct and continuous subordination of women healers or nurses to medical men, an image common in the popular imagery of the twentieth century.

Brightening the Distant Shadows: Women Healers Reclaimed

That the presentations of some nursing and most medical histories are fundamentally incomplete or inaccurate is addressed by Margaret Connor Versluysen (1980) in Celia Davies's anthology *Rewriting Nursing History.* Davies briefly introduces Versluysen's article by saying that the author "sees existing history as history from a male viewpoint" (Davies, 1980, p. 175), which has devalued and trivialized women's work. Versluysen sought unnoticed alternative sources on women healers that should have been central to any history of nursing. She used these sources to assess the writing of Ehrenreich and English (1972), whose thinking, according to Davies, is polemical and not detailed historical scholarship. In contrast, Versluysen believes their work is important in creating a better programmatic base for rewriting nursing history. If Ehrenreich and English and other feminist theorists are taken seriously, Davies admits that historians must start further back than the nineteenth century, asking about, and not taking for granted, early gender divisions of labor and analyzing the differential treatment of men and women. Because so many nurses are women, there are few comparative cases, says Davies, so "we fail to see and appreciate the difference this makes. Critiques such as this [Versluysen's] can help keep us alert" (Davies, 1980, p. 175).

Alternatively, we might claim that some historians have not grasped the *structured* gendering of the whole of patriarchal culture; thus, it is not merely a question of comparative cases, or of simply being alert. Rather, the analysis of gender requires a different perspective, just as the analysis of racist society does. Few serious thinkers would consider the historical situation of African Americans in Western cultures without reference to the racist structure of these societies. Similarly, competent thinkers can no longer merely be alert to the differences in the treatment of women; analysts of women workers, such as nurses, must see the gendered social arrangements inherent in the cultures in which they have worked. Versluysen understands this, and, in agreement with Ehrenreich and English, she states that women have *always* been the main healers in European, and particularly British, society, a fact conveniently excluded from some nursing and most medical histories. This exclusion is not simply a factual error, but a failure to embed the particular in the general; therefore it produces an inadequate and inaccurate theoretical understanding of nurses and nursing. It should be, for example, relatively easy to show statistically that women have done most of the healing, not only in British but in most Western and many non-Western cultures. Versluysen claims that women "have delivered babies, rendered first aid, prescribed and dispensed remedies and cared for the sick, infirm, and dying, both as a neighborly service and as paid work. Yet, aside from histories of nursing, the vast range of women's past healing work is virtually absent from the annals of written history" (Versluysen, 1980, p. 175). This is hardly a polemical position; it is probably a commonsense fact, observable in many societies even today.

Versluysen argues that women must explicate the implicit biases in the basic frame of reference of history, uncritical acceptance of which has induced historians to ignore a large amount of data on women's roles in the management of health and illness. She turns to overlooked scholarly works to provide evidence of the extensive female healing roles in the past, which to her are "very different from those we know today" (p. 175). From these sources, Versluysen concludes: "This evidence suggests that conventional distinctions between doctoring and nursing, amateur and professional medicine, orthodox and unorthodox healers may be less relevant for an analysis of the past than distinctions between men and women" (pp. 175–176). If this theoretical assertion is correct, and we believe it is, then the whole of medical and nursing histories cannot continue to be accepted without radical reconstitution of the role terminology and distinctions upon which they are based. If gender is the key to distinctions in functions, then what constitutes the presumed differences in healing activities?

Indeed, Versluysen and other women historians have had to reconsider what history is. To them, it is not the past as such, but an intellectual operation that reconstructs the past through interpretation of fragmentary written residues. Restricted to available resources, the historian selects from these in accordance with her or his own implicit social and intellectual values and schemata. Obviously, prior intellectual assumptions and categories always cause history to be both selective and value-laden, never "a theoretical, neutral collection of 'facts,' since 'facts' only become history via the intervention of individual historians" (p. 176). In this sense, history is only "objective" in the presentation of analysis and findings in a way amenable to the critical scrutiny of others.

Despite presumed scholarly detachment, most history is unidimensional, presented from the male point of view, reflecting men's interests, values, and concerns: "Our legacy is a literature in which vast tracts of the past seem to have been populated (quite remarkably) exclusively by men!" (p. 176). We can sometimes "catch sight of female shadows in the distance, but devaluation and trivialization of women's lives . . . have excluded systematic and sustained analysis" (p. 176). The recent growth of the histories of childhood, family, and women are forcing history open, but even this scholarship "is a tiny drop in a vast ocean of disinterest and apathy" (p. 177).

Critically important is Versluysen's assertion that the thoroughness and consistency of the historical devaluation and exclusion of women are not purely accidental; instead they reflect a society that has developed "an elaborate set of beliefs to justify its consistent ranking and rewarding of male interests and activities more highly than comparable female interests and activities. . . . If we look into the mirror of history, we find a systematic interpretation of past health care practice in a way which assigns positive value and superior status to male healing work, and little or no value and subordinate or marginal status to female activity" (p. 177). This is only one interpretation of the past and does not represent absolute historical truth.

Indeed, Versluysen asserts that history has reflected the narrow, gendered exclusivity of organized medicine, the story of a socially privileged group of male healers, and further narrowed the story to the "great men of medicine," the presumed agents of social progress, based on the idea of history as intrinsically progressive. This, in turn, assumes an egalitarian society in which benefits are extended to all regardless of class, race, or gender—a highly questionable premise. To Versluysen, great physicians of the past did not make history alone and certainly did not achieve the contemporary health system by a supposed triumph of male medical rationality over quacks and masses of illiterate "old wives." This gendered selective perspective is an "extremely partial view of the past" (p. 178). Indeed, physicians have dismissed persons and ideas outside their control as insignificant and inconsequential. Unfortunately, "[h]istorians have generally accepted this dismissal with great alacrity and little criticism" (p. 178), viewing nonmedical personnel as marginal amateurs.

Not every medical historian, however, has ignored the contributions and achievements of women healers in the past. One of the few who has recently attempted to redress the medical gender-selective perspective is William L. Minkowski (1992). In contrast to other medical historians, he acknowledges that healing has always been considered the province of women, noting that in the Middle Ages they served as herbalists, midwives, surgeons, barber-surgeons, nurses, empirics, and traditional healers. Because women were excluded from academic institutions, Minkowski concludes that they did not have the opportunity to contribute to the science of medicine, and thus, being "untutored" in medicine, they used botanical therapies, home remedies, purges, and herbal medications and also learned from observing physicians.

However, given the roles listed and functions enumerated by Minkowski, one must ask what was left that early physicians did differently. Furthermore, was learning only one-way? Did physicians such as Paracelsus never learn anything from women in their varied healing roles? Indeed, Minkowski admits that the scientific study of human illness was largely missing and that incantations and amulets were used by *all* practitioners, including physicians. We must ask then what did the women healers, particularly those who worked full-time in their communities, observe physicians doing that was substantially different from or better than the women's own practices? Indeed, were there even any physicians present in their communities for the women to observe?

It is quite easy to prove that before the eighteenth century few physicians existed, and these were mostly in urban centers; thus, the majority of "amateurs" were women, but these, Versluysen claims, have been dismissed as illiterate old wives. Historians have simply ignored or dismissed the extensive system of home-based care. But a wide range of sources exist: diaries, memoirs, letters, housewifery manuals, herbal compendia, popular health manuals, local records and activities, popular works on health and illness for women, midwifery texts written by women, and so forth. This potential evidence has "hardly been tapped, since historians have assumed, quite incorrectly, that women's healing work constitutes the mere trivia of history" (Versluysen, 1980, p. 179), relying instead on past medical writers, who had a vested interest in the derogation of women's healing skills.

Versluysen hypothesized a causal connection between medical misogyny and the closure of medical occupations to women, and asserts that physicians' pejorative value judgments about women healers have been accepted as historical fact because historians have ignored other sources, preferring to rely on medical references. When they have dealt with women, there is a stereotyped triptych: "illiterate old wives, exceptional wives, exceptional heroines or saintly ministering angels whose mystical aura contrasts starkly with the apparent rationality of male medicine" (p. 179). Women healers as a social collectivity are missing; the individualization of female healing excludes the widespread healing roles of the masses of women. Emphasizing the few exceptions as unrepresentative and atypical excludes any systemic understanding; thus, even these "exceptional" women are forced into stereotyped molds.

Historical interest in midwives and birthing assistants has, until recently, also been almost nonexistent, probably because their functions were not part of organized medicine until the end of the nineteenth century. This denies historical fact; British records of royal midwives can be traced to the fifteenth century and ecclesiastical licensing of professed midwives to the sixteenth century, but "Despite considerable source material, the first comprehensive social history of English midwives was not published until 1977" (p. 181). Jean Donnison's *Midwives and Medical Men* (1977) traced the history of interprofessional rivalries and women's rights, firmly connecting gender and professional roles in her analysis. The only major British study previously published was by an obstetrician, James Hobson Aveling (1872), who concluded that rational management of childbirth was invented by medical men. Why has this version held sway? Because, claims Versluysen, myths of male rationality and expertise are so deeply entrenched that myths about female ignorance and incompetence are rarely questioned.

To his credit, Minkowski (1992) attempts to correct some of these myths and medicine's biased account, admitting that midwifery was clearly the women's "medical" monopoly. (If medical men were seldom involved in midwifery, it is unclear how the monopoly can be termed "medical" unless, of course, one accepts the idea that "medical" equals "healing" and also "nursing.") According to Minkowski, physicians believed that their "dignity and self-esteem were diminished by the manual nature of care for the pregnant patient; for them, medicine was an intellectual exercise" (p. 292). In addition, male contact with female bodies could lead to scandal. Guy de Chauliac, a fourteenth-century surgeon, was even unwilling to discuss midwifery because it was dominated by women.

Monica Green's 1989 research on the obstetrix (the original Latin term for midwife in the thirteenth century, subsequently changed in France to *sage-femme* [wise woman] or *ventrière*) proves that midwives actually played a wider healing role than simply delivering babies. Varying by time and place, midwives or sage or wise women were often involved in the whole of women's health as well as the well-being of entire communities, some of which bestowed upon them special privileges, tax exemptions, or pensions, and at times even passed prohibitions against midwives leaving the towns, so valued were their services. Minkowski, on the other hand, asserts that the medieval women's health roles were "wholly unspecialized" and involved more of a custodial than therapeutic character. Certainly this can be questioned, but what is not debatable from Green's research is that "women did perform varied medical functions beyond those of empiric and midwife; they served as physicians, apothecaries, surgeons, and barber-surgeons. . . . Evidence for their involvement in these more specialized areas of practice comes from the feminine endings of nouns descriptive of their healing work, from guild societies to which they belonged, and from legislation regulating their professional activities" (Minkowski, 1992, p. 292).

Not only were women "practicing medicine" in obstetrics, gynecology, and pediatrics, they were also involved in all other areas of medicine. Sophia Jex Blake (1886), for example, one of the first British women physicians in the modern period who, with other women, faced virulent opposition as a "petticoat physic," responded to her critics by publishing a treatise that proved that women had historically practiced medicine. Her work was followed by the pioneering study of Alice Clark (1919) on the working life of women in the seventeenth century; the research on women practitioners in the Middle Ages by Eileen Power (1921); the history of women in medicine from the earliest historical period to the start of the nineteenth century by American physician Kate Campbell Hurd-Mead (1938); and the work of Muriel Joy Hughes (1943), later republished in 1968, which focused on female healers or empirics, nurses, and physicians.

The question of what title or term should be used to describe women healers forced Hughes, for example, to use the term "empiric"; the evidence on female physicians further substantiates the existence of female healers but leaves the problem of boundaries unclear, since historians have traditionally accepted male definitions of physicians. If such definitions rest on formal training from which women were excluded, almost all women would automatically be omitted, regardless of training. In this sense, we may ask whose historical account is polemical. Is it the abbreviated version by Ehrenreich and English that insists on the full history of all women healers? Or the typical medical history that largely excludes women healers of all kinds? Or more recent histories of nursing that often limit women healers to the restricted definition imposed on nurses from the mid nineteenth century onward?

The Dividing Line: Gender, Not Function

It should be obvious by now that the truncated version of nursing history as it emerged in the late nineteenth century is not properly embedded either in women's general history or in the more specific history of women as healers. Further, it is clear that formal education cannot be the key to a definition of female healers. In addition, most healing has been historically undertaken by women, often without any labels applied at all, other than familial terms. If these facts are accurate, then the so-called polemical version of feminist nurses and non-nurse historians must be reconsidered. It is highly likely that gender, not function, has been essential to role definitions and distinctions. It was not until the *widespread* adoption of scientific theory and method by physicians in the late nineteenth century that functional distinctions could be clearly delineated. This assumes, however, that nurses were not equally influenced by science. This, too, is at least partially incorrect. In fact, it was often physicians who wanted to exclude nurses from scientific knowledge, but nurses kept insisting on *both* theoretical and practical education. Even without it, they were forced to use scientific methods, for better or worse, in their daily work. Thus, even the functional distinctions based on science are blurred at best.

There is sufficient historical evidence to assert that women's past medical and nursing work has been varied and extensive in scope, involving women of all social classes, "from the wise women skilled in the use of herbs and ointments, to the chatelaine in her castle, and the woman selling her skills as physician and surgeon in the open market" (Versluysen, 1980, p. 183). The array of evidence is so substantial that "it is quite false to assume that women are capable of little else but the simplest nursing" (p. 183). For example, Hughes (1943; 1968) found that women from the eleventh to the fifteenth centuries had the main responsibility for medical and nursing care of the sick, of first aid, and of attendance on servants and guests at home and patients in secular and convent hospitals. Healing duties were obviously within the sphere of women's activities, whether the women were highly literate and educated ladies, fictional heroines, or women of other classes. Growing and administering medicinal herbs, dispensing remedies, healing wounds, setting bones, managing community health needs—these were all functions of women healers, who were often quite successful in their multiple roles and, even though excluded from formal training, compared favorably with physicians. It should be stressed again that all healers, regardless of gender, were subject to the superstitions of each period; thus, the use of charms, prayers, and so on were not limited to either women or men.

In Ardent Defense of Women and Their Accomplishments: Actions of Early Women Healers and Nurses

What exactly were medieval women healers, nurses, and physicians or, more generally, empirics doing as portrayed in the literature of the time? Educated women of the Middle Ages wrote of their work, but "Not many women committed either their experiences in healing or their observations on the subject to paper, but those who did represent a widely scattered group of women belonging to different social levels" (Hughes, 1968, p. 37). Again, although largely excluded from formal education, many of these women could at least read and some had "as thorough a training in the arts and sciences as it was possible for women to acquire" (p. 37). For example, Princess Anna Comnena, author of *The Alexiad,* a chronicle of the reign of her father, the Byzantine Emperor Alexius I (1081–1118), alluded frequently to sickness and health, and demonstrated thorough training, extensive reading, and intelligent application of medical knowledge.

Comnena grasped "truths in advance of the doctrines and beliefs of her day . . . and suspected other causes of illness than those accepted by physicians" (p. 37). She asked, for instance, whether climate and diet, rather than the four humours (blood, phlegm, yellow bile, and black bile), advocated by physicians, might not be the actual causes of illness. Indeed, the empress, Comnena's mother, ordered her daughter to be present at meetings of physicians at her father's last illness "to adjudge the physicians' arguments" (p. 39). The empress and Comnena evidently had a low opinion of most of these medical men and sided with only one physician, who argued for purgatives. The other physicians disagreed, however, and "made an incision at the elbow, . . . to relieve the patient's asthmatic breathing" (p. 39). When this did not work, they tried an antidote of pepper that Anna thought made her father worse, and finally tried cauterization, which also failed.

Comnena discussed battlefield wounds and commented positively on her father's consideration for wounded soldiers and captives and his construction of a hospital for the ailing. She noted that his army stopped at the sound of a trumpet when a captive woman gave birth or when someone died. Comnena observed that Byzantine women's chief healing functions were carried out by nursing at home, where they alone cared and cured, using physicians only when absolutely necessary. The empress herself did most of the nursing of the emperor, who was also attended by Anna: "Because she was so competent, she was slightly contemptuous of the diagnoses and services of the doctors. She was far more satisfied with her own and her mother's efforts to alleviate the distress of the Emperor by taking his pulse, massaging him, and preparing digestible foods for him" (p. 41). It is clear that Anna was very knowledgeable in both medicine and nursing. It is not at all clear that the distinction between the two can be made except in retrospect, following the gendered differentiation of functions.

Indeed, early feminist Christine de Pisan (ca. 1364–1429), daughter of Thomas de Pisan, astrologer and physician, wrote in the fourteenth century that women received insufficient credit for their contributions to home and society and, more particularly, "the ingratitude of men who criticized women even though women spent their lives as nurses either to their children or to their husbands" (p. 41). Pisan, who "won renown for her ardent defense of women and their accomplishments" (p. 37), stressed that women should learn not only household arts but sciences. She would not, said Hughes, have accepted a published, contemporary conduct book in which a man instructed women on the details of household management: "It is obvious that a woman did not write the book, for the section on cookery contains only a few simple remedies for the sick, and in no other section are other than general remarks made on the subject of care" (pp. 42–43). Indeed, he even included an incantation for the bite of a dog or other mad beast that involved writing several words on a crust of bread.

Much more useful are letters written between women in which they ask each other for advice, exchange measures taken and remedies given, and detail the results of experiments with them. Hughes stated: "In cases of severe illness, they summoned physicians, with whose services they were not always pleased" (pp. 45–46). In the fifteenth century, two English women, Agnes and Margaret Paston, involved in the management of large households of relatives and servants, assumed "the roles of nurse and physician in caring for children, bandaging wounds, setting bones, and treating colds and other complaints" (p. 46). The Paston letters discussed herbal medicines and cures in the form of ointments, plasters, and potions; emphasized diet for cure; and expressed fear of foul air as a cause of disease.

While their menfolk were away conducting business in London, the Paston women wrote and asked them to buy fruit or spices for medicinal supplies or preventive remedies. Indeed, "The Paston men placed great faith in the advice and the medicines of the women of their family" (p. 48). When Sir John, while in London, suffered pain in his heel, he was urged to come home, and he responded, "I would full fain be hence" (Gairdner, 1900–1901, Letter No. 212; cited in Hughes, 1968, p. 48). Years later, the younger Sir John wrote to his wife asking her for a plaster remedy for his friend, the king's attorney, and urged her to tell him "hough it shold be leyd to and takyn from hys knee, and hough longe it shold abyd on hys knee unrenevyd, and hough longe the plays-ter wyll laste good, and whethyr he must lape eny more clothys about the playster to kepe it warme or nought"(Gairdner, 1900–1901, Letter No. 898; cited in Hughes, 1968, p. 48). Hughes surmised that Sir John's wife's plaster must have created wonders at home or her husband would not have wanted it for the king's own attorney!

No matter how competent, neither women nor men healers could stop the plague—all medicine and nursing failed. Margaret Paston wrote that they knew not where to be so it was better to stay at home. For very severe illnesses, a leech or doctor was sometimes called from the closest town and shared by families. But, as Hughes noted, in many cases of sudden illness, "the immedi-ate assistance of doctors was of no avail" (p. 50). Indeed, "The experience of the Paston family with doctors led the women to become as skeptical as Anna Comnena of any real benefit to be derived from their ministrations" (p. 50). Margaret warned her husband in 1464 to beware of medicines and physicians, whom she would never trust after their failures with her husband's father and her own uncle.

"She Was a Noble Surgion": Legendary and Fictional Accounts of Women Healers

Hughes also researched and analyzed the fictional romances, lais, and chansons for the healing knowledge and practice of women, finding that these, like factual sources, presented women as skilled with herbal medicines and the care of wounds. For example, "In Malory's *Morte Darthur,* the Irish King placed Tantris in the care of his daughter, La Belle Iseult, 'because she was a noble surgion.' The daughter of the king in the ballad 'Sir Cawline' was called 'a leeche full ffine" (p. 51). If wounded, knights were removed from combat to a castle, hostel, or religious house, where heavy armor was removed in order to examine wounds. The steps in healing wounds were outlined in *The Siege of Jerusalem:* women by torchlight looked at the "hurtes . . . waschen woundes with wyn" and with "wolle stoppen," and "with oyle & orisoun, ordeyned in charme" (Kölbing and Day, 1932; cited in Hughes, 1968, p. 53).

It is important to note that the skilled man or woman in fictional accounts was ascribed the *same* healing powers as physicians. Indeed, in one story a knight maltreated by Salernian physicians is rescued by a woman healer and her precious ointment. In caring for their soldiers and armies, royal leaders such as King Mark sent for "alle maner of leches & surgens bothe unto men and wymmen" (Hughes, 1968, p. 59). The nurses, who performed innumerable medical and nursing services near the battlefields, are less frequent in fiction because they were taken for granted. On the capture of Jerusalem, however, one writer said, "If the women had not been there, the host would have been in a bad plight" (Richard, 1868; cited in Hughes, 1968, p. 59). Women not only administered fluids and potions but also set broken arms and dislocated shoulders: "Aucassin's dislocated shoulder offered no great problem to Nicolette, who reduced it with her own hands, and then applied a poultice of flowers and leaves" (Hughes, 1968, p. 59).

Hughes found that fictional women healers treated the same complaints and ailments that were seen by physicians. Fantastic cures of leprosy or of insanity, for example, appeared in fiction, but neither physicians nor women healers could in actuality do more than send lepers to hospitals, where women often took care of them. Hughes concluded that medieval women had from experience a good deal of sound knowledge of the treatment of wounds and souls; knew the importance of rest and sleep, the efficacy of hot baths and herbal concoctions; could treat dislocated or broken bones—"[a]nd most of them were not bothered by the erudite hocuspocus which was the stock-in-trade of their professional brethren" (p. 61).

The "Nursing Saints": Medieval Female Nurse-Physician-Infirmarians

During the twelfth and thirteenth centuries, there was an outburst of women's energies as women founded secular nursing orders, worked in the proliferating hospitals, or cared for the sick in homes and orphanages. Minkowski acknowledges that many women's actions were attempts at "some measure of independence from a constricting social system" (Minkowski, 1992, p. 289). With the emergence of larger numbers of nursing orders, nurse-physician nuns increased in number and represented one group of women healers. A second group consisted of those hired by the upper class, whose families employed nurses to take care of their children and their sick. "More spectacular were the women who came mainly from the ranks of nobility and who 'sacrificed' themselves in the cause of charity and won distinction as 'nursing saints'" (Hughes, 1968, p. 114).

From the eleventh to the early thirteenth centuries, European hospitals and charitable institutions grew to 19,000; these often offered specialized care for the sick, old, blind, and leprous, and for pilgrims and unfortunates of all kinds. The Black Death in 1348 was so grave that many women from all societal strata became healers, establishing orders of secular nurses. Some joined small orders that served certain types of patients while others were in large organizations that cared for all types of illnesses and patients. Minkowski notes that in German hospitals the women made all essential purchases, kept precise accounts, supervised all housekeeping and kitchen personnel, evaluated the need for further inpatient care, and admitted and released patients based on diagnoses and prognoses. Minkowski twice emphasizes that the women performed these activities without any medical preparation; however, it is more accurate to say that they often had no *academic* medical training in specific institutions. What is clear is that German women in hospitals cared for the sick, the mentally ill, children, and even livestock. If a physician was present, any care of women patients that required touching breasts, abdomens, or female genitalia was done by the women. In pesthouses used to isolate people with contagious diseases, the women nurses-healers sustained the total care of people struck by the plague and other communicable diseases.

The Benedictine order set the pattern in women's orders of active service combined with the contemplative life, where the practical life of the abbey was not neglected and abbesses were respected for their administrative skill. "In the twelfth century, abbesses such as Euphemia and Héloïse gained distinction . . . while Hildegarde won fame as a healer and as a writer on the phenomena and nature of the spirit" (Hughes, 1968, p. 117). Euphemia, abbess of Wherwell from 1126 to 1157, administered the care provided to the sick and the necessities of life in health and sickness for the sisters; she built an infirmary, under which was constructed a watercourse to carry off refuse that might contaminate the air, and created gardens and vineyards.

Héloïse (d. 1164) followed Abélard's rule for the monastery, which established the conduct of the nuns' life, but advocated leniency for the sick, saying that the law was not made for the sick, who should receive whatever their illnesses demanded. Abélard further claimed that "medical training was a primary need of an infirmarian" (p. 119). In addition, some of the nuns should be experienced in phlebotomy and bleeding, so that it would be unnecessary for "a man to enter among the women for this purpose" (p. 119).

Some abbesses wrote scholarly books. In 1167, Herrad of Landsperg in Hohenburg wrote an encyclopedia of knowledge, *Hortus deliciarum*. Hildegarde, although lacking university training, "won renown for her intelligence and knowledge of medicine," and "spread a zeal for learning. There is no doubt that Hildegarde was known as a healer" (pp. 120, 121). Her mystical treatises, for example, the *Scivias* (1141–1152), established her original and beautifully written books on the universe, on humankind and nature, on birth and death, the sun, moon, wind, the humours, the soul, and the nature of God. In addition, she produced two medical-nursing works, the *Subtilitatum diversarumque creaturum libri novem* and *Causae et curae*; both of these reflected twelfth-century medieval knowledge; however, "most of her cures were the usual herbal compounds" (p. 123). Whether the remedies published by physicians were any better than the herbal and other treatments commonly used by nurses or other women healers is highly questionable. Whether physicians derived some of their treatments from women's experiential knowledge seems possible. Certainly, we can no longer assume that women derived *all* their learning from physicians, who apparently *never* learned anything from women healers.

It is clear that the women ran their own convents and separate infirmaries, advocating a common area for patients with ordinary maladies, but special houses for the lepers and the mentally ill. It is important to note that beyond being gentle, good-tempered, kind, compassionate, and able to give affectionate sympathy, skill was necessary and "a knowledge of medicine sufficient to enable the infirmarian to manage her department with efficiency and to effect cures in the cases which came under her care" (p. 125). There is no evidence that cure and care were separated. Furthermore, the abbess ruled the infirmarian, and she was responsible for the lay sisters who washed patients, changed bedding, and kept the building orderly.

Most of the biographical accounts focus on "nursing saints," the women who did not join either religious or secular orders, but engaged in charitable work and, in the medieval period, developed a new kind of social service: "European history contains constant references to women founding churches, schools, hospitals, and convents" (p. 131). Because the medieval women were socially prominent or later canonized, their lives were recorded, but their followers' names, "though perhaps legion, died upon the lips of those who profited by their generosity and kindly attentions" (p. 131).

Mathilda, wife of Henry I of England (1100–1135), cared for lepers in her home, tended them, provided food, washed and dried their feet—this during a time in which lepers were shunned and isolated outside of cities. Without physicians' permission, Mathilda founded in 1101 the Hospitale of St. Giles outside London for forty lepers, the first such institution in this area. In Silesia, Bohemia, and Hungary, other nursing saints provided health care: Hedwig (1174–1243); Anna of Bohemia, who founded a hospital in 1253; and Agnes, princess of Bohemia, who spent several years at Hedwig's convent, remained to care for the sick rather than marry Frederick II, and in 1253 founded a nunnery and hospital. Elizabeth, daughter of King Andreas II of Hungary, built a hospital and founded two infirmaries, one for sick or orphaned children whom she cared for so well they called her mother.

Medieval Women Empirics

Although too brief glimpses are afforded of medieval women in nursing and medicine, they were as actively engaged in healing the sick and caring for the distressed as their modern sisters. Even though "they labored under the terrible handicaps of ignorance and superstition, . . . history and literature alike pay tribute to their practical wisdom, especially in herbal medicine; to their dexterity in administering treatment, no matter how suitable or baleful their remedies might be; and to their willingness to do whatever they could to alleviate human suffering" (Hughes, 1968, p. 135). With few exceptions, women were excluded from the front ranks of medicine and were not admitted to medical schools, doing most of their work as "empirics, midwives, or, of course, as nurses" (p. 135). Though they may have been ignorant of medical principles, they, according to Hughes, mixed traditional love and practical common sense, and some, such as French empiric Jacoba Félicie, were more successful than physicians.

Again it must be stressed that Hughes had to use the term "empiric" to classify women healers, since many were not specifically called barbers, physicians, surgeons, or even nurses. The classification as nurse probably involved much of what subsequently became gendered and, in retrospect, may have influenced the improper split between cure and care. The empirics who administered their herbs and potions were as successful as "scientific" healers; however, it is very difficult to assume that any genuine medical science existed during much of the Middle Ages. The accounts of actual women healers are strongly supported by their counterparts in medieval literature: "the chief difference between the ladies of fiction and the ladies of history was not in the scope of their activities, but rather in the almost invariable success which attended the efforts of the former" (p. 136).

Did the large and important role that women enacted as nurses, healers, or empirics with physicians' functions increase their status in medieval society? Did their work win respect and gratitude? Hughes concluded: "Despite the dog-in-the-manger attitude of the professional physicians, the skill of women in the relief of suffering was widely recognized, and was sometimes contrasted favorably with that of their male rivals" (p. 137). In fiction, for example, Chaucer satirized a male Doctor of Physic, but wrote positively of female ministration to the sick in their homes (Robinson, 1957). However amateurish or even mistaken by modern standards, the ministration by medieval women was "sufficiently successful to win them the gratitude, the devotion, and the respect of their contemporaries" (Hughes, 1968, p. 138). Evidently, the gratitude, respect, and devotion also gave women more power than the medical men and clergy would allow.

Physicians' Motives in Banning Medieval Women Healers

With the founding of universities, the medical faculties began to demand medical licensure as a prerequisite to practice. Since no women could attend a medical facility, no women, as previously noted, could be certified; thus, all women were "practicing medicine without a license." Obviously, if one uses this definition of a physician, then few women healers would appear in medical histories. And yet, claims Minkowski, these women "performed a service virtually indistinguishable from the one so zealously cherished and aggressively defended by academically trained male physicians" (Minkowski, 1992, p. 289). To Versluysen or Ehrenreich and English, the women's healing activities were distinguishable because they were probably superior to those of physicians, in part because the men's academic training was more philosophical than clinical and was based on grossly inaccurate explanatory or theoretical systems.

Were physicians' motives for licensure based on an altruistic concern for their patients or on sexist elimination of women healers as competitors? To answer this question, Minkowski (1994) examined in detail the court records of the trial of Jacoba Félicie in the Bishop's Court of Paris in 1322. Two church rulings in 1131 and 1139 and a papal decree in 1213 extended restrictions that prohibited clerics from giving health services to people outside of monasteries. This created an even greater demand for community-based women healers, who had been the preeminent health-care providers for centuries. Organized medical faculties were a new phenomenon, emerging in the later thirteenth century and the fourteenth century. So was the idea of medical licensure, which was finally enacted under Frederick II, the Holy Roman Emperor, who required candidates to swear to never consult with a Jew or with illiterate women. In 1271 the medical faculty of the University of Paris used a questionable 200-year-old statute to forbid any Jew or Jewess to operate surgically or medically on anyone of the Catholic faith. Using the same statute, all other women, whether educated or illiterate, were entirely excluded. Thus, the faculty essentially claimed a monopoly.

Minkowski noted that physicians were totally immersed in a classical liberal arts curriculum of theology, philosophy, logic, and the writings of Hippocrates and Galen that gave them no real clinical advantage. Physicians had not yet learned to dissect the human body; physical examinations of males were conducted but not of females; these were done by women examiners, who conveyed their information to the medical men. Clearly, the attack on women and Jewish healers could not be based on superior knowledge, skill, or therapeutics.

Minkowski further questioned medical "idealism" since claims for better patient care were based on what physicians wrote about themselves, "a device that surely creates conflict between truth and self-service" (Minkowski, 1994, p. 87). Indeed, when King Philip VI commanded the Paris medical faculty to take measures to deal with the devastating Black Plague of 1348, the professional action of the physicians, said Minkowski, is still unknown. However, according to Hughes (1968), the physicians fled the city in fear, but the sisters of the Hôtel-Dieu in Paris remained courageously at their post. Clearly, the physicians' assertions that they would protect patients by university licensure and medical monopoly are highly questionable. Nevertheless, they enlisted the aid of the Bishop's Court when women healers continued to violate the self-proclaimed medical policy that banned all unlicensed practitioners. The two-century-old regulation on which the physicians based medical authority was never produced in court cases. Indeed, the medical faculty did not even exist at the time of the earlier issuance of the regulation. Nevertheless, in collusion with the Church, fines, imprisonment, and excommunication were imposed and citizens were urged to report healers who violated regulations. Such reports were given secretly and under oath to the dean or faculty, who were not required to supply the names of informers to the accused.

Since she was one of the most famous women healers of the medieval period, Jacoba Félicie's prosecution as an illegal practitioner has received considerable attention. In 1322 she stood trial in the Bishop's Court and was punished by excommunication, which she appealed. The king's surgeon, John of Padua, the most illustrious witness, said that the law prohibiting "illegal" and "ignorant" healers had been in effect for sixty years and that it was approved by both the Church and the king. Félicie had defied the law despite being "unlettered" and not judged competent to treat her patients' diseases. Since the legal system also forbade women from practicing as attorneys or being witnesses in criminal cases, they should be barred from offering healing services since they had to prescribe medications for diseases, which might lead to death and involve criminal charges.

Félicie's attorney first denied the validity of the statute because it did not meet the even older law that required all parties affected by a corporate act to be informed and invited to discuss any new law. Obviously, the medical faculty had made no attempt to seek approval or even discussion of the prohibition from any of the groups of healers affected by it. Second, the defense attorney asserted that Félicie had been instructed in healing and medicine and her competence was widely respected by her patients, male and female. Indeed, she had "successfully cared for many sick people whom master physicians had failed to cure" (Minkowski, 1994, p. 90). For example, a friar at the Paris Hôtel-Dieu said that the prescriptions of masters at the Faculty of Medicine had not relieved his symptoms, but Félicie's treatment had cured his illness. Several other patients also claimed that the physicians had failed to cure them but that the woman healer had successfully dealt with their illnesses. Despite a moving appeal to sanction the right of wise and experienced women healers to care for other women, Félicie was found guilty as charged, heavily fined, and excommunicated. A panel of physicians brushed aside her eloquent appeal for women to serve other women, and all witnesses were arrogantly dismissed: "her plea that she cured many sick persons whom the aforesaid masters [physicians] could not cure ought not to stand and is frivolous, since it is certain that a man approved in the aforesaid art could cure the sick people better than such a woman" (p. 92).

What were the physicians' motives? It appears that they were not only clearly sexist but, in the exclusion of Jewish men and women, anti-Semitic and racist as well. Evidently, "Medicine could only be learned from books, even those more than one thousand years old" (p. 93). Why, asked Minkowski, were defense witnesses in the Félicie case not asked questions to uncover any errors in diagnoses and treatments? Why was nothing said of the failure of licensed physicians to deal with illnesses that Félicie subsequently successfully treated? If academic training was so important, "why did neither prosecutor nor the medical faculty resort to the obvious expedient of testing the defendant?" (p. 93). If women were unable to comprehend medical complexities because of intellectual inferiority and lack of formal education, why were they considered competent in midwifery? If the physicians were so concerned about their patients, how did the thirty-eight medical practitioners in medieval Paris intend to care for 200,000 inhabitants? Minkowski could not reconcile the faculty's declared goal of improving health care with the decimation of the people's primary health-care providers. The complicity of the Church directly contributed to the suffering of the poor, who were unable to pay for or even have access to licensed physicians. For Minkowski, the Church's motives were related to its negative attitudes toward women; the majority of the healers were viewed as temptresses, even Devil's disciples, whose charitable work and health care were merely expiations for women's original sin. The male academic physicians "could not have chosen an ally more supportive than the Church" (p. 95). Minkowski concluded that the medical faculty acted duplicitously under the guise of improving standards of health care when they actually had no significant advantage over women healers.

Is Minkowski right in asserting that the Church was a supportive ally in controlling women healers? There is evidence that the theology taught was indeed antifemale and that the actions taken by male religious authorities were aimed at restricting and controlling women. The bishops in 1212 had ordained the smallest number of nursing sisters possible, and Innocent IV (1243–1254) decreed that they follow the rule of St. Augustine and become cloistered, thus confining nurses behind convent walls. Even with the severe limitations placed on the nuns, Hughes noted that their work was appreciated by such contemporaries as William of Nangis (fl. 1285–1300), who wrote that the devout sisters, "not fearing death, worked piously and humbly, not out of regard for any worldly honor. A great number of these said sisters were frequently summoned to their reward by death" (Géraud, 1843; cited in Hughes, 1968, p. 116).

In the twelfth and thirteenth centuries nunneries flourished, but in the next two centuries, they became increasingly poor, and "nuns frequently complained of the lack of lay sisters and of the added burden of work they were obliged to bear" (p. 125). By the fifteenth century, in one example, one nun alone attended the elderly nuns, nursing them day and night, doing all the work of the lay women. She dealt with "attacks of fever, . . . intolerable toothaches; sharp gouty spasms; affections of the brain, the eyes, the throat, the spleen, the liver, and pains in divers parts of the body" (p. 126), as well as those who were in "frensy," and who "nowe syngethe, nowe cryethe" (Aungier, 1840, p. 395; cited in Hughes, 1968, p. 126). In addition, she cared for the crippled and the deaf girls who came to live at the nunnery.

There is little doubt that restrictive church rulings continued throughout the following centuries. In the anthology *Pioneer Healers* (Stepsis and Liptak, 1989), Carlan Kraman acknowledges that religious houses provided opportunities for study and training for women who were unhampered by the constraints of marriage and family and less encumbered in their pursuit of wisdom, sanctity, and learning. However, "all too often, active ministries which they also chose, such as the care of the sick and the instruction of the ignorant, were denied by the rule of the cloister that was imposed upon most religious houses for women from the sixth century onward" (Kraman, 1989, p. 18).

By 1298, strict cloister for all religious women was required by directive of Pope Boniface VIII. Women were forbidden to do nursing work outside the cloisters except during disasters or epidemics. Some abbesses and prioresses permitted exemptions for nurses to care for the needs of neighbors; but after the Council of Trent in 1563, Pope Pius V in subsequent years reinforced the required strict cloister, despite women's desire in all periods to go outside to serve the sick, poor, and ignorant. According to Kraman, "Attempts to do this were consistently obstructed by church law and the control of the hierarchy" (p. 18).

In Italy, Angela Merici established in 1535 an activist congregation, the companions of St. Ursula, but a generation later Milan's archbishops changed the group to a cloistered community. In France, Jane Frances de Chantal founded, in 1609, the Order of the Visitation to minister to the sick and needy in their homes, but, again, in 1618 the Bishop of Lyons changed the rule to exclude *external* works of mercy. In England, Mary Ward in the early 1600s founded a noncloistered group of women, but "her ideas were regarded as dangerously novel . . . by 1631, her institute was suppressed" (p. 18). Thus, evidence is clear that despite continued efforts to care for the sick, poor, and ignorant, women in sisterhoods were increasingly restrained and controlled by the male-dominated Church hierarchy.

An Unremitting and Bitter Contest: The Sisters of the Hôtel-Dieu

The Sisterhood of the Hôtel-Dieu in Paris was the oldest of the religious nursing orders and suffered some of the most vicious controls by clerical and civil powers. Decades before Kraman's and Hughes' analyses, Nutting and Dock discussed at great length the nursing order of the Hôtel-Dieu, which originated in the mid seventh century; here the poor, infirm, and sick were sheltered by women in an attached nunnery. To Nutting and Dock, records of the order document "the unremitting and bitter contest which for centuries was carried on by the clerical and civil powers over the administration of the important and extensive institution. In this, as in every similar contest, the nursing service was the chief storm centre, and to gain control of the nursing staff the main point of vantage sought" (Nutting and Dock, 1907, vol. 1, p. 294). The protracted struggle attests to the elemental importance of nursing to hospitals. For twelve unbroken centuries, the women cared for the sick, but the sisters were excluded from university and professional training, and Nutting and Dock laid the blame for this exclusion squarely on the men, who authored and executed the constitution imposed on the order. As noted previously, in 1212, the bishops in council decreed that to economize, "just as few nursing Sisters as possible should be maintained in each hospital" (p. 297). Nutting and Dock note that the policy of heaping work on women's departments is "a naive and simple expedient which has not entirely disappeared from modern institutions" (p. 298).

The rule under which the nursing sisters were forced to function specified the time of rising, retiring, and praying; the daily rounds; the number of meals and kinds of food; the clothing; the comings and goings; and the punishments for offenses. These were all initially imposed by male religious authority. However, the prioress assigned nurses to wards; gave them permission to go outside; managed the midwives; purchased all supplies; controlled linen and storerooms, bandages, surgical dressings, housekeeping supplies, drugs and pharmaceuticals, laundry, and clothing of patients; and directed patient services.

Clerical control, challenged by the sisters for over four centuries, was finally transferred to secular directors, but "they encountered in the ancient nursing order a determined and baffling antagonist, requiring edict after edict from Parliament [the French legislature] itself to quell it" (p. 310). The overworked sisters refused to reveal their exact numbers: "The Sisters had to get the work done, and there is a limit to human endurance" (p. 311). Nutting and Dock further said they "fail[ed] to find any trace of a humane treatment of the nurses such as the directors claimed for the patients" (p. 312). When they requested to be relieved of their laundry duties, the women, burdened with 3,600 patients, were accused of "always trying to do nothing" (p. 313); they were "seditious and 'cast contempt on the Board of Directors'" (p. 314); they "changed the patients from one ward to another" (p. 315). The women resented interference in ward management and were unwilling to submit to the medical authorities, who were not yet in complete control of patient admissions.

By the end of the eighteenth century the physicians had total control of the hospital, but charges leveled against the sisters continued, even when they no longer had control over the secular directors and the "scientific" physicians, who, after a prolonged period of power, still had not substantially improved the hospital conditions:

If in three hundred years' time the directors had not been able to correct such hideously insanitary conditions as those existing in the water-closets and clothes-rooms, or to see that the physicians admitted and classified the patients properly and separated the infectious from the non-infectious cases, it is hard for even the most staunch supporter of civil government to see wherein their administration was superior, from the standpoint of hygiene, to that of the clergy, especially when it is known that conditions in other French hospitals were measurably better. (pp. 333–334)

The situation was desperate for the women: "Little by little the sisters had lost much of their former territory. The clothes-room, the sale of patients' belongings, the pharmacy, laundry, and much of the housekeeping had been taken out of their hands, and now their field of activity was still further restricted by the introduction of paid nurses, and a steady diminution in their own numbers" (p. 326).

The women lost control, not only in Paris but throughout Europe, which led to, as Nutting and Dock said, "The Dark Period of Nursing . . . a period of complete and lasting stagnation after the middle of the seventeenth century . . . Solely among the religious orders did nursing remain an interest and some remnants of technique survive" (pp. 499–500). The result was a level of nursing far below that of previous years. Nutting and Dock asked, "Was it by chance, or was it the logical result of a definite cause, that this state of things was coincident with a subjection of women in general, so little questioned, so entrenched that it might almost be called absolute?" (p. 500). They answer, "The latter conclusion is irresistible. . . . All the history of this time shows women reduced by the slow pressure of masculine domination to their lowest terms of self-expression" (p. 500). Except for small groups of privileged women in each country, women's education was infantile, their occupation absolutely linked "to the four walls of private life and domestic service, in legal relations weaklings and dependents" (p. 500). With women forbidden the right of free initiative and excluded from shaping the social order, a complete and general male supremacy prevailed: "At no time before or since have women been quite without voice in hospital management and nursing organisation, but during this degraded period they were all but silenced" (p. 501). Control of nursing staff, duties, discipline, and conditions of living were taken from women; even the nursing leader was a figurehead with little power to alter conditions. The strong feminism of Nutting and Dock should be heard in their own words:

The state of degeneration to which men reduced the art of nursing during this time of their unrestricted rule, the general contempt to which they brought the nurse, the misery which the patient thereby suffered, bring a scathing indictment against the ofttime reiterated assertion of man's superior effectiveness, and teach in every branch of administration a lesson that, for the sake of the poor, the weak, and the suffering members of society ought never to be forgotten—not in resentment, but in foresight it should be remembered: Neither sex, no one group, no one person, can ever safely be given supreme and undivided authority. Only when men and women work together, as equals, dividing initiative, authority, and responsibility, can there be any avoidance of the serfdom that in one form or another has always existed where arbitrary domination has been present, and which acts as a depressant, effectually preventing the best results in work. (pp. 501–502)

Ironically, this feminist analysis and interpretation was often missing from later analyses of nurses and women healers. Even Hughes (1968), who emphasized the importance of women healers, did not stress their struggle to exist within male-dominated systems.

By the second half of the twentieth century, the emphasis on proving that women healers existed and were respected *and* the feminist concern about the subordination of them expressed by Nutting and Dock were clearly missing in, for example, Eliot Friedson's 1970 sociological analysis of the history of medicine. Friedson used the contentious relationships between the Augustinian nuns at the Hôtel-Dieu and the physicians and surgeons to illustrate the "inevitable" shift from religious to secular control in health care. According to Friedson, this shift was due to the ascendancy of scientific technique over religious dogma. He did not recognize or acknowledge the issue of female versus male control, or the economic threat of women healers to medical authority and dominance. A decade later, Louis Greenbaum (1980) also omitted such issues in his analysis of nurses and doctors in conflict at the Hôtel-Dieu on the eve of the French Revolution. Operating under a new reform code, approved in July 1787, the Hôtel-Dieu was to be a major health center for the treatment of acute and chronic diseases. All diagnostic and therapeutic procedures, as well as admissions and discharges, were to be controlled and managed by staff physicians and surgeons, to whom the nurses would now be responsible. Needless to say, such regulations of the new code were unacceptable to the Augustinian nurses. Greenbaum agrees with Friedson that the battle was between religion and science; neither gave any serious consideration to the possibility that it was a gender-based conflict. Greenbaum admits that for twelve hundred years the hospital had been a house that belonged to women as a shelter for charity and consolation. Indeed, the nuns claimed that they had been "sovereign custodians of the sick, without intermediaries" (Greenbaum, 1980, p. 248). They considered themselves superior to physicians and surgeons, who were "strangers who sold their services and who lacking holy vows, could not be genuinely committed to the welfare of the sick" (p. 248). The sisters had contempt for the "inexperience, the arrogance and dubious remedies of the medical team, which was now to supervise their every move" (p. 248). That the fight was actually between women and men is clear in a statement of the nuns: "It is to women and especially to those who by their vocation are devoted to the continual care of the sick to whom is reserved that empire so sweet that nature and religion give them over the sick, that Providence confers on them. Whom better than they know how to console despair, to temper chagrin, to calm anxiety . . . constantly at bedside talking, consoling does she not more often influence healing than the application of medicines that almost never aids nature" (p. 248).

The Augustinian sisters went to court to block the new code following the French Revolution—which, like the Enlightenment writings, such as Rousseau's *Emile,* brought no greater *liberté* or *egalité* for most women. Imposing a central, hierarchical structure based on that of military hospitals, the physicians outlawed frequent snacks, soup, and cookies and forced the women to accept the control of men in diet, medication, and treatment. Again, it must be emphasized that the scientific bases for medicine had not yet fully emerged at this time. The scholarly espousal of science by the few was not and is not equivalent to the clinical application of practical research findings by the majority of practitioners.

The women were deprived of their management, of determining which patients the physicians would be allowed to visit, and of executing only verbal orders. They lost control of the pharmacy, kitchen, and laundry. The men performed surgery to the point that more operations occurred at this hospital than at any other in Europe. The new surgeon general merged the four wards, and demolished partitions and the chapel. The male physicians eliminated the women's principle of charity, and through all these changes the nuns' defiance supposedly impeded surgical treatment, since the sisters continued to supply food to the patients.

The women wrote letters to the male authorities of the Church, to the male authorities in the legislature, and to the King's first ministers, protesting that their thousand-year right to control the hospital had been violated. When the king refused to help, they eventually turned to the Parliament. They accused the physicians of disrespect, of degrading surveillance, a dictatorial approach, immorality, neglect and cruelty to patients, professional incompetence, and malpractice. The nuns contemptuously addressed the physicians as "businessmen," accusing them of falsifying financial records and of causing in a short time the dramatic increase in mortality from one in six to one in four deaths. The tyrannical despotism of the surgeons, who discharged patients uncured, was decried. The physicians, the nuns said, rushed through their rounds, spent eighteen to twenty seconds per patient, and "altogether failed in their obligation to prescribe adequate treatment" (p. 252). The sisters further claimed that the hospital administration was not superior to their own. The prioress stated that some wounds now took months to heal whereas before they had taken no more than one week. The surgeon general had, according to her, caused more patients to die in the last three years than in the last ten under the administration of the women.

According to Greenbaum, the women deplored the intolerable noise of four hundred to five hundred surgical students, for whom the surgeon general had advertised in the newspaper. They specifically charged that women patients had been forcibly brought to the surgical amphitheater and had died as a result of violence. On appeal, the men in government supported the men in religion, who supported the men in medicine. The prioress, after exhausting all appeals, notified the authorities that her nuns would physically prevent the entrance of any workmen into the wards.

Although Greenbaum perceives the fight as one between the spiritual and the temporal control of health and illness, it is obvious that women healers were subordinated to the men in medicine. To the women, each act of care for the patient was an act of spirituality. To the men, each act brought financial remuneration. Ironically, Greenbaum admits, "It would be difficult to exaggerate the hard life of the Augustinian nurses and the unspeakable conditions . . . under which they worked" (p. 256).

Parliamentary Edict: No Women May Practice "Fisyk"

Was the situation of women healers and nurses any better in England than on the continent? Eileen Power (1921) provided evidence that English physicians, like their European colleagues, were also actively moving to exclude or control women healers. The medical men brought a petition to Parliament demanding that no woman engage in the practice of "Fisyk" under pain of long imprisonment. In 1421, the men in the English Parliament turned down a request for a license from a woman physician, and issued the edict demanded by the physicians. Obviously, gender was the key factor. Few could argue that the scientific base of English medicine was so advanced in the fifteenth century that medical functions were based on superior knowledge. Certainly, the situation was not improved by the dissolution of religious orders following Henry VIII's break from Catholicism; few adequate substitute organizations developed. Indeed, Nutting and Dock concluded that "it might almost be said that no [institutional] nursing class at all remained during this period" (Nutting and Dock, 1907, p. 502). Eventually, most women were forced to practice medicine, surgery, and nursing as domestic arts; thus, a housekeeping manual dated 1700 stressed that women, as part of their daily business, have a competent knowledge of "Physick and Chyrugery" to help their maimed, sick, and indigent neighbors. Importantly, Clark (1919) showed, from memoirs, letters, family and local archives, and account books of boroughs and parishes, that some seventeenth-century women performed their healing tasks as *paid* work.

According to Versluysen (1980), the evidence of paid work as a basis for professional standing in the community is important, but more relevant is the wide extent of unpaid healing work in the female community as a whole, which "seems to have been characterized by a considerable degree of mutual aid and support" (p. 185). University-educated physicians of England's Royal College, a tiny elite, were deliberately restricted to only thirty-four members in 1618, and, states Versluysen, the numbers of urban-based groups of organized male apothecaries, druggists, and barber-surgeons were very small and did not begin to multiply rapidly until the late seventeenth and early eighteenth centuries. The evidence suggests that before the later years of the seventeenth century, "the male impact on the everyday healing experiences of most people was minimal . . . women in the past . . . were society's unofficial health care experts" (p. 185), particularly since midwifery and the care of infants and children were exclusively female preserves. Thus, medical functions—diagnoses, prescription of therapy, supervision of the sick—are not intrinsically "masculine" tasks. Even though physicians have historically claimed these for men, they could only justify women's exclusion because of gender by eliminating them from formal training and orthodox knowledge; thus, their ideas and practices were also automatically "unreliable" and "dangerous."

Such charges against women healers are highly suspect, given the fact that the assumed historical coherence and homogeneity of most medical groups was not actually achieved before the mid nineteenth century. Prior to the 1858 Medical Registration Act, few British physicians possessed university degrees. Indeed, surgeons were regarded as craftsmen and apothecaries as tradesmen, and the unqualified were legion: "Even at the beginning of the nineteenth century, it was still possible to obtain medical qualifications from no less than 18 different, independent licensing bodies, and to purchase illicit medical degrees from less salubrious sources, or simply hang out a sign calling oneself a doctor" (p. 186). When physicians finally unified, the previously separate and predominantly male groups, apothecaries, and barber-surgeons were incorporated. As Versluysen states: "If sex were not the main criterion of professional membership, it would be necessary to explain why certain categories of relatively uneducated men were included in the profession, whilst more highly educated upper-class women were not" (p. 186).

The allegation that British informal healers gained their knowledge in a haphazard way can also be contested. Knowledge of healing, like other domestic skills was passed from mother to daughter, and it was "not uncommon for widows to take over their husbands' 'barber surgeons' or 'apothecaries' practices, whilst some professed midwives in London had served a seven-year apprenticeship" (p. 186). Even without formal licenses, and despite the jealous accusations of physicians, there is historical evidence that patients had considerable confidence in women healers.

Clark also found the general standard of physicians to be very low; indeed, "the chief work of the country practitioner [was] the letting of blood and the wise woman of the village may easily have been his superior in other forms of treatment" (Clark, 1919; cited in Versluysen, 1980, p. 187). Philosopher Thomas Hobbes, for example, "preferred an experienced old woman [to] the most learned and inexperienced physician" (p. 187). Despite medical discoveries, "it was not until the end of the nineteenth century that male medicine could claim any rigorously scientific orthodoxy for its therapy" (p. 187). Medical decisions were often based on arbitrary and conflicting theories of disease causation; thus, "it is extremely dubious to impute standardised knowledge and expertise to the medical group and mere superstition and ignorance to female practitioners" (p. 187). Although some physicians were experienced and skilled and some women healers were ignorant old wives, the issue is the "falsity of making unconditional generalised assumptions which oversimplify the merits and skills of either sex" (p. 187).

Is there, for example, an eternal unchanging link between female nature and nursing the sick? No, states Versluysen: healing roles change through time and gender-typing of certain skills and therapies as nursing responsibilities is a relatively recent historical product of social change. Before the eighteenth century there was "little formal distinction between what were thought of as 'doctoring' and 'nursing' tasks" (p. 188). Instead, the differentiation was between classical academic medicine and women healers, and mostly male barber-surgeons, apothecaries, grocers, and druggists. Medieval nursing orders could be male or female. Apart from midwifery and wet-nursing, Versluysen, in agreement with Clark, concludes that the poorly paid, low-status employment allocated to women did not emerge until the seventeenth century. Indeed, Clark concluded that the medical male takeover was mirrored in all professions.

The earlier exclusion of women from guilds, from church priesthood and authority, and from colleges and universities laid the base in patriarchal society for their later exclusion from the public sphere. The use of gender as the basis of cultural organization *preceded* the emergence of capitalism, which is simply another reorganization of patriarchal power, more severe, perhaps, in consequence for women healers, but certainly no abrupt departure from previous centuries of male power: "even in the early eighteenth century, women were not necessarily pushed into nursing work, and healers were still often classified according to specific skills rather than sex" (p. 188). Versluysen argues that rigid distinctions between curing and caring functions were not clearly established until the nineteenth century, and that these were derived from Victorian ideological stereotypes of "femininity" embodied in the respectable, obedient wife-mother of the middle-class family. The passive female role provided a symbolic base for the subordinate position of women healers and cast the male physicians in the heroic role of savior of the sick. Indeed, the nurse's role today "derives from an historically specific value system about sex roles" which prescribe male and female behaviors toward the sick, but are not "empirical descriptions of healing roles that had always obtained nor factual statements about the intrinsic 'natural' properties of men and women" (p. 189).

Clearly, an alternative history of women healers, and thus of nurses, must be created: health care is not "a neutral site for the benevolent care of the sick," it is "an arena in which the sexes have historically competed over who should control and deliver healing services" (pp. 189–190). Male domination has required female devaluation, but women's historical healing skills must be recognized: "we can insist upon a positive rather than a negative status for women in history" (p. 190).

Evidence is still limited and fragmentary, but more will not be created if women's healing work is dismissed and trivialized. Versluysen calls for a mapping of the terrain of women healers and recommends more detailed questions on "which tasks were performed by whom, and for which patients" (p. 190); on the historical differentiation of women's multiple healing functions and the reasons for gender stereotyping; on the extent to which gender differentiation arose from developments in care for the sick, changing attitudes to illness, or societal changes; on the effects of gender differentiation of personnel in fields of work, social settings, markets, institutions, and social classes; and on the interaction between occupational and family changes in relation to the social position of the sexes—in short, the sum and substance of how and why women in the past lost control of healing to the male medical profession.

Versluysen commends Ehrenreich and English (1972) for providing a history of health care from "below," rather than "above" as in orthodox medical histories. Since the authors connect women's exclusion with that of other underprivileged groups, such as racial minorities, they, according to Versluysen, make a good case that the control of health-care services mirrors the aspirations of social and political movements and cannot be understood in isolation from social issues.

> We should not forget that throughout the ages women have willingly cared for the helpless, infirm, and socially dependent, but that the reward for this valuable social service has too often been indifference, scorn, or the status of a servant class. We do not know why this has happened with such consistency, nor why women's caring has been so devalued in our society, but perhaps history could provide some answers from the past and suggest an alternative for the future. (p. 197)

To understand the devaluation of women healers, we must focus on nurses, the largest group of women caregivers today, in relation to the development of a medical monopoly based in part on the use of patriarchal privileges to obtain economic and political advantage. From this perspective, nurse-physician relations, as described in subsequent chapters, can be differently configured. Indeed, today's nurses are certainly not recent interlopers into healing activities, which are erroneously presumed to have always been the sole province of male-dominated medicine. If the facts presented in this chapter are supported by further research, it is physicians who must answer for their intervention into the traditional healing activities of women and who must be held responsible for the elimination of female competitors.

Nursing must also be considered from a different perspective—one that is not derived from traditional medical history. No one would deny the medical successes that have resulted from applying advances in the physical and biological sciences to health practices in the twentieth century. Nor would anyone deny the many individual acts of cooperation between specific nurses and physicians. But we can analyze the systematic exclusion of women scientific healers and nurses from scientific knowledge and technology; consider the ways in which their cooperation was obtained and enforced; and question in subsequent chapters whether the medical monopoly was or is good for people's health or whether it is an historical hangover that hampers the provision of the best health care and should therefore be altered by fostering the independence of today's nurses in providing at least primary health care.

2 | "She Hath Done What She Could"

Reforming Nursing as Physicians Tighten the Medical Monopoly in Great Britain, 1800s to the Early 1900s

Medical control over women's healing activities in Europe, particularly in Great Britain increased during the eighteenth century, becoming a reality by the mid to late nineteenth century, despite the fact that university-educated physicians were a distinct minority among health-care practitioners. Indeed, there continued to be a variety of ways, until at least the 1860s, to claim to be a physician, including obtaining an illegal degree or possessing no degree at all. Nevertheless, the medical monopoly that excluded women was strengthened, even though many medical treatments lacked scientific bases and unanimity on the efficacy of specific scientific theories was yet to be achieved in medical practice. Indeed, treatments that were deleterious to people's health, such as leeching and bloodletting, were common. Despite these facts, British physicians had largely achieved direct or indirect control of health-care facilities by the nineteenth century; however, the quality of care in these institutions did not necessarily improve as a result of medical dominance. In fact, it was usually safer to remain at home than to go to a hospital for care. It is generally agreed that frightful conditions and appallingly high death rates prevailed in many British hospitals, almshouses, and other similar institutions. Given the earlier closure of all Catholic convents in England, institutionally based nursing and medical care by women had been severely curtailed, leading, in Nutting and Dock's (1907) view, to a dark period of nursing stagnation.

By the late eighteenth century some physicians were forced to recognize the need for something other than potions and surgery as necessary to cure. Several nursing manuals were published, and in Germany, Franz May's manual (1784) even recognized the fact that nurses needed "good treatment." Women should not be treated as slaves or lazy day laborers; instead, their interest and loyal cooperation must be aroused. However, the nurses (called "attendants" by some manual writers) continued to be bullied by stewards and clerks, often had no practical teaching in the handling of patients, slept in miserable accommodations, ate poor food, worked inhuman hours, and received small pay with no opportunity for advancement. Not surprisingly, such substandard institutions often failed to draw enough women to nurse the sick, although the women continued to provide most of the health care in their homes and communities.

In the early nineteenth century, women's relief societies in the Napoleonic

Wars led to the revival of the Kaiserswerth Deaconesses, an ancient order whose nursing work had never quite died out. The resurrection of the order, although usually attributed to a man, the Reverend Theodor Fliedner, originated in the work of early feminist Amalie Sieveking, who rebelled against the doctrine that marriage was the only destiny of women, and who wrote two feminist *Commentaries on the Bible,* for which she was strongly castigated. It was from her Protestant Sisters of Charity that women leaders were recruited for the Deaconesses, a model which was subsequently brought to England by Elizabeth Frye and later studied by Florence Nightingale, who then led the women's revolt against the inhumane conditions and high death rates in both military and civilian services and facilities.

In this chapter, we present evidence for increasing medical control in Britain from the nineteenth century to the early twentieth century, focusing first on events at one English hospital to determine whether the institution's rules and policies were in the best interests of nurses, patients, or the institution itself. We also question whether the nurses or attendants were ignorant, incompetent, and immoral women from the worst backgrounds or were uneducated but well-intentioned women working and living in difficult, if not impossible, conditions. We turn next to comparisons of male medical and female nursing perspectives on the emergence of "modern" nursing in England from 1840 to 1897 to prove that divergent perceptions of the same events had emerged by the end of the nineteenth century. We consider next the extent to which gender issues influenced the development of "modern" nursing is clear, particularly in the transposition of traditional family roles from the private to public sphere. This transposition was based on a theory of naturalism—the idea that the division of work was biologically inherent or "naturally" a result of differences in reproductive functions. Obviously, this "theory" sustained physicians' power, despite the efforts by Florence Nightingale and other early nurses to justify women's reform of nursing by promoting the idea that nursing was women's work.

Efforts to establish a parallel structure of nursing controlled by women and expressing a female value system were thwarted by the impact of the 1858 Medical Registration Act in Britain, which gave physicians complete control over diagnoses and access to patients. All women were excluded from medical licensure, even midwives, who had obtained their own licensure by the sixteenth century; however, male barbers, who functioned as surgeons, and male apothecaries were included. Nevertheless, nurses initiated major changes. For example, Nightingale's experience with physicians in the Crimea led to her reforms of the British medical military service and, on her return from the Crimea, reforms of hospital and public health institutions in England. Given the sometimes terrible conditions for health care, it is clear that male medical dominance was often not in the best interests of patients. We analyze Nightingale's own attitudes toward medical men, who as individuals were sometimes acceptable, but whose monopolistic organizations were unacceptable because of the horrific conditions they created or failed to change for both patients and nurses.

Research on the Nightingale Training School from 1875 to 1890 is presented, as well as the degree of its success in creating a nursing structure in which women had power over nursing. We also analyze the extent to which feminism influenced nursing reforms; and the rejection or acceptance by physicians of Nightingale nurse reformers. In analyzing the conflict which ensued at two London hospitals, it is clear that physicians viewed nurses as only subordinate assistants, decried their education as dangerous, and directly attacked the women and their leaders. The men insisted on the primacy of their patriarchal roles based on scientific authority, which they did not intend to share, except in a highly diluted form necessary to order taking. Although the women fought back, they, as further research shows, eventually lost their direct link to the boards of directors or trustees and were subject to bifurcated lines of authority in hospitals and to dependent relations in public health organizations. Nevertheless, they still worked to reform these institutions. By the 1890s the nurses had moved to create their own professional organization, but again had to struggle with physicians, who rejected the nurses' efforts or tried to control the women from within their own organization, even opposing nurses' registration, which nevertheless was achieved following World War I. This chronology of conflict and control is hardly a story of nurses and physicians struggling together to achieve the best health care for the people. Rather, it is a story of physicians fighting to monopolize health care and of women fighting to reform it. Certainly, some medical men actively supported women nurses, but the overall trajectory was toward increasing medical control and decreasing nursing autonomy.

"For the Good of the Patient?" Conforming to a Rigid Regimen

By investigating primary documents from one provincial hospital, the Royal Devon and Exeter Hospital in Southwest England (commonly known as Exeter Hospital), Ruth Hawker (1987) questions whether the power of the trustees and, increasingly, that of physicians was in the best interests of the patients. Founded in 1743, the hospital cared for the sick poor, usually those not employed by affluent families in which the women organized care for their own employees. At the ceremony to lay the foundation stone, the wealthy were told they had a duty to help the sick poor, who, in turn, had a duty "to be obedient to their superiors, and grateful to their benefactors" (Hawker, 1987, p. 144). Indeed, each patient at discharge had to give thanks in prayer before a hospital official. This hospital rule remained in effect until 1912.

The rules set by the hospital board of governors were strictly enforced: any patients breaking a rule were discharged; their names were written on a black-list on the wall, and they were subsequently refused readmittance for any reason. Nurses and other employees were also subject to ruthless, strict discipline, and those who transgressed the code of conduct were quickly dismissed. Patients were expected to help with domestic tasks; physicians decided who was well enough to do these, placing a red *P* above each of their beds. Even reading material was controlled from 1829 onward by a group of five clergymen, who selected sources from a list approved by the Society for Promoting Christian Knowledge.

From 1743 into the early nineteenth century, nurses at Exeter Hospital were often drawn from the same ranks as their patients. Although some nurses were dismissed for breaking codes of conduct, many seemed to be kindly, well-meaning women, who had "a homeliness about them that made the patients, especially the old folk, feel at home in the hospital" (p. 148). Instead of deploring the difficult working conditions, Hawker states the women could, because of their common social class, enter into the troubles of their patients; indeed, the nurse-attendants slept in a partitioned section of the ward, ate with their patients, and shared domestic chores with them.

Although in earlier times women in religious orders had founded and taken charge of entire hospitals, the prereform nurses at Exeter Hospital were limited to assisting physicians, for example by fetching warm water to help with dressings, applying bread or linseed poultices, and giving a variety of therapeutic baths. By the 1830s surgical and casualty patients had increased, and in 1835 a surgical nurse was appointed.

By the mid nineteenth century, apothecaries were replaced by physicians at Exeter Hospital, and young, unqualified men began to be replaced by those trained in medical schools. The women took on more duties, increased their workloads, and extended their workdays; however, formal nurses' training did not begin until 1888, although an educated new matron had been previously appointed. Gradually, "new" nurses replaced the old-style attendants and created a more disciplined schedule and routine. The post–nursing reform eras produced a "'better class of nurse with more general information and power of perception'" (Harris, 1922; cited in Hawker, 1987, p. 148). However, in this process, the nurses at Exeter Hospital became more distanced from their patients.

In the second half of the nineteenth century, the notion of "for the good of the patient" was put forward as the reason for most of the changes at Exeter Hospital; however, the good of the patient and the good of the organization could not be easily disentangled. Indeed, Hawker claims that nurses were increasingly expected to produce greater conformity from both patients and their visitors. However, two or three of the sick escaped each week, and relatives created "a great tumult" outside the hospital about limitations on visiting hours. Any nonconforming patients and nurses were dismissed, the latter without compensation: "The needs of the institution, then, were paramount, despite those few occasions when the Governors appear to have acted in the interests of the patients" (Hawker, 1987, p. 151).

In the early nineteenth century, hospital life was similar for patients and nurses: "Both had to submit to a rigidly disciplined regime, but because of their shared social status they had a common understanding which drew them together and apart from the institution" (p. 151). The new nursing system in the mid nineteenth century, presumably for the good of the patient, may have actually increased the control of patients by nurses and physicians and decreased the governors' direct control, but Hawker does not analyze the ways in which physicians increasingly used trained nurses as their agents of control over patients. To her, the hospital system was gender-stratified and the employment of Nightingale nurses did not alter this organizational pattern of gender-defined subordination. Whether or not the changes were for the good of the patient, they certainly did not redistribute labor and its rewards between the sexes.

Whose History? Gendered Perspectives on the Development of Modern Nursing in England

Hawker did not analyze the identities of her sources by gender; thus, it is unclear whether her account is primarily derived from public records that were mostly produced by male administrators or physicians. In contrast, Katherine Williams (1980) in her study of English hospital nursing systems from 1840 to 1897 purposely searched for alternative accounts, which could be used to understand the ways in which biases serve the interests of different occupational groups. To Williams, history is more than facts; indeed, these are expressed through the minds and interpretations of historians. Unfortunately, she, unlike Versluysen, does not overtly acknowledge the fact that the majority of historians have been men, or that their view of history has prevailed, or that perceptions of nursing history have been influenced by the patriarchal cultures in which medicine has had not only the occupational but the gendered power to name reality. Nevertheless, a gendered occupational analysis is indirectly achieved in her comparison of a female nurse's perspective on nursing history to that of a male physician.

Williams compared Margaret Breay's historical account of nursing, published in 1897 in the *Nursing Record and Hospital World,* to the historical perspective presented by an anonymous medical author in the 1897 *British Medical Journal.* When Queen Victoria ascended the throne in 1837, there were, said Breay, neither skilled nor trained nurses; women who nursed did so because they were not fit for anything else: the "'nurse of the day was not only ignorant, but dangerous to the sick upon whom she was supposed to attend'" (Breay,

1897; cited in Williams, 1980, p. 43). Breay recognized that novelists such as Charles Dickens may have exaggerated the nurses' disrepute. A nurse such as Sarah "Sairey" Gamp in *Martin Chuzzlewit* may have been a fictional character, but she was also a "person who disgraced one of the noblest callings to which womankind can devote themselves" (Breay, 1897; cited in Williams, 1980, p. 43).

To Breay, Elizabeth Frye, a benevolent and farsighted Quaker woman who founded the Institute of Nursing Sisters in 1840, was the first pioneer reformer of nursing in Great Britain. Well before Nightingale, Frye founded a training program connected with St. John's House to educate trustworthy women to be well-trained private-duty nurses, primarily for the sick of richer classes in their own homes; the program produced women of character and efficiency to take over from nurses of the day, who were "represented as so hard and cruel that the very name of 'Nurse' was held in horror and contempt" (Breay, 1897; cited in Williams, 1980, p. 43). It was Nightingale who created the modern *system* of nursing. Using money from the Nightingale Fund, created in 1855 by public contributions to enable her to start a nurses' training school, she established the principles of hospital nursing and of nurses' relationships with other workers at St. Thomas' Hospital.

Did the medical historian writing in 1897 acknowledge the change from unskilled and untrustworthy women to those who were useful and efficient? Yes, but he concluded that physicians were less than satisfied with the outcome. Although agreeing with Dickens' portrayal, the physician perceived Frye, not Nightingale, as having founded "sick" nursing in Britain when she established the Protestant Nursing Sisters and her Nursing Institute.

In neither the medical nor the nursing perspectives do accounts appear of organized religious orders for nurses in previous centuries, or of the impact on nursing that the dissolution of such orders had in England. Nor is there any description of community women healers—not even a reference to the nursing activities of licensed or lay midwives. Nor is the prevalence of Dickens's fictional nurse Sairey Gamp actually determined according to any standard of historical or sociological research. Indeed, there is no account of how and why institutional nursing had reached its presumably deplorable state. There is no analysis of the impact of feminist thought or political actions in the nineteenth century. Instead, the medical historian traced "modern" nursing to the investigations of the treatment of men wounded in battle in the 1830s. These inquiries "forced upon them [physicians] that if they were to do the best possible for their patients, they wanted hands, gentle, skilful, and sympathetic, which would work with them and for them at the bedside" (*British Medical Journal*, 1897; cited in Williams, 1980, p. 44). To the medical author, old hospital "methods" had "accepted any rough, incapable, and sometimes disreputable female as an attendant on the sick" (p. 44). Evidently, hospital "methods," not particular administrators or physicians, had hired and accepted these women. The inadequacy of these "methods" forced physicians to consult with leading male philanthropists to find a remedy. Ironically, there is no acknowl-edgment or evidence presented on how the physician could remedy the low quality of *medical* training and practice. In this account, there were evidently no disreputable, incompetent physicians.

To the medical author, Nightingale and her trained nurses and ladies went to the Crimea because of the "sad tales" of soldiers' and sailors' suffering, but evidently not because of inadequate medical care. Of the nurses sent, eleven were educated in the nursing program established by Elizabeth Frye in associa-tion with the physician founders of St. John's House. No credit is given to Nightingale's pioneering work in hygiene, nursing practice, education, or hos-pital reform. Nor is Nightingale's training at Kaiserswerth credited, or her work as superintendent of the Home for Invalid Ladies on Harley Street, both institutions founded by women. Instead, the medical historian focused on the physicians at St. John's House, who he credits with starting hospital reform. For example, physician William Bowman, who wanted to improve nursing at King's College Hospital, enlisted nurses from St. John's. St. Thomas' Hospital also enlisted "trained" nurses, who were supervised by Mrs. Wardroper. This chronology seems to imply that the men were critical in establishing nursing education, which presumably scarcely existed in any hospitals prior to this time. For this medical author, the nursing, hospital administration, and do-mestic medical activities of women in previous decades and centuries were simply nonexistent. Indeed, Williams concludes that even in the Victorian pe-riod, "We are given a view of the proper definition of nursing as already estab-lished and of Florence Nightingale as its student" (Williams, 1980, p. 47).

Although Breay also omitted several hundred years of women nurses, heal-ers, empirics, and hospital administrators, she at least credited Frye, Nightin-gale, and women leaders in nursing with establishing the principles of modern nursing care, conduct, and arrangements. Indeed, nurses were moving to adopt the three-year system of training, which, "after a long discussion, and strong opposition, [was] practically admitted to be necessary both for the wel-fare of the sick, and . . . of the training schools" (Breay, 1897; cited in Williams, 1980, p. 46). In contrast, the medical author saw nurses' education as produc-ing unsatisfactory results: the training was overdone, too specialized, too theo-retical, and too similar in style and method to medical training, which had "not proved equally suitable to the sick nurse, whose work is essentially practi-cal and whose efficiency depends more on skillful handling and observation than on acquaintance with the minutiae of physiology or anatomy. A bad style of nurse has resulted from this false training and it is on the increase" (*British Medical Journal,* 1897; cited in Williams, 1980, p. 46).

To Breay, systematic training had led to a higher standard of education, which would "inevitably result in probationers becoming more and more re-garded as pupils and less and less treated as servants of the Institution" (Breay, 1897; cited in Williams, 1980, p. 48). Indeed, better nursing education would secure professional status that would lead to registration and recognition by the state. In contrast, the medical author saw nursing beginning with women in their homes, who then penetrated hospitals and took on the rank of skilled workers, attracting numbers of women of culture, position, and education. He claimed that nurses were divided on the need for registration, and until they agreed, it was unprofitable to discuss the issue.

These two historians focused on the same events and the same issues from 1837 to 1897; however, they differed markedly in their perceptions, even on the pioneer status accorded to Elizabeth Frye and Florence Nightingale. In Breay's view, Frye established institutes *outside* of hospitals based on selective recruitment and explicit preparation to establish a standard for *private* nursing; she did *not* reform hospital nursing. It is Nightingale who, as the chief pioneer in hospital reform, established not only the conduct of nursing but nurses' relationships to other hospital workers and, thus, transformed the status of women from servants to educated pupils and then to professional caregivers. To the medical historian, Frye and her philanthropic nursing institute were important, but the essential point was that women who became hospital nurses retained their womanliness, *not* that they introduced new knowledge and practice. From this perspective, medical knowledge and an understanding of environmental factors constituted the treatment of the patient; these, in turn, created the change in the character of hospital nurses.

Williams concludes that physicians wanted to "retain the status of nursing as it was already established—a set of practices deriving mainly from medical knowledge, and not as the set of principles introduced into hospitals through the Nightingale Fund at St. Thomas" (p. 51). Any change was attributed to the right kind of "womanly character," and this change was credited to physicians, as, for example, the man who first requested the introduction of the St. John's Sisterhood into King's College Hospital. This "first" hospital reform produced "womanly" nurses, who were then introduced into St. Thomas' Hospital. In the medical view, these changes preceded Nightingale, who merely extended existing principles and was, therefore, not the true founder of "modern" nursing.

To the nursing historian, modern nursing did not emerge simply from a familiarization with hospital practices, but from the introduction of new principles, which required redefinitions of institutional arrangements and thus created a different occupational identity. In contrast, the medical historian stressed the need for different training of nursing and medical students. To him, the central issue was medical control of both the women and the theories of practice on which their nursing would be based. The physicians who referred to nursing as a skilled profession did so in terms, states Williams, that accepted changes in the *character* of nurses but no alterations in their status or work, "which did not stem from a medical definition of nursing" (p. 53).

Which historical interpretation is correct? By obtaining evidence on the actualities of British nursing services in the nineteenth century, Williams hoped to answer this question. However, she seems to have accepted the predominantly male medical evidence of what nurses were actually supposed to be doing. If the medical and nursing views of general historical events differed so substantially, how could one rely on the men's perceptions of the actual work done by women? Unfortunately, Williams relies on available public records, such as medical journals, which were almost exclusively edited and written by physicians. Lay magazines were also usually controlled and written by men. The women possessed "no magazine or journal that was exclusively theirs, and between 1840 to 1870, made practically no contribution to public debate" (p. 54). Clearly, Williams needed to seek private sources, such as the hundreds of letters written by Nightingale, to determine women's contributions to the debate. Since Williams restricted her research to public evidence and to the debate conducted primarily by male philanthropists and physicians, it is difficult to accept that these data provide objective evidence as to what women nurses actually thought and did. By now, the biases in masculist history have been made so obvious by the work of women's studies scholars that they are almost unremarkable. Thus, one cannot assume that physicians' descriptions of nurses' functions in the nineteenth century were any less biased toward women than those of men external to medicine. Nevertheless, it is at least useful to consider what the men had to say about nursing.

The Status of Nursing: A Set of Duties Defined by Physicians or the Creation of Radically Different Structural Arrangements by Nurses?

From lay authors, good nurses are portrayed as the ideal of woman—patient, gentle, and devoted. Sarah Gamp may have been a fictional caricature, but her likeness to some nurses, according to one writer in *Frazer's Magazine* in 1848, was obvious. Ironically, no actual evidence for the prevalence of disreputable nurses is provided. In 1852 the *Medical Times and Gazette* stereotyped the paid nurse of the old school as "a hard-minded, ignorant and lazy woman, who sleeps when she should be awake and is cross when she should be patient" (*Medical Times and Gazette*, 1852, January; cited in Williams, 1980, p. 54). Where is the statistical evidence for such a woman? If physicians and politicians eventually wrested control of most hospitals from women, and, in England, destroyed most of the nursing sisterhoods, then we are still left with the question of why the so-called scientific men created such horribly "unscientific" care of patients. Furthermore, since most nursing and medical activities were still carried out by women in their homes, what change in women's character had to be accomplished? Why would Harriet Martineau in 1858 recognize that mothers and daughters provided good nursing based on common sense and affection?

Williams tried to understand the differences in historical perspectives on the emergence of modern nursing, but from the medical perspective; she used evidence from only two hospitals (St. Thomas' and Guy's) and two male physicians (Dr. John South and Dr. Steele), both of whom described old-style nurses as practically the lowest servants in the institutions. This status shifted to probationer and pupil in a nursing system in which the daily work of sisters, nurses, and ward maids were directed by a matron, but she and all the women were under close medical control. By 1880, this system was widespread; for example, John South at St. Thomas' Hospital stressed that both sisters and nurses should report to a specific attending physician or surgeon, and, in their absence, to the apothecary or house-surgeon. He did acknowledge that in severe cases the sister should attend to patients, "which, but for her unremitting care and womanly aid would not attain successful issue" (South, 1857; cited in Williams, 1980, p. 59).

During this period, the same nursing positions were described at Guy's Hospital, and the sisters, as the medium of communication between patients and medical staff, were selected from "respectable females . . . particularly from upper servants" (p. 60). At St. Thomas' Hospital the day nurse or ward maid performed the duties of a housemaid, cleaning and bedmaking, making poultices, and attending to the wants of patients. By the late nineteenth century the nurses' conditions were presumably improved in accommodations, food, sleeping arrangements, remuneration, and promotion. The recruitment of a class of "women of good character" to go through a period of probation led to a closer approximation of nurses to sisters, both of whom did fewer domestic chores and had better ratios of patients to nurses. It is peculiar that the role of nursing leaders in changing these conditions is not noted. Instead, South emphasized that the probationary sister had much to learn, "which can only be attained in the ward, by the kind and patient assistance and guidance of the physician or surgeon to whom she is attached" (p. 63). To him, the sort of attendant the nurse became depended "mainly on him" (p. 63). Indeed, he used his long-standing relationship with the ward sisters, and through them he "controlled the status of nursing as a set of practical duties to be defined by him" (p. 63).

Williams also relied primarily on accounts by South and Steele in describing nursing institutes and nurses' religious communities. In the 1840s Frye's Institute of Nursing Sisters had an active staff of nearly a hundred women; of these, usually two probationers worked at the hospital for two months on medical, surgical, and obstetric wards, and, according to Steele, an average of twelve women received instruction. South stated that two or three of them were trained at Guy's Hospital. He admitted that initially he was not in favor of this arrangement because he feared inconvenience and interference. The women, however, turned out to be attentive and observant. Indeed, said South, the apparatus for making the best sisters existed and experience shows "that we do make them" (South, 1857; cited in Williams, 1980, p. 65). Again, the role of nurses in "making" other nurses is not mentioned. Neither is the influence of the women from the Institute of Nursing, or the women's actual nursing in private homes.

When Williams turned to the women's own description of the arrangements at St. John's House Sisterhood, she found that in 1848 they had their own council of management, sanctioned both by the physicians from King's College Hospital and by Anglican bishops. Obviously, in patriarchal societies, men must retain control, but in the archives, the lady superintendents wrote that their system differed from King's College Hospital nursing in three ways: first, all nurses were churchwomen of respectable character; second, all had a full year's training; and, third, all worked from lowest to highest positions. The women allowed no separate and lower grade of persons, for example, for night nurses. The system was organized as a career with rewards of higher status in the sisterhood rather than the permanently subordinate status of the ward sisters. The superintendent stated: "A St. John's House nurse is not regarded by her superiors as a drudge, who is to be worked for the convenience of others until she can work no longer and then cast aside as useless" (St. John's House Sisterhood, 1874; cited in Williams, 1980, p. 67). Domestic and nursing work were restructured and scientific knowledge integrated into nursing. Indeed, the St. John's House nurses "imported radically different structural arrangements into King's College Hospital" (p. 68). Attempting to explain their work and structure, they produced only a four-page pamphlet and published no written theory of nursing. The pamphlet used military images: the nurse on duty was the "sentinel" to keep watch and protect human life against sudden "assault" and warn the "garrison" of the approach of danger.

Williams argued that nursing was defined as a set of practical duties in a system which was formulated by physicians and communicated to ward sisters, who had "no source of nursing knowledge that was external to the sphere of the ward" (p. 69). However, if these nurses are considered in the context of all women, most of them must have been responsible for at least some nursing and doctoring at home. Did the women who became institutional nurses learn nothing from their sisters, mothers, and grandmothers? Williams does argue that, at St. Thomas' Hospital in 1861, the nursing system shifted to create nurses as pupils in principle and in practice; thus, they were removed from the control of ward sisters to that of women administrators external to the ward. Instead of crediting Nightingale, however, Williams referred to Henry Bonham-Carter, Nightingale's cousin by marriage and secretary to the Nightingale Fund.

At St. Thomas', training was formalized and set down in writing. Students were provided information on their duties and these records were reviewed in the matron's office. Critically important was the annual review of student records by the committee of the Nightingale Fund, which provided the money for the nurses' training "and was not in any respect subject to the scrutiny of the hospital's lay management" (p. 71). The removal of women's funds from direct hospital or medical control was a step forward; indeed, women's control of the training and practice of other women as nurses originated with Nightingale, who stressed that women must control their own work in nursing.

Clearly, Nightingale thought male medical and hospital authorities, who chose uneducated women to serve as obedient servants and work for little pay, caused the problems associated with the old-style nurses. It is still unclear how women, who often gave good nursing and medical care at home, would, on entering hospitals, forget their "good sense" and "affection" and become the terrible females, who by 1865, were characterized as gossiping, ignorant, and full of mischievous superstition and fancies. Such lay opinions, presented by Williams, support the usual historical view, but there is actually little evidence from the women themselves. Nor are there analyses of the effects of male control on them. Nor is there comparable evidence on the very inadequate state of medicine in the nineteenth century, now more than amply reported, particularly in the treatment of women patients.

Despite the shaky state of medical knowledge, physicians, claims Williams, continued to want not reform but simply the improvement of nurses as women. However, in 1857 South rejected public perceptions of nurses as ward maids, who, like housemaids, required "little teaching beyond that of poultice-making, which is easily acquired, and the enforcement of cleanliness and attention to patients' wants" (South, 1857; cited in Williams, 1980, p. 56). To him, women of "better station," given increased remuneration and certainty of promotion, could be appointed as nurses or ward servants. In 1871 physician Steele said nurses were previously "little removed from the ordinary class of domestic servants" (*Guy's Hospital Reports,* 1871; cited in Williams, 1980, p. 56). These women, usually between 20 and 40 years of age and from a good class of domestic servants, rarely left their work, but were sometimes discharged for drunkenness, or, more frequently, for staying out without leave, or neglect of an important duty, or incompatibility of temper. Nursing tasks were loosely defined, and actions to deal with "patients' immediate wants" were often not specified. Given these facts, Williams concludes that Sarah Gamp was a *literary* character, and the use of her as a characterization of hospital nurses had to be explained by more research. What, she asks, were the reasons for nurses to be publicly accorded the reputation of the irresponsible Sairey Gamp? She concludes that philanthropists' claims for reforms were based on different ideals and social relations that forced reputation rather than fact to become the central issue.

It is important to emphasize that Nightingale stressed the centrality of women's control over women's work and refused to allow physicians to take direct control of nurses' training. Williams believes that this freed pupils from the ward sister's arbitrary allocation of duties, but no reference is made to freeing nurses *as women* by placing their education and practice under the control of women. Williams referred to Bonham-Carter, not Nightingale, as meriting the credit for insisting on the separation of the matron's nursing and domestic duties in actual hospital arrangements. Indeed, Williams argues that the definition of nursing as a set of practices did not change as a result of Nightingale; what changed was the source of control of nursing practices in different social relations. For Williams, what was achieved was not freedom from total male control of the prereform nurses, whether caricatures or not, but removal from the control of another woman, the ward sister, the conduit for physicians' orders. Without an analysis of the sex-stratification system and the very real, legal subordination of women in the nineteenth century, Williams cannot adequately explain the subordinate role of the ward sister or relate this to the system of male medical and lay control; thus, the importance of Nightingale's demand that nurses' training be led by women is lost.

It is important to hear Williams's conclusion: nursing history is not objective. According to her, a greater degree of objectivity between observer and observed may be obtained if the everyday practice of nursing is studied in the wider context of the hospital. How will this "objectivity" be achieved if the gendered nature of patriarchal society is peripheral to the analysis? Or if the primary sources relied upon are men's, both medical and lay? Whose perceptions of the "actual" work of women should predominate? Those of the women workers themselves, or those of the men who controlled them? Whose leadership should be considered? Women such as Nightingale? Or men such as Bonham-Carter, who were acting on Nightingale's vision and directives? Finally, if Williams had taken a longer historical view, as described in chapter 1, perhaps it would be clear that the medical monopoly begun in the thirteenth and fourteenth centuries had largely been achieved by the mid nineteenth century, forcing women into a subordinate but at least a gendered parallel structure by the end of the century.

Biological Naturalism? Nursing and the Gendered Division of Labor

How does Williams's analysis, which is more concerned with occupation than with gender, compare to research specifically focused on the influence of gender on the emergence of "modern" nursing in the nineteenth century? Eva Gamarnikow (1978) researched the determinants of the gendered division of labor in Britain from 1860, the year Nightingale opened the Nightingale Fund School of Nursing at St. Thomas' Hospital, to 1923, the year when British nurses elected their first General Nursing Council.

Her perspective, like Williams's, is also limited because she does not consider women healers who were external to institutions during the nineteenth century or women's healing activities in previous centuries. Nevertheless, for the period covered, Gamarnikow found that the patriarchal character of the gendered division of labor was clearly apparent: first, in the subordination of nursing to the medical profession since, by the nineteenth century, the latter possessed the primary right to decide who would be defined as a patient; second, in the ideological comparability between nurse-physician-patient and mother-father-child relationships, particularly in the role of physician as father; third, in the identical moral characteristics of the "good nurse" and the "good woman"; and fourth, in the use of familial authority relations to justify domestic labor, which, even when redefined, gave cleanliness and hygiene a central but problematic role. Taking a longer historical perspective, starting from well before 1860, we might interpret these factors as descriptions of how women healers dealt with the erosion of their healing functions, or at least consolidated these in different terms by the later nineteenth century.

Clearly, the division of labor in the nineteenth century was thought to be biologically caused or "natural" and associated with reproductive functions. The theory of "naturalism" characterizes labor, both in the family and the wage sectors, as "masculine" or "feminine" and specifies tasks and allocates jobs by biology or by analogy. Alternatively, a division of labor may be explained by technological processes; however, biological determination usually underpins such technological explanations.

Exploitation of all women workers, including nurses, is located in the family, where women exchange unpaid labor for upkeep, although their reimbursement is usually less than the value of their services. Historically, the man has controlled the woman's labor, goods, and services; thus, they could not be exchanged or sold on the market because they belong to the man as husband. To Gamarnikow, the traditional marriage contract is a labor contract in which the husband controls the wife's labor, the domestic mode of production, which differs from the capitalist mode of production. The latter depends on the free sale of labor, not the transfer and ownership of the labor of women as wives, who have no direct access to raw materials or to the means of production.

The subsistence level that presumably sets wage rates in the capitalist market is not paralleled in the domestic market, where there are no socially determined subsistence levels. Instead, the wife, as domestic worker, is dependent for her upkeep and consumption on her husband's class position and income. According to Gamarnikow, patriarchal exploitation of free domestic services is transferred into the nonfamilial labor market where all women are treated as potential wives-mothers, dependent on men because they are biologically female. This emphasis on gender differences, rather than on human similarities, legitimizes the hierarchical differentiation between the labor of men and women. As a mode of work organization, the gendered division of labor identifies *all* women, whether married or not, as subordinates and allocates functions and tasks accordingly.

To Gamarnikow, the "maleness" or "femaleness" of a task is not inherent in the operation itself, but in the ideological identification and distribution of tasks and jobs as gender-specific; thus, some women may enter "male" jobs or men enter "female" jobs without these jobs losing their gender specificity: "rather, this becomes an individualized act, frequently resulting in contradictory and difficult work relations—female executives and male nurses being cases in point" (Gamarnikow, 1978, p. 101).

In the nursing literature, Gamarnikow found not an economic analysis of gendered labor, but a sociological model of professionalism. For example, historical coverage of nurses' battles over registration seldom recognizes that the conflict was *not* about changes in the occupational hierarchy, but about definitions of work and authority between nursing and medicine within the already established hierarchy. In Gamarnikow's view, differences among nurses over class, educational background, and length and type of training have occurred within *identical models of the subordination of nurses to physicians.* Although this is in part true, we could argue that the political organization of women, their insistence on formal training, on state recognition of women workers, and women's development of public leaders, speakers, and lobbyists were all forms of rebellion against their subordinated female status. Further, it could be argued that the extensive rejection of these actions by physicians is evidence of their understanding that women were moving beyond the domestic sphere and creating changes in the public arena.

Ironically, Gamarnikow's evidence for the similarity of arguments for and against nurses' registration is initially derived from two physicians: Dr. Bedford Fenwick and Dr. Sydney Holland. Dr. Fenwick, proregistrationist and husband of Ethel Gordon Fenwick, described nurse-physician relations in a way similar to Dr. Holland, antiregistrationist and chairman of the London Hospital. In 1904 Dr. Fenwick stated that technical knowledge was essential if the nurse was to carry out the duties entrusted to her by the doctor and to report symptoms efficiently to him between his visits. A week later, Dr. Holland testified to the Select Committee on the Registration of Nurses that registration would cause nurses to see themselves as creating a profession, to think of themselves as colleagues to physicians instead of women who carried out physicians' orders; thus, nurses would become pseudoscientific persons.

Gamarnikow observed that both men placed nursing as subservient to medicine. Indeed, she argues that nursing was "an occupation united by a common recognition of the existence and nature of the boundaries between itself and medicine" (p. 102). Although this is debatable, she is certainly correct in asserting that the dividing line between the two occupations is not a primarily technical but a flexible one, both historically and across institutions in any given period; thus, the two unequal spheres are primarily based not on technological factors but on gendered differentiation of laborers, patterned on the prevailing patriarchal power relations, whose legitimacy is derived from a form of biological "naturalism."

In Gamarnikow's view, nursing reforms in the nineteenth century did not directly attack the gendered system of health care. Instead there were two aims:

one, to establish a single stratified occupation to direct the organization and management of patient care; and two, to introduce this occupation into existing institutions and reform nursing modalities, as established by Nightingale. It is possible to argue that these two aims were also related to a third: to change some aspects of sex-stereotyped labor relations. Indeed, Gamarnikow admitted that nursing reform was associated with the development of an organizationally autonomous nursing hierarchy located in a separate department. Although she does not see this as changing the gendered division of labor, it is clear that any development of female autonomy, once religious nursing orders in Britain were largely destroyed, represented a partial shift away from total exclusion or very peripheral status in public institutions. Nightingale vested the whole responsibility for discipline, training, and management of nurses in the female head of the nursing staff, who reported directly to the governor, not to physicians, and to the matron. Clearly, there was an implicit, if not explicit, threat to total male medical control if there was a separate female hierarchy with a matron in charge of all the women in the hospital. Unfortunately, the separate authority of women answerable only to the board of governors or directors was contested and the Nightingale model was modified to reflect a gendered division of labor, which was not neutral or based on equal contribution and participation: "Instead it created stratified health care and interprofessional inequality" (p. 107). Eventually, many nurses would come to see their own subordination as natural. For example, one nurse in the journal *Hospital* said: "We nurses are and never will be anything but the servants of doctors and good faithful servants we should be, happy in our dependence which helps to accomplish great deeds" (cited in Gamarnikow, 1978, p. 112).

Why would any woman assert this? In part, because female subordination was considered "natural," but also in part because the division of labor was increasingly located in science, which had provided a new rationale for female subordination. Diagnosis presumably originated in science; women's treatment simply followed men's scientific judgments. Thus, female obedience was the "logical" correlate. Indeed, one surgeon at the Free Hospital conjoined science with the military model, saying that the nurse's duty was to obey: "Rightly or wrongly, we cannot have every subaltern of genius discussing his superior's orders. Only one battle has been won in a century by the disobedience of orders. But let not the nurse think herself a Nelson!" (Hawkings-Ambler, 1897; cited in Gamarnikow, 1978, p. 108). Not only was the nurse not an admiral or a general, she definitely was not supposed to be a scientist. Ironically, new scientific ideas were only slowly incorporated into medical practice. There was great variability in the incorporation of scientific techniques until late into the nineteenth century. Nevertheless, in the journal *Hospital* in 1894, Louis Vintras stated that the nurse must recognize the physician as her *scientific* chief and maintain a rigid discipline not even second to the soldier's: "A sense of duty, an absolute obedience to orders, a thorough comprehension of these orders, are the fundamental principles of nurses" (Vintras, 1894; cited in Gamarnikow, 1978, p. 109).

Extending Home to Hospital: Nurse as Mother, Physician as Father

The ideological reconstruction of gendered relations depended on the transposition of family structure to health care by representing the nurse-physician-patient triad as mother-father-child. Thus, the nurse must have the indulgence of a mother to the child and if firmness is needed "She can always invoke the physician's orders for the refusal of any unreasonable request" (Vintras, 1894; cited in Gamarnikow, 1978, p. 110). How the nurse could be both mother and soldier is certainly worthy of deeper analysis.

The family analogy became a major motif in nursing literature. Although this motif recurred, Gamarnikow did not attend to countervailing themes: the continual demand for adequate education, including scientific knowledge, and for independent control of nursing as a body of women controlled by women, even if subordinated to male institutional authority. These conflicting themes are not considered by Gamarnikow, but they are necessary for a full analysis.

Some nurses did seem to accept the family analogy. Sister Grace, for example, in 1898 recognized that the house-surgeon and sister must work well together for the sake of patients. As in a marriage, the responsibility for this relationship rested chiefly with the woman, who was told: "Never assert your opinions and wishes, but defer to his, and you will find that in the end you generally have your own way. It is always easier to lead than to drive. This is a truly feminine piece of counsel, and I beg you to lay it to your heart" (Grace, 1898; cited in Gamarnikow, 1978, p. 127). Gamarnikow relied heavily on the male-controlled journals, such as *Hospital;* thus, it is not clear whether such pronouncements were typical of the private opinions of most British nurses. Certainly, such advice was found occasionally in nursing journals, but it was contested by numerous other articles that insisted on standards, registration, education, scientific knowledge, and control of these by nurses themselves. Nevertheless, to Gamarnikow, the key struggle was not to change the hierarchical structure of health care, but to create paid women's jobs instead of Victorian female charity; thus, Nightingale's goal at St. Thomas' was to train as many women as possible, to certify them, and "to find employment for them, making the best bargain for them, not only as to wages, but as to arrangements and facilities for success" (Nightingale, 1867, p. 2; cited in Gamarnikow, 1978, p. 112). Nightingale wanted to "give the best training we could to any woman, of any class, of any sect, 'paid' or unpaid, who had the requisite qualifications, moral, intellectual, and physical, for the vocation of a Nurse" (Woodham-Smith, 1950, p. 483).

According to Gamarnikow, early reformers were heavily influenced by early protofeminist theory, for example, that of A. B. Jameson, who in 1856 demanded equal participation in nondomestic work, but accepted a "natural" division of labor, based on the extension of women's traditional work. Jameson believed that women in public jobs could bring a better balance between the elements of power and love and incorporate family sympathies into all forms of social existence to ameliorate evil and suffering. Although laudable aims, the initial powerlessness of women resulted in an all-woman occupation that was justified by the social structure of the family. This produced a contradiction: "it gave women access to a non-industrial job, but at the same time deferred to medicine in setting it up and defining its limits" (Gamarnikow, 1978, p. 114). Established and defined as women's work, nursing was situated in the patriarchal structure in which science and authority belonged to physicians and caring and the application of science to nurses.

Health care, said Gamarnikow, was based on alleged gender-specific personal qualities and virtues, which were found in long lists of qualities predominately related to personality and subordination, not to skill and technical knowledge. Terms related to nurses' subordination included "patience, endurance, forbearance, humility, unselfishness, self-control, self-sacrifice, self-abnegation, self-effacement, service orientation, self-surrender, devotion, loyalty, discipline and obedience" (p. 115). Whether *all* these terms mean subservience is questionable. Other common terms focused on personal qualities, which ranged from quiet, neat, orderly, punctual, dutiful, and chaste, to persevering, self-reliant, principled, and courageous. Again, whether all those terms suggest womanly subordination is debatable. Terms pertaining to relations with others include kindly, gentle, generous, and courteous, but also thoughtful and firm. Terms for attitudes to patients, such as love, sympathy, pity, and comforting, seem even more sorely needed a century later. Terms such as accuracy, watchfulness, success, reliability, and truthfulness were used to describe the observing and reporting of symptoms. Here, there seems a clearer case for assuming subordinate status, since independence in action is not described. However, technical competence and skill required nurses to be ingenious, ready, quick, intelligent, alert, keen, sensible. Nevertheless, Gamarnikow concluded that character was linked to "femininity," and in turn to womanly moral attributes.

By the end of the nineteenth century the close link between nursing and "femininity" as a combination of moral qualities that supposedly differentiated women from men shifted from personal virtues to tasks; these were linked with family-based factors best found in good training of daughters by mothers for domestic labor and mothering. Gamarnikow claimed that tasks most similar to housework were relabeled hygiene, which came to occupy a key but difficult position in nursing, one that was presumably derived from Nightingale's earlier emphasis on hygiene as the scientific basis for nursing. However, Gamarnikow did not discuss Nightingale's differentiation between nursing and domestic labor, which also formed the basis for subsequent debates on nursing and menial labor. Indeed, Nightingale insisted that nurses were not mules, that they had important patient care functions that must take priority over those related to housework. Furthermore, it is also important to recognize, as Nightingale did in the Crimea, that filthy conditions killed people. Asepsis was, and is, scientifically important—possibly an extension of womanly housework at its best. It is also the basis of public health. Indeed, most of the health advances by the turn of the century can be attributed to environmental changes in everyday life, not to specific medical cures or treatments in hospitals. Thus, the importance to women of "hygiene" as the basis for advances in health matters requires more thorough analysis.

Compromise versus Control: Nurses Strive for Reform, Physicians Tighten Authority

Heavy emphasis on structural work relations sometimes excludes the content of reforms demanded by women nurses and non-nurses and their actual achievements. Certainly, Nightingale's reforms of the British military system of medical care and of hospitals were no small accomplishments. Much of this relied on principles of hygiene and resulted in a very substantial reduction in death rates. However, as she moved from private and from district or public health to hospital nursing, the nurse-hygienist was increasingly confined to providing or supervising nursing care that was usually connected to medical interventions.

Despite her contention that the gendered division of labor was not challenged by nursing reforms, Gamarnikow did recognize that efforts to enhance female autonomy provoked fear among physicians, who from 1860 to 1880, a period of major health-care reform in Britain, had taken control of diagnoses, achieving their monopoly through the 1858 Medical Registration Act. Physicians and even some women feared that women's institutional and educational autonomy and their state-sanctioned organizations would lead to occupational independence. Even Elizabeth Garrett Anderson, early British woman physician, opposed nurses' independence, using the experience with apothecaries as "evidence" of "imperfectly educated practitioners." Medical dominance was maintained because physicians controlled access to patients by monopolizing the initial intervention that designates the person as patient. Thus, said Gamarnikow, both independent nursing processes which focused on hygiene and those that depended on enactment of men's orders remained under medical control. By the end of the nineteenth century, physicians were warning nurses that they had no certificate to diagnose or to judge the severity of illness; therefore, they could not decide who were patients or admit them to hospitals.

Because access to patients continued to depend on prior medical intervention through diagnosis, nursing shifted to a primary identification with patient care, rather than with hygiene in its broad societal sense or even in the more narrow sense of housework; thus, "Nursing practice became even more closely subordinated to medicine" (p. 120). The ideology of motherhood and housework furthered the patriarchal relations between nursing and medicine.

Gamarnikow concluded that the development of the female nursing occupation had to be accomplished within an area of labor *already* controlled by men; thus, success in establishing paid jobs for women depended on "situating and defining these jobs in a way which would pose no threat to medical authority" (p. 121). The result is a gendered division of labor in almost pristine form that cuts across the usual social class boundaries. Thus, technological determinism as the ideological basis for the division of labor between nurses and physicians is *not* supported. Rather, the ideology of naturalism, with interconnections among femininity, motherhood, housekeeping, and nursing, is central to situating and subordinating nurses. Clearly, any "pure" form of socialist or sociological analysis that emphasizes technology as the material basis for the functional divisions in health care is insufficient. Overriding this theoretical and "commonsense" view is the overwhelming evidence that patriarchal dominance allowed physicians to obtain control of the functions of women healers, who then had to compromise in order to establish their public roles in health care.

From Gamarnikow's point of view, nurses in the nineteenth century did not essentially crack the gendered work structure, but only forced open public, paid work for women. This perspective focuses heavily on hospital nursing and not on other areas in which nursing reformers were very involved. It also downplays the actual reforms in working arrangements and relationships; in methods, processes, and procedures; in institutional structures; in the institutions themselves; and ultimately in the health care received by people in and out of institutions. Certainly, Gamarnikow's focus on gender, when compared to Hawker's (1987) and Williams's (1980) analyses, does provide a better theoretical basis for explaining what happened to women healers and nurses, particularly in the later decades of the nineteenth century. Unfortunately, sociological and historical analysts of nursing too often lose sight of the actual work nurses did, the very real changes they produced in how their work was to be conducted, how health-care practices changed, and how institutions were altered to achieve better care of people.

Who Were the Ignorant and Incompetent? Early Nurses Struggle against Physicians' Hostility

A central contradiction in constructing women's history, as discussed in the overview, is related to the problem of power and powerlessness in women's lives. Gamarnikow is quite correct in her evaluation of gender as central to the subordination of women nurses, but focusing on what they achieved *despite* their relative powerlessness provides a more balanced perspective. Many of these achievements are associated with Florence Nightingale, who did not accomplish her reforms alone. Because of the central importance of Nightingale to most historical accounts of nursing in the nineteenth century, it is appropriate to consider her achievements in some detail and to stress that her reforms were often achieved in cooperation with other women, many of them nurses. (For a fuller analysis of Nightingale, see Roberts & Group, *Feminism and Nursing*, 1995, chapter 1.)

Unfortunately, "The Nightingale literature has too often presented this remarkable woman as a stereotype within a stereotype" (Versluysen, 1980, p. 180). Of the more than fifty biographies about her, many published in her lifetime, most have focused on her Crimean period or on her founding of modern nursing, achievements that could be more easily fitted into the expected stereotypes of a Victorian lady. According to Versluysen and many other recent Nightingale analysts (e.g., Baly, 1986; Monteiro, 1987), her other intellectual achievements as medical statistician, radical reformer of the British Army Medical Corps, political expert on imperial India, and creator of the Indian Sanitary Commission do not sustain the conventional myths of femininity and thus they have often been overlooked or minimized. But this has happened to nursing history in general, not only because it has attracted, until recently, only a small number of serious scholars, but because the actual reforms achieved in work and institutional arrangements have been overlooked or trivialized by those who accept the medical historical perspective. In addition, it is very difficult to estimate the quality and quantity of changes in the nineteenth century when the history of women healers in previous centuries is missing, trivialized, or stereotyped. Indeed, it is still unclear how competent or incompetent women attendants or nurses were even in the eighteenth and early nineteenth centuries. And these institutionally based women are yet to be adequately distinguished from or embedded in the broader context of women healers in families and communities.

Certainly, Hawker's account of pre-Nightingale nurses does not agree with those of some other scholars. In sharp contrast, for example, is nurse Susanne Everett (1974), who cites Nightingale as accusing hospital administrators and physicians of hiring only those women who "'had lost their characters, i.e . . . [they] should have had one child'" (p. 14). Presumably, the men wanted women who had lost their "innocence," but were less clear about their clinical standards since, according to Everett, the old-style nurses had a "staggering ignorance of even the simplest medical duties." Even if knowledgeable, the nurses of the 1840s had to function in hospitals that were "places of unimaginable wretchedness and squalor," where victims of cholera or other diseases common in slums and tenements "arrived filthy and remained filthy" and were placed into beds that were covered with sheets from previous occupants and located in large, gloomy wards "crammed with fifty or sixty beds less than two feet apart" (p. 14). Clearly, Everett, as both nurse and historian, is less sanguine than Hawker or even Williams about the possibility that any old-style nurse, no matter how competent, could provide good care in such environments.

If civilian institutions were appalling, were military conditions any better for attendants and their patients? If the medical historian in Williams's account was accurate about physicians realizing the need for better nursing from their survey of military conditions in the 1830s, change was certainly not evident by the 1850s from the horrendous factual accounts of medical and military incompetence. In 1854, for example, Howard Russell, the first war correspondent for the *Times* (London), reporting on the Crimean War, said there were no dressings or nurses available to the soldiers, no linen to make bandages, no preparation for the commonest surgical operations, not even the appliances commonly found in workhouse sick wards. Russell charged that "the men must die through the medical staff of the British Army having forgotten that old rags are necessary for the dressing of wounds" (Russell, 1854; cited in Everett, p. 15). In the same year, Nightingale and her nurses left for Scutari, and on their arrival faced a "hospital," an artillery barracks, which was vast, filthy, and dilapidated, containing four miles of beds under which were large sewers from which "rats and other vermin swarmed over the rotten floors" (Everett, 1974, p. 18). Indeed, the "hospital" had no kitchen, food, medical equipment, laundry facilities, beds, basins, soap, brooms, mops, trays—not even plates, knives, forks, or spoons. This situation was overseen by the purveyor's department and the medical department, with twelve clerks under Dr. Andrew Smith, the director-general of the British Army Medical Service. Between these groups, relations were confused; their respective powers were unclear if not obscure.

Nightingale "found herself not only strongly resented by the doctors, who viewed her appointment with disgust (they called her 'the Bird' behind her back) but without the meanest facilities at her disposal" (p. 19). Despite these conditions, the London *Times* Fund, monies donated by the public to send to Nightingale to help pay for bandages and medical supplies needed in the Crimea, was opposed by Dr. Menzies, the chief medical officer of the hospital at Scutari; the British ambassador to Constantinople, Lord Stratford de Redcliffe Canning, recommended using it for a Protestant church, but he finally did put it at Nightingale's disposal. Although officially condoned, Nightingale had no position in the male political, military, or medical power systems. Her strategy was to do nothing unless requested by doctors, but this decision sustained a gender-segregated subordination and institutionalized nursing system which might operate under the control of women but was always subject to medical authority.

Dealing with the Mean and Selfish: The Women Rebel against Medical Incompetence and Authority

Everett's analysis of Nightingale's achievements is clearly supportive of Breay's 1897 perspective, discussed earlier. According to Everett, Nightingale's nurses "rebelled against waiting for an official sanction before attending to men obviously dying from lack of food and medical care" (p. 20). Finally, with more men coming and a supply ship destroyed in a hurricane, the harassed physicians had to turn to Nightingale, who had the money and government authority to act. She quickly became unofficial hospital purveyor, procuring 200 scrubbing brushes, installing boilers, and arranging for laundry by soldiers' wives. She supplied 2,000 socks, 500 drawers (underpants), slippers, plates and utensils, and screens to block views of surgery. After refitting an entire regiment with warm clothing, she wrote home that she was clothing the British Army!

Nightingale and her nurses established the kitchen, provided special diets, cleaned the wards, administered daily dressings, managed compound fractures, and started a lying-in hospital. Despite medical opposition, she never let a man under her care die alone; working on her knees in dressing rooms for eight-hour stretches, she and her nurses eventually produced a tremendous reduction in death rates. Reading and recreation rooms were set up for the men, again over the objections of military authorities, who accused Nightingale of spoiling the "brutes" and also objected to her reform of helping soldiers to send home their pay. Becoming the army's banker, she sent large sums to families each month, proving that men would not drink up their money if it could be sent home safely: £71,000 was sent back to England in six months. Clearly "hygiene" was only one part—although an extremely important one— of Nightingale and her nurses' reforms.

Nightingale's Aunt Mai visited her in Scutari in September 1855, appalled at Florence's physician condition and "horrified by the web of intrigue, the petty thwartings, irritations and discourtesies" (cited in Everett, 1974, p. 22) with which Florence was forced to deal. Her aunt claimed that the quantity of talking and writing was the weary work for Florence, "the dealing with the mean, the selfish, the incompetent" (p. 22). In 1856 the War Office finally issued a statement that supported Nightingale's demands. Yet Nightingale, writing to Sidney Herbert, said: "There is not an official who would not burn me like Joan of Arc if he could, but they know the War Office cannot turn me out because the country is with me—that is my position" (cited in Everett, 1974, p. 22).

Back in England, Nightingale worked for immediate reform of the army medical system, which had produced a 73 percent mortality rate from disease alone. As Everett noted, Nightingale wrote letter after letter to men in power, but they were inclined to think her attitude "overwrought." Only after she presented to Queen Victoria and Prince Albert a plan for total military reform of hospitals, organizations, education, and administration of the Army Medical Department was Nightingale taken seriously. She clashed, however, with Lord Panmure, who delayed issuing a warrant for an investigative commission (the Royal Sanitary Commission) and refused to accept her negative opinion on the partially finished Netley Hospital, which subsequently proved, as she had predicted, unsatisfactory.

By 1857, an extraordinary number of reforms were produced by Nightingale, who, as a woman, could not serve on the newly formed Royal Sanitary Commission but had to rely on its chairman, Sidney Herbert, to enact her reforms. On his death, Nightingale said that he took her work, the object of her life, with him, because his death took away her means to do it. Still, she did not stop; she moved to create reform in India, becoming directly concerned with sanitary circumstances of natives, meeting again with "raised hopes, delays, and finally constructive plans fading away for lack of administrative cooperation" (p. 25). By 1872, Nightingale said she went out of "office" and could do no more, but she then established the Nightingale Training School for nurses and entered into still other conflicts.

Proving Women's Worth: Early Nurses' Struggle against Stereotypes and Male Control

Were reforms of hospital nursing necessary? Certainly, Lee Holcombe's (1973) historical analysis in *Victorian Ladies at Work* agrees with Everett's views. Although the old-style nurses may have been, as Hawker (1987) says, generally decent, lower-income women, the hospitals, controlled by men, were often unsanitary, with wards that were poorly heated, lighted, and ventilated, overcrowded with beds that were often dirty and infested with vermin. Matrons were treated as head housekeepers, and few, said Holcombe, had experience in nursing, therefore, they often left the supervision of nurses to the medical staff. Sisters or nurses were often relegated to the performance of domestic duties, while physicians and medical students assumed the skilled nursing care that had previously been provided by women.

Holcombe soundly condemned the nurses' working conditions, in which they normally served fourteen to fifteen hours at a stretch, sleeping in basement rooms, cupboards, or the wards, receiving salaries so insubstantial that few women would wish to choose nursing as a means of support. Essentially, the role of women in the broader society defined the role of women in nursing, allowing them only the most menial tasks at the lowest rates of pay. Even worse conditions prevailed in workhouse infirmaries, considered "'receptacles for pauperism' rather than places of healing for the poor" (Holcombe, 1973, p. 70). In these institutions, the "seriously ill and the convalescent, acute and chronic cases, the contagious and the non-contagious, lying-in cases and mental cases were all jumbled together in the same crowded and dirty accommodations" (p. 71). Much of the nursing was done by the inmates themselves. In middle- and upper-class families, patients were, as noted previously, cared for by women in their homes.

Unlike Hawker's, Holcombe's view is in accord with that of Everett, who accepts the idea that incompetents were too often found among pre-Nightingale nurses. Unfortunately, the conditions in hospitals and infirmaries seem sufficient evidence that nurses were also degenerate. To Holcombe, the salvation of nursing came from the development of science in medicine and the call to women to serve as handmaidens to physicians. Once again, it is important to note, although Holcombe did not, that the elimination of women's religious orders, the exclusion of women from formal medical education, the takeover of the functions of women healers and eventually even midwives, and the insufficient funding of institutional social and health services all contributed to the stereotyping of early nurses. As noted in chapter 1, Nutting, Dock, Ehrenreich, English, and Versluysen would all say that classism and sexism provided the bases for the destruction of nursing as a legitimate and honorable activity for women in their communities. Instead of dealing with these factors, Holcombe pointed only to the revival of the Kaiserswerth Deaconesses as the model for modern nursing and ignored the reasons that led to a need to revive a religious order for women nurses.

What exactly were the factors that caused both lay women and sometimes those in remaining religious orders to work in unsanitary and often poverty-stricken conditions? In Holcombe's view, the friction between hospital and spiritual authorities increased over time, and nurses in religious orders became outdated because of the scientific developments in medicine. Although this is a traditional interpretation—later used, for example, by Friedson (1970) and Greenbaum (1980), as noted in chapter 1—a feminist analysis suggests that women were caught between the men in power in religion and in medicine. From this perspective, many women healers were forced out of spiritual, compassionate work and out of competition for any lucrative lay roles within health-care systems. By excluding women from university education, the medical monopoly maintained its control over a *potentially* scientific approach (which, we reemphasize, was not actually widespread among most physicians until well into the nineteenth century) that could eventually be the basis for the diminution of the role of women nurses in religious orders.

The exclusion of women from all public roles by the mid nineteenth century made Nightingale's efforts to help women "break through the conventional shackles binding them to idle, useless lives" (Holcombe, 1973, p. 73) laudatory. Holcombe continued the traditional interpretation of Nightingale as shaping the nursing profession with her own image: "strong and pitiful, controlled in the face of suffering, unself-seeking, superior to the considerations of class and sex" (p. 74). She demonstrated on a grand scale what the feminists always claimed: "the great good that could be done in society by trained and dedicated women" (p. 74). Clearly, the feminist vision also included fair economic remuneration, reasonable working conditions, a degree of autonomy, and appropriate status for women. These have yet to be fully achieved.

As noted previously, Nightingale had to compromise on what she wanted for women. She initially wanted a separate training school under the direction of women, but was forced to establish her school at St. Thomas' Hospital. Unlike Gamarnikow, Holcombe stressed that Nightingale's most revolutionary proposal was that the nurses would not be subject to control by men in hospital administration or medicine. Instead, "they should be under the absolute command and control of the hospital matron, who would both oversee their training and supervise their nursing work after they were trained" (p. 75). Nursing was women's work and women must reform it.

What was the reaction from the "fraternity" of medical men? According to Holcombe, men in medicine "did not always look with favour on the training of nurses" (p. 77). In sharp contrast to Williams, Holcombe cited South, the senior surgeon at St. Thomas' Hospital, as one example not of objectivity but of opposition. His 1857 pamphlet stated that the proposed training school for nurses was unnecessary. He rejoiced that of 173 doctors in seventeen London hospitals, only five from two hospitals had subscribed to the Nightingale Fund. Many physicians were afraid the women would no longer consider themselves subservient, but more nearly the men's equals. For example, at Guy's Hospital, the trained nurses were considered "impossibly conceited and completely unwilling to heed the doctors' orders" (Holcombe, 1973, p. 77). However, Holcombe asserted that the men's fears that women would reject male authority proved to be unfounded. Unfortunately, this assertion is correct: to this day obedience by nurses is still usually expected and often obtained.

"Careful Not to Arouse Animosities": Florence Nightingale's Attitudes toward Physicians

By now it should be clear that most men as physicians have historically not supported the independent organization, practice, and professionalization of women as nurses. How then did the early nursing pioneers deal with these physicians? Zachary Cope (1958), in *Florence Nightingale and the Doctors,* depends on Nightingale's correspondence with physicians to answer this question, but it is probable that the views she expressed to physicians were not the same as those she expressed privately to other women. Indeed, Nightingale was in writing "careful not to arouse animosities" (p. 12). She extracted all possible information from her visitors and made copious notes, often concealing her identity and hiding her activities. As a woman, it is clear that she believed that she could not be known as the initiating force in many of her activities; thus, she often conducted her work behind the scenes. While superintendent of nursing, Nightingale had proposals brought to committees without informing the members that they came from her. Caught between two sets of authority, she manipulated the situation so as to effect change. After the physicians had approved one such proposal as their own, Nightingale said in a letter to her father: "It was a bold stroke but success is said to make an insurrection into a revolution" (Nightingale, December 3, 1853, cited in Cope, 1958, p. 18).

Cope asserted that Nightingale did not have a high opinion of the curative power of professional medicine; however, she was loyal to individual physicians in the Crimea. Had she not accepted male medical authority, perhaps modern nursing would not have emerged as it has. Loyalty was mandated by the subordinate status of women in the general society. But she attacked the military medical organization as a disaster. She was equally critical of medical groups, understanding their "professional prejudices." She also had little respect for the opinions of physicians regarding their affiliated hospital situations. Early in her career, according to Cope, she learned that physicians, like other people, had many weaknesses.

Because Nightingale had visited and studied every major hospital in Great Britain and most of the large ones on the continent, she was recognized by some physicians as being an unrivaled expert in hospital planning. Although not university trained, Nightingale was often critical of the ideas expounded by physicians, but in her public statements she conciliated the men, "knowing their power." However, she believed that "'The sick are the most credulous of human beings. They will believe anything the 'Doctor' (whether allopathic, homeopathic, or hydropathic) says to them. For their sake let us be most careful to carry the 'Doctor' with us" (Nightingale, September 16, 1860, cited in Cope, 1958, p. 21).

In her nursing school, Nightingale did not favor teaching too much "pure medicine," because she felt that nurses would become intolerable "from airing their knowledge or miserable from seeing methods adopted which were not in keeping with [those] ... they had been taught were the best" (p. 23). The subordinate and relatively powerless role of women is clearly implicit in this assertion. Although she favored women doctors, she did not want to see nurses become "medical women." In this, given the blurring of functions at the time, she probably restrained nursing from the development of greater autonomy. However, she herself did not hesitate to evaluate medical treatments and prescriptions. Cope implied that Nightingale was beyond her sphere; but in her *Notes on Nursing* (1859), it is clear that she was ahead of some physicians, who were still using "heroic" methods such as leeching, severe purgatives, and other invasive procedures. These make some of Nightingale's recommendations on hygiene seem a model of sanity.

The Nightingale Training School to Carry Out Her Ideas

In 1986 Monica Baly published her research on the Nightingale Training School from 1875 to 1890, focusing on nursing politics and the Fund Council, which started with Sidney Herbert to administer the Nightingale Fund, and, under Nightingale, was more a symbol than an actual working group. Indeed, Nightingale claimed "the doctors on the Council had an absolute administrative incapacity and the three civil doctors are perfect infants in administrative matters" (Nightingale, 1859; cited in Baly, 1986, p. 187). Given Nightingale's influence, she, without formal membership, actually controlled the expenditures and considered using capital to set up "a school of our own" (p. 188). This did not occur. Both Nightingale and the council recognized the need for clinical training, but were concerned that they were subsidizing the hospital; they doubted the quality of training; and disliked the exploitation of probationers: "The Fund Council agonized over the problem for years, but they did not solve it and it remains largely unsolved" (p. 191).

According to Baly, Nightingale did not appoint a woman to the council, although she had influenced the Metropolitan Board to appoint women: "There is something a little illogical about the insistence of putting 'all power (in nursing matters) into the hands of one female head' and yet excluding women from the governing body" (p. 192). Certainly, Nightingale understood the limitations on female power and appointed influential men to the Fund Council, but only those who would support the causes she espoused. Indeed, Baly observed "that the Council used Emily Faithfull's Victoria Printing Press, which was founded in 1876 as a Women's Printing Society, to provide work for women" (p. 193).

Baly nevertheless concluded that the absence of women on the governing board was because Nightingale preferred working with men, not women, about whom she did not have a high opinion. Even her favorite women, said Baly, sooner or later fell out of favor, unlike most of her men favorites. However, Nightingale's relations with women were far more positive and complex than this (see Roberts and Group, 1995). It is more likely that Baly's second reason for Nightingale's failure to include women is the more relevant: "she wanted a Council with influence in high places, which was something women did not have" (p. 193). Indeed, this explanation seems even more likely since fund members wanted to be represented on the Court of Governors of St. Thomas' Hospital, positions that would surely have been denied to women.

Baly connects the demand for longer and more scientific and rigorous training of nurses to feminist pressures for opening inexpensive high schools to girls and for the establishment of institutions of higher education for women. By the 1880s some nursing leaders, Eva Lückes, for example, were graduates of new girls' schools, such as Cheltenham College, and many women sought higher education. Nightingale, according to Baly, rejected longer periods of training because she feared this would mean longer hospital exploitation of nurses: "If the Fund Council would not stop this, what hope had hospitals without a fund?" (p. 195). Indeed, a wide variety of earning and learning schemes existed, said Baly, with "more emphasis on earning than learning" (p. 195). Women students often followed a schedule from six in the morning to ten at night; for this they were paid nothing if in training, or a pittance if they were "trained" nurses. In return for their training, they were bound to the hospital nursing school, filling any nursing post needed for a specified period of time.

The nurse training schemes, claims Baly, did wrest some power from physicians, because the nurses were under female authority and moved from ward to ward for experience. This removed them from the direct control of a few physicians on one ward. Indeed, some nursing leaders, such as Ethel Gordon Fenwick, were strong proponents of suffrage; nevertheless, Baly sees nursing as not touching the women's movement until the 1880s, but this assertion is debatable. On the other hand, Baly sees the conflict between nurses and physicians as one in which "not all the new-style nurses used their independence tactfully" (p. 195). One might reverse this and question why so many women in nursing were so "tactful"? Indeed, Judith Moore's (1988) perception (considered next in this chapter) of the women's struggle at Guy's and King's College Hospitals is quite different from Baly's. Baly reported that Margaret Lonsdale, a former probationer at Guy's, with reforming zeal wrote an article in the *Nineteenth Century Journal* in which she accused physicians of opposing the nurses' changes because they feared medical malpractice would be exposed by cultured and refined women, whose criticisms could not be brushed aside as easily as those from less-educated, poorer women: "If talked of by the old nurses no one took any notice" (p. 196).

Instead of lauding Lonsdale's courage, Baly saw the article as unfortunate, and one that was dismissed as ridiculous by physicians in their correspondence to the *British Medical Journal*. To these writers, physicians alone should give orders and guidance, although a woman superintendent was needed to report nurses' dereliction of duty under the physician's charge. Baly perceived Lonsdale's article and the subsequent correspondence about it as stirring up a hornet's nest and "a great deal of emotional irrelevance which indicated the professional insecurity of both doctors and nurses" (p. 156). One could, instead, see the conflict as an effort to expose the sex-segregated differentials of power and, as such, a very important test of women's capacity to direct nursing and their public work. Baly did recognize that "After 20 years the principles enunciated by the Fund Council were by no means fully accepted" (p. 196).

Baly rejected Lonsdale's account, but accepted an article by nurse Pringle, supported by surgeon Joseph Bell and published in the *Edinburgh Medical Journal* as a "reasoned" statement. Obviously, any article approved by physicians both before and after publication would not necessarily represent a radical feminist's or even a moderate reformer's position. Certainly, few could deny Pringle's point that the conditions for nurses in the past had been so appalling that it was understandable if they fell asleep or were unable to do their work. Nurses were, nevertheless, often "clever, dutiful, cheerful and kind, endowed above all with that motherliness of nature which is the most precious attitude of a nurse" (pp. 196–197). To Pringle, good conditions, although needed, were insufficient to make good nurses.

In Baly's view, Pringle dealt with Lonsdale's complaints with "sagacity." Pringle stated that her experience with physicians had been different and that nurses received the behavior they themselves attracted or merited. Why Baly sees Pringle's "blaming the victim" as sagacious and reasoned is unclear. Indeed, surgeon Bell, called Don Quixote by Baly, approved the movement of nurses from ward to ward, but concluded that "the real object of the nursing staff is to help the physicians and surgeons to care for the sick poor" (p. 197). Articles by such physicians and by Pringle led Baly to conclude: "Such words of wisdom should have quelled the controversy" (p. 197). From her perspective, it, unfortunately, "smoldered" on. From a feminist perspective, disenchantment with the subordination of nurses continues, quite appropriately, to blaze over a century later.

The Escalating Struggle for Nursing Reform

In contrast to Baly, Judith Moore (1988) in her fine book *A Zeal for Responsibility* details from a feminist perspective the trials of nursing reformers in two English hospitals in the nineteenth century. Moore's work represents the fusion of women's and nursing's history and the reconstitution of medical history. As in Versluysen's analysis (1980), it typifies the best of the new research on nursing; heavily influenced by feminism, it represents a consistent analytic integration of gender, class, and profession. Moore analyzes women in conflict with male physicians and hospital administrators at two prestigious London teaching hospitals: King's College Hospital in 1874 and 1883 and Guy's Hospital in 1880. The nurses struggled to achieve autonomy, independence in decision making, and power in the hospitals' hierarchies. The nursing sisterhood of St. John's House, an Anglican organization that developed, as noted previously, to fill the gap left by the collapse of religious nursing orders, was central to these conflicts. According to Moore, the prevailing assumptions about women's biological inferiority were used by medical and administrative men to justify their subjugation of nurses. But the nurses, now drawn from the middle and upper classes, confronted the men, fighting for their own rights and those of their patients.

Detractors of nursing, said Moore, have at different times—and sometimes simultaneously—claimed that women either had an inborn gift for nursing, needing no additional training, or that, without practical instruction, they were "at best a nuisance, at worst a danger, to their patients" (p. ix). In reality, educated nurses were a threat to physicians, who feared women's autonomous judgment on the men's presumption of a scientific and moral knowledge base that was often inadequate. Indeed, Moore asserts that women such as Nightingale were determined to use every weapon they possessed, "charm, social pressure, and almost blackmail" (Abel-Smith, 1960, pp. 19–20; cited in Moore, p. xiii). Nurse Agnes Hunt even sent smallpox patients to voice their complaints to members of a hospital committee.

Physicians insisted that "Nurses must always be *servants,* and they cannot safely be permitted to rise above that position in society" (*Lancet,* June 4, 1881; cited in Moore, 1988, p. xiv). Respectability must not interfere with obedience. In contrast, Sister Dora Pattison, sister in charge at Walsall Hospital, insisted on conservative surgery and conducted postmortems to increase her knowledge. In the absence of a house-surgeon at Walsall, the nurse in charge acted as surgeon in emergencies. Moore makes the case that Sister Dora's audacity was fueled in part by her intense religious convictions, typical of sisterhood nurses who publicly challenged medical complacency, even cruelty. These nurses, Moore pointedly claims, did not simply complain to each other or use "feminine" tact and patience, but confronted the men, risking their jobs and livelihood. Clearly, Moore contests the idea that nurses' foremothers were "limited ladies." In fact, she turns upside down the usual nursing history: it is *today's* nurses who, in contrast, seem reticent and fearful. Centrally important is the trivialization of women's history that, according to Moore, and Versluysen before her, has created a traditionalism in nursing curriculum so pervasive as to exclude the truth of women's own history, relying instead on a bastardized form of masculist medical history and thus excluding the feminism basic to the rise of "modern" nursing.

In the 1870s the gendered division of labor was centrally important. The medical profession's social prestige was rising, but was still inferior socially to that of military officers, clergy, and barristers. The number of physicians was rising so rapidly that newspaper accounts feared they were "doomed to languish in poverty and obscurity" (London *Times,* Oct. 3, 1884, p. 9; cited in Moore, 1988, p. 40). The reality was quite different: most physicians achieved some degree of success. Nevertheless, the men attacked not the increasing number of women but their change in status from domestic, a position into which they had been earlier pushed by physicians who assumed control or excluded women's religious orders. The physicians' blockage of midwives and district nurses, claims Moore, provided evidence that both urban and rural areas were to be controlled by the men. On the other hand, educated nurses had made hospitals places fit for wealthier patients and a source of income for hospital administrators and physicians. It was nurses who made hospitals possible, not hospitals that made nursing a reality.

The solution to the gendered occupational conflict was to force women's submission. By relying on societal sexism, physicians could demand faithful assistants from the lower classes, who could not regulate medicine. For example, physicians refused to allow nurses to know the contents of bottles of medicine, even removing labels and instead putting numbers on them and, subsequently disallowed nurses the use of simple instruments. The *Lancet* recommended that physicians "lock away beyond their [the nurses'] reach every particle of medicine" (Moore, 1988, p. 46).

The usual claim that the women possessed only enough information to be dangerous was refuted by the nurses themselves. In actuality, the nurses were often neither illiterate nor lacking in knowledge. In fact, Moore claims that nursing provided the basis for women to enter medicine, not, as is usually understood, for medical women to open up nursing.

Over the years, the men gave no ground and continued to reiterate the same strictures: "Every scrap of information she possesses beyond the mere routine of sick-tending is not merely useless but mischievous" (*Lancet,* Dec. 11, 1880, pp. 946–947; cited in Moore, 1988, p. 48). The primary role was assistant to the physician, but women, as Moore notes, "could and did form strong bonds to each other in public as well as in private settings, even across the class lines separating nurses from sisters" (p. 50). The issues of authority and knowledge were fundamental during the crisis at Guy's Hospital. Moore believes that this conflict has been buried in nursing history because it was seen as an embarrassment. How could subsequent nurses under the domination of men admit to their foremothers' disobedience?

Margaret Elizabeth Burt, educated at St. John's House and previously superintendent at the Leicester Infirmary, was appointed matron at Guy's Hospital in 1879 by Edmund Lushington. Burt tried to introduce a system of nursing that had been successful at King's College Hospital. She did not introduce her own or any other sisterhood to Guy's. Nevertheless, physicians used religion as a criticism of her administration. On attempting reforms, Burt was subjected to every kind of indignity; for example, libelous statements were published about her supposed abuse of patients and caricatures of her "gross character" were mailed to her.

Relying on the reports of Margaret Lonsdale, who championed Burt's cause, and according them greater veracity and courage than did Baly, Moore described the fight over the nursing reforms as a typical struggle by the physicians to return to the use of untrained women, whose main task was to study the characters and "fancies" of the medical men. The physicians' opinions were represented by Dr. J. Braxton Hicks, who did not want a central nursing system or a matron or superintendent responsible for nursing, as this system would allow the women to band together in opposition to medical wisdom and authority.

The nurses, who were referred to by the name of their wards (e.g., Miss Clinical), were expected to be loyal subordinates. In the ward system, the medical residents, according to physician John Neale, were made more "confident in themselves" (p. 59) if they had a woman on whom they could rely. The matron in a central system, on the other hand, *"reigns supreme . . . free from fear* of losing her comfortable home, and may even go so far as to have the audacity, when occasion presents, of making open or underhand reports about the medical staff" (p. 59). As Moore reported, a women's system of "espionage" was to the men particularly problematic, since women presumably lacked judicial minds and were, said Neale, easily "swayed by prejudice" (p. 60).

Clinical training in several types of nursing, movement among wards according to patients' needs, and even written records were, as Moore states, dangerous innovations according to physicians, who even rejected the women's use of a thermometer. The struggle at Guy's Hospital went on without an external audience until Lonsdale publicized it and subsequently had to defend herself. Again religion was raised, but this was not the central issue; more likely it was a screen from behind which women and class could be attacked and trivialized. In reality, Burt's innovations, as Moore claims, were *structural*, designed to concentrate nurses' work on nursing itself, to create an esprit de corps among the women, and provide a new scale of remuneration and an equity in sharing duties. The only religious requirement was to attend morning and evening prayers at the hospital.

The military model was used as an analogue, with the nurse as the regimental officer who, even though she knows the whole plan of campaign is a blunder, still carries out the orders. What, asks Moore, did patients think of this "Charge of the Light Brigade" policy? She answers: they were never asked! The fundamental value conflict over whose interests are to be promoted and protected is still critical in debates on nursing ethics today. The care of patients was central to the women's reforms. Lonsdale claimed that before Miss Burt's appointment patients were neglected, covered with sores, and dying. These assertions were completely rejected and ignored by Dr. Walter Moxon, who simply accused Lonsdale of being a liar. However, Moore agrees with Lonsdale's accusations: "It . . . seems unlikely that thirty-two critically ill patients under the care of no more than three nurses would be entirely free of bedsores even without 'rough and rude' treatment" (p. 73).

In 1880 the Guy's Hospital board of governors issued a committee report that was favorable to Burt; her reforms were reported by the committee as an honest endeavor to supply properly trained nurses in "due subordination" to the medical staff, whose orders had not been obstructed. Then, as now, the committee recommended improved communication between physicians and nurses. Nevertheless, Dr. Samuel Wilks denounced the report in the *Times*, as did the *British Medical Journal.*

The conflict between Burt's reforms and the physicians at Guy's Hospital became even more public over a manslaughter charge against nurse Pleasance Louisa Ingle, who was accused of causing the death of a consumptive patient by giving her a bath. This incident became purposely entangled with the fundamental issue of the nurses' independence and self-reliance. In the *Times*, Dr. S. O. Habersohn claimed: "The painful death of a patient during the last few days is the best illustration of this kind of nurse" (p. 79), referring to women who acted independently of physicians' directions. At the trial, nurse Ingle stated she had not been informed of the patient's diagnosis; she believed it to be hysteria. Subsequently, Ingle was convicted, largely on the hostile testimony of Dr. F. W. Pavy. During the trial, Dr. William Gull contested Pavy's testimony, saying that the nurse had not caused the death of the patient since tubercular meningitis was sufficient to cause death. Burt was not called to testify, although she was available. Permission to bathe the consumptive patient was given by a nurse, who was neither trained nor hired under the new system, but the incident was still attributed to Burt's nursing reform policies. Thus, the conclusion was that physicians must have complete control.

Subsequently, the governors still failed to unearth real weaknesses in the nursing system, or diminishment in medical authority, and specifically warned the medical staff that the governors' "painful duty" would be to take action if the struggle for power continued. The physicians protested the report, and two, Habersohn and John Cooper Forster, were then asked to resign. The medical staff withdrew its letter of protest and the governing board withdrew its request for resignations.

The *British Medical Journal* criticized the physicians at Guy's for being unable to sustain their unanimity and for allowing the governors to "dictate to them the terms on which they shall meet the matron" (p. 88), who they hoped would be removed if the men could find any reason to get rid of her. The rumor mongering by physicians continued in print with the closure of ten beds attributed to nursing problems, not to the decline in revenues which was the real cause. Habersohn and Forster, both nearing retirement, resigned, but they were treated as martyrs. The physicians sustained their harassment of Burt, her system, and the new nurses, and implied that her subsequent resignation was caused by pressure, though it was actually occasioned by her marriage. Burt's reforms survived, but so did the power of physicians to demand obedience, reduce women's education to a minimum, and use the free services of student nurses. Burt's epitaph on her memorial tablet read, "She hath done what she could" (p. 169), and Moore concluded that it was "less, certainly, than she must have hoped, but more than the hostile medical staff and their supporters in the press had ever been willing to admit" (p. 169).

Although the status of nursing as a profession began to rise, the physicians, as Moore notes, continued to see "themselves as by rights patriarchal rulers, undervalued and mistreated if they were asked to cooperate with nurses" (p. 172). Medicine, the "most beneficent profession that has ever existed" (*Medical Times and Gazette*, Aug. 16, 1880, p. 463; cited in Moore, 1988, p. 174), now claimed scientific authority. For women this claim was astonishingly premature! The functions of the ovary and fallopian tube were not known; the menstrual cycle was incompletely understood; with the development of the speculum, the uterus was considered to be the source of all women's problems. Unfortunately, medical ignorance was used to substantiate "scientifically" the subordination of women, particularly in education and employment. Nurses were expected to comply with stereotyped, presumably scientific medical pro-nouncements. Nurses who criticized physicians were disruptive *and* unfeminine *and* unnatural: "a conventional understanding of gender rather than any abstract principle of equity or even of efficiency in the workplace was at the center of the period's disputes between nurses and doctors" (p. 177). The physicians' attack against nurses extended to all women, particularly suffragists.

That professional autonomy was and remains the issue is obvious. Moore accurately sees the work of Amitai Etzioni (1969; 1980) and other current medical sociologists as a latter-day effort to explain that nurses are *semi*professionals. If they would only give up their inauthentic aspirations, the dysfunctional consequences of their attempts to pass as full professionals would disappear. If the women only understood that independence and collegial authority are inappropriate, then they could be happy as *semi*professionals. Moore claims that the evidence from the Victorian nurses proves the opposite: the women were already or potentially full professionals. It is precisely this fact that caused the men to attack them. If women could be excluded from scientific knowledge, then their claim for professional authority could be denied and physicians' control would be strengthened and solidified.

The Result of Increasing Medical Monopoly

By the end of the nineteenth and the beginning of the twentieth century, women in England were still expected "to take up their work in a missionary spirit for the good of the community, without regard to their own comfort or health" (Holcombe, 1973, p. 78). There was, of course, a strong tendency, as Nutting and Dock stated earlier, to overlook the material well-being of the nurses, whose salaries were dependent on endowments or taxes. In 1890 a government commission heard nurses complain of working eighteen-hour days for minimal recompense. Despite recommendations, changes were slow in coming; nevertheless, one guide to careers noted that a nurse was "not the unconsidered hard-worked woman she used to be" (p. 79). The commission also noted that pay did not increase with more education or experience, a theme that is echoed by nurses today. Nursing salaries, however, rose little in the years following the commission's report. Nurses were physically "used up," with no provision for pensions at the mandatory retirement age of fifty years. Finally, a pension fund paid into by nurses was established; it was inspired by a nurse who contracted typhoid in the wards and became permanently disabled, later to die penniless in a workhouse. However, it was not until after the Second World War that most British nurses were to receive any reliable monies upon retirement.

Again, two wars forced attention to the British nurses. The South African War found women dumped into field hospitals where they faced male orderlies who refused to do menial work; thus, the women were forced to do their own work and the men's as well. Following the war, Dame Sidney Brown headed a new nursing organization in Britain, and the status of the profession improved, ironically as a result of war.

The Poor Law Nursing Service, developed as a result of Nightingale's influence on the philanthropist William Rathbone, led to changes in the notoriously bad conditions. The largest single group of nurses in regular public employment in Britain by the late nineteenth century were in this service, but nurses "have only just been rescued from the workhouse" (Versluysen, 1980, p. 181). Although conditions were bad, Rosemary White (1978) noted that Poor Law nurses were not necessarily drunken, incompetent, passive, or uncaring, but sometimes had high standards of care and even defended patients against male officials. Nevertheless, some conditions were so awful that few women could have provided good care. For example, in the Liverpool Brownlow Hill Infirmary, *two* paid but untrained women were employed to care for *twelve hundred patients.* Most of the nursing care was done by pauper attendants and policemen. However, in 1865, William Rathbone, a friend of Nightingale's, and Agnes Elizabeth Jones, the first superintendent of nurses at Brownlow Hill, began an experiment with twelve Nightingale nurses and seven probationers that changed the entire system. The experiment ran three years and was to prove the value of trained nursing in public workhouses. The experiment was very successful, proving trained nurses' worth in providing care for the poor, but unfortunately, Jones contracted typhoid fever and died, only one woman of many who courageously entered situations of peril to prove women's worth in the renewed profession. Even though some nurses died to create the changes necessary, they were still not included in, for example, the Metropolitan Poor Act of 1867, which had no provisions for nursing care and applied only to London, not the rest of England. Finally, Nightingale and others forced legislation that would provide nursing care in poorhouses (the Poor Law Nursing Service). By then, however, women were found to be a sound investment, since it was cheaper to use nurses in training to replace both the pauper attendants and the paid but untrained women. Thus, even with increased influence, nurses still suffered the economic fate of other women in the general society: the misuse of their labor at penurious wages.

Nurses were caught between the authority of workhouse administrators and that of physicians, leaving their duties ill-defined. The bifurcation of lines of authority left nurses without the authority to do their jobs. The medical resident officers spent minimal time with patients who could offer little remuneration. According to Holcombe, the nurse was left without the authority of the physician and without the physician himself. The women could not obtain the medicines, foods, and appliances they needed for their patients. Working at low pay, they, as now, often had inadequate staff to support them. Nevertheless, the women took on dangerous jobs, with some forming the Fever Nurses Association in 1908 to deal with infectious cases.

The beginning of public health nursing or district nursing in England extended logically from the workhouse reforms. According to Holcombe, there was little control over the work of early nurses, which led to "slovenly care and neglect of patients, and little communications between the nurses and doctors, which led to the nurses' usurping the doctors' functions" (Holcombe, 1973, p. 90). Given the analysis of the medical takeover of women healers' roles and their exclusion from formal education, Holcombe's assertion is highly questionable.

What is clear is that the nurses' work was arduous; often on bicycles, the nurses served scattered populations, working fourteen hours a day, with a half day off every three weeks. Yet one woman wrote: "Here I realized for the first time the tremendous scope and power of a nurse's life. One went into those homes, not as 'my Lady Bountiful,' but as a fellow human being, a friend to give personal help, to teach and to serve" (p. 92).

Most nurses still went into private homes; however, the nurses often received only a small proportion of the fees, which were collected by the men in hospitals that, incidentally, assumed no legal risk for the nurses they supplied. This structure forced women to rely on physicians for referrals to avoid the hospital exploitation. Finally, the women formed their own associations, leading to British nurses' thirty-year war for state registration. As noted previously, Ethel Gordon Fenwick led the battle, even in opposition to Nightingale. Organizing the British Nurses Association in 1891, for the first time women formally associated together for self-government. Ignoring the medical men would have caused havoc, so physicians were allowed to join the association and were represented in governance. Despite the considerable control by men, any independence of women seemed unacceptable to the hospital administrators and physicians. Registration, controlled by women in their own organization, was totally unacceptable. Instead of devoting themselves to their "onerous duties and noble ends" (p. 98), physicians claimed the nurses would make a trade union, reducing work, increasing pay and pleasant conditions. Nurse supporters said, "As working women, nurses have a right to run on their own responsibility . . . they ought to be free to make their own conditions and not to be at the beck and call of institutions" (p. 98).

In contrast to Gamarnikow's assertion, registration was not the key gender issue; rather it was the establishment of an independent association of women, who would control their own occupation. Such an association was unnecessary, according to physicians, because the men themselves could decide whether nurses were sufficiently well-trained. In 1893 British women won a charter to list but not register nurses; finally, the men in the association placed themselves on record as opposing registration! Outraged, Fenwick and other nursing matrons realized that nurses and physicians in joint organization could lead only to "disastrous" results: "'We must be free to organize ourselves; the relation of man to woman complicates the situation; the relative position of doctor and nurse makes it impossible ... though we do not claim independence of the medical profession, we claim freedom to discuss our own affairs, to make our own laws, to decide on common principles of work'" (cited in Holcombe, 1973, p. 100).

It took the heavy casualties and severe injuries of the First World War to demonstrate the need for fully trained and *registered* nurses. In 1919 the women finally won registration. They had achieved the right to organize together and to define their own purposes in consort with each other and to regulate their own occupation. However, registration, as Gamarnikow pointed out, did not solve the gendered division of labor that caused the problems the nurses would continue to face in the twentieth century in both Great Britain and the United States.

3 | The Search for American Nursing Origins
Differing Approaches to the History of Nursing and the Medical Monopoly in the United States, 1800s to the Early 1900s

The extent to which the long history of women healers and the experiences of European, particularly British, nurses, have influenced the development of American nursing and nurse-physician relations has not been studied in depth. Instead, a number of American researchers have focused on nurses in a women's world, particularly from the late nineteenth century onward; thus, the long view of women healers is often missing and the development and impact of the medical monopoly is not fully explicated. However, as noted in the overview of this volume, perceiving women only in relation to men may exaggerate the victimization of women and limit understanding of their strengths and weaknesses within their own networks. So it is important to consider research that is primarily focused on nurses before continuing in subsequent chapters with a more direct analysis of nurse-physician relations.

Each researcher focuses on different groups of women, some in religious orders, some in domestic medicine and nursing, some in wartime endeavors, others in women's hospitals, and still others in health-reform activities, early hospital nursing schools, or public health nursing. Research also varies in the time periods covered and even in the interpretation of events within the same time periods. There is variation in the degree of emphasis on gender and on the interrelations among feminism, nursing, and women healers more generally, thus providing quite different interpretations of early nurses and nursing leaders. And finally, research also varies in the degree to which the women's world is perceived in the context of a cultural patriarchy. Thus, some researchers give limited attention to sexism, to the patriarchal privilege of physicians, and to their efforts to gain a monopoly by subordinating nursing and blocking health-care reform or supporting it when needed to promote medical interests.

In this chapter, we begin with the impact of European religious orders on American nursing and health care. Although there has been a lack of integration and synthesis between religious and secular nursing histories, it is clear that, despite church restrictions on women's religious orders, both European and indigenous American nursing sisters often independently founded hospitals and together created a vast network of health and social welfare services. We turn next to research that locates the emergence of hospital nursing not in the importation of Nightingale's reforms but in the context of women's work and thought in their own American communities, in which the rights of slaves and of women were central concerns. Though Nightingale's work in the Crimea did create a model for wartime nursing, the origins of military nursing in the United States can be traced to the colonial period; however, the emergence of "modern" American nursing is often traced to the nursing/medical activities of women in the American Civil War. Central to these analyses are the opposition of male physicians and surgeons to women nurses and the gross inadequacy of medical care.

Modern nursing in both Europe and the United States developed in the feminist context of widespread and influential health reforms led in large part by nineteenth-century women. In the American context, some researchers elaborate on the reforms and reformers, but do not specifically detail the role of nurses as participants in this movement; however, the research findings do establish the inadequacy of medical practices, the sexist medical treatment of women, and the need for alternative therapies, and provide a context for the development of "modern" nursing.

In both the United States and Great Britain, the nineteenth-century women's movement influenced not only health reform, but also the emergence of women physicians and the founding of hospitals for women. Clearly one offshoot of feminism, these women and institutions provided nurses' training, but the manner in which gender and professional roles interacted is still unclear. What is readily apparent in our consideration of the research is that both British and American women physicians and nurses could and did successfully create their own women-oriented hospitals despite the opposition of some physicians.

Some research traces the development of American nursing and a nursing ideology not to feminist reforms but to the importation of Florence Nightingale's model, which, as adapted in American hospitals, is presumed to have created a system of subordination and an ideology of obedience that was subsequently reinforced by the nurses themselves. This research does not in general incorporate a systematic analysis of what physicians did to force nurses' compromises and is, therefore, relatively weak on nurse-physician relations. This approach is in sharp contrast to the research on American women nurses in public health nursing, which comes to quite different conclusions, emphasizing not the compromises but the courage of early nursing leaders and groups in taking on male-dominated institutions. From this perspective, nurses fought, often successfully, a pattern of medical domination by reaching out to help women, children, and families, thus achieving social change even if unable to stop the growth of a medical monopoly of health care. Obviously, the emphases of the researchers discussed in this chapter vary on the specific components of women's healing activities and their emphasis on feminism and attention to gendered relations with physicians. Until they are integrated into a unified whole that systematically incorporates nursing, nurses, and their relations with physicians, we can only contrast and compare types of research to provide a sense of American women's work in health care in the nineteenth century and into the first decades of the twentieth century.

The Impact of Women's Religious Orders on Early Health Care in America

It is clear that most American nursing histories have not achieved a long historical view on nursing. As discussed in chapter 1, what accounts we have of earlier periods are often abbreviated, or their authors have been too unaware of women's general status to provide much clarity. Therefore, the domestic medical and nursing activities of women are briefly acknowledged but omitted from subsequent analyses. Similarly, the influence of feminism is noted, but often the precise interconnections are missing. In addition, accounts of the impact of different religious orders on nursing are only briefly considered, primarily in the European and not the American context, and the story then proceeds without blending the religious and secular histories. The actual impact of gender on *both* secular and religious nurses and their organizations is still unclear because there is no *integrated* analysis of attitudes toward and actions taken on female status or gendered subordination, particularly in relation to male-dominated medicine.

How did the control of European women's religious orders in previous centuries affect American women healers in their orders? As documented in chapter 1, the adverse church rulings on women's religious orders in Europe had particularly restrictive effects on their nursing and medical activities. Carlan Kraman (1989) asserted that this history of sustained reversal made the efforts of St. Vincent de Paul and St. Louise de Marillac exceptional because they succeeded in founding a noncloistered order in 1646, after thirteen years of service in Paris. It is their order which became the American model for Catholic women. The importation of this model was possible in part because there were very few American doctors in the seventeenth century and only some almshouses for the indigent in the eighteenth century that sometimes provided help for orphans, the mentally ill, and control of criminals. As discussed in the previous chapters, treatment of the sick usually occurred at home, where women provided better care. Kraman stresses that there were shocking abuses in the almshouses, although somewhat better conditions in voluntary hospitals were evident by the mid eighteenth century.

During America's Revolutionary War the colonists first had contact with Catholic sisters, who cared for the wounded of both armies, for example at the Hôtel-Dieu in Quebec. By the early nineteenth century indigenous sisterhoods emerged that provided service to the sick and poor; one was founded by African American women, for example, in 1829 in Baltimore. Other European-based congregations were also founded, often to deal with immigrants from France, Germany, and Ireland. St. Elizabeth Seton's Sisters of Charity was the first order to engage in hospital work and provided care at the Baltimore Infirmary, connected with the University of Maryland. Few records from the women survive, but a Johns Hopkins physician later wrote that their nursing was excellent; indeed, many sisters were of great intelligence and, for the period, of superior education. He concluded: "They did what the good nurse of the present day does—carried out the doctors' orders with promptness and intelligence" (Doyle, 1929, p. 782; cited in Kraman, 1989, p. 23).

In contrast to this physician's recollection, it is clear from Kraman's account that the nursing sisterhoods in America from the early nineteenth century on did not simply follow men's orders, but actually *created* hospitals, as women had done in Great Britain and Europe. For example, the Sisters of Charity of Nazareth organized a new congregation on the Kentucky frontier. Starting first in a log cabin, they visited the sick on horseback, and, two years later, they founded St. John's Hospital and an orphanage in Nashville, Tennessee. When cholera hit Louisville, Kentucky, in 1832–1833, they established a new facility, St. Vincent's Infirmary, which later became a hospital. Despite poverty, insufficient funds, and anti-Catholicism, the women's orders—for example, Seton's groups, which were known after 1850 as the Daughters of Charity of St. Vincent de Paul—expanded to more than twenty locations, founding the Mount Hope Retreat, the first Catholic mental hospital in the United States, and St. Vincent's Hospital in the Bronx, New York. An offshoot, the Sisters of Charity, organized Cincinnati's St. John's Hospital. In 1865 four young women traveled to Santa Fe, New Mexico, and set up a hospital in an adobe building with mud floors; visiting the sick and poor, they even begged for funds from the mining camps. In the Indian Territory of Kansas, still another group opened St. John's Hospital in Leavenworth in 1864, and members of the same Sisters of Charity of Leavenworth went to Last Chance Gulch, now Helena, Montana, and opened another hospital; this was followed by two more, one in Butte and then another in Denver.

To these American women's groups were added European orders; for example, in 1836, the French Sisters of St. Joseph of Carondelet, after a journey that included a seventy-day sea voyage, arrived in St. Louis, where they opened a hospital in 1849, mainly for fever-stricken Irish immigrants, then another in Wheeling, Virginia, and another in St. Paul, Minnesota. The Irish group Sisters of Mercy, founded in 1831 by Catherine McAuley to serve working women, moved to Pittsburgh, where they converted the Old Concert Hall into a hospital; within thirteen months it had admitted 254 patients. They then moved to Chicago and in 1852 started Mercy Hospital. Another group of this order came from Ireland; arriving in San Francisco in 1854, they immediately dealt with a cholera epidemic. Renting a vacant building, they named it St. Mary's Hospital, the first Catholic hospital on the Pacific coast of the United States. Additional sisterhoods from France and from Germany arrived and also established hospitals; some, such as the Hospital Sisters of the Third Order of St. Francis, sought refuge from religious persecutors, and opened a Springfield, Illinois, hospital in 1875 that was, according to Kraman, initially so primitive that the women slept on the floor with their cloaks their only cover.

Kraman also described the efforts of Protestant sisterhoods; for example, in 1849, Lutheran deaconesses from Kaiserswerth founded hospitals in Pennsylvania, Wisconsin, and Illinois. Episcopalian sisterhoods from England, such as the Sisters of St. Luke, took charge of hospitals in Baltimore, New York, Boston, and other cities and towns. The Community of St. Mary, originating in New York in the early 1860s, created women's shelters, orphanages, a hospital for children, and a hospital and infirmary. Kraman concludes that these women entered a society that had not developed a coherent strategy to care for the sick, poor, and abandoned; yet they took on the challenge and organized what later became "a vast and efficient network of hospitals, orphanages, and homes for the destitute and elderly . . . contributing specifically to the development of health care in the United States" (p. 38). Kraman's work focuses on women and does not detail gendered occupational interrelations. Male support is implied, but little information is provided on the direct or indirect involvement of medical men. However, Kraman's account does provide clear evidence that women founded and directed their own hospitals, even though more research is needed to explicate the actual power relations that prevailed. Furthermore, how the nursing sisterhoods interacted with community women healers has yet to be fully understood.

The Domestic Roots of American Nursing Schools

The impact of the British experience on the development of American nursing is still unclear, particularly since few researchers have investigated the origins of American nursing prior to the mid nineteenth century. However, the results of detailed research on the *domestic* roots of lay nursing in at least one city, Philadelphia, were published by Patricia O'Brien in 1987 and in 1993 (as Patricia O. D'Antonio). The traditional written history of "modern" nursing begins with Nightingale's heroic achievements and her subsequent influence, and continues with "moving stories of strong and resourceful women, supportive and generous men, prestigious and well-loved institutions" (O'Brien, 1987, p. 12). The prior activities of women in religious orders and their hospitals, as discussed by Kraman, are missing from this perspective, and so are detailed data on pre-Nightingale women healers. To O'Brien, the traditional story overshadowed "a more important story played out in an earlier era and in a different historical context" (p. 12).

The usual historical account, for example, in Pennsylvania, begins with the appointment of Nightingale superintendents trained at St. Thomas' Hospital to the Philadelphia Hospital and the University of Pennsylvania Hospital, where successful nurses were produced: for example, Mary E. P. Davis, founder of the *American Journal of Nursing;* Jane Delano, important in the American Red Cross; Linda Richards, central to the establishment of nursing schools across the country; and Lucy Walker, a founder of the organizational forerunner of the National League for Nursing. In contrast, O'Brien begins her story in the 1830s, when nursing was perceived as the natural, loving duty of women and mothers, and traces the way in which "these domestic roots shaped contemporary thinking" (p. 12). From her research, O'Brien traced the current tension between the images of ministering mothers and scientific professionals to the domestic origins of nursing. More importantly, O'Brien moves the history of nursing into the broader realm of the history of women and of labor.

Moving toward a revisionist theoretical framework, historians of women are no longer "compartmentalizing women's work into a sphere separate from their family and domestic life, they are coming to see both as inextricably intertwined" (p. 12). Some suggest that women saw "their work not as freedom from domestic ties, but as extensions of them" (p. 12). However, such extensions for women textile factory workers, among others, are not clear. In contrast, O'Brien claims that nurses' accommodation between home and work was very different from that made by women in factories: "Rather than breaking that link they extended it" (p. 13).

In nineteenth-century Philadelphia "the burning social issues of the day were abolition and rights of women" (p. 13). Quaker women were involved in antislavery societies, the Underground Railroad, and the first women's rights convention at Seneca Falls in 1848, where Philadelphian Lucretia Mott's equal rights resolution was passed. It called for the overthrow of the monopoly of the pulpit and for women's equal participation in all trades, professions, and commerce.

The cult of the lady emerged, but was far from the reality of most women's lives. O'Brien notes that nursing was associated with home and domestic life, and mothers, daughters, and sisters nursed and doctored their families. Some women neighbors were considered born or professed nurses. By the mid nineteenth century, books and magazines for women were being published, and some of these even promised to make family members their own physicians. Quaker physician Joseph Warrington's book, *The Nurses Guide* (1839), and his organization, the Nurse Society of Philadelphia, sought to provide an alternative to both the traditional hospital and the midwife. However, Warrington's Philadelphia Nurse Society Home and School, which opened in 1850, trained women to be responsible to physicians, not to create an independent calling. As O'Brien notes, Warrington's primary concern was, in his own words, to impress on women "the importance of understanding their relations with a class of men who devote years to the acquisition of the *science*" of medicine

(Warrington, 1839, p. 2; cited in O'Brien, 1987, p. 13). Warrington essentially wanted to provide a group of women to span temporarily the gap between midwives and the emerging obstetricians. Thus, women would no longer be responsible to other women, particularly those in childbirth, but to men, who were in the process of establishing the legitimacy of allopathic medicine, especially obstetrics.

To get rid of the competition, physicians had to get women who nursed to take orders, rather than "presume to oppose their own opinions to those of the physician" (O'Brien, 1987, p. 14). In contrast, the "irregular" practitioners emphasized domestic medical and nurturing self-care, not subservient hospital or home nurses. Warrington had prepared women for home care under medical control, but Ann Preston, pioneer woman physician and founder of the Female Medical College of Pennsylvania in 1850 and the Woman's Hospital of Philadelphia in 1861, was concerned with training not only women physicians, but also nurses to work under medical direction in the Woman's Hospital, where women's and children's diseases and care were central. O'Brien claims Preston publicly played down rigid hierarchy and stressed intelligent cooperation, but privately thought she could get rid of chambermaids since nurses could also do many of the domestic tasks. Following Nightingale's 1859 *Notes on Nursing*, Preston (1863) published a book on nurses and their training, hoping to recruit nurses from among her readers, but O'Brien notes that nurses in training at the Woman's Hospital of Philadelphia rarely exceeded one or two each year in the 1860s. Preston's lectures were, nevertheless, very popular with "ladies of leisure," who paid $2 for a course of ten lectures. O'Brien concludes that there was "little to differentiate the instruction of mothers from that of paid workers. . . . To practice it [nursing] in the home was to fulfill the calling of 'true womanhood.' To practice it for a wage kept one within the domestic sphere, a world where the only pertinent analogy was to 'chamber maids'" (O'Brien, 1987, p. 14).

Yet, other forces, particularly the heroic work of women in the Crimean and U.S. Civil Wars, were legitimizing nursing. Wealthier women who had struggled against dirt, disease, and medical indifference or callousness during the Civil War formed boards of lady visitors to inspect city hospitals, and these women reported on the squalor and stench of such institutions. For example, Pauline Henry, a wealthy invalid, offered $1,000 to the new University of Pennsylvania Hospital for nurses' training. The men refused her money so Henry gave $3,000 in 1875 to the Woman's Hospital to send their trained nurses to other hospitals. In 1876 six of these nurses went to Philadelphia Hospital, where the squalor, food, and supplies were almost intolerable to the women. Undaunted, Henry also tried to place trained nurses in the Jefferson Hospital department for the insane, but men balked at providing even a minimal monthly salary of $10 and a separate dining table for the nurses. Eventually the Pennsylvania Hospital accepted the trainees, who later, in 1884, established the Pennsylvania Hospital Training School for nurses.

By tracing women's actions and the historical events within Philadelphia from the early nineteenth century, O'Brien could conclude: "In essence, then, 1885, the date traditionally associated with the emergence of trained nursing in Philadelphia, becomes less a milestone and more the gradual culmination of decades of indigenous experimentation" (p. 15). Why is this date still important? Because it marked the introduction of Nightingale's influence. In response to a request from the male president of the Philadelphia Hospital Board, Nightingale sent Alice Fisher, a St. Thomas' graduate, to set up the nursing school at the University of Pennsylvania Hospital. However, as O'Brien states, the Nightingale nurses were late on the scene: "The Woman's Hospital nurses trace no direct line to Florence Nightingale. Their roots were indigenous to their own historical time, and their role carved from their own personal experiences and from a rhetoric blending the ideology of domesticity with that of medical science" (p. 15).

By 1885 the Woman's Hospital nurses had already established a network of trained and influential nurses not only in Philadelphia, but in Wisconsin at a Quaker mission for Indians (1869); in New York City at Bellevue (1871); and at the Connecticut Training School for Nurses in New Haven (1872). The latter claimed to be the first of the Nightingale schools. In O'Brien's view, the Nightingale imagery was used to legitimize paid work for women, linking home and work in a calling and providing physicians with obedient and disciplined female subordinates. The nurses' status and prestige were associated with Nightingale, lending an "aura of legitimation to the quest for professional authority, to the structure of current nursing interventions, and to the extrapolation of a body of unique nursing knowledge. . . . [However] the emphasis on Nightingale and on the Nightingale legacy to modern nursing obscures more than it clarifies" (p. 16). The search for American nursing origins in Nightingale is wrong, claims O'Brien, because nursing's roots are in the home, in the domestic environment, in the linkage between home and hospital. Nurses have overlooked these because of the medical emphasis on rationality, objectivity, and autonomy above intuition, subjectivity, and interdependence. It is to O'Brien's credit that she positions nursing in the context of women's history. However, she does not provide many specific details on what medical and nursing functions women actually performed in their homes and neighborhoods.

In 1993, O'Brien, now publishing under her married name of D'Antonio, again stressed that domestic nursing and medicine preceded the establishment of formal nursing education. Women were central to practice. This fact is obvious, for example, in the lists of therapeutics they prepared for domestic medicine cabinets. Most physicians attacked community practitioners, especially midwives, as quacks, even blaming the women for practices originally instituted by the physicians themselves. According to D'Antonio, given the similarity in techniques, the physicians could often only accuse the women of being "outdated." Underpinning such charges was the threat the women posed to physicians' practices, particularly since the independent midwives freely gave their opinions and openly expressed disagreements with medical men. They refused to refer patients' questions back to physicians and even refused to assist physicians whose proposed treatments they disapproved.

Paid nurses generally entered families with their own experience and therapeutics, although family members still did most of the nursing and doctoring without hired nurses. Middle-class nurses, whose family ties made physicians' claims of superiority questionable, were the greatest threat to physicians, whose "authoritarian highhandedness" and insistence on obedience to orders rested on shaky grounds. Physicians attacked by saying that "professed nurses were 'ignorant'; middle-class women who nursed 'misguided'; working-class women who nursed threatened the nurse-physician relationship through their 'prejudices' while middle-class women did so through their misleading 'affection'" (D'Antonio, 1993, pp. 236–237). Physicians tried to ally themselves with mothers to correct the "misguided" and "ignorant" professed nurses, who "needed" to be supervised by medical men. As D'Antonio observed, the alliance of women across classes could only be broken if middle-class women's belief in the value of professed nurses' care was eroded. To do this their experience and competence had to be attacked. One physician, for example, said that in the lower ranks of society, no habit was so little cultivated as attention: "Thousands pass from cradle to grave without seeing correctly a single object which passes before them" (D'Antonio, 1993, p. 238); thus, hired nurses could not be trusted with the domestic management of the sick. To observe correctly required formal education, but even educated mothers were inadequate because they did not have the "right" kind of experience; thus, all women, regardless of education or experience, needed to be supervised by physicians.

Physician Ann Preston tried to recruit middle-class women but was largely unsuccessful, probably in part because she, like Warrington, emphasized a "hierarchical therapeutic alliance" even though he, unlike most of her male colleagues, emphasized "enlightened and refined" women nurses (p. 239). Lectures at the new Woman's Hospital were well attended by both women nursing at home and those nursing in hospitals: "Apart from sporadic ward supervision by Woman's Hospital physicians and a differing fee structure . . . there was little to differentiate the instruction of mothers from that of their middle-class sisters in the hospital" (p. 239).

D'Antonio concludes that the hierarchical ordering of physicians as educated superintendents of middle-class nursing women in the domestic sickroom eventually created a female managerial role that "devalued the physical aspects of nursing care . . . now the domain of the hired help, the working-class woman" (p. 240). Again, D'Antonio emphasizes that the reforms associated with Nightingale simply reframed "menial tasks" into a higher form of service into a "calling," making it respectable for middle-class women who could mesh their desire for paid work with the societal female image. D'Antonio emphasizes that nursing histories usually begin with the formal training schools in the late nineteenth century, but by then the framework for American nursing had already been established: "In exchange for this domestic authority, the hierarchical ordering of relationships remained sacrosanct" (p. 242). The physician gained "absolute" command of clinical care. The cost was the loss of the traditional alliance of women healers from all classes.

Not Even Common Courtesy: Nurses' Struggle against Physicians' Abuse during the Civil War

Many women were in fact doing much healing work beyond the physical boundaries of home and neighborhood. During the Civil War, when women extended their nursing and medical activities beyond their local communities, these were often seen as acts of competition with physicians. Marilyn Mayer Culpepper and Pauline Gordon Adams (1988) trace the emergence of women as a vital force during the Civil War, but, unlike D'Antonio, they connect this to Nightingale's activities in the Crimea, where she presumably legitimized work outside the home for women of quality.

Were American military physicians and surgeons more welcoming to nurses than their British colleagues? Evidently not, since the women aroused the ire of many medical men. Nurse Georgiana M. Woolsey wrote that hardly a surgeon treated women with even common courtesy. Unable to close the hospitals against women because of government policy, the men "determined to make their lives so unbearable that they should be forced in self-defense to leave. . . . Some of the bravest women I have ever known were among this first company of army nurses. They saw at once the position of affairs, the attitude assumed by the surgeons, and the wall against which they [the nurses] were to break and scatter; and they set themselves to undermine the whole thing" (Dannett, 1959, p. 88; cited in Culpepper and Adams, 1988, p. 982).

Even after the war, the physicians and surgeons concluded that women had been best at cooking special diets, washing and ironing the laundry, and providing linens. Culpepper and Adams note that the 1864 Sanitary Commission bulletin condescendingly approved as nurses only those women who were strictly obedient, conforming, docile, and respectful of the superior knowledge and authority of the surgeons. Again, it is important to emphasize that at this time most physicians had minimal education and there was little standardization of even the six-month to two-year education they *may* have achieved. What did the women actually do? They worked "16-hour days, sleeping on top of baggage on the hospital boats or among boxes in supply rooms. Still clad in their blood-stained skirts, they forgot to eat, anguished over the inexorable march of death" (p. 982).

Many women had been activists for the emancipation of slaves and for women's rights, and they persevered in the miserable conditions of war with slaughter so great that many wounded men waited overnight unattended and some waited three to five days before seeing, even briefly, a doctor, who often had a "scant knowledge of first aid and few pain killers" (p. 983). In surgery, ether, chloroform, or whiskey—anything with fast action—was used since speed was important. According to Culpepper and Adams, "All efforts failed to keep nurses' quarters, their patients, and themselves clean" (p. 983). Hannah Ropes, hospital matron in Maryland, told her daughter not to join her because the nurses got dirty and full of lice: "We run the gauntlet of disease from the disgusting itch to smallpox" (Brumgardt, 1980; cited in Culpepper and Adams, 1988, p. 983). Within the year, Ropes died of typhoid pneumonia, which also cut short Louisa May Alcott's nursing career at the same hospital, forcing her to go home. Before Ropes's death, she, like Alcott and many other women, were outspoken about the physicians' incompetency or corruption: "Ropes refused to condone the chief surgeon's arrogant manner with patients and his general disregard for them. She was appalled by the steward's efforts to feather his own nest by starving the patients, stealing their clothes, and selling their rations" (p. 984). Initially, Ropes failed to get Surgeon General William A. Hammond to listen, even when the steward locked a patient in a dark hole off the cellar. She then went to Secretary of War Edwin McMasters Stanton, who confirmed her accusations and sent the surgeon and steward to prison. Contrary to physicians' statements following the war, the capacity to obey did not make the best of women the best of nurses. In fact, as in the case of Ropes, the opposite was, and probably still is, true. (For an extended discussion of nurses' experiences during wartime, see Roberts and Group, 1995.)

To Purify Society: Women Health Crusaders in Nineteenth-Century America

The context from which nursing emerged in Great Britain and America included not only the military but also the women's health-reform movement. Researchers such as Regina Morantz (1977) provide evidence that the work of medical scientists and advances in bacteriology and medical therapeutics do not tell the whole story. Indeed, the revolution in health care was far more pervasive, created by a large constituency of ordinary lay advocates of new practices through self-help in health, public hygiene, dietary reform, temperance, hydrotherapy, and physiological and anatomical knowledge. A large number of women's rights advocates and abolitionists were connected to health reform. However, Morantz and other researchers have not clearly identified the interrelations among feminists, health reformers, Civil War nurses, domestic medicine and nursing, and the institutionalization of nursing. Certainly, we know that these trends in the nineteenth century coexisted within the context of women's demands for equality. Even without knowing all of the specific connections, it is important to grasp the wider influence of women on health reform. To connect this explicitly to the work of women in nursing is a task for future researchers.

To Morantz, the reformers shared a fundamental enlightenment—rationalism—calling for self-help based on sharing the laws of hygiene and physiology. Traditionally, "medical historians . . . have emphasized . . . the decline of heroic medical therapeutics" and the rise of health reform since reformers usually rejected the "bleeding, purging, and dosing" favored by medical men (Morantz, 1977, pp. 491–492). These explanations exclude the correlations between changes in women's status and their interest in the health movement: "Former accounts have only briefly acknowledged and never analyzed women's participation. Yet a number of the most outspoken of the health crusaders were female, and women swelled the ranks of the new movement" (p. 492). The connection between health promotion and women's roles is clear in an 1837 resolution of the Boston-based American Physiological Society: "woman in her character as wife and mother is only second to the Deity in the influence she exerts" (p. 492). Therefore, her education should qualify her to further the physical, intellectual, and moral interests of humanity. In the Northeast, Ladies Physiological Societies appeared, and women lecturers taught enthusiastic women the "laws of life." To Morantz, the "profound changes in women's roles underlay their active interest in health reform" (p. 492).

The cult of the lady, the indolent, leisured wife who was often weak, dependent, and sickly, was rejected by health reformers and women's rights advocates, who favored instead women's superior moral and spiritual responsibility to elevate the domestic sphere, particularly health and hygiene. The health-reform movement readjusted female roles to the traditional values about women's place, but simultaneously eroded these sentiments by offering female leaders a way out of the home and an active role in social change. As Morantz noted, "Good health became a prerequisite to woman's new place in the world" (p. 495). Dress reform became a symbol of women's new aspirations. The reformers' refusal to be immobilized by impractical clothes became a moral issue: "They called upon women to liberate their world by freeing their bodies from the harmful effects of tight lacing and long, heavy unhygienic skirts" (p. 495). Mary Gove Nichols warned that little could be expected of women if their daily labor was to simply carry about their clothes. How would a woman in long full skirts ever become a geologist, botanist, or a mythologist? asked Edith Denner.

Lecturers attacked women's widespread ignorance of their bodies, relying heavily on anatomy and physiology in their talks. Advice on pregnancy and childbirth was "strikingly prophetic of today's feminist critique of professional obstetrical practice," with physicians' treatment seen as "unnatural and often outrageous" (p. 496). Regarded as invalids, pregnant women were bled, given paregoric, magnesia, and minerals, and poisoned with inappropriate substances, "just as though they were going through a regular course of fever," instead of engaging in a natural process (Trall, 1850, p. 121; cited in Morantz, 1977, p. 497). In matters of sex, reformers urged restraint, particularly from husbands' sexual abuse that caused female ill health and infant mortality. Excessive childbearing endangered women and babies, so birth control (i.e., family planning) was publicly advocated.

The idea that humans could affect the future by manipulating environmental conditions was, said Morantz, a modern view that involved a belief in progress and the abandonment of passivity in dealing with life's problems. Reform ideas about personal cleanliness, public health, and family hygiene were part of middle-class culture by the end of the century. "For a minority of brave, ambitious and talented women, health reform also provided an outlet and an escape from an intolerably narrow and confining role. . . . They understood that to purify society, women would have to enter it" (p. 500).

The emphasis on educated motherhood and scientific domesticity helped make women modern, but not necessarily equal. Indeed, Morantz concluded that female moral superiority as a source of power should not be confused with liberation and that the excessive concern with women's maternal role still confined women to a separate but unequal sphere. To what extent, and in what ways, women in nursing influenced the health reforms and the changes in women's roles remains unclear. What is clear is that the institutionalization of modern nursing did not occur in a vacuum apart from women's public efforts to create social change in health care.

Women Physicians, Nurses, and Women's Hospitals

We know that some of the nineteenth-century American and British health reformers were women physicians, but their historical relations with women nurses are still far from clear. Vern L. Bullough (1983) claims that many women physicians and nurses in the late nineteenth century were closely allied: Elizabeth Blackwell and Marie Zakrewska are, for example, two physicians who presumably supported nursing. Since women physicians were usually excluded from medical organizations and hospitals, they sometimes served as nurses in the Civil War. Bullough examines the experience of one woman physician, Ida May Wilson (1864–1955), in relation to nursing. Between 1894 and 1896 Wilson attended the Ohio Medical University in Columbus, where there was no entrance exam; the only requirement was the ability to read and write. Indeed, Bullough could find little difference between nursing and medical education at that time. When Wilson graduated, there were no jobs for her, so she, without any nursing experience, became a hospital superintendent of nurses, work she liked sufficiently to return to Columbus to enter nursing school. Bullough notes that Wilson's brother, also a physician, took her to task for deserting medicine; after three years of medical study, why, he asked, would she want to be on duty as a nurse twenty hours in each day: "In medicine you make a visit and leave your orders and let the others take the worry" (p. 4). He admitted she would not make a fortune, but offered his office, books, and drugs for her use. Wilson followed his advice and practiced medicine until she was in her eighties. From her autobiographical notes, Bullough concludes: "Nurses worked harder and took orders from physicians who knew little more than they did" (p. 4). Equally important, he states: "It also indicates something about the tenuous nature of a woman in medicine since she and probably many others felt far more at home among nurses than physicians" (p. 4).

According to John Gabel (1978), in 1902 Wilson helped organize the Women's Medical Club of Columbus to promote medical women. She later marched in a suffragist parade, "wearing a purple and yellow sash and carrying a 'Vote for Women' banner" (Gabel, 1978, p. 66). However, in 1941 in a newspaper article on Wilson's fifty years as a woman "medic," the reporter noted that Dr. Wilson and other female physicians would "not discuss nor admit discriminations. They seek no favors and resent women who do. . . . They see no objection to the small percentage of girl students accepted each year" (Columbus *Citizen*, 1941; cited in Gabel, 1978, p. 65). The phenomenon is common: "I'm not a feminist but . . ." or "I've never been discriminated against, but I remember the time . . ." To refuse to identify with the subordinate group against the dominant, and to repress any negative experiences, makes it easier to identify with men and escape their negative evaluations and those of other women who are connected with them. Clearly, it was difficult for Wilson to join nurses, to go "down" in status after her medical training. Subsequently, *if* the reporter was accurate, her identification with physicians required the repression of the discrimination she actually experienced and even detailed in her own writing.

Women physicians who identify primarily with male physicians can hardly make common cause with women nurses. However, some female physicians did create their own hospitals in which nursing could be defined and supported. As previously noted, women established hospitals in Philadelphia, and in Boston the New England Hospital for Women and Children was founded in 1862 by Marie Elizabeth Zakrewska. As described by Laura Punnett (1976), the hospital was to offer medical aid for women in sickness or in childbirth, provided by competent physicians of their own sex; to assist educated women in the practical study of medicine by providing professional instruction; and to train nurses for the care of the sick. The nursing school, one of the earlier formal institutions of this kind in the United States, was begun in 1871. Thus, women in medicine were supporting the education of women as nurses.

Unfortunately, there remained problems and inequities in role definitions and expectations. The superintendent of nurses required that nurses observe gynecological examinations, but the women physicians refused permission, citing the modesty of the patients. The "curiosity of nurses" could not be satisfied due to the embarrassment of the woman patient. Economic differences were also apparent between the two groups of women. A female resident physician in training received about $800 a year; the nursing students were paid up to $3 a week ($156 a year), from which they were expected to pay for their simple calico uniforms. After graduation nurses received between $14 and $18 per week. Although denying nurses' involvement in some clinical situations, medical women affirmed nursing by supporting their education and by paying fairly decent wages, given the tenuous circumstances of any totally female-controlled and newly founded institution.

The debate about the innate weakness of women and their tendency to be sickly was considered a false issue; women were employed in part to prove that they were capable of hard work. In short, the women rejected the idea of female frailty. In addition, instead of keeping women ignorant of anatomy, the women physicians spoke to gatherings of women in "such a frank and direct way" that it "startled and shocked them," even though being of "lasting benefit" to them (Punnett, 1976, p. 8). The women physicians and nurses at New England Hospital did not view pregnancy and childbirth as a disease but as a normal event; thus, they placed little emphasis on abnormality. They attacked puerperal sepsis, taking seriously the theory of the infectious origin of disease. These attitudes contrast sharply with those of some male physicians at the time. To minimize infection, the women separated the maternity and surgical wards in different buildings. Unlike some male physicians, the women informed their patients of the presence of venereal disease. The hospital received some male support, but patronizing attitudes were not accepted. Punnett concluded that the hospital reflected the tensions of the time, exemplifying the burgeoning women's movement in an attempt to achieve equality.

In contrast to Punnett, Reverby (1987) claims that disputes were common at the New England Hospital, and, since the medical and nursing staff were all female, she reasoned that having gender in common did not lessen the conflict between doctors and nurses: "the power structure, not the specific sex of the individuals, shaped the encounters" (p. 74). But who shaped the medical women? To what power structure did they give their loyalty? Bullough (1983) and Gabel (1978) revealed how at least one woman physician, Ida May Wilson, was pressured to reject nursing and, as a member of a very small minority of the medical profession, adapt in order to practice. In what ways did socialization in medical education and practice in patriarchal American and European cultures influence gender conceptions of labor and specifically women's labor? To what extent did women physicians, whether trained in European or American medical schools, need authority even more than men, precisely because they were denied it by men?

As noted earlier, if feminist consciousness of the common plight of women as a subordinated group was missing or secondary to professional membership, then we would expect women physicians to behave like their male colleagues. Indeed, their peripheral status might make them even more concerned with their own achievement and authority than men, who were under no similar pressure as anomalies in a woman's world. In patriarchies, when women step beyond their usual subordinate roles and do so without a feminist consciousness of female commonality, the interactional dynamics can be expected to be biased in the direction of the accepted reference group—in health care, male physicians. Even if female physicians identified themselves as feminists, the institutional power structures they learned in training would shape subsequent encounters between women as nurses and women as physicians, since all of them were initially shaped by the patriarchal culture in which they developed and were trained.

There are still insufficient social psychological data on *current* interactions between female physicians and female nurses or female or male physicians with male nurses. As noted in the overview to this volume, a formal model of comparisons among *all* types of gendered relations cannot be created without much more research. Therefore, Reverby's reference to the refusal of Dr. "Zak" (Zakrewska) to allow the nursing superintendent to join women physicians on their rounds provides only one useful example of female-female interaction in which the male medical reference group is more salient than the female group. As Reverby notes, Dr. "Zak" thought the nursing superintendent would have too much authority. The nursing committee backed down, leaving the nursing superintendent in a less powerful position since she could only visit patients after the physicians had visited.

The practice of "male-only, physician-only" rounds was often the norm learned in medical training, which did indeed prevent nurses from learning new knowledge as well as observing the mistakes of physicians. In a distinct gendered system, we would expect a sharply differentiated communication system in order to maintain the illusion of superiority of one sex-typed occupation over the other. How this transferred to the New England Hospital is a topic requiring much more extensive systematic and thorough research than is available in the brief four paragraphs allotted to this topic in Reverby's analysis. What is clear, as Punnett noted, is that laywomen proved that together they, like their religious sisters, could run hospitals efficiently and provide competent health care in their own institutions. Over time, unfortunately, such hospitals, under economic and social pressures, usually merged with male-dominated institutions.

The Dilemma: How to Care by Order

Despite continuing efforts by women to achieve reform and their successful efforts to establish a paid occupation in institutions, nurses were in the peculiar position of being, as Reverby (1987) said, "ordered to care," which to her was the dilemma of American nursing from 1850 into the twentieth century. In contrast to O'Brien (1987), who traced organized nursing activities in Philadelphia to women's concerns and efforts as early as the 1830s, Reverby tracks modern nursing to Nightingale's American edition of *Notes on Nursing*, which was well received, for example, in 1860 in *Godey's Lady's Book*. Reverby does state that nursing for working-class women was not a new experience and that middle-class women had nursed family members or neighbors, but not for wages. However, she did not give evidence, as Paul Starr (1982) did, of the extent to which most nursing and medical functions, paid or unpaid, were commonly provided by women of all classes. Nor does she acknowledge, as Eleanor Flexner (1970) did, that women healers were paid as early as the colonial period.

If nursing and medical activities were *both* part of women's work with families, friends, and community, then presumably *both* were an important expression of love for others and "integral to the female sense of self" (Reverby, 1987, p. 199). Unfortunately, Reverby's deemphasis of women's medical activities leads her to stress nursing as caring, not curing. By the late nineteenth century nursing as labor is seen as separated from caring as familial love, although "The permeable boundaries for women between unpaid and paid labor allowed nursing to pass back and forth when necessary" (p. 199). Institutional demands made caring more difficult for hospital nurses, and, though some nurses did try to seize some form of power to define their caring, "the lack of a defined ideology of caring undermined their efforts" (p. 200). Although paternalism was noted by Reverby, the full expression of gender discrimination is not explicated, leaving a sense of ill-guided fatherly benevolence, rather than the use of gender to create or sustain institutionally structured occupational class systems based on a gendered division of labor.

To Reverby it was Nightingale's reforms that provided a theoretical explanation for the duty to care and an associated "political base from its female hierarchy" (p. 200). However, Reverby's view of Nightingale is fairly traditional: an upper-class reformer concerned with efficiency and moral order in military and civilian health care, and with training nurses as women of character and discipline to create health and order in both homes and hospitals. As Reverby sees it, Nightingale's model was "built on an uneasy alliance among concepts drawn from the sexual division of labor in the family, the authority structure of the military and religious sisterhoods, and the link between her moral beliefs and medical theories" (p. 41). This view of Nightingale and her model is open to debate. Whether American nursing should be traced to Nightingale is also debatable. However, since she is often used as a symbol of worldwide "modern" nursing, the varied perceptions are still critically important to current explanatory systems. (For an extended discussion of Nightingale's views and perceptions of her, see Roberts and Group, 1995.)

Reverby does point out that Nightingale did not see womanhood itself as sufficient to qualify someone to be a nurse. Neither did she believe that a lady disappointed in love or a workhouse drudge desperate for money would automatically qualify as a nurse. Indeed, as noted previously, Nightingale saw women's control of nursing as central to her reform, but to Reverby, women's relatively independent authority represented no gain: "Nursing did not present a direct challenge to physicians' authority because it was structured around a hierarchy of its own, with a separate arena of concern" (p. 42). However, the *public* organization of women was itself an act of independence, and the demand for education or training was also controversial—for women to be educated for public work roles was highly questionable to many. Furthermore, the state of medicine at that time was not sufficiently different from the state of nursing to allow men to feel unthreatened by educated women nurses. For the female hierarchy in the hospital to be separate from men's direct control was not acceptable to many physicians, even though the nurses might be loyal but not servile to the physicians. Although Reverby seems to trace the order to care to Nightingale, she herself said, "True loyalty to orders cannot be obtained without the independent sense or energy of responsibility, which alone secures real trustworthiness" (Nightingale, 1893; cited in Reverby, 1987, p. 42).

To Reverby, Nightingale's emphasis on sanitation matters—order, ventilation, clean drains and sewers, and decent diets—was not central to medical and surgical interventions. However, given the state of medicine at the time, the importance of these factors can hardly be underestimated. Indeed, the sharp reduction in the mortality rate in the Crimea after Nightingale's intervention tends to support the critical importance of her sanitation concerns to *both* nursing and medical cure.

Reverby further characterized Nightingale as replacing sexuality with motherly authority, not out of the fixation of a sexually repressed woman, as asserted by some writers, but rather as "an attempt to limit any male claim on a woman through the sexual exchange . . . [and] to place nurses above the suspicion that sexual interest motivated their desire to care for male patients" (p. 43). To Reverby, the gendered division of labor, combined with models from religious sisterhoods and sanitation ideals, linked together duty, obligation, and order. Although Nightingale sought to free women from the bonds of familial demands, she, according to Reverby, re-bound them in a new context.

In this account, there is no corresponding model of power as espoused by medical and hospital men; thus, it is unclear whether Nightingale's presumed model is an adaptation to patriarchy or an independent assertion from the female world or some variation of each or both of these. Nor is there any way to determine the extent to which the physicians forced nurses into another form of subordination by modifying Nightingale's model to reinforce medical, not nursing, authority. Certainly, Reverby's own data suggest direct opposition, at least in wartime, to women nurses. For example, Reverby notes that during the Crimean and Civil Wars, women faced "the overwhelming filth and stench of the barracks' hospitals, the disorder of the military procure-ment system, the cries of wounded and dying strangers, and the intransigence and hostility of physicians unwilling to accept the aid of 'meddling women'" (p. 44). Indeed, the American women "perceived the authority of the physi-cians and the surgeons as their biggest problem" (p. 46). In the face of inade-quate care, which was protected by professional etiquette, "some women quickly replaced their meekness with indignation and outrage" (p. 46). Obvi-ously, tensions were high between women healers or nurses and male physi-cians. Nevertheless, Reverby concluded that womanly professionalism based on the authority of the mother could not counter surgeons' authority; without support and orders from higher authorities, "such qualifications did not give women the basis for an organized assault on male power in the army hospitals" in which they faced "disdain and abuse," not "'courtesy and kindness'" (p. 46). Alternatively, one could say that the women faced overt patriarchal privilege and power and confronted blatant sexist rejection.

Reverby saw little change in hospital nursing following the Civil War, but noted that a small coterie of urban upper-class women had learned that their feminine virtues and organizational skills had forced change. This led them to reform the terrible conditions in hospitals and to aid the small-town girls who in the 1870s were migrating to cities for jobs because of depressed economic circumstances. Reverby does not clearly connect nursing to the emergence of the women's health-reform movement prior to or after the Civil War, or to feminism in general. In contrast, O'Brien (1987) clearly saw feminist and racial issues as central to societal debate and important to the development of nurs-ing, at least in Philadelphia. Reverby does credit women reformers for laying the plans for the opening in 1873 of Nightingale-inspired training schools in New York, Boston, and New Haven. But if O'Brien is correct, at least the New Haven school was originally staffed by women nurses trained in Philadelphia, not by Nightingale nurses. Clearly, O'Brien's research on the pre-Nightingale era and her stronger emphasis on feminism force a different interpretation of events and change the more traditional historical interpretations based on the Nightingale model. In Reverby's analysis, the feminist history of women seems peripheral or even at times oppositional to nurses' actions.

Whose Domain? Physician Authority over Hospitals and Nursing Widens

Reverby does note that physicians were reluctant to accept another trained person in the sickroom. "Just as many physicians feared 'medical women,' they saw trained nurses as yet another female intrusion into a male domain" (Re-verby, 1987, p. 48). Given the evidence, for example, of European and Ameri-can women in religious orders, who actually founded hospitals, it is appro-priate to ask at what point in time and in what way did physicians come to believe that hospitals were *their* domain? Given a longer historical view, physicians' reactions can be differently interpreted, as, for example, at the Hôtel-Dieu in Paris as described in chapter 1.

In Reverby's view, feminists placed women's rights at the center of their struggle; this presumably made nurses' call to duty, as a model for female authority, seem derived from an "increasingly antiquated language . . . [a] collective female grasping for an older form of security and power in the face of rapid change" (p. 200). The obligation to care and the associated female character to act on this duty "required sacrifice on the altar of altruism" (p. 200). Altruism did not provide either a justification or rationale for nurses' rights or the ideology needed to gain control over nursing organization. Indeed, bedside duty was translated by medical and hospital men "as duty in the broader political arena as well" (p. 200). While struggling to define itself, nursing was subject to conflicting class positions over definitions, strategies, and even the meaning of womanhood: "Commonalities of the gendered experience could not become the basis for unity as long as hierarchical filial relations, not equal sisterhood, underlay nurses' lives" (p. 201). Reverby did not discuss how the united forces of male domination from medical, hospital, legal, and political institutions negatively affected the women's unity.

Reverby did, however, note that some nurses created "the very special safety and comfort of a women's culture" (p. 201), but separate women's institutions could not be sustained without economic and cultural power, making "difficult the collective transition out of a woman's culture of obligation into an activist assault on the structure and beliefs that oppressed them" (p. 201). Again, the overt actions by men in power to destroy such efforts were not explicated. To Reverby, some nurses "were not merely silent in the face of these difficulties . . . [they] pressed in different ways for increasing autonomy and power" (p. 201). However, "the demand for autonomy based on the duty to care could not provide them with the ideological formulation needed" (p. 201). When women nurses used the strategies of male groups—for example, unionization—there were different consequences because of gender and class ideological experience. Again, Reverby did not detail the differential power used by men to reinterpret and to block the nurses' strategies.

Given Moore's (1988) analysis (see chapter 2), Reverby is probably too sanguine when she states that many physicians quickly understood the importance of the trained nurse to patient recovery and health. It is true that physicians' materia medica was limited; patients' lives *did* depend, as Reverby says, on their food, care of their dressings, careful observation for danger signs, and baths to control fevers. It is probably more correct to say that the men needed the women's help, but would not fully accept it until the women were subordinated and controlled. Certainly, medical acceptance of nursing increased *after* the cheap or free labor of student nurses produced higher incomes and better patient outcomes at little additional cost to the hospitals and physicians. Yet even with the women supposedly under control, the men continued to stress obedience throughout the nineteenth and into the twentieth centuries.

To Reverby, the key difference between the "old" and "new" nurses was the character of the woman herself. A womanly woman, carrying the basic values of her gender, made the ideal nurse, one who expressed submission, self-sacrifice, and altruism, not independence and individualism. As noted in chapter 2, Williams's (1980) nineteenth-century medical historian would have agreed with this assertion, but Breay, the early nurse-historian, would *not* have agreed, stressing instead the introduction of new nursing procedures, processes, and relations. Reverby qualified her assertion by saying that neither Nightingale nor American nursing reformers wanted mindless supplicants, but tried instead to "define a role for women in the service of humanity in which women trod softly and tactfully between the equally dangerous poles of total deference and outright defiance to accomplish their tasks" (Reverby, 1987, p. 51). Nevertheless, in practice "loyalty and deference to the physician, rather than independence, were stressed" (p. 51). This was evidenced in physicians' speeches at nurses' graduation exercises. In these, loyalty and deference were extolled in endless homilies. What did nurses think of these speeches? As Reverby noted, nursing leader Lavinia Dock called the talks wearisome rubbish—perennial platitudes, already taught in the models of hierarchy in which duty and discipline were stressed with little respite from work. How widespread were such reactions? If widely held by a number of nurses, we must question who was stressing deference and in what ways.

In agreement with Gamarnikow's (1978) analysis of British nurses, Reverby said that if the military model of obedience proved insufficient, the patriarchal family model was held out to the young women, assuring American nurses that they were not really wage earners but part of a hospital family in which, as one person said, they were "cared for as a father cares for his children" (p. 52). Discipline was reinforced with uniforms, badges, pins, caps, and ceremonies: "moral order, ethical rules, and technical competence were confounded" (p. 53). The nurses' ideology, claims Reverby, justified gender subordination and the reality of the work made it necessary since inexperienced students, without mature skills and judgment, came to constitute practically the whole nursing staff of a hospital. Not only were there economic advantages to women's free labor, there were also benefits to medical authority from the use of young, inexperienced women students, who could not easily mount an organized assault for autonomy on their institutional "home" and hospital "family."

The school's departmental independence from the hospital, the power of the nursing superintendent, a separate female hierarchy—none of these could fully protect the integrity and education of students. Although nursing leaders understood the importance of separate women-controlled institutions, hospital schools were *not* separate, forcing nursing superintendents to demand conformity since they obtained little advantage from defending students: "At some of the larger institutions, more powerful and heroic women were able to extract a greater degree of authority from trustees, superintendents, and physicians. But . . . [the nurse superintendent was] constantly pressured to serve the institution's and physicians' demands before the needs of her students" (Reverby, 1987, p. 75). After struggling for nursing parallel autonomy, some nursing superintendents began to wonder if something were wrong with them—were they, for example, too quarrelsome? Indeed, one asserted that nursing leaders must be made of heroic stuff to surmount the difficulties. To Reverby, such women, when confronting medical and hospital power, learned to proceed slowly and cautiously in making innovations, and the growing power of physicians increasingly undercut the nurses' alliance with trustees.

Physicians and administrators recognized the threat from an administratively distinct nursing department and a powerful nursing superintendent, particularly if she reported directly to hospital trustees. Such an arrangement "would be an ever-present threat to their own positions and to the use of pupils as workers" (p. 70). It would undermine deference and power; thus, the position of the nursing superintendent was a subject of continuing conflict, which the physicians eventually won because of their total control over the admission of paying patients and the increasing value placed on medical care. Eventually, hospital trustees' moral decisions were displaced by physicians' medical decisions. By the early twentieth century a dual authority structure had emerged: hospital administrators, "often in alliance with the physicians, moved to assure that the nursing school and its female superintendent remained dependent on *both* physician and hospital superintendent authority" (p. 71).

Reverby concludes that ultimate control over nursing was taken out of the hands of the majority of nursing superintendents. The resulting dilemma was that hospital demands took priority over nursing authority and education: "And because the nursing work force was made up almost entirely of women, altruism, sacrifice, and submission were expected and encouraged" (p. 75). To Reverby, exploitation was inevitable, particularly since the nursing authority structure had no independent power base. She concludes that because of the subordination of women, the hospital's authority structure, and growing physician power, "the nursing authority structure, rather than protecting the student, became the mechanism through which she experienced her oppression" (p. 76). Female subordination is, of course, *not* independent of hospital authority structure, nor of physician power; thus, these are not three separate causes but rather interrelated aspects of the overall patriarchal culture which is organized in *all* its aspects around gender differences.

In her 1979 work, Reverby paid little attention to the efforts of physicians to obtain a monopoly by excluding and subordinating nurses. She stated: "Recent works in nursing history suggest that sexism, male greed, and women's passivity explain nurses' subordination. But nurses must not be seen solely as victims or heroines in a male-dominated system. We must understand both why certain nursing leaders chose the direction they did and how and why their rank and file responded" (Reverby, 1979, p. 219). Reverby called not for one strong voice, but a chorus of historical voices expressing varied explanations. It is readily agreed that women do not all sing soprano parts. What is less acceptable is the rejection of a gendered analysis within a medical culture that has been blatantly and obviously sexist, not simply paternal. Without a finer-tuned analysis of causality of nurse-physician interrelations, the chorus of women's voices cannot be fully heard. Indeed, the focus on the *internal* nursing world and the exclusion of male-dominated medical and hospital dynamics can lead to blaming the victims, not the victimizers.

Fortunately, Reverby's 1987 analysis presents a more balanced view that better incorporates gender. She refocuses nursing as caring, defined not as individual traits but as work formed by power and ideological relations. To her, the ethics of care and the effects on morality were not the critical issues for nurses, because they were expected to conform to a set of rules based on the acceptance of orders. The duty to care was actually more complex, and conflict continued between nurses, physicians, and others; "however, the duty to care became translated into the demand that nurses merely follow doctors' orders" (Reverby, 1987, p. 203). How physicians achieved this hegemony is not sufficiently explained; nevertheless, women's obedience to duty as ordered mostly by men left nurses, according to Reverby, hesitant to speak about their rights, or create a vision of caring, or "the power to give that vision substantive form" (p. 203).

Liberal feminism does provide a political language, a basis for caring focused on values and equality: "The demand for the right to determine how to care challenges deeply held beliefs about gendered relations in the health care hierarchy and the hierarchy itself" (p. 207). However, the individualism and autonomy demanded by liberal political feminism may be insufficient to deal with collective social needs: "those who claim the autonomy of rights often run the risk of rejecting altruism and caring itself" (p. 207). By conjoining autonomy and connectedness, Reverby postulated that conditions for caring might be created, without self-immolation, and that this might lead to a new political understanding for caring and the power to implement it. However, nurses' dilemma, said Reverby, is too much tied to gender and class in the broader society to expect one occupational group alone to resolve the problem. Nurses and non-nurses need to create a new vision of how to link autonomy and altruism and to gain the power to forge this new unity. This would benefit everyone by resolving some ambivalences about the meaning of womanhood and untangling the conflicted metaphor of nursing. Caring would be no longer narrowly conceived or subject to obedience to medical authority. Whether Reverby's emphasis on care as opposed to cure would trap nurses once again in a powerless position, unable to incorporate both aspects into a single coherent philosophy of nursing, remains a question.

One is left, at least in part, with the impression that the victims of sexist subordination were responsible for their subordination through a nursing ideology that stressed strict discipline. As Reverby sees it, character gave way to conformity, order slipped into rigidity, and caring was subordinated to medical orders. This evaluation leaves little room for the ongoing efforts by at least some nurses to escape from the control of both medicine and hospital administration. Indeed, from the perspective of gender subordination, at least some nurses never gave up the struggle for some autonomy. Without a continuous and strong women's movement to support their efforts, the going has been rough.

Quietly yet Determinedly Feminist: Early Nursing Leaders Continue the Struggle

In contrast to Reverby, Doris Daniels (1976) clearly recognized both the critical contributions of early American nursing leaders to the continuing struggle for relative autonomy and nursing's interconnectedness with women's status in society. Indeed, some of these leaders were in close contact with British nurses, and together they created a worldwide network of nurses and an international organization to unify their efforts. These women clearly understood the need for a feminist perspective. Nurse leader Lillian Wald, for example, knew that "the nurse question had become the woman question" (Daniels, 1976, p. 39). That organized nursing was "a gauge and an inseparable part" of the "eternal women's movement" (Wald, 1912a; cited in Daniels, 1976, p. 40). And, according to Lavinia Dock, to uplift the nurses' cause was to do a genuine bit in the wider world of feminism. Early nurse leaders knew that Nightingale's plan to take nursing out of the hands of men and give it to women was a major effort to give women control of their own work. As noted previously, the majority of physicians initially opposed such control. One physician saw the nurse as only a servant, one who should be middle-aged when she began nursing and "somewhat tamed by marriage and the troubles of a family" (Nutting and Dock, 1907, vol. 2, p. 201). Again, in contrast to Reverby, Daniels stressed that American women who entered early nursing schools rejected such taming, seeing themselves instead as pioneers. Nurse leader Annie Goodrich said, "I look back upon those two years at New York Hospital as the happiest of my life. Undoubtedly, the most important factor was the superintendent of nurses, Irene Sutliffe" (Goodrich, 1950, p. 598). Another nurse urged her colleagues to "grow in the belief of the sisterhood of women, and help each other by appreciation . . . learning to work together in a noble harmony" (Speakman, 1902, p. 182). Clearly, there was a strong feminist consciousness for many of the earliest students.

Daniels claimed that these early nurses also learned to fight together; indeed, Dock said that most of them got started on their militant careers even *before* they finished training (Daniels, 1976, p. 43). These courageous feminist nurses battled the public and medical establishments to prove that nursing education was essential; they fought to prove that the methods of teaching should be "worked out by the brains, bodies and souls of . . . women" (p. 43) and must be left in their hands. As Daniels noted, they struggled to obtain equipment, libraries, laboratories, and classrooms; they demanded that standards of excellence in training and performance be established and defined by nurses themselves; they worked against the stigma of being only housemaids and insisted on professional status. Clearly, Daniels's view of the internal nurses' world contrasts quite sharply with Reverby's.

Both Dock and Wald published their belief that nursing could not advance more rapidly until women's education and status were elevated. Isabel Stewart claimed that nurses were "interested in anything that had to do with the elevation of women, and with giving them the tools with which to work, and giving them a chance to develop their minds" (p. 44). In reflecting on the nurse pioneers, Dock said the "leaders . . . were quietly yet determinedly Feminist" (Dock, 1929, p. 221). Daniels noted too that "all nurses were not in agreement on the women's movement, but those who were not feminists seemed to be rare. Both Wald and Stewart were able to remember only one or two who stressed femininity rather than feminism" (Daniels, 1976, p. 63).

In contrast to Reverby's image of nursing leaders, Daniels depicts Wald, Dock, and others as close friends who took joy in each other's company and in their pioneering work. The most committed was, of course, Dock, who was reared in a Quaker family that held liberal views on the "underdog." Unlike Wald, Dock was a plainspoken woman who did not temper her language or suppress her feelings: "The enemy was clear to Dock—the medical men" (Daniels, 1976, p. 45). Dock minced no words in writing to one doctor: "'[It seems] particularly unseemly and ungrateful for physicians to talk about 'fighting' nurses. Why, you owe seven tenths of your success and prestige to nurses. And here you are trying to beat down . . . the very women on whom your success depends. If you do not think this is shabby, I do'" (Dock, 1909a; cited in Daniels, 1976, p. 46). Dock also called doctors selfish and stupid, unable to recognize what was in their own best interests: good education for women in nursing, without which patient care and hospitals would slide back in short time to a state of general degradation.

Dock believed that no one but a few doctors wanted nurses to be women servants. In the battle over nurses' licensing, Dock wrote to Wald that she feared they were done for: "There is some deep laid villainy—it means, body, soul and mind under the doctor's heels if it goes through" (Daniels, 1976, p. 46). She grudgingly recommended compromise by admitting a couple of physicians to the board rather than losing all. Younger nurses, such as Isabel

Stewart, had imagined and stereotyped Dock as tall, angular, and intellectual; but found her to be a small, short person with curly hair. After attending a suffragist meeting, Dock gave a lecture to nursing students while still wearing "Votes for Women" on her hat and the same on a banner across her chest. Through these actions, she became a heroine to many younger nurses.

According to Daniels, Mary Adelaide Nutting, Dock's collaborator on *A History of Nursing*, focused on the moral obligation of nurses to be intelligent, not simply good, sweet women. Through Wald, Nutting obtained from Helen Hartly Jenkins an endowment of $200,000 to sustain the first collegiate course in nursing at Columbia University. Nutting stressed the importance of women, and particularly nurses, engaging in intellectual issues and thinking about their responsibilities and progress. Indeed, both Nutting and Wald lobbied to educate physicians, fought for registration, organized professional groups, and supported women's appointments to executive positions.

An old girls' network developed, said Daniels, at least in the Northeast, and the requirements for membership were "talent, personality, adaptability and spirit" (p. 49). Younger women, such as Stewart, called Wald the great promoter, who was well aware of her power: "if an official did not 'do his duty' she did not hesitate to 'put a little more pressure on him'" (Wald, 1930; cited in Daniels, 1976, p. 52). A high priority for Wald and Dock was nurses' autonomy. Dock claimed that doctors had made a mess of nursing and women no longer quite trusted them. Wald agreed, saying, "When medicine gained control, almost complete control of the nursing orders and organization, it did not reflect credit on either branch of the healing art" (p. 54).

Wald's public health nurses worked in the field without direct medical supervision, although they were nominally under physicians' orders. According to Daniels, Dock warned Wald of the opposition from physicians, who expressed strong disapproval because Wald's nurses carried ointments in their bags and even dispensed pills. The physicians believed it was wrong for district nurses to function in any way except under the strict control of physicians. But Wald did not back down. She continually spoke and wrote, encouraging people to send for her nurses because in many cases skillful nursing was of "greater value in preserving human life than the best medical advice" (Wald, 1930; cited in Daniels, p. 55). Wald's nurses carried the findings of the scientists and laboratory to the people, making them intelligible to ordinary folks: "What a change . . . from the priestly secrecy of the . . . medical practitioner" (p. 55).

Lillian Wald knew that any woman with a commitment to the profession understood that nurses must stay in control: "There may be some souls so humble and so meek that the old time position of women nurses—namely that of blind obedience in the treadmill—is all that they desire" (Wald, 1912a; cited in Daniels, 1976, p. 55). However, she and many other nurses wanted more than subservience and being dictated to by physicians. Agreeing with

Dock, Wald stressed that the male takeover of nursing and the exclusion of women from any control of their work would cause the character of the work to deteriorate. It is this view that some early leaders, such as Wald and Dock, extended to the international sisterhood of nurses, which was always linked to the women's movement for better living and working conditions. Dock, of course, observed nurses in many nations—women who were bitter over their exploitation and lack of recognition. The drive for registration and adequate education for nurses, for example, took place throughout several Western nations, exposing women in nursing to many apathetic or hostile public officials.

The picture painted by Daniels is of brave, embattled women whose feminist consciousness was high and who understood what their pioneer work, if successful, could mean for nurses and all other women. In contrast to Daniels, Reverby perceives nursing superintendents as essentially losing the power struggle with physicians and hospital authorities.

Toward a Multifaceted Conceptualization of Nurses' Place in Women's History and in Medical History

Clearly, nurse-physician relations cannot be understood without an analysis of both groups and their interactions. The origins of "modern" nursing in the United States cannot be fully understood without a longer historical perspective and broader analysis of both nursing and medical functions provided by a variety of women caregivers. Such a longer and broader historical perspective must also take into account patriarchal privilege, particularly in the medical profession, and must deal with the reality of gendered restrictions on women as a subordinated group, grasping the very real difficulties that women reformers, both nurses and non-nurses, faced. This latter task may be very difficult for historians who do not know women's or, more particularly, feminist history or have not themselves been involved in efforts to create social change for women in their own era. In addition, social scientists' lack of direct experience with and knowledge about the work nurses were and are actually doing can create more problems. Thus, readers may get accounts of early nurses' "compulsive" concern with cleanliness that do not deal with the very real need for hygienic care and facilities, as noted in this chapter and chapter 2. Indeed, these accounts may make nurses' activities seem somewhat silly, rather than essential to patients, particularly in periods devoid of "miracle drugs," such as sulfa and penicillin. Nurses' work with the sick and dying may also be lost in social scientific analyses, which may focus on social relations among the women, almost as though they were engaged in nothing more than secretarial or social work.

Despite interpretive difficulties, in the future we look forward to a blending of the several research approaches described in this chapter. Such a multifaceted conceptualization will obviously require modifications of each approach, but in this process women healers and nurses can be better placed in relation to women's history and to medical history. Thus, we can more easily understand the centuries-long efforts of physicians to achieve status by creating a medical monopoly through the exclusion or domination of women healers, nurses, and female physicians. And we can better grasp the equally long history of some women's refusal to be excluded and dominated and even their eventual rejection of their previous compromises. To eliminate long-term, gendered perspectives of the relations between nurses and physicians is an exercise in futility that can only create a caricature of nursing and nurses as the main culprits in their own subjugation. Indeed, the gendered basis of nurse-physician relations becomes even clearer as the continued efforts by medicine to control nursing and all health care in the late nineteenth and early twentieth centuries in America are examined in the next chapter.

PART
II

*The Purposeful Move toward
Dominance: Subordinating Nurses and
Achieving a Medical Monopoly*

4 | "For Their Own Good"
Physicians Manipulating, Trivializing, and Coercing Nurses, Later 1800s to the 1920s

This chapter focuses on the continued efforts by physicians in the United States to achieve a monopoly in health care in the mid to late nineteenth century and into the first two decades of the twentieth century. From previous chapters, it is clear that physicians over several centuries were determined to create a gendered monopoly, but it is equally clear that women continued to provide most of the health care in their homes and communities, and in the hospitals, clinics, and other institutions they founded. As organized feminism emerged in the mid nineteenth century, women reformers were increasingly critical of traditional medical practices and created alternate therapies and practices. They reformed military medical services, and a few breached the all-male barricades to enter medical schools and engage in medical practice. Together, laywomen created their own hospitals for women and children, following the tradition of their nurse sisters in religious orders. At the same time, hospital nursing schools were established and hospital and public health nursing were developed as paid and public occupations for women. All of these activities and achievements were part of the demand for women's rights and constitute clear evidence that women did not easily relinquish their historical centrality in healing.

Despite the women's efforts, physicians extended their monopoly, not only by the continued exclusion of women from science and higher education but also by the destruction of alternative "irregular" schools of medicine—homeopathic, eclectic, and "lay"—that did accept women and by the incorporation of women healers' functions into medical practice. It is important to re-emphasize that the extension of physician control occurred at a time when the practice of medicine could hardly be classified as fully scientific. Only gradually did researchers discover causes of pestilent diseases and practitioners begin to use anesthesia and aseptic and antiseptic methods. These, along with better diagnostic procedures, laid the basis for a complete medical monopoly.

In the United States, physicians absorbed other men from "irregular" practices, incorporating surgeons, but limiting dentists and chiropractors to a restricted range of practice. By the late nineteenth century, at women's insistence, a few female physicians were being admitted to medical schools; for example, a group of wealthy women contributed $500,000 to Johns Hopkins University in exchange for the admission of women to the College of Medicine (Starr, 1982). Subsequently, women students were restricted at most medical schools, often to just 5 percent of the total number of students accepted. The remaining irregular schools were dissolved; thus, women healers were excluded from any alternative formal education. Physicians tried to limit nurses' education, constrain their practice through legal restrictions, subject their patient care to paternalistic or military-style authority, and make their work dependent on obedience to medical orders. The degree to which women themselves submitted to the men's actions requires much more refined research that acknowledges women's very restricted legal, political, and social rights and opportunities during this period.

Increased specialization of physicians, associated with the formalization of scientific advances in medical education, eventually created an intellectual basis for a medical monopoly, but only if women nurses could be kept minimally educated and limited to relatively powerless roles. In the basic sciences there were several developments: in bacteriology, with the discoveries of Pasteur and Koch in the 1860s and 1870s; in antiseptic techniques in surgery; and in the development of immunology in the 1880s to fight against tuberculosis, cholera, and typhoid. These developments intersected with innovations in instrumentation: the stethoscope in 1816, followed over many decades by the ophthalmoscope, the laryngoscope, and the microscope, then X-rays, chemical and bacterial tests, the spirometer, and the electrocardiograph (Starr, 1982).

Physicians' efforts to exclude women from knowledge emerging from the basic sciences, and their refusal to let nurses use new instrumentation sustained women's subordination in nursing, although many nurses themselves continually and actively sought greater scientific knowledge and techniques and incorporated these into their education. Nevertheless, the relatively powerless position of women in the general society allowed physicians to achieve the subordination of nurses and other women health workers. The scientific justification for professional authority also created the conditions for medical consensus. In 1900 the American Medical Association (AMA) had a membership of 8,000, or approximately 7 percent of a total of 110,000 physicians. By 1910, 50 percent of all physicians belonged to the AMA, and by 1920, 60 percent (Starr, 1982).

Cultivating the Image of Learned Professional: Physicians Strengthen Their Control over Nurses

Prior to the latter part of the nineteenth century, the intellectual, clinical, or moral bases for physicians' authority, although claimed by them, could certainly not be central to their attempts to subordinate women nurses and healers. Medical historian Paul Starr (1982) noted that from colonial times onward domestic medicine and lay healers *predominated;* as in Europe, medical care by physicians in America was limited. Joseph Kett (1968), for example, could say that as late as 1818 medical care in New Jersey belonged almost entirely to women (cited in Starr, 1982, p. 49); therefore, many women who entered nursing certainly did not lack experience. During the colonial period, books written by physicians for the masses were self-consciously political; others confessed that professional knowledge and training were unnecessary for most diseases, since the best that could be done was to "assist the healing powers of nature" (Starr, 1982, p. 31). Since nurses were much more central to the hourly and daily provision of such assistance, the women's nursing contributions to nature's process could hardly be less than those of the physicians. Nor could the men's objections derive from more sophisticated explanatory theories; many physicians, as noted in chapter 1, still subscribed to the classical idea of four humours until French thinkers from 1800 to 1830 rebelled against these vague "systems" and began to formulate at least some clinical methods. Testing the previously accepted methods revealed they had no therapeutic value; however, there were presumably no viable alternative therapies to replace them. In the United States, physician Benjamin Rush at the University of Pennsylvania Medical College told his students in 1796 that there was only one disease in the world, the "morbid excitement induced by capillary tension" (p. 42), and it had only one remedy: the lancing and letting of blood, and purging—emptying the stomach and bowels. It was not until about 1850 that this "explanatory system" began to fall into disrepute because of alternative explanations from "irregular" practitioners.

Physicians' objection to nurses and other women healers could hardly be based on superior medical training, since this consisted of only three to four months in each of two years, with no graded curriculum until after 1850. The majority of physicians simply had little or no formal training. By 1840 medical school graduates in different states represented only 20 percent to 35 percent of those practicing. In 1874 the meager educational requirements made it easy to secure a diploma, and physicians were often little more knowledgeable than their patients; from 1800 to 1850, only 8 percent of graduates from the leading colleges and universities became medical doctors. Indeed, J. Marion Sims's father exclaimed over his son's decision to enter medicine that there was no reason for his college education, since medicine had "no science in it . . . no honor to be achieved in it; no reputation to be made" (Sims, 1889, p. 116; cited in Starr, 1982, p. 82).

The apprenticeship needed by physicians in training was conducted by preceptors over whom there was little if any control. It was not until the 1890s that the sciences of physiology, chemistry, histology, pathology, and bacteriology were formally incorporated at Harvard, Pennsylvania, and Johns Hopkins universities. By 1906 an AMA-sponsored survey, which was never published, found large numbers of substandard medical schools; some were possibly "redeemable," others beyond salvage.

Despite these obvious limitations, physicians cultivated the image of the learned professional while often simply taking over the functions of others, usually women healers and nurses. One physician, D. W. Cathell, told his colleagues in 1881 that attitude was critical; if physicians acted in too "convivial" a way, they might be perceived after all as only "ordinary" people (p. 86). The premium was on manly, quick, bold action and heroic methods. The association of medicine with maleness excluded any identification with the subordinate group of females. Obviously, objections to nurses could not be based on better therapeutics since the physicians' heroics were not only inadequate but often dangerous. The rejection of women nurses could not be based on morality since the medical code of ethics was more concerned with occupational imagery and power—for example, keeping secret from patients any medical differences of opinion. From the seventeenth century to the late nineteenth century, medical objections could not have been based on licensure. First attempted and rejected in New York City in 1760, medical licensing laws were not widely enacted or enforced until the end of the nineteenth century.

How then did physicians come to control women in nursing? Certainly, if nurses were members of a subordinated gender, it was possible to keep them in their places. Furthermore, the centrality of women to domestic medicine began to subside because of reduced costs for medical services, smaller household size, the changeover to manufactured from homemade goods, migration to urban centers, and changes in transportation, making medical care more accessible and encouraging displacement of community women healers by urban physicians. These factors, according to Starr, intersected with the accumulation of patients in hospitals; this happened first in mental asylums, which were the precursors for medical control in the subsequent rise of general hospitals. In 1873, for example, there were fewer than 200 hospitals in the United States; by 1920, there were more than 4,000, and by 1920 more than 6,000 (Starr, 1982, p. 73). By controlling patient admissions and hospital privileges, physicians could also control access to alternative healers, specifically nurses. In fact, the control of a large class of obedient subordinates was itself a necessity if physicians were to achieve a monopoly and a higher social status. Massing patients in hospitals could not alone account for the increased prestige and power of physicians. Hospitals had to be staffed, but not by men who might challenge medical monopoly; even minimally educated women were a threat to the consolidation of male professional authority. Any identification with members of a subordinate gender, such as women physicians, was also vigorously opposed, and these unwanted persons were subject to severe ostracism and ridicule.

The battle over the education of women in general and of women as nurses was waged throughout the nineteenth century and into the twentieth century. Thus, women, mostly excluded from medical schools and driven from alternative institutions, were left with hospital training of an apprenticeship type, directly or indirectly controlled by male hospital administrators and physicians. By 1912 nursing leaders, such as Mary Adelaide Nutting, emphasized the need to move nursing away from the control of hospital men. By the 1920s the Goldmark Report (1923), a comprehensive analysis of nursing in hospitals and health facilities, proved the gross inadequacy of instruction for nurses in hospital programs. Slowly, throughout the twentieth century, women in nursing moved the profession into universities, hoping for greater control of education and, through this, legitimization of their work.

The struggle for relative nursing autonomy has been blocked by hospital administration and organized medicine at every point in the historical past. This is documented in the literature on nurses' education and employment (see Roberts and Group, *Sexism and Nursing,* publication pending) and on power and leadership in nursing (see Roberts and Group, 1995). It is documented in the political relations between the two occupations within the system of gender subordination (see Roberts and Group, *Gender and the Nurse-Physician Game,* publication pending). It is documented in the treatment by physicians of women as midwives and as patients in a number of American and British sources and in specific historical research studies. It is documented by several nurse researchers, best articulated by Jo Ann Ashley (1976) in *Hospitals, Paternalism, and the Role of the Nurse,* a study of the gender-based medical subordination of nursing in the later nineteenth and early twentieth centuries. Unlike other researchers, Ashley did not focus on women's relations *within* nursing, with little reference to the medical world or the patriarchal culture in which the "women's world" existed. Instead, she analyzed and critiqued the impact of organized medicine on nursing. Unfortunately, Ashley has been described as too "angry" by at least one historian (Reverby, 1987). It is as though emotion and intellect cannot fuse—as though women historians cannot express moral outrage or even indignation without being considered too "subjective," even though their facts and their arguments are essentially accurate. Does combining *thinking* and *feeling* make their work and conclusions any less accurate? We would assert that *connected* thought, integrating both reason and feeling, is probably more, not less, honest.

Building on Ashley's earlier work, some nurse-historians, such as Mariann C. Lovell (1980), have specifically researched physicians' motives for controlling nurses and creating a medical monopoly. Traditional medical histories stress that such control was in the best interests of patients. But as Hawker (1987) found in her English study (see chapter 2), the interests of patients were not necessarily improved by increased medical control. Nor were American patients' best interests the sole objective of physicians' move toward a monopoly in health care, a fact amply demonstrated in Lovell's research, *An Historical Study of the Development of the Medical Profession as a Business.* She found that the medical profession was preoccupied with profits and male privileges and asserted that sexism in medicine was *not* inadvertent or merely a reflection of the broader society.

Failure to establish a medical monopoly by the 1840s led physicians to form the AMA in 1847 to control supply and demand and to influence legislative actions. The AMA lobbied for legislation "to raise the level of competence of physicians and lessen competition from other healers as well as to increase the power and status of the profession" (Bullough, 1986, p. 350). After such bills were passed in Texas in 1873 and in West Virginia in 1881, the Supreme Court in 1888 ruled that occupational licensure was a valid exercise of state power. Medical licensure spread rapidly through all states, but the fact that it came first and claimed all-inclusive powers meant that nurses' licenses later became, in effect, "amendments to the medical practice acts" (p. 350).

Nevertheless, through the organized efforts of nurses, even when most U.S. women did not yet have voting rights, many state legislatures were lobbied, and in 1903 North Carolina became the first state to require nurse registration; by 1923 all other states had followed suit. However, in none of these early acts was nurses' scope of practice specified, only that the registrant be someone of good character who had completed a nursing program and passed a broad examination.

By 1902 the men had sufficient power to achieve state laws that made practicing medicine without a license a crime. Once "licensure, artificially high standards, and certification rules" (Lovell, 1980, p. 15) established sufficient control, the AMA won its first major political battle against national health insurance following World War I. Organized medicine, said Lovell, opposed even the "mildest and most constructive . . . intrusions" (p. 16), such as compulsory diphtheria inoculations and smallpox vaccinations, mandatory reporting of tuberculosis cases to public health agencies, establishment of public venereal disease clinics and Red Cross blood banks, Blue Cross and other private health insurance programs, government subsidies to reduce maternal and infant death, and free centers for cancer diagnosis. Interference with the sacred American home, a sexist appeal to patriarchal privilege, was a key charge leveled by the AMA lobby.

The coercive power of the AMA prior to World War II included membership as a requirement for specialty board certification. Dismissal from the AMA, or unwillingness to join because of conflicting views on practice or attitudes toward compulsory health insurance, influenced specialty "merit." Any physician with the strength to disagree could "face a genuine economic threat" (p. 18). Even if no coercion existed, physicians were likely to join because of positive benefits, most importantly, cheaper malpractice insurance for members and access to other physicians as expert witnesses in litigation. Uniformity was maintained even in the *Journal of the American Medical Association*, which disseminated approved political information that kept out divergent viewpoints on political and economic issues.

The AMA Code of Ethics: Controlling Patients and Withholding Information

In Lovell's view, the AMA code of medical ethics, which was adopted in 1847, established oppressive commercialism: patients were to answer all questions, avoid all but their family physicians (not even friendly visits or passing the time of day with other doctors was acceptable), and take no action on health without consulting the physician. Physicians must not advertise or offer free advice, not even to the poor. Respectful obligation and legal immunity for MDs were expected from the public. Lovell believes that this paternalistic "ethical" code established physician ownership of patients, unquestioning devotion to physicians, patient dependence with loss of self-confidence, physician control of information, discouragement of competition, cultivation of paying clients only, and patients' belief in the "magic" cures of physicians.

Over time, a coercive or oppressor consciousness tended to "transform everything surrounding it into objects of domination. Everything, including human life, is reduced to the status of objects" (p. 112). "The power relationship which results, whether it is between physician-patient, doctor-nurse, father-child, husband-wife or any two groups or individuals along the medical hierarchy, constitutes oppressive violence" (pp. 113–114) because it objectifies and therefore dehumanizes. To Lovell, subordination of female nurses by paternalistic medical deception leaves unquestioned the right to coerce and manipulate for "their own good."

Paternalism and the Preoccupation with Profit, Privilege, and Control

Although the medical profession was preoccupied with profits, male privileges, and control over others, organized medicine professed only "pure," not economic, motives and certainly did not admit to the sexist subordination of nurses. But physicians did employ all the prevailing gender stereotypes and the model of the Victorian family to control women and keep them in "their place." Indeed, Lovell charged that these stereotypes were central to the success in creating the medical citadel.

In agreement with Gamarnikow's British research (1978; see chapter 2), Lovell (1982) asserted that American nursing and medicine were based on the metaphor of a holy marriage in which physicians, like husbands, assumed that nurses, like wives, were legal, subservient partners, who were expected to further the men's careers. Conceptually, such paternalism involved "one person caring for another and guiding another in a fatherly way . . . *Pater* means father, possessor, or master . . . *family* comes from *famel,* which means servant, slave, or possession. *Paterfamilias,* therefore, means owner or possessor of slaves" (p. 210). From the patriarchal order of the private household came the structural basis for the American physician-nurse relationship in the public workplace. Thus, women as nurses were to care loyally for the "hospital family," meeting the needs of all and keeping everyone happy, particularly the men, who as physicians could come and go as they pleased. To sustain the paternalistic hospital "family," control mechanisms to create fear and ignorance were used to obtain power over nurses and maintain social and professional inequality. Controlling and withholding information were and still are powerful tools of deception that rely on ignorance. Many physicians hoard their knowledge, using it as property to be sold as a commodity. Thus, healing skills are not spread but instead are concentrated in an elite medical group, who, said Lovell, use Latin words, a few scientific terms, and a chemical formula or two to impress patients and even nurses and force them into silence.

Manipulation of information is based on the fear of competition with nurses, whose knowledge could undermine medical stature, authority, and jobs. If, however, the physicians could dupe nurses into believing they belonged to a subservient group that had insufficient knowledge to control its own education, they could be convinced they needed the guidance of the "superior" male profession. To ensure this, physicians purposely withheld information and ignorance became a reality. Pioneer nurse Linda Richards recalled that nurses were forbidden to read the medical histories of patients. Numbers and not names were even placed on drug bottles so that nurses would not know what medicines they were giving to patients. In 1906 an article in the *Journal of the American Medical Association* laid out the methods to keep nurses ignorant and therefore under physician control: Any "initiative" by nurses should be reproved by physicians; nurses' education should be strictly limited only to "indispensable matters"; instruction should be "entrusted exclusively" to physicians, who would judge what the women needed to know; medical instructors should emphasize the "dangers of the initiative" of nurses to keep them from "inconsiderately stepping out from their proper sphere" (*Journal of the American Medical Association,* 1906; cited in Lovell, 1982, p. 217).

As proposed by Bok (1979), paternalistic deception, the intentional communication of messages meant to mislead women who are made to believe what the deceiver does not believe, is accomplished not simply by lying, but through gesture, disguise, action or inaction, and even silence. Historically, deception may outrank force as a means of subjection, compelling people to accept degrading work ostensibly because it is done in the best interests of others. Masquerading under altruistic purposes, the medical monopoly was presented as in the "best" interests of women and their patients. To Lovell, organized, paternalistic medicine has "carefully cultivated deception throughout its American history . . . honesty and truthfulness have been left out altogether from medical oaths and codes of ethics and are often ignored in the teaching of medicine" (Lovell, pp. 212–213).

Women have existed as a caste within every class and racial group, serving "as the domestic servants of society, freeing the male for the work day by bearing all the auxiliary and supportive chores" (Bianchi and Reuther, 1976; cited in Lovell, 1982, p. 213). If allowed into the work world, women were "generally structured into the same kind of domestic services and auxiliary support systems of male executive roles—as nurses, secretaries" (Bianchi and Reuther, 1976; cited in Lovell, 1982, p. 213). Thus, women provide the support system for male work and mobility and, through female domestication in the private sector, also provide the rest, recreation, and erotic life that keep men from being alienated from their public work. When applied to the health-care industry, women as nurses have been controlled in order to increase the power and identity of the medical patriarchy, which has "suppressed these women into a subservient category that works for but does not profit from the business of medicine" (p. 213).

Dominant groups view themselves as "naturally" the normal and provide rationalizations for the demeaning and demoralizing treatment that is often expressed in medicine as "we know what is best" for women as nurses or patients. If the "normal" is the "man's world," then this becomes the "real world," and this, as Lovell notes, makes patriarchy equivalent to the general culture. Any woman who objects to the "normality" of this view is silenced. Even Florence Nightingale (1928) was advised not to publish her strongly feminist work *Cassandra,* written in 1859, and she followed this advice, silencing her very negative critique of the status of women, leaving only her more conservative words for future generations of nurses, most of whom still do not know of their founder's feminism.

The muffling of strong women advocates creates silences that split women apart; through interior colonization, women can, as feminist Mary Daly (1978) said, be controlled by silent "remote control"; women who feel they are free from fears and therefore are "liberated" quickly collapse under the "unacknowledged power of these fears" when confronted by more powerful men. Fearing disfavor, the nurse gives in rather than incurring wrath or being ignored or dismissed as "ungrateful" or "unfeminine." Thus, paternal control, once it is embedded internally, will effectively keep women nurses in their "proper place."

Lovell provided evidence of physicians' stereotyped perceptions and their deceptive efforts to control nurses. In an 1897 speech, for example, physician Sir William Osler commended nurses for making life easier for physicians, but omitted the fact that the women had also made medicine more profitable for the men. For Osler, a woman could have no higher mission in life than nursing, reaching the ideals of her soul and the longings in her heart from which no woman could escape. Obviously, women, ruled by hearts, not heads, could hardly be economic competitors. Nor could they compete if they believed another physician who, in 1913, urged nurses to undesirable areas of work because of their "instinct of the eternal feminine for sacrificial service," which was the woman's "sole saving grace," constituting "the guiding light of her star of undoubted destiny" (Beard, 1913, p. 2149; cited in Lovell, 1982, p. 215). Certainly nurses could not compete if they were limited, as G. Torrence suggested in 1917, to caring for the poor, feeding invalids, and bettering conditions in very densely populated areas. To keep nurses serving physicians, platitudes about their being "good girls" were needed as medicine guided nursing toward sacrificial service: "With nurses caring for 'God's poor,' physicians are free to serve God's rich and to make a handsome profit at nursing's expense" (p. 216).

The Purposeful Use of Gender Discrimination to Achieve a Medical Monopoly

Evidence from crosscultural research supports Lovell's interpretations of her American data. In 1987, Phillip Darbyshire, British nurse-researcher, also traced the gendered and class-defined history of nurse-doctor relationships in Great Britain and concluded that these were *systemic* and culturally determined, not simply the accumulation of individual ideas and actions. Thus, current problems between nurses and physicians are not resolvable simply on the individual level. Although comforting, it is, according to Darbyshire, naive to assume that the collaboration and mutual respect portrayed in today's pulp novels and career brochures actually exist. Present relationships could be traced to physicians in the nineteenth century who purposely created a legally restricted "White, male, middle-class occupation"; however, class, as a divider between nurses and physicians, seems "positively opaque when compared to the sexist basis of medical domination" (Darbyshire, 1987, p. 32). To Darbyshire, British medical literature is "replete with overt (and not so overt) abuse of women as nurses" (p. 32). Early articles by physicians accused trained nurses of being too conceited and unwilling to be subordinate to medicine. Furthermore, nurses' instruction should be exclusively given by physicians since they were the only ones who knew what the women should learn. The focus on gender was clear in another physician's belief that nurses represented the "eternal feminine," devoted to sacrificial service.

Darbyshire warned: "It is tempting to dismiss such views as merely the deranged meanderings of individual doctors, but this is to miss the point: that the sexist domination of nursing by medicine was not haphazard or accidental but structured and institutionalized, designed to ensure the continued subservience of nurses and to reflect the dominant power relationship within society" (p. 32). To Darbyshire, the independence and clinical freedom of physicians— the lone physician solving society's ailments without help from other health-care professionals—are images from the past. After medicalizing numerous social problems, physicians were forced to keep up with constantly changing scientific and technological advances and also try to deal with a vast amount of social knowledge. Despite the overload, physicians have continued to reject other health professionals, who have increasingly insisted on being consulted and involved; nevertheless, "the notion persists among some [physicians] that teamwork is merely a group of people doing what they say" (p. 32). Thus, the medical monopoly continues to take priority over people's health.

No Nursing Domain Is Free of Attempted Medical Control

Researchers such as Ashley, Lovell, and Darbyshire were clearly morally outraged by organized medicine's unfair and discriminatory use of gender to obtain control over nurses and the ceaseless and unrelenting drive by physicians to create a medical monopoly. This monopoly negatively affected nurses' efforts to enact their own values in preventive and holistic health care, to provide quality care in hospital bureaucracies, and to achieve some semblance of relatively independent education, licensure, and practice. Throughout the decades researched, there are some critical transition points that mark the increasing domination of medicine and its eventual monopoly. But over the years, *no* nursing domain has been free of physicians' indirect or direct efforts to control it, including nurses' relation to the state in licensure and practice laws and to the public in nurse registries, agencies, clinics, and actual practice; nurses' access to patients both inside and outside of hospitals; nurses' education, including the location, length, and content of programs; nurses' access to and use of scientific knowledge, technological advances, and new instrumentation; nurses' specific functions, activities, and even standards and ethics of practice; nurses' exclusion or inclusion on private and governmental boards and ruling bodies. Medicine's efforts extended even to the development and internal functioning of professional nursing organizations, the choice of nursing leaders and the breadth and depth of their authority. The fluctuations and problems in nurses' identities have been created by medical and administrative imposition of "subnurses" and the spin-off of nursing functions to other specialists, which have caused a multiplicity of bureaucratic problems. The recruitment of nurses, their employment and salaries, and their shortages have been medically influenced. Finally, physicians have tried to control even the characters, personalities, demeanors, and interaction styles of nurses, both as women and as workers.

In short, there is very little that physicians and their medical organizations have not tried to control. Therefore, nurses have had to establish their occupation and their professional status, consolidate their organizational power, define their roles, provide good patient care, and work to achieve these goals while constantly facing continued pressures and frequent opposition from organized medicine. Given their gender subordination, nurses have had a difficult struggle, particularly since scientific justification of a medical monopoly was a widespread reality by the beginning of the twentieth century. If the primacy of women healers in previous centuries, as discussed in chapter 1, is accurate, than what is evident in this chapter is the culmination of centuries of medical takeover. What is also obvious is the constant refusal by some nurses to accept totally subordinated roles. Given the multiple, sometimes contradictory, and often changing perceptions of women's roles, it is not surprising that nurses have varied in their own views of nurses' roles and relationships with physicians. Indeed, nurses' political unity has been difficult to achieve partly because of the subordinated status of women. In contrast, the predominantly male physicians, historically members of the superordinate gender group, have had a distinct political advantage that is implicitly derived from their patriarchal privilege and partially validated by their control of scientific knowledge, which is often the explicit justification of their gendered monopoly.

A "Convenient" Reconstruction of the Evolution of Nursing and Medicine

Is there evidence that physicians were deceptively silent about the history of women healers? Did they intentionally or unintentionally create a self-congratulatory medical history that conveniently excluded or trivialized or condemned women in health care? Did physicians, as Lovell contends, use historical silence to justify their coercive treatment of women nurses and patients? Let us consider two commencement speeches given by physicians to nurses, the first by E. D. Ferguson in 1901 and the second by Woods Hutchinson in 1905.

In a two-part article derived from his speech, Ferguson (1901a; 1901b) traced his perceptions of the history that led to scientific, but not professional, nursing; indeed, he doubted the desirability of the latter term. He began by focusing on the development of hospitals, referring to the temples of Hygieia and Aesculapius (Asklepios) in Greece, where priests prayed (no priestesses are mentioned), discussed the rules of life, and provided medicinal measures (no nursing measures are mentioned). He then discussed Hippocrates, the "father" of medicine, and then Egypt, where medicine obtained a high grade of specialization, although hospitals were presumably nonexistent. Thus far, women healers, other than Hygieia, and midwives were not mentioned and presumably could not have evolved if they did not exist! Turning to Roman sources, Ferguson did credit one woman, Fabiola, a Roman matron, with founding the first Christian hospital, but this institution he downgraded to an almshouse. He described monks' activities in monasteries where separate structures were erected for the sick. Again, any reference to women healers in homes or hospitals was missing. Even nurse nuns in their own orders and convents were not mentioned.

Ferguson credited "Mohammadan" theocracy with the spread of hospitals, but he ignored the Middle Eastern nurses and women healers. Thus, their evolution was also somewhat difficult to assess. Continuing with Christian hospitals, Ferguson claimed that these were characterized by the "sordid motives" of administrators and an absence of scientific knowledge. The hospital medical officers were blameless since they lacked influence and supposedly were unable to affect the administrators. In addition, physicians, presumably more then than now, were interested in the commercial aspects of medicine. Still, no reference was made to nurses or to women healers, unless some administrators could be assumed to be women. Eventually, claimed Ferguson, the bad conditions aroused physicians to reform the degraded hospitals and management, but no women healers or nurses are mentioned as part of the reforms. Their presence is implied, however, and thus their responsibility for the foul conditions may also be inferred. Indeed, the coarseness in care was due not to physicians but to the hospital attendants, who were neither orderlies nor nurses. Thus, physicians presumably were obliged to deal with Sairey Gamps, there evidently being no women nurses at all prior to the mid nineteenth century. The nursing sisters were seemingly only involved in "sentimental" ministrations, absorbing their "little" knowledge by observing physicians. Finally, Ferguson mentioned nurses, but both lay and religious women were denigrated or trivialized. However, he commended Elizabeth Frye, a nineteenth-century "Quaker wife and mother" who worked with prisoners at Newgate prison against the male authorities' desires and transformed the situation: "without aid and only a woman's strength [she] accomplished almost a miracle" (Ferguson, 1901a, p. 468).

In his second article, Ferguson focused on Florence Nightingale, who met Frye in London, where Nightingale studied the hospital conditions and then visited other institutions on the continent. Ferguson noted that Nightingale became a pupil of Pastor Fliedner, who attempted to dissuade her from nursing and then insisted she begin by scrubbing floors. Clearly, Ferguson attributes to Fliedner more influence on Nightingale than she credited to him. On her return to England, she was not able to break the tradition of a "conservative people," or those connected with hospitals; therefore, she reformed a sanatorium for sick women. In Ferguson's account there is no evidence that physicians opposed Nightingale or that societal sexism toward women existed at all. Indeed, when Nightingale went to the Crimea, Ferguson claimed that it was the government and the army, not specifically medical authorities, who were responsible for the gruesome state of affairs. Since some training of nurses had begun, Nightingale, given the support of the Roman Catholic bishop of London, had access to some experienced women. But if the older nuns gave only "sentimental" and unknowledgeable care, how then did their presence help

Nightingale? Ferguson's trivialization of nursing sisters created a peculiar illog-icality in his historical account.

Ferguson did admit finally that the conservative English surgeons exhib-ited prejudice against women nursing male patients, particularly in army ser-vice during wartime, where the women were seen as representing a "heretical" and "ungodly" intervention. Instead of dealing with the long, difficult, and humiliating situations caused by physicians, Ferguson said that Nightingale quickly overcame all sentimental and even boorish opposition and, since she was "careful that nursing should never interfere with the surgical and medical supervision . . . a cordial relation soon existed" (Ferguson, 1901b, p. 624). It is clear that Ferguson saw nurses' evolution really starting with Nightingale only when she, out of necessity, subordinated nurses' work to the control of physi-cians. So much for the long view of women healers' "evolution"! To Ferguson, technical training was absolutely necessary for nursing to obtain the best "medical" results (not nursing or even health-care results).

In his speech, Ferguson warned student and graduate nurses that their usefulness depended on dealing with the conditions in sickrooms without "ob-trusiveness or sentimental nonsense." After denying or denigrating women healers prior to Nightingale, Ferguson said, "There is no sex in good works, and men and women alike are quietly, steadily, and efficiently working that her development may continue" (p. 626). Ironically, Ferguson provided more than ample evidence of gender bias in his account, allowing only fifty or sixty years for the "evolution" of women healers and nurses. Thus, Lovell's research conclusions about silences, derogatory put-downs, and even deceptive inter-pretations by physicians are documented in this graduation speech and in sub-sequent publications.

Ferguson's perceptions were not atypical. In a commencement oration on the origins of nursing and medicine, given to graduating student nurses at the California Hospital in Los Angeles, Woods Hutchinson, MD, admitted that the origins of medicine were "often not particularly flattering to our pride" (Hutchinson, 1905, p. 148). Indeed, tracing the history of even illustrious medical institutions often led to the very humblest of antecedents. Including nurses as devotees of medicine, Hutchinson tracked their origins not to wise women or priestesses but to medicine men and shamans, who presumably believed in demonic possession and administered "bitter, nauseous, and other-wise abominable messes" (p. 149). He further claimed that current household medicine consisted of horehound, chamomile, and "other abominable teas," all "clear survivals of demonism" (p. 149). Hutchinson attacked women herb-alists whose teas and tonics had the sole virtue of a bitter taste. In fact, the "whole edifice of even modern medicine is riddled through and through with traces of its origin from pure magic" (p. 150).

Hutchinson admitted that the modern surgeon originated with barbers and corn-cutters. The physician, at least in Great Britain, was a gentleman, but the surgeon, even at the turn of the century, was still referred to as "Mr.," not "Dr." Bloodletting by surgeons or leeches was, said Hutchinson, also traceable to the release of diseased demons and was, along with purging, due to "ghastly, degrading, and utterly harmful superstitions [that] did harm, and little else but harm" (p. 151). Indeed, such practices contributed to the contempt for and dislike of physicians in fictional and historic literature apparent even within the previous fifty years. He admitted that even "Shakespeare seldom refers to the leech or the surgeon except in such terms as might be applied to a footman or groom . . . [and] evidently regards them as rank impostors dealing with charms and spells and practising upon the credulity of the people" (p. 151). To "modern" physicians, such attitudes were painful and humiliating. Up to this point, Hutchinson, unlike Ferguson, did admit the humble origins of medicine, but he dealt with predominantly women healers and herbalists in homes and communities by satirizing, trivializing, or denigrating their medicine and therapies. Thus, Lovell's research generalizations are again supported.

Somehow from the barbarism and ignorance of the past emerged the present-day trained nurse, who had not, until recently, been recognized as the peer of medicine, even though nursing originated further back in antiquity, traceable to the maternal affection shown to the young before nurses or physicians existed. To these mothers human survival could be attributed. Nevertheless, Hutchinson separated the nurse from the physician. According to him, only nurses had culled no deadly poisons and brandished no bloody scalpel, but relied on nature, which was to be trusted, not hated or despised. And now, claimed Hutchinson, nursing had become the third foot of a tripod with medicine and surgery, which made these fields "as firm as that of the everlasting hills" (p. 154). Indeed, in the future, every child would have surgical housecleaning by seven or eight years of age—tonsils trimmed out, appendix removed, gall bladder excised, and, if the child was female, the fifth toe removed to enable fashionable shoes to be worn, and perhaps even the "excessive mobility of the linguistic organ of the gentler sex" (p. 155) could be surgically corrected.

In the meantime, physicians and surgeons, once "monarchs of all we surveyed," now faced the nursing profession, "our most dreaded critic and our most valued assistant" (p. 155). Physicians, said Hutchinson, were often unjustly praised by patients and families for recoveries the physicians had nothing to do with, or they were unjustly denounced for losing impossible cases. Now with modern nursing had come another influence. "This person, the only one that we are afraid of, is the nurse. She does not say much, but her look can express volumes" (p. 155). When physicians make fools of themselves, they know the nurses know it, even without saying anything: "When the nurse says we have done well in a case, we know we have, but when she maintains a polite reticence . . . we shudder to our very backbones" (p. 156). Hutchinson said that physicians were now under the dominion of women not only at home but at the office and hospital—an assertion he knew was untrue. Nevertheless, he warned nurses not to be too sure of diagnoses; he advised them to use their own judgment and to avoid the drill-sergeant form of precision. It is clear that Hutchinson, although more honest than Ferguson about medicine's origins, used ridicule and satire to trivialize the history of women healers and nurses. In fact, he was never really able or willing to analyze nurses' history and evolution. And, of course, the "fears" that physicians had of nurses certainly did not stop them from continued efforts to control them.

Do other data support the contention that physicians have tried to control nursing domains? Exactly how did physicians respond to the development of "modern" nursing in the United States? What did they say about nursing in American journals? Do their published statements support the feminist analysis by some nurse-researchers that physicians used gender-based subordination to achieve a monopoly in health care? Thelma Ingles (1976) traced physicians' views of nursing in published statements from 1873 to 1913 and concluded that nurses and non-nurses do not understand the often negative role that physicians have played in the development of the nursing profession. In an understatement, she noted that the first schools of nursing in the United States were not "whole-heartedly supported by physicians" (p. 125). Many looked with dismay on women entering "their" domain—which, it must be noted again, physicians had probably taken, at least in part, from women healers in previous centuries.

For Ingles, the question of the "trained" nurse was coupled with the larger issue of women's rights. Surprisingly, until the 1970s few nurses had made this connection as clearly and succinctly. She further speculated that many of the early nursing leaders might have been "Amazons," and their characteristics may have been sharply incongruent with the stereotyped nurse-as-mother image. It is unfortunate that Ingles used an almost homophobic stereotype to describe some early women leaders. What precisely is an "Amazon"? Obviously, any woman deviating from the Victorian model of "femininity" could automatically be seen as aberrant. Just how aberrant is evident in the men's thought on women nurses, not only in the medical journals but also in nursing journals, where physicians published many editorials, graduation speeches to hospital nursing students, and "philosophical" treatises on the education and practice of nurses. The presumption that physicians could define another profession marks the development of nursing as a profession distinctly different from the emergence of "male" professional groups. The territorial boundaries of a "woman's" occupation were considered to be *within* the domain of the medical "profession." Whether justified or not, the right of physicians to control women was implicit or explicit in their writing.

Over- or Undertaught? Physicians Debate Nurses' Education

Ingles found interesting regional differences among the men who wrote on nurses: physicians from New England were sometimes more supportive, but those in New York wrote "diatribes of a destructively critical nature" (p. 126). A few unsung heroes, such as Dr. Richard Cabot, could conceive of a woman's "liberal profession." Indeed in Boston in 1874, one physician said: "The longer we live and practice, the less faith we have in mere medicine, and the more curious do the old rules appear which point to medication, and say nothing of diet, manner of living, pure air, or *nursing*" (p. 127).

After nurse training schools had been in existence a while, there was some agreement among physicians that at least hygiene in hospitals had improved. Although what was written was often, as we shall see later, incongruent with what was practiced, at least one physician noted: "Under the new regime, by placing the sick in the care of a school, results have been secured, good nursing and care insured, the mortality diminished, an improved moral tone and prestige won for the hospital" (p. 128). Note, however, the extent of gender stereotyping of the nurse associated even with these more positive comments:

> She has a quick perception of what is needed, and she readily and cheerfully does it, no matter how repulsive the task may be. . . . The work the nurse is doing steadily and faithfully, and the information she brings me is invaluable. The only wonder to me is how I got on with these cases without a woman's help. She visits from morning to night, seeing that my medicines are given as directed, inaugurating and enforcing much-needed sanitary measures, often making with her own hands articles of clothing for the sick. (pp. 128–129)

It is clear from such an accolade in defense of "trained" nurses that they were seen as extensions of the physician, bringing him information, and that they were extensions of the traditional volunteer women, who provided "objects of their own making," presumably on their own time and without pay.

In 1870 the *Philadelphia Hospital Report* confirmed that by using trained nurses the mortality from puerperal fever had been substantially reduced. By 1906 even the *New York Medical Journal* accepted the fact that the training school had become "an essential feature of the modern hospital" (p. 130). Although these were positive comments, it is equally clear, although unstated, that physicians in the hospitals could not conduct their business without the unpaid or poorly paid labor of women, primarily nursing students rather than graduate nurses.

It is morbidly fascinating to observe the extent to which physicians felt it was their prerogative to debate and to control the curriculum, education, and types of nursing schools. Some wanted training for housekeeping; others advocated drilling with no formal theoretical instruction; some wanted the curriculum under hospital control, some under physician control, and a few under neither. Some physicians saw nursing schools as educational centers, while others saw them as training centers for hospital employees. What is central is the assumption that it was the physicians' prerogative to define the meaning of occupation or profession for another group of human beings. Implicit in their thinking was that woman functioned as an aid to the man. Dr. John Packard wrote: "Another most important function of the nurse is the watching of the patient, and to give the physician a clear and faithful report of what takes place between his visits" (Packard, 1876; cited in Ingles, 1976, p. 131). Here one could easily replace the word "nurse" with "wife" and "patient" with "child," making obvious the sex-stereotyped transposition of familial roles into the workplace. How were the men to get the women to produce reports? Packard continued: "Now all of these matters can be taught by steady, patient drilling. . . . In the vast majority of cases it would be idle to begin the training of a nurse with lectures in anything. . . . We do not want a scientific person; we do not want a person with theories of her own, or with a smattering of other peoples' theories" (Packard, 1876; cited in Ingles, 1976, pp. 131–132).

What is somewhat ironic is how physicians, who previously took their knowledge, at least in part, from women, could now reverse the process and attempt to create a woman who had no explanatory system of her own, not even one derived from others. It is wise to remember, as noted in chapter 1, that Paracelsus threw away his medical books and learned, as he stated, all he knew from the sorceress or wise woman in the forest. To another physician, however, "trained" nurses, even with their "admirable training in explicitly obeying the physician's orders, lack that minimum of culture . . . there is a kind of roughness and disagreeable abruptness . . . due to hospital life" (Otis, 1883; cited in Ingles, 1976, p. 133). Otis called for a better class of women, who exhibit "tenderness, gentleness, delicacy of step and touch" (Otis, 1883; cited in Ingles, 1976, p. 134). In short, the nurse was seen as a woman defined by the standard stereotypic notion of the female role. In fact, Ingles noted that many of the comments might have been made yesterday; certainly, variations on the same themes have been repeated throughout the twentieth century.

In Support of "Wholesome Ignorance"

Perhaps the full extent of sexist pressures can be best ascertained by analyzing Sir William Osler's 1891 speech to the Johns Hopkins graduating class of nurses, republished in *Aequanimitas* in 1932. Admitting the greater antiquity of nursing, he said: "If, Members of the Graduating Class, the medical profession, composed chiefly of men, has absorbed a larger share of attention and regard, you have, at least, the satisfaction of feeling that yours is the older, and, as older, the more honourable calling" (Osler, 1932, p. 16). Osler then proved the antiquity of nursing by citing examples of female-tending-male images, such as Eve with Enoch and Elaine with Lancelot. Shifting to evolutionary theory, Osler defended the division of labor in the "incessant warfare in which man is engaged" (p. 17). Individually, "man," the unit, the microcosm, inherits the taints of "blood and brawn," but nurses continue, "judging not, asking no questions, but meting out to all alike a hospitality worthy of the Hôtel Dieu" (p. 17). Thus is ignored the determined struggle of the nursing sisters against physician control at the Hôtel-Dieu, as documented in chapter 1.

Osler personified nature as the traditional female, saying: "We have not yet risen to a true conception of Nature . . . we can no more upbraid her great laws than we can the lesser laws of the state. . . . The pity is that we do not know them all; in our ignorance we err daily, and pay a blood penalty" (p. 18). Ironically, Osler believed that male physicians, not female nurses, must seek out the laws of Mother Nature, of female being.

In a second speech in 1897, also republished in 1932, Osler asked: Is the nurse an added blessing or an added horror? The nurse, he claimed, had overturned the inalienable right of mother, wife, sister, friend, and old servant: "You are intruders, innovators, and usurpers, dislocating, as you do, from their tenderest and most loving duties these mothers, wives and sisters" (p. 150). Nevertheless, the nurse made the practice of medicine easier and saved the apothecary's bill; in fact, she was an analogue to the slave ant in Darwin's work on instincts, which "put all to rights." Still, the nurse might be a "source of real terror" to a wife who feared the nurse's involvement with the husband. Of course, the nurse could also be a "source of misery" to a husband, whose sick wife might become overly dependent on the nurse. In fact, there might even develop an "occult attraction between women" (p. 151), of the weak for the strong. To reduce all these possibilities, Osler warned: "Do enter upon your duties with a becoming sense of your frailties" (p. 152). He further cautioned the nurse to state: "I will keep my mouth as it were with bridle" (p. 153). Above all, nurses were not to discuss particular infirmities with patients. Of course, the women simply could not escape the "perils of half-knowledge of pseudo-science" (p. 154). They would "involuntarily catch the accents and learn the language of science, often without a clear conception of its meaning" (p. 154). With apparent sympathy, Osler stated: "It must be very difficult to resist the fascination of a desire to know more, much more, of the deeper depths of the things you see and hear, and often this ignorance must be very tantalizing, but it is more wholesome than an assurance which rests on a thin veneer of knowledge" (p. 155).

Ignorance may be blessed, but "inconsistency so notorious in the sex" (p. 155) must not lead women to barter away their heritage for a hoop of gold. Marriage is necessary, but he advised nurses to "abstain from philandering during your period of training" (p. 156). Following all these injunctions, Osler claimed that the nurse had always been a member of the trinity with physician and priest. After being enthroned in the medical godhead, she was reminded of her superfluity in the unemployed ranks of women nurses, partially caused by those women who "will not or cannot fulfil the highest duties ... [of] Nature" (p. 157). Assuming that women became spinsters at age twenty-five, Osler warned that single women might become a "dangerous element"; this was followed by a veiled allusion to Sappho and lesbianism. On the other hand, she might fritter away her life as a do-gooder. These women might become unpaid Deaconesses who would not need training schools, which were not really giving proper education anyway. In any event, hospital nurses should withstand the erosion of their sympathy by institutional corrosion. Osler concluded: Women who do "noble deeds amid the pestilence . . . we love" (p. 158).

Physician Authority in Selecting Nursing Leaders

In 1913 Osler recalled in still another graduation speech two remarkable Nightingale-trained women, Fisher and Hawley (no first names were given), who, in the late nineteenth century, took charge of the Philadelphia City Hospital, which was at the time a byword for political corruption and hospital inefficiency. Both women came from England, where they presumably had not had to deal with ward politicians or a hopeless hospital without a proper system of arrangements. Nevertheless, "The first thing they did was to get complete control of the politicians, and that is never hard for a tactful woman to do" (p. 74). (If this were so, why were women still unable to vote?) Osler continued, "Next they got the medical staff, which is an easier thing for a tactful woman to do" (p. 74). What exactly the women "got" was not stated.

That these English nurses were requested by the male administrators at Philadelphia City Hospital is clear. But did physicians have similar control over hiring American nursing leaders? Indeed they did! After the Johns Hopkins Nursing School was established, there were eighty applicants for the directorship position. The women's credentials were reviewed by five men, including Osler and two other physicians; no nurses or women from any other background were mentioned as being part of the review board. Of the five final candidates, Isabel Hampton (later Robb) "entered the room looking like an animated Greek statue" (p. 75). According to Osler, all the men smiled at each other, knew the appointment was settled, looked at her certificates in a perfunctory manner, and selected her. Obviously, her appearance, not necessarily her credentials, was initially critical to the men, who also assumed they had the unilateral right to choose the woman who would lead the nursing staff.

To Osler, nurses' training was "only a little less arduous, and a little less extensive than that given to a medical student, and indeed is more extensive than was given to medical students in former days" (p. 76). Whether there was too much education and too little training was an issue Osler would only discuss privately with the superintendent. According to him, many paths were open for nurses, for example, becoming the "righthand man [*sic*] of the county health officer" (p. 78).

As in previous graduation talks, Osler linked nursing and nurse leaders to gender stereotypes. First, the "protective mechanism" of tact, without which no woman could be a success, and which was "instinctive" with most women, enabled them to always do the right thing at the right time. Indeed, a tactless woman was, to him, a calamity. For example, one nursing superintendent, well-trained, with a splendid presence and a good record, tried to create a "revolution" in training. The members of the hospital's board of trustees were antiquated, obstinate, and self-opinionated; nevertheless, according to Osler, the woman's lack of tact caused all the problems and difficulties she encountered.

The second virtue, neatness, was the essence of nursing work and the "prime duty of a woman of this terrestrial world . . . to look well" (p. 79). The third virtue, as emphasized in Osler's past lectures, was taciturnity, which he interpreted as silence: nurses needed to remain quiet about all matters pertaining to patients and their care. The fourth virtue was sympathy, but Osler advised the women to withhold it, giving it only sparingly. The fifth virtue, gentleness, Osler believed was nurses' birthright. And sixth, cheerfulness, was one of "the chief functions of all cultivated women" (p. 81). The last virtue, charity, was a nursely attribute. At no point was intelligence or knowledge or clinical competence mentioned as critical to nursing care; gender stereotypes were the bases for defining nurses and their leaders.

The tactful, neat, silent, sympathetic, gentle, cheerful, charitable woman, even if loved for doing noble deeds amid pestilence, should not aspire to medical knowledge. However, in 1889 one physician warned: "The day has gone by when the physician can afford to keep nurses in utter ignorance of what medicines they are administering, and what effect they desire to obtain from such medicines" (*Boston Medical and Surgical Journal*, 1889; cited in Ingles, 1976, p. 135). From a time when women were the primary herbalists, they had reached a position of medically imposed "total ignorance" of the medicines they gave to their patients. Fortunately, Lavinia L. Dock (1890) published a textbook specifically on drugs, so that nurses could be knowledgeable about the medications they administered to their patients.

An Unsatisfactory Dictum: Loyalty and Obedience to the Physician

In sharp contrast to Osler is Dock's (1900) thoughtful consideration of ethics. Dock was warned by a "liberal-minded" man against developing a nursing code of ethics. In medicine, it had been a cause of contention, therefore, he advised, "Be good women but do not bother with a Code of Ethics" (Dock, 1900; cited in James, 1985, p. 37). Dock rejected his suggestion, saying this physician did not take nurses seriously. To her, it was necessary to distinguish between ethics, etiquette, and the unreasoning reverence for statutes, fines, and punishments. For example, if the nurse does not rise when a doctor enters, she commits a breach of *etiquette,* not ethics. This distinction may not be understood by physicians; indeed, in their graduation speeches to nurses, Dock heard few ethical considerations; their grave words were "unflavored mental pablum," platitudes that the same men the next day would not recognize. Dock asked, "What do they teach us of ethics? Well, this,—as yet the extremest that we have heard,—the nurse's whole duty, loyalty, and obedience begins and ends in subordination to the doctor. Beyond this there is no horizon and outside of this she has no reason for existing. Ponder over this dictum and acknowledge that there is something unsatisfying in it" (pp. 40–41). Was there no more than this? Dock responded that the nurse must be "allowed the same amount of independence as any other moral being" (p. 41).

Suppose, asked Dock, nurses were taught to value, first, loyalty and justice as living principles. In nine out of ten cases, this might be consistent with loyalty to physicians. What of the tenth case? There might be circumstances that "make it wrong for her to obey and remain subordinate to the doctor . . . her loyalty might be due, not to the doctor, but to the patient" (p. 41); or even to the family, or friends, or the public. Dock claimed, "There is an obedience which is slavishness and a subordination which is moral cowardice" (p. 41). Although it was difficult to draw the line, knowledge of obligations and duty to all, not just one class of people, was needed. As a class of working or professional women, nurses were deficient in this knowledge. There was, she said, a vast world of duties and responsibilities of which nurses had heard scarcely a whisper.

Dock urged nurses to enter the world beyond physicians and patients and engage in voluntary association with others. In an analogy, Dock claimed that the average women's club often begins with self-culture, rather timorous and self-exclusive, until it gets into the subject of general education, when it becomes more democratic, casting artificial social distinctions aside and entering into "the thick of public school work, public amusements, municipal housekeeping, public hygiene, the housing and condition of the poor" (p. 45). In this process, the whole world opens to the obligations and responsibilities to all people.

Similarly, Dock wanted nurses to enter into relationships with people outside the profession to learn of life: "If one has simply learned her responsibilities to the medical profession, another may be able to balance that one-sidedness by a knowledge of duties to other working women or to the cause of better education in general" (pp. 46–47). To Dock, some nurses held doctrines that do not admit the accumulated advantages accrued through the labor of all previous workers; however, nurses must learn the history and status of their work in relation to that of other workers.

Before all else, said Dock, nurses have the obligation to establish independence of outside control in their personal and professional lives. She reported that some nursing associations "are almost entirely controlled by the medical societies"; that the nurse registries were "managed by boards of managers of training schools," which excluded nurses from making rules, selecting officers or disposing of income (pp. 48–49). Nurses who accepted such conditions ignored "the first duty of inhabitants of a free country, namely to *be* free" (p. 49). Dock stressed that unnecessary and belittling subordination held back all nurses. She found it strange that medicine, presumably "free" from a commercial spirit, should be willing to conduct small business enterprises, such as nurses' registries, taking the modest incomes they had not earned to apply to medical libraries. But what of the women, who "might stand independently, but . . . prefer contributing to those who do not hesitate to take advantage of them?" (p. 49). She believed most physicians did not want this relationship, but why should nurses "encourage the less considerate by allowing them pecuniary advantages which the more thoughtful would not condescend to ask for?" (p. 50).

Dock asked nurses to consider the struggle and the strain endured by those in charge of training schools to win and hold the advantages now assumed or even criticized. Should not their problems be shared? Was there not an ethical responsibility? In contrast to others, nurses, said Dock, had outgrown the old form of lifelong dependence but had "not yet arrived at the spontaneity of free, voluntary, enthusiastic support and interest shown by college graduates to their schools. We are, in this respect, a tame, colorless anomaly" (p. 53).

All of these issues, Dock said, led back to the professional and ethical culture and to the community status of nursing. Was nursing education a success or were student nurses "a money-saving device? Even in our probationer year we do an immense amount of work for considerably less cost to the hospital than the wages of untrained domestics would amount to" (p. 53). Presumably, women do this to get an education, but, asked Dock, what if they do all the work and get only a smattering of education, "enough to deceive ourselves and, to a certain extent, other people" (p. 53). Dock claimed that nurses must not only understand their ethical responsibilities to others, but the ethical responsibilities of others *to nurses* as well. If not, they lose dignity and spirit, and are imposed upon unfairly. She insisted that nurses learn self-expression: "In the past we have been a silent sisterhood . . . we have heretofore stood aloof, looked askance, and spoken in monosyllables . . . as a profession we have not had sense of unity until very lately" (p. 55). And even this was shaky.

Dock believed that obedience must be for a worthy cause, not merely submission to winding spools forever without knowing what the spools are for! Nurses needed to clarify whether the work or the individual was most important. If the work, then the individual should be subordinated. To her, each was equally important. She advocated that nurses wear obedience as they wear uniforms: to accomplish a piece of work. If nurses did not adopt obedience as a law for the soul, they could avoid pointless and uncalled-for tractability in general affairs. To Dock, ethical development had no end: from cruelty to slaves, to refusal to hold slaves, to insistence on the equality of slaves. Similarly, nurses could develop ethically; not content with the little duties of yesterday, today they could focus on their duties to other nurses, but tomorrow their duties "will be to all human beings" (p. 57).

An Epidemic of Medical Criticism and Disapproval

The difference between Osler's and Dock's perceptions of nurses seems to represent an impassable gap. Osler's praise of the self-sacrificing woman seems far removed from Dock's concerns; Dock's position was probably not read by most physicians. Indeed, in 1901, the *Journal of the American Medical Association* published an editorial comment reprimanding a nurse or nurse superintendent (the writer was not sure of her status) who spoke before a nurses' convention, deploring physicians' incompetence in administration. This nurse was branded as one of those objectionable kind of "parasites that bite their hosts and benefactors" (p. 982), referring to the statement once made by Dr. Malcolm Morris that the trained nurse was a "parasite" on the medical profession.

Other physicians, such as George P. Ludlam (1906), superintendent of the New York Hospital, recalled observing the growth of nursing to a dominant position in the hospital and to a controlling influence on business and routine. According to Ludlam, physicians had observed the "simple" nurse transformed into a professional woman. The struggle for existence had happened "without any noisy or boisterous demand for recognition, but with a quiet, persistent, unintermittent development" (p. 851). To him, the physicians were silent but interested spectators. There seems little to support this assertion. Ludlam's primary interest was the control and organization of training schools, which, he believed, should emphasize over and over again the intimate, harmonious, and complementary relation between nurses and physicians. To achieve this, superficial medical knowledge should be eliminated, and practical knowledge of nursing stressed. He urged a closer relation between the nursing school and the attending staff of physicians and surgeons. The current "divorce" was unfortunate; the nurse should look "to him who has professional charge of the patients in her ward" (p. 852).

Ludlam was not simply a silent but interested spectator of nursing; he was an active and outspoken advocate for medical domination. Control of the nurse training school, he said, should be subordinated to an executive authority, who would be a physician. Indeed, an independent department of nursing was "unfortunate and revolutionary" (p. 852). Relying on male military models of authority, Ludlam stated: "The tendency of the training school is more and more in this direction of independence" (p. 852). He noted among the women a restlessness under control and a desire to be self-governing. He advised careful selection of the woman head, who should be free of interference but "distinctly subordinate and amenable to the general executive authority of the hospital" (p. 853). How this woman leader could be free of male interference but at the same time subordinated, even amenable, to men in power is not clear!

Ludlam's position may be contrasted to Lavinia Dock's views of hospital organization (1903). She noted that several papers dealing with authority over nurse training schools had appeared in medical and nursing journals, one even referring to nurses as "women folks." In one paper, physician Stephen Smith advocated that the hospital superintendent should be appointed by the medical board; the board would also select the matron, who should also be the superintendent of the nurses' training school. Furthermore, Smith wrote, the medical board should exercise full authority over the training schools: "It should prescribe rules and regulations governing the school, arrange the course of instruction, select the instructors, appoint the superintendent of the training school and examine the candidates for graduation" (cited in Dock, 1903, p. 10). To Dock, this meant that nursing would revert back to total subservience; indeed Smith's plan would entirely destroy Nightingale's goal of women being in charge of women.

Why, Dock asked, should a person who does not totally understand the work of nurses expect that a male superintendent or medical board could adequately represent a nurse to the board of trustees? Dock claimed that it was easy to name autocratic hospitals that had failed to obtain and retain women; indeed, one nursing superintendent was so hampered that "she was obliged to spend time in carrying pins around to the wards, which she should, instead, have given to reorganizing and supervising the nursing service" (p. 14).

In 1906 Dock sent a warning to British nurses:

> Do you see that nurses are just now undergoing a withering course of criticism from certain members of the medical profession? There is really quite an epidemic of disapproval and criticism in the medical press . . . much of it ill-natured, narrow-minded, and intolerant. . . . I do not regard this as a medical unfriendliness pure and simple, but as a part of the general masculine jealousy and alarm over the progress of women. They are full of irritation at the thought of women standing beside men on an equal plane. (Dock, 1906, p. 487)

Not all nurses would have agreed with Dock. Indeed, divisions in the ranks of nurses on gender were basic to differences in nurse-physician relations. Compare Dock's letter with an excerpt from Grace Holmes' 1907 poem "The Doctor As the Nurse Knows Him":

> And he—as with a woman's gentle touch—
> Closes the dull eyes, folds the lifeless hands.
> . . . He's gone—His silent hand clasp seemed to say
> "You need the Great Physician for *this* pain." (p. 182)

In fictional accounts as well as poems, nurses without a feminist perspective could inadvertently reinforce nurses' subordination. For example, nurse Mary Sewall Gardner, in addition to writing the first major text in the field, *Public Health Nursing* (1916), later published three fictional works focused on the lives of early public health nurses. After retiring in 1931 as director of the Providence District Nursing Association, Gardner later published her first novel, *So Build We* (1942), which focused on the life of a director of a visiting nurse association. Her second novel, *Katherine Kent* (1946), portrayed a woman who was a public health nurse for thirty years. Lois A. Monteiro (1987) analyzed both of Gardner's novels and found that a central theme was nurse-physician conflict. In her second novel, Gardner posed the conflict as a question of ethics: Will Nurse Kent act as the physician's or the patient's agent? In 1906, working out of no office, with no fee, no set hours, and no uniform, Kent receives her referrals from physicians, who leave information for her at the pharmacy. While in the phone booth one day, Kent overhears a local physician, Brandt, telling the pharmacist that his business is rotten and that the visiting nurse is probably passing his patients to other men. After Brandt departs, the pharmacist tells Kent that the physician probably has been losing patients ever since his first case. The townspeople do not like Brandt because he refused to help a woman in childbirth one stormy night and the woman died. The pharmacist advises Kent to stay away from Brandt.

When Brandt goes out of town temporarily, he leaves five patients for Kent, who finds one in very bad condition. She calls another physician, who hospitalizes the patient. On his return, Brandt expresses his anger over Kent's actions and she experiences his hostility as a form of persecution for which she has no redress. Brandt continues sending patients to Kent, but harasses her over many petty details. Though no charges are made, Kent is finally fired by her agency. She asks another physician what she could have done to prevent this crisis. He replies that she should have forced Brandt to give proper orders and directions about his patients.

Monteiro noted that Brandt is depicted as incompetent and an alcoholic, but that Gardner gives her heroine no words or actions to deal with these issues. The focus is on the unfair treatment of Kent for her protection of Brandt's patients; she does not protest her firing. Monteiro claimed that these fictional accounts in the 1940s fit with Gardner's own early textbook, in which she advises nurses not to diagnose, prescribe, recommend a particular doctor or a change of doctor, or suggest a hospital without a doctor's approval, and never to criticize a physician, verbally or nonverbally. Such recommendations, said Monteiro, have led some feminist critics to point out "nursing's submissiveness to authority, particularly in the hospital nurse's response to administrators and physicians, as one reason for the profession's failure to reach its full potential as a political force in health care" (Monteiro, 1987, p. 68). Monteiro recognized these forces at work in Gardner's fiction: Katherine Kent is not praised for her work on behalf of patients, but she "is portrayed as someone who is immature, unwise about the proper way of getting things done, and at fault for not looking to others for advice" (p. 68).

Submission to authority is a more complex issue and involves problematic contradictions. Nevertheless, feminist nurses still adhered to the Nightingale dictum and, as restated in 1908, it was critical to them:

> The undivided control of nurses in all that relates to their teaching, training, and discipline must lie in the hands of women. . . . Whenever the principles of Miss Nightingale have been accepted nursing has made wonderful progress . . . wherever her principles are ignored, and we find men (no matter whether medical or lay) in charge of the discipline and education of nurses, conditions are either as bad as they ever were, or are steadily declining . . . to that state of degradation where nursing was when she rescued it. . . . This is not a petulant expression of revolt. . . . It is simply a plain statement of fact. (*American Journal of Nursing*, 1908, p. 334)

Warfare in the Hospital "Family"? Putting Nursing under a Single Authority

As supporters of Nightingale's demand for women to control nursing, Lavinia Dock, Lillian Wald, and other early feminist nurse leaders continued to criticize men's efforts to exert patriarchal control. For example, in the late nineteenth century, George H. M. Rowe, superintendent of Boston City Hospital, called for a "unal" plan to put nursing under a single authority, the hospital administrator. However, nurses knew that would mean a loss of independence. Dock believed that Rowe's plan would be devastating: "underneath their arguments lay nearly a century of 'female institution building' and the political sensibility that understood the necessity for separate institutions run by women" (Dock, 1949; cited in Reverby, 1987, p. 72).

Lillian Wald also fought institutional subordination of nurses. For example, she presented a minority report to the New York State Conference of Charities and Corrections decrying the loss of nursing authority. If the nursing superintendent were appointed by physicians, she would overdo her responsibility to them and slight her other grave responsibilities. Nevertheless, the majority approved, giving final authority over nursing to a medical board.

On feminist grounds, Dock directly attacked Rowe's unal or single-authority plan, denying the validity of "his old-fashioned patriarchal ideas, likening his views on hospital organization to that of the traditional vision of the family as headed only by a man" (p. 72). In her strong feminist voice, Dock claimed that Rowe's plan made the *man* the unit, but the modern family had *two* heads—"on the principle, I suppose, that two heads are better than one"

(Dock, 1903; cited in Reverby, 1987, p. 72). Certainly, if nurse, medical, and hospital administrators *all* reported to the trustees, then the women would have equal footing. To Dock, blundering and interfering men, failing to understand women's work, created friction, but better this than "dull acquiescence in all sorts of improper arrangements" (Dock, 1903; cited in Reverby, 1987, p. 73). Clearly, physicians' modification of Nightingale's model was apparent to Dock, and she rejected it.

In Reverby's analysis, Dock's language is considered to be more overtly "antimale" than that of other nurse leaders; however, Reverby admits that Dock was articulating the shared view that nursing brought moral and technical order to hospitals. Indeed, Dock rejected the idea that women should be subordinated at the bedside or in the boardroom: furthermore, she expected that the advice of women and men would be treated equally by trustees. It is peculiar that naming the gender of an adversarial group and objecting to its attempt to subordinate another gender-defined group is described as antimale. This belittles Dock, making her seem to be involved in petty spats with individual men rather than in criticizing the restriction of nurses' relative independence in hospital structures. Simply put, feminist assertion is *not* equivalent to being antimale. Indeed, men *were* meddling in women's work for the specific purpose of gaining power over the work *and* the women.

Unfortunately, the trustees of Boston City Hospital sided with the physicians and hospital administrators, making the nursing superintendents more vulnerable and thus easier to attack. Eventually a medical monopoly was enhanced by the destruction of the key element in Nightingale's reform: the right of women nurses to control their own system, select their own leaders, and to report directly to trustees, not to physicians or administrators. Essentially, they also lost the right to decide appropriate and proper nursing procedures. This shift in organizational structure was a significant milestone in the development of medical monopoly.

A Purely Ancillary and Parasitic Existence?

Not only were nurses' training, practice, and organization topics of concern to physicians, but nurses' salaries and the question of whether nursing was a profession were hotly debated by physicians. Richard Cabot was one of the few to espouse positive and supportive ideas about nursing that have only recently been tried. Of medicine, he said: "Out of the trade of the barber and the apothecary we are . . . developing something worthy of the name of the liberal profession" (Cabot, 1901; cited in Ingles, 1976, p. 136). He saw a similar evolution in nursing, making a clear distinction between the training and the educating of nurses. Cabot's refreshing honesty is in sharp contrast to the tone of his colleagues writing in the *Journal of the American Medical Association,* in which one physician stated that the nurse was "purely ancillary" with an existence that is entirely parasitic and "dependent on the medical profession" (*Journal of the American Medical Association,* 1901; cited in Ingles, 1976, p. 140).

From still another editorial, this one in the July 1903 *Boston Medical and Surgical Journal,* it is obvious that men feared that women would claim the privileges which were linked to a "liberal profession." Raising the fear that is today even more apparent, the editor warned: "'physicians would become consultants and . . . nurses would become, essentially, practicing physicians'" (cited in Ingles, 1976, pp. 143–144). The editor asserted that such a role goes far beyond "our conception of nursing."

Francis Denny, MD, in the June 1903 *Boston Medical and Surgical Journal,* elaborated on the need for nurses to understand the principles of what they were doing. The repercussions from his "radical" piece included an editorial in which it is clear that the physician was not ready to lose a woman who was willing to do the "hard, menial, disagreeable work, which after all constitutes the essence of their calling" (*Boston Medical and Surgical Journal,* 1903; cited in Ingles, 1976, p. 142). According to one physician, the occupation needed speed, not salaries, wages being limited by "well-recognized conventions." It is clear that those conventions were based on women's debased salaries and status in general.

To some physicians, hospital control of nurses had had disastrous effects. According to R. L. Larsen (1904), in a letter to the editor of the *New York Medical Journal and Philadelphia Medical Journal,* the hospital had turned loose "female nurses who are as unfit to properly and scientifically nurse a sick human being as an infant is unfit for the task of constructing a twenty story skyscraper" (p. 235). He deplored the use of nurses to scrub or mop floors and then handle sterilized instruments or materials. Further, he said that there was no other term than graft for the practice of sending students out to care for patients when "the fee for nursing the patient is transferred to the institution's coffers" (p. 235). This graft was not hidden; indeed, hospitals even advertised that "undergraduates can be secured by patients at an expense of twelve to fifteen dollars a week" (p. 235).

In the same journal issue, Charles W. Kollock (1904) also deplored hospital graft, but advocated no more than two years of nurse training: "too much time is spent in attempting to teach them subjects which are not necessary. . . . This [will] displace important practical work, and perhaps, have a tendency to make them wiser in their own conceit and inclined to criticize the physicians under whom they serve" (p. 235). Drudgery is inherent in the job, but there is evidently even a "right" way to do a drudge's work.

As early as 1892, Dr. J. H. Emerson indicated that nurses do best with patients in hospitals and in private homes, and if their numbers increased, then competition would lead to a substantial reduction in their wages (cited in Ingles, 1976, p. 149). Dr. Alfred Worcester (1887), hardly an advocate of nursing education, claimed that nurses' salaries were higher than they should be and that women's education should proceed under the direction of physicians, particularly when dealing with patients in private homes (cited in Ingles, 1976, pp. 149–151). Today, the education of nurse clinicians under the preceptorship of physicians can be seen as a variation on the earlier views of physicians. These efforts to obtain direct control were fought by fledgling organizations of women in nursing, only to be reintroduced under different guises decades later.

Dr. Frank Allport (1909) addressed how nurses could be secured for poor people. He proposed six months of nurses' training in work outside the hospital, at a small fee, with or without room or board. The nurses' fees would be paid either to the hospital or to the nurse, who would then reimburse the hospital. Nurses were to pay for their training, receive small remuneration, and then divide their fees with the hospital, essentially providing almost free services to the poor (cited in Ingles, 1976, p. 151). Of course, the physicians retained their rights to more substantial incomes and to control both poor nurses and poor patients.

Ironically, at the same time that the "high wages" of nurses were deplored, an editor of the *New York Medical Journal* suggested that a ward be set up for older nurses who did not have medical insurance or earn enough money to care for themselves when sick. In England the need for pension funds for older nurses was advocated by Ethel Gordon Fenwick, who stated in 1900: "For the sake of the sick it is the duty of the people and the State to hold the balance of power between the associated professions of medicine and nursing, so that the economic independence of the one from the other . . . may be maintained as an essential principle. The evolution of the trained nurse in the future depends upon the evolution of the woman" (Ingles, 1976, p. 155). Fenwick clearly understood that the status of nursing depended on the general status of women; she strongly espoused the rights of nurses to organize to advance their own professional and economic causes.

In contrast, Dr. George M. Gould in a 1889 graduation speech to the John Hopkins School of Nursing advised against the organization of the nursing profession since "Majorities are tyrants and democracies are as tyrannous as any other type of government" (cited in Ingles, 1976, p. 155). Evidently, organized men could accept "tyrants," but they deplored majority rule for women! Gould proclaimed:

> [B]y nature woman in her use of social power and organization is a "born tyrant!" In the purely personal relation she is grace divine, but whenever put in authority over others, and especially over other women, she usually manages to make herself as hateful and hated as human ingenuity will permit. . . . The commercial doctor is bad enough; do not add the commercial nurse to the terrible burden under which humanity must suffer. If the spirit of trade-unionism gets control of your societies and organizations, I hope they will be quickly blown to smithereens. . . . I beg you will keep the financial relations to

your patients utterly out of reach of your laws and by-laws and resolutions. (cited in Ingles, 1974, pp. 156–157)

It is fascinating that the AMA, then and now one of the most powerful "unions," has successfully sustained financial relations with patients as a central concern of its predominantly male organization. But nurses were advised against organizing and to refrain from any financial considerations.

Not only did physicians feel they had the right to define the organizations, the education, the curriculum, and the identity of nursing as a vocation or profession—they also believed they had the right to determine women's relationship to the state. For example, in 1904, the *American Journal of Nursing* published an article by physician Francis Schill, who supported state registration of nurses and recommended better nursing standards and the restriction of nursing practitioners to those who were qualified. For the medical profession, these changes would give the physician assurance of a "supply of fairly uniform nurses, upon whom he can rely to carry out his instructions" (Schill, 1904, p. 34).

In contrast, Malcolm Morris, the physician who referred to women in nursing as parasites on physicians, thought that state laws on registration of nurses were "positively harmful." In the *Southern California Practitioner,* he asserted that physicians realized that hospital nurses "claim too much. They are often overbearing and dictatorial and require too much attention and waiting upon" (Morris, 1907; cited in Ingles, 1976, p. 157). If state registration laws were passed, he said, it would "only be a little while before doctors will refuse to employ such nurses and will turn to those with less pretentions [*sic*] but of greater usefulness" (p. 158).

Noting that nursing was the best-paid occupation for women—a deplorable assessment given the low salaries of women in and out of nursing at that time—Morris believed that any increase in wages meant that women were putting down physicians and patients. The editor of the *Southern California Practitioner* agreed and recommended that physicians should affect the nursing world "with appropriate attitudes" and "instill . . . a spirit of self-sacrifice" (cited in Ingles, 1976, p. 158). Evidently, men were to work for money, but women were to work for the glory of humanity.

"We Must Reprove Every Attempt at Initiative on the Part of Nurses"

One measure of medical respect for nurses and their leaders is the extent to which their thoughts and opinions were published in medical journals. Unfortunately, Ingles found *only two* articles written by nurses in the medical journals during the entire forty-year period she researched. Nursing leader Isabel Hampton, at Johns Hopkins University Hospital, and Mary Samuel, superintendent of nurses at Roosevelt Hospital, are the only two women whose writings appeared in medical journals (Hampton, 1889; Samuel, 1906). In her article, Samuel exemplified the required tact so valued by Osler: "The many avenues now open to women in the nursing profession make a broader education essential. . . . It is surely well-known that the more reliable, efficient and highly qualified a nurse may be, the less likely is she to overstep the bounds; much more often is it the uneducated, the unrefined, inefficiently trained woman who thus brings discredit on her profession" (Samuel, 1906; cited in Ingles, 1976, p. 161). Ingles's data and analysis seem to parallel Lovell's, indicating that many men in medicine were increasingly threatened by women in nursing and acted to control them, striving to erase any semblance of autonomy that might emerge.

Indeed, as Jo Ann Ashley (1976) documented, sexism in the "hospital family" continued unabated in the 1900s, reinforcing the idea that the role of women was to serve men's needs and convenience. Stereotyped as less independent, creative, and intelligent than men and as lacking initiative, nurses were increasingly controlled by medical and administrative men who claimed the right to ensure that nurses would remain "ideal" women. Physicians continued to exert their control over hospital training schools, and they repeatedly expressed their views that nurses existed solely to assist physicians and hospitals. Physicians continued to fear nurses' independence from the medical profession. Since the physicians were educated, a nurse did not need to be. She could rely on her "womanly qualities." Indeed, William Alexander Dorland (1908), physician and professor at the University of Pennsylvania, told the 1908 graduating class of the Philadelphia School of Nursing that they must accept their intellectual inferiority—a little knowledge is a dangerous, even "fatal" thing. Too elaborate a professional education would hamper nurses or even render them useless. For him, a capable nurse was born, not made.

In 1906 the *Journal of the American Medical Association* published "Nurses' Schools and Illegal Practice of Medicine," in which physicians and administrators were urged to reprove "[e]very attempt at initiative on the part of nurses" (*Journal of the American Medical Association*, 1906; cited in Ashley, 1976, p. 78). Furthermore, instruction should be "limited strictly to the indispensable matters" and avoid everything that would "lead them to substitute themselves for the physician" (p. 78). To ensure this, only physicians should teach nurses. These steps were justified as "a matter of simple justice" (p. 78).

As Ashley emphasized, the nurses were attacked not simply as nurses, but as women. In 1908, for example, Ludlam attacked the excessively "comprehensive" teaching of dietetics to student nurses: knowledge of "proteids, carbohydrates, starch, dextrin, minerals, and salts" (Ashley, 1976, p. 80) was unnecessary. Instead, the women needed to know how to serve a piece of steak or a chop before the gravy had congealed. In 1909 Henry Beates stressed the need for nurses to receive only the bare essentials of medical knowledge. Their training was too absurdly comprehensive and would lead them to "usurp the functions of physicians" (p. 80). A woman should *never* appear learned or of great importance; rather, she should render intelligent obedience to the physician. More particularly, Beates asserted, head nurses should be "*especially,* the subjects of intelligent official control" (p. 81). Realizing that nurses were moving to professional status, physicians moved to stop them and force them to meet the needs of physicians.

Ingles noted that physicians in New York publications deplored the "'overtrained nurse . . . [who] frequently presumes . . . to sit in judgment of physicians . . . in a meddlesome and sometimes offensive manner'" (Ingles, 1976, p. 147). In 1906 Dr. W. Gilman Thompson stated the problem succinctly: "The whole question is this: Is nursing a subordinate profession to medicine, or is it a separate distinct and independent profession?" (Ingles, 1976, p. 147). To which he responded, "The work of the nurse is an honorable 'calling' or vocation, and nothing further" (p. 147). The good physician suggested that payment of tuition for nurses' training, which had been proposed as a way to provide support for "women in distress," would be improper, since women were unlikely to work more than ten years. This attack on women's educational needs and aspirations was the same as the broader assault on women in general, based on an erroneous set of assumptions current then and still alive in different guises today.

In 1910 physician Francis Denny wrote a surprising article on the need for instruction in nursing as part of medical education. Denny recognized that in the cure of acute disease, "There remains a small number of doubtful cases where life hangs in the balance" (p. 596). In these, nursing is recognized as critical. For alleviation of suffering, Denny affirmed the use of opium and other drugs, but thought the work of the nurse stands "high in comparison."

The really critical problem to the physician was that he could not supervise the nurse intelligently (or control her) if he did not know her methods. Denny stated that physicians needed to know nursing in order to prescribe treatment; for example, they might see the discomfort of patients and the number of disturbances caused by physicians' demands. Medical students were urged to have one or two months of nursing experience, particularly at nighttime when patients' conditions vary. Although objections could be raised that poor nursing of patients would result, Denny claimed that male medical students were stronger than nurses so patients would not be delayed getting to bedpans, etc. There seems little comprehension that the nurses might have objections to this assertion! Although positive to nursing, Denny was still interested in control. Curiously, he did not realize that his plan originated with a nurse, who had different motives for unifying nursing and medicine. In a tactful but pointed editorial in the *American Journal of Nursing* (*AJN*), it is suggested that Denny had essentially "stolen" the idea from a nurse, Miss Davis: "our criticism is that Dr. Denny does not seem to know that the plan is three years old, that his plan originated in the brain of a trained nurse. . . . Surely Dr. Denny must have been taking a long nap. . . . We welcome every helping hand in this work, but we reiterate that the two professions of medicine and nursing must be united in their efforts before either can expect to accomplish much for good in the way of nursing advancement (*American Journal of Nursing*, 1910, pp. 1000–1001).

A Hint of Things to Come: A Physician's Proposal for Two Classes of Nurses

In sharp contrast to the direction nursing was taking at this time was the experiment in nursing education proposed by William O. Stillman (1910). Speaking to a medical association in 1909, he advocated the need for two classes of nurses, presumably in order to serve larger numbers of patients from the poor as well as middle and upper classes. The cost of fully trained nurses was presumably too high. However, the income differential between physicians and nurses was not mentioned. Nor was it suggested that the higher cost of physicians should lead to the creation of two classes of MDs.

Nevertheless, Stillman asserted that previously domestic nurses were "as a rule densely ignorant of the fundamental requirements of good nursing, and largely controlled by superstitions, prejudices, and laziness" (p. 111). Visiting nurses were useful, but not for long-term attendance. Furthermore, Stillman felt it was impossible to develop such nursing on a sufficiently large scale, because endowments were not available to offset the inadequate fees from poorer patients. It is interesting that he did not conceive of state-funded free clinics, later proposed and enacted in the Sheppard-Towner Act (see chapter 5), which organized medicine vigorously opposed. Indeed, Stillman rejected increasing the knowledge of physiology and hygiene through public schools, another part of the Sheppard-Towner Act, embodied in nurses' education of mothers and children in clinics and homes.

In contrast to the nurses' own solution—using state-sponsored clinics and home visitations—Stillman's proposal was to produce less thoroughly trained nurses; this would set up competition among the women, which would ultimately reduce the wages of trained nurses and create a hierarchy in the nursing profession. Stillman claimed that the alternative was for trained nurses to reduce their fees for poor patients, as physicians presumably did. Given the male-female income differential and the relative absence of physicians caring for the poor, this suggestion was highly questionable.

Stillman decided that physicians must take over the training of the second class of nurses in a six-month course that did not "overtrain" or cause the women to consider themselves as even approaching the grade of registered nurse. Stillman found a number of excellent women among those who were desperate, having been suddenly thrown upon the world or left with a dependent family. Clearly, in a gender-stratified society, such women would hardly have many, if any, options. This was the real basis of Stillman's solution to the "nurse problem." Although he made the point that "his" women would not compete with fully trained women, "Our nurses are encouraged to take nursing magazines and continue their studies after graduation. We require them to wear a nurse's cap and distinctive nurse's dress" (p. 112). These women were expected to work for $12 to $15 a week. Obviously, no matter how well-intentioned this proposal, the fact remained that physicians were taking over the education of nurses, reducing their training to a bare minimum, and creating a class of women who would eventually directly compete with fully trained nurses.

The "Nursing Problem": One Physician's Attack on Nursing Leaders

Another physician who saw nurses as "the problem" was AMA president Theodore Potter (1910). In his speech to the AMA, Potter claimed there was no medical opposition to the modern nurse; however, he complained that nursing textbooks, to which he gave little attention in his address, had evolved into "treatises upon the practice of medicine" (p. 995). Seeming to contradict himself, he lauded physicians for giving some of their time to provide nurses with lectures very similar to those in medical schools. Unfortunately, he failed to mention the severely limited number of lectures and the lack of theoretical materials available to nursing students, or that they were overworked as free laborers in hospitals.

According to Potter, physicians had "endorsed, complimented, gallantly flattered, and gratefully almost petted the trained nurse, with her neat cap and gown" (p. 995). At no point did he recognize physicians' misuse of women students, or their rejection of nurses during the Civil War, or their historical attempts to limit or control nursing education and practice. Indeed, in his view, physicians had "gladly aided nurses in almost anything which they thought desirable and have been easily persuaded to endorse and cooperate" (p. 995).

After ignoring historical facts and applauding what good fellows the physicians had been, Potter arrived at his main point: nurses are largely under the direction, even domination, of a few leaders, who had accomplished radical changes, but these did not qualify nurses as professionals. Indeed, complained Potter, the management and control of nursing schools had become quite independent of the medical profession and were being used "to advance the political interests and plans of the organization politicians" (p. 995). He distinguished these political nurses as different from those of ability and force of character. Some nurses had even affiliated with the American Federation of Labor! On the other hand, some "organization politicians" advocate nursing as a profession (p. 995). Condescendingly, Potter acknowledged that the term "professional" could refer to a horseman or even a thief, but the term was usually associated with two qualities, autonomy and independence: "And neither of these belongs to the vocation of the nurse" (p. 996). The physician gathers truth from all sources but at the dictation of no one; he formulates principles, plans of action, and applications "as he pleases, as he thinks best, subject only to his own reason and moral sense and the law of the land" (p. 996). But this is not true of nursing, which is "essentially subordinate" (p. 996).

To Potter, the fundamentals of the sick or operating room were "expressions of the needs, wishes, and scientific demands of physicians, not of nurses" (p. 996). Even diets, baths, douches, enemas, mechanical agents of record keeping, and physiological observations were the essentials of medicine; therefore, "the individual physician must be supreme, independent, the individual nurse subordinate and dependent though by no means servile" (p. 996). The appeal to personal worth and rights and the useful and honorable necessity of her calling—these had no direct bearing on professional status. That nurses engaged in scientific study was inconsequential. The nurses' "earnest, sometimes indignant, repudiation of a servile position" (p. 996) was irrelevant.

The nursing leaders, "organization politicians," were a "necessary nuisance to be endured as long as possible" (p. 997). So much for women like Dock or Wald! To Potter, politically active women were concerned about positions, log rolling, getting themselves and their friends on the platform. The other type of women leaders were thinkers, teachers, and educators, who, even though they were irrational about being professional, still deserved sympathy. Potter did grant them professional status, but only as educators, not nurses. As educators, Potter admitted they did have some qualities of autonomy and independence.

Nurses striving for official and professional positions presumably did not want to meet the higher requirements of medical licensure. According to Potter, they had pushed hastily forward "in connection with the general movement for 'the emancipation of women' and with some forced and artificial features, which, it seems to me, will need critical but broad minded revision" (p. 997). The route for any dissatisfied nurse was not to become a contemptible "near doctor" but a physician.

Potter also attacked nurses' fees, their "excessive commercialism," and the "close corporations of graduate students" (p. 997). This from medicine! Indeed, nursing textbooks, which now covered the whole field of medical science and practice, were, said Potter, caused by commercial motivations. If he were a nurse, Potter said, he would "contemptuously throw such books into the fire" (p. 998).

The domestic nurses ranged from the "bumptious and dirty ignoramus," to the "well meaning but crude amateur," to a "limited number of really responsible and capable nongraduates" (p. 998). Potter claimed the *nurse* autocracy caused patients to dread expenses. As expected, he believed that nurses' training was much too long, and he supported Stillman's proposal to produce two distinct classes of nurses.

Although it would be "uncharitable" to criticize, Potter said that nurses must conquer misconduct: "[b]ribery, graft, unchaste word and action or worse, unkind humiliation or weakening flattery and adulation" (p. 998). In addition, nurses should not pet or coddle rich patients, or use silly endearing terms. Finally, Potter, in agreement with an unnamed but "eminent" British authority, charged that "the trained nurse has stolen a birthright of the medical student" (p. 998). So much for the history and predominance of women healers in previous centuries! Their origins and contributions were totally ignored and denied by Potter.

Potter called for the AMA to review the "problem" of women in nursing. He assured his audience in his presidential address that he had not tried to excite the physicians to anger, malice, or unreason; indeed his words would not, he was certain, lead to an attack on the nursing "vocation" or individual nurses. Potter claimed to make no recommendations, he simply posed them as questions—a Machiavellian strategy that could not help but incite his physician audience to further hostility toward nursing.

Objections to Educated Nurses Are Trivial and Childish!

In contrast to Potter, a few physicians, such as Henry M. Hurd (1910), supported educated nurses. In a commencement speech (he had given one every year since 1891), Hurd honored the fiftieth anniversary of the St. Thomas' training school and the ninetieth birthday of its founder, Florence Nightingale. Hurd credited Nightingale with major influences on the medical profession and with bringing order out of the Crimean chaos of official incompetence, although he did not discuss her struggle with physicians.

Hurd understood that a medical order may state what should be done, but a nurse's training tells her how to do it: "Telling the nurse what to do is not enough and cannot be enough to make her work perfect" (p. 72). Nightingale's emphasis on educated observation and reflection for women led Hurd to ask, "Has any instrument of precision ever been put into the hands of physicians which has begun to do as much for the advancement of true medical work as the trained intelligence of the educated nurse?" (pp. 72–73).

While nurses might question whether they want to be instruments in men's hands, most could agree with Hurd's assertion that the current objections over the "so-called over-educated and over-trained nurse" (p. 73) were trivial and childish. Directly taking on gender stereotypes, Hurd deplored "the laudations heard even now in the year of our Lord 1910 of the natural-born nurse who 'mothers' her patients, who needs no training and who only follows her heaven-born impulses and her womanly intuition" (p. 73). Hurd asserted that physicians should be thankful for Nightingale's insistence on training because they can expect and demand the intelligent and skilled assistance which have "contributed immeasurably to the success of medical and surgical practice" (p. 73).

Such public commendations of nurses by physicians were rare in the early twentieth century. Even MDs who encouraged broader education for nurses continued to view them as subordinates. For example, Richard Olding Beard (1913) stated at an AMA meeting in Minneapolis that nurses were essentially handmaids to medicine, but they did need university-based education. Although medicine was the habitual critic of nurses' development, Beard believed this was logical because physicians were the only ones appropriate to judge nurses' fitness. He did not suggest, however, that nurses were the only appropriate judges of physicians' fitness. As a "human commodity," the nurse was the most helpless and, because of unfitness, the "most hopeless factor in the evolution of her own class" (Beard, 1913, p. 2150). Poorly prepared, imperfectly trained, even in essentials, hurriedly pushed into an alien world, the female nurse was "a half-baked product . . . [the] instinct of the eternal feminine for sacrificial service has been her sole saving grace, the guiding light of her star of undoubted destiny" (p. 2150).

Despite this stereotyped perception, Beard nevertheless supported university education for nurses, who, at the University of Minnesota, received their degrees on the recommendation of the medical, not the nursing, faculty. Beard criticized hospitals for making nursing education their own economic salvation by using the free labor of nursing students and by overworking them. He called for the elimination of substandard hospital schools of nursing or their affiliation with university medical schools. However, "The schools for nurses should be under the direction of the medical faculty or should have a special faculty affiliated with the medical school, on which a number of medical educators should sit" (p. 2151).

Beard objected to the proposals made by Stillman and other physicians to create different "classes" of nurses. He argued for standardization of nurses for *all* people, a goal still sought by professional nursing today but too often opposed by organized medicine. Although regarded as a friend of nursing, Beard nevertheless still saw nurses as women to be directly or indirectly controlled by physicians. He seemed mainly concerned with which group of men had the "right" to nurses and nursing. Involved in the struggle between physicians and hospital administrators over the control of nursing, the "ever-extending commodities requiring male ownership" included social groups, which were "human commodities. . . . To these groups, the profession of nursing women belongs" (Beard, 1913; cited in Lovell, 1982, p. 216). Beard claimed that the hospital had become the "creative agent" of the "trained nurse" and was now attempting to become "the maker and molder of 'the thing created'—its 'foster mother'" (cited in Lovell, 1982, p. 216). Note the complete and deceptive silence about Florence Nightingale, Clara Barton, and the many women who actually created "modern" nursing. After erroneously crediting administrative and medical men with the creation of nurses, Beard then asserted physicians' "rightful" ownership of nurses. Even though physicians had been only "advisors" over the birth of "modern" nursing, medicine had been the "habitual critic of her development" and "rightly so" because only the physician could competently judge a nurse's fitness and unfitness (cited in Lovell, 1982, p. 216). Thus, physicians, not hospital administrators, should control and own nurses.

To Lovell, this oppressive paternalism was and still is "violent and abusive": nurses were dehumanized, even referred to as "it." Nursing input was not considered; nurses were treated as objects to be acted upon, not as human beings able to take action. The medical "right" to coerce and manipulate nurses was simply assumed to be the prerogative of the physician, who presumed to exercise his authority for the nurse's "own good." If medicine could control nursing education, then nursing would come more directly under the authority of physicians. Beard recommended that the profession of medicine, the "natural ally" of nursing, should provide its "wisdom" to the women, who must determine, but only with the help of the medical profession, whose handmaids they were.

The Neutering of Women? Physicians' Views of Feminism and Nurses' Independence in the Early Twentieth Century

The "wisdom" of physician ownership was clearly threatened by some nursing leaders, who were labeled "organization politicians," particularly those who espoused suffrage and who were attacked in a 1915 medical critique of women's liberation. Its author, Arthur C. Jacobson, MD, asserted that feminism was a misnomer. To him, "neuterism" was the more appropriate term. If feminism differentiated the sexes by intensifying the feminine character, then the name was "appropriate." However, if feminism declared that "sex ought not to be considered in art, literature, science, business, or politics, would it not seem to be opposed to such differentiation?" (cited in *Medical Times,* 1972, p. 71). Jacobson could or would not conceive of any other gender template for women or men; they were two kinds of people with very different characteristics. He could not conceive of women taking on "masculine" characteristics, but even if this were conceivable, he concluded: "It is possible for women to cease in part to be women, but it is not possible for them to become men in any degree" (p. 71).

Jacobson warned that higher education and economic independence might result in "fewer marriages, fewer children, lack of the maternal instinct, relative inability to nurse children, and lack of interest in the elementary sex impulse and purpose" (p. 71). Since these were a denial of "feminine" attributes, then feminism was misnamed. To Jacobson, it was a fact that feminists, who were more austere than saints, would "abolish wholly the sex appeal in its age-long form or in any other form" (p. 71). Feminists, "more respectable than angels," had an "instinctive aversion" to a woman who lives "a full feminine life" (p. 71). Without the slightest awareness of the irony, Jacobson thought feminists incapable of comprehending a George Sand. (In actuality, some feminists had claimed her—Aurore Dudevant—as an example of a creative woman who chose her own lifestyle.)

Jacobson believed that the feminist was at war with femininity, more than with man and his world. Indeed, woman's sphere was, to a feminist, man's sphere. Note again the sharp division into two separate globes of action. To Jacobson, feminism was not feminine because it excluded, limited, or ignored the woman's special sexual functions, suppressed the sex instinct, created sterility, and presented any child born with a dry breast. In his view this dry-breasted creature considered sex a nightmare and the act of love, a crime. Given these definitions, Jacobson concluded that "there must be but few real feminists in the world" (p. 72). If these few were successful, there would be a world "peopled in large part by frigid, sterile, economically capable and academized (not educated) neuters, akin to the workers set apart by certain departments of the insect world" (p. 72).

Jacobson claimed that he could tell a "feminist" by her adeptness in dodging a woman's sphere; she should actually be called a "neuter" (perhaps even an insect!). How could nurses deal rationally with physicians such as Jacobson? Did he include nurses in his "neuter" category? He wrote for a medical audience who might easily transpose his categories to women in nursing. Any assertive nurse could be seen as going beyond woman's "natural" sphere and thus be labeled a neuter. Jacobson's view is a chilling example of medicine's determination not only to control and define nursing and nurses, but to define the essence of femaleness as well.

The impact of such pronouncements, given the societal subordination of women in general, was potentially severe. The degree to which women nurses incorporated such "medical" views of women activists and of independent nurses is unclear. However, some nurses, such as Sarah E. Dock (1917), almost apologized for the monopoly of nursing by women: "It is about the only thing we are allowed to do without the blame of trying to take away the work from the poor men" (p. 394). Deploring a lack of nursing applicants, Sarah Dock blamed this on lack of training for obedience: "No matter how gifted she may be, she will never become a reliable nurse until she can obey without question. The first and most helpful criticism I ever received from a doctor was when he told me that I was supposed to be an intelligent machine for the purpose of carrying out his orders" (p. 394). For this nurse, strictly formal, professional relations were required, although greater clarity was needed on whether and when a nurse could act in an emergency. "Naturally the doctor is or should be the nurse's chief instructor" (p. 395). Time for relaxation must be provided, because "Even a machine needs rest and repair" (p. 396). And, of course, if the "machine" was not functioning properly, it should be replaced by another one.

Ironically, it was the traditional, not the feminist, nurse who had become a machine, a neutered or at least a neutral object, almost an obedient robot. Clearly, the antifeminist propaganda of Jacobson and other physicians had produced the desired effect in at least some nurses. Others were, however, more outspoken and progressive.

"The Fine Figure of an American Nurse"

As the United States entered the First World War in 1917, many nurses volunteered their services, despite the opposition and disapproval of male military conflagrations by nurses such as Lavinia Dock and Lillian Wald. As in the Spanish-American and Civil Wars, the nurses, even though now better organized, still retained an ambiguous status. They continued to receive less than honorable treatment. (For a fuller discussion of nurses in wartime, see Roberts and Group, 1995). Nevertheless, the need for nurses became critical; many served and some received public recognition for their efforts.

In 1919 Brigadier General W. S. Thayer gave the eulogy for nursing leader Jane A. Delano in Philadelphia. For Thayer, Delano belonged to that group of women who had become the right arm and a necessary branch of the medical profession. Thayer claimed that one of the greatest advances in medicine had been the perfection of nursing methods. Having subsumed nursing, medicine could now take credit for it as "the most important element of treatment" (Thayer, 1919, p. 188). To him, gentle women had always nursed the sick. What was new was the standardization of nursing, which he now attributed to medicine's influence. Laborious nursing tasks required physical strength, but also intelligence, stability, and strength of character: "Relatively few women are adapted to the career of a trained nurse" (p. 189).

Reflecting on the prejudice expressed toward women nurses in 1891 among the male medical officers in the Spanish-American War, Thayer admitted these biases continued; however, Delano was credited with establishing the Army Nursing Corps and Red Cross Reserve. Recounting the horrors under which the nurses worked, Thayer praised them effusively, and he commended Delano: "She was a fine figure, the figure of an American Nurse" (p. 192). Unfortunately, such high praise did not lead to officers' commissions with full power nor to full military benefits for nurses. These did not come for decades.

Despite prejudicial treatment, nurses can be credited with organizing military nursing and struggling to provide decent care in both the Spanish-American War and the First World War. It is also to nursing's credit that through the decades of the late nineteenth and early twentieth centuries, while physicians were consolidating their power in health care, individual nurses and some of their leaders continued their difficult struggle to attain more education and the right to educate and supervise the members of their profession, and to organize themselves into a body of respected graduate nurses. Throughout these decades, nurses had to deal with many physicians and hospital administrators who trivialized and demeaned nursing's contributions to health care, who supported the societal gender stereotypes of women as subordinate to men, less intelligent, and unworthy of collegial respect. As documented in previous chapters, centuries of competent health-care practices by women healers were forgotten, ignored, or denied. Medicine's propaganda even wrested from the women the historical, factual public health-care initiatives developed by them, leading the public to believe that physicians had always been the primary healers, always possessed superior medical and pharmaceutical knowledge, always had their patients' best interests at heart, and always had these, not economic gains, as their sole concern.

Medicine's monopoly of health care solidified during the late nineteenth and early twentieth centuries due in large part to gains in knowledge derived from the basic sciences. In addition, this period fostered societal perceptions of women as "naturally" weaker than men and biologically inferior. These forces destroyed many attempts by nurses to achieve a higher status for their profession. Still, despite medicine's hostility toward nursing and its fear of economic and professional competition, nurses continued their efforts to achieve professional recognition while at the same time working for social reform in many areas critical to health care. As will be seen in chapter 5, nurses continued to be a problem for organized medicine and physicians were more determined than ever to consolidate their power and achieve a total medical monopoly.

5 | "The Exclusive Guardians of All Matters of Health"

The Consolidation of Medical Monopoly in the 1920s and 1930s

By 1920 the Western world had been through a terrible war, in which close to 550,000 Americans were killed, including 300 nurses who had served overseas. World War I not only claimed a horrible toll in human life, it also served as a catalyst to swell the ranks of qualified graduate nurses. Although some nurses, such as Lillian Wald and Lavinia Dock, were deeply opposed to war, many nurses volunteered their services, and the importance of nursing to the war effort was recognized by virtually every segment of society.

To satisfy demands for nursing personnel, nursing schools and their leaders scrambled to provide sufficient numbers of qualified graduate nurses, not only for service overseas but for the civilian population as well. As in other wars, nursing's popularity and status rose during America's involvement in World War I, and so did physicians' status and power. However, when the war ended, nurses returning home were expected to marry or revert to the more subordinate role associated with civilian nursing. Physicians, on the other hand, took active steps to consolidate their power and monopoly in health care.

By 1920 feminists had finally succeeded in gaining suffrage and political enfranchisement for women; they had reformed a wide spectrum of laws, practices, and attitudes, forcing open colleges and universities, occupations, and professions to women. But as the women's movement declined or shifted away from clear-cut women's issues to broader social concerns in the later 1920s and 1930s, medical power and control were being consolidated. Thus, women in nursing experienced declining support from feminists and increasing domination by physicians. After gaining control of hospital nursing, physicians exerted their influence over public health. Though nurses and other health reformers fought for and supported the federal Sheppard-Towner Maternity and Infancy Protection Act, designed to improve women's and children's health, organized medicine opposed the act and eventually caused its demise, which slowed or stopped the national network of clinics it would have established.

Nurses researched and documented the inadequate and unsatisfactory state of nursing education and practice and struggled valiantly to create uniform standards and training based on state licensure. Most physicians, however, opposed the nurses' goals, in part because by the 1920s nurses were the only remaining viable competitors to physicians on every front. Physicians continued to admonish nurses, including those in public health, to be obedient to medical authority. By the 1930s the American Medical Association (AMA) had established a set of committees on nursing that tightened its control. Medical domination was made easier, too, by the severely difficult circumstances caused by the Great Depression. The working conditions and economic status of nurses declined significantly during this period, while the economic and social status of physicians remained constant or even improved.

The debate on whether nursing was scientific work or a nurturing ministry veiled nurses' actual work and their inventive efforts. Often gender, not science, determined the degree to which a particular technology was considered scientific. The male-controlled media, now including the radio and motion pictures, created and reinforced the images of the nurturing, loyal nurse and the sacrificing, scientifically competent country doctor. In subsequent decades, these images were continued, in more urbanized, sophisticated form, by television. Some nurses, such as Elizabeth Kenny, defied these images, questioned medical power, and created their own therapeutic techniques, only to fall victim to severe medical censure. Whether the censure of these nurses and the medical monopoly of diagnosis, prescriptive authority, and practice were in the patient's best interest is highly questionable. In this chapter, we continue to trace the gendered struggle between organized medicine on one side and nursing and women health reformers on the other, and consider the work of nurses during the 1920s and the 1930s.

The Consolidation of Medical Power

The consolidation of medical power was largely accomplished by the 1920s. In 1904 the AMA established the Council on Medical Education; it formulated a minimum standard of four years of high school, an equivalent period of medical training, and a licensing examination. By 1910 the grading of medical schools, according to requirements of state licensing boards, had reduced by one-fifth the number of medical schools in the United States (Starr, 1982). Lengthening the required educational period produced a long-term decline in the number of medical students. The increased cost of modern laboratories, libraries, and clinical facilities forced mergers with private or state universities. The AMA Council on Medical Education sought funding from the Carnegie Foundation. Abraham Flexner, the foundation's representative, surveyed medical schools and found libraries with no books, laboratories that consisted of a few test tubes in cigar boxes, and reeking corpses caused by failure to use disinfectants. Even Harvard University had no physiology laboratory before 1870.

Flexner's investigation led to closure of several schools and thus enhanced the market position of the smaller number of physicians that resulted. The AMA's power increased as it became the only accrediting agency for medical schools. By 1922 only 81 medical schools remained; these produced 2,529 graduates in that year. Thirty-eight states now required two years of preliminary college work before entrance to medical school (Starr, 1982, p. 121). By 1936 the Rockefeller Foundation gave $91 million to medical schools, with two-thirds going to seven institutions. The intent was to wed research to medical practice; thus, medicine cashed in on the increasing reverence for science and technology. Nevertheless, the widespread aversion of some physicians to basic science was still apparent in the battles between old-line practitioners and the new research scientists.

Eventually, homogeneity and cohesiveness of the profession resulted, with greater uniformity in values and beliefs. The first listing of hospital internships, open to some medical school graduates, was published by the AMA in 1914; by 1923 these were available to all graduates. Deliberate discriminatory practices against women, Jews, and African Americans promoted greater social homogeneity, reversing the somewhat more liberal policies during earlier periods when feminism was stronger (Starr, 1982, p. 124). The declining number of women physicians was caused by outright discrimination, sustained for most of this century by quotas which limited women to only 5 percent of medical school admissions, as noted in chapter 4. Only nurses were left as potential competitors to physicians.

By the 1920s the distribution of physicians was related to the per capita income by region, resulting in geographical and urban-rural inequities. Physicians had forced out other competitors—for example, osteopaths and chiropractors—by denying access to hospital privileges or the right to prescribe drugs. The fight over authority to prescribe drugs was led by the AMA, and by the 1920s the drug manufacturers could deal only with physicians. Ironically, it was the physicians themselves who had misused many drugs, such as laudanum in the nineteenth century. These misuses, especially of psychotropic drugs, have been in large part directed toward women.

The logic of the AMA's regulatory system was simple: "withhold information from consumers and rechannel drug purchasing through physicians" (Starr, 1982, p. 133). Even baby food and milk substitutes were channeled this way. With no feeding instructions provided for mothers, they were forced to go to physicians, who often gave them faulty information based on manufacturers' misleading claims.

Public health advances, particularly the isolation of organisms responsible for infectious diseases and immunological breakthroughs, were far more successful in the late nineteenth and early twentieth centuries than were the rest of medical "therapeutics" or the drugs used to treat diseases. Nurses were directly involved in these public health advances, but eventually they lost their control over the bureaucracies that evolved. Nevertheless, evidence suggests that the great decline in mortality rates around the turn of the century was due primarily to changing lifestyles and to general public health hygiene efforts.

Actually, reductions in mortality from specific diseases occurred *before* effective prophylactics or therapies were in the hands of physicians. Neverthe-less, they took much of the credit for the work of nurses, women reformers, and public health advocates. Dr. Paul Ehrlich's salvarsan, for the treatment of syphilis, the first major chemotherapeutic agent, was not improved upon until sulfa drugs were developed some twenty-five years later. Antiseptic techniques and anesthesia increased the prestige of surgery. Here, nurses were originally central as early anesthesiologists, but again they subsequently lost ground. New diagnostic techniques were also prohibited to nurses. Just as thermome-ters were initially denied to women, so each new instrument was denied; then, as newer technology became available, the women were sometimes allowed to use the older methods. As Starr noted, these new procedures, such as the X-ray, enabled physicians to view and discuss what they saw at a distance from both patients and nurses, thus contributing to professional disparity and med-ical dominance over diagnoses.

With monopoly, physicians' income and prestige rose. Between 1900 and 1928 their annual incomes doubled from a range of $750–$1,500 to a range of $1,500–$3,000. Their average net income in 1928 was $6,354. From 1929 to 1934, during the Depression, their average income was still three to four times higher than those in other occupations (Starr, 1982). These figures cannot be accounted for by increased costs of education alone. The barriers that re-stricted entry to medicine were also responsible: by the 1930s, medical schools were rejecting 45 percent of their applicants. Before 1900, admission rejec-tions, noted Starr, had been virtually unknown. By 1925 occupational prestige rankings rated physicians third, behind bankers and college professors, and just ahead of the clergy and lawyers. Subsequent rankings have consistently placed them in top positions.

Collective mobility of the medical profession was accomplished by system-atically subordinating threatening competitors, such as nurses, and denying them knowledge, autonomy, and power. Medical authority, arising from nurses' and patients' deference and institutionalized forms of dependence, en-couraged the public to see medical interests as similar to their own (Starr, 1982). It is doubtful this could have been accomplished to the same degree if nurses had achieved independent status and deprived physicians of large num-bers of deferential female followers.

Nurses Rebel: Want More Control over Education and Working Conditions

By the turn of the century and continuing to the end of the 1930s, nurses in major cities increasingly complained of overcrowding on hospital wards, limited training opportunities, overwork, and repressive hospital and medical control of nursing registries and private duty work. Historian Susan Reverby (1979) recognized that the graduate nurse was in an ambiguous situation: a professional expected to do servant's work; an independent worker paid a standard wage and subject to busy and slow seasons like a factory worker; a skilled worker but one with no financial incentives, training, or supervision to improve skills.

Although Reverby claimed that the nursing schools had become "stunted matriarchies," she admits that by 1910 nursing leaders had moved strongly against overcrowding and lack of training. Some nurses even engaged in sporadic strikes and limited union organization. Hospital administrators had to agree to some upgrading because they were losing control over their workforce as more patients refused care by untrained student nurses, bringing their own private-duty nurses to hospitals instead. Hospital administrators still did not understand how to determine their own costs or measure productivity. By 1914 efficiency experts such as Frank Gilbreth criticized the lack of standardization and the haphazard organization of hospital work.

By the 1920s administrators were "refurbishing their nineteenth-century paternalism in order to obtain a more loyal work force" (Reverby, 1979, p. 213). To achieve loyalty from within required training to identify with the hospital "family," but institutional personalities were not readily forthcoming; therefore, hospitals were "constantly searching for workers who could be relied upon to be loyal, self-motivating within set limits, imbued with the service ethic, willing to accept low wages and their place in the hierarchy, and yet able to transcend normal work loads when emergencies (defined by the administration) or shortages occurred" (p. 214). In other words, women workers were wanted because they could be forced to take lower salaries, were socialized to give service, and blocked from upward organizational mobility. In her analysis, Reverby lumped together nursing and hospital administrators, who presumably together resolved the "nursing" problem by creating subsidiary nursing workers as demanded by physicians' committees. However, even in the 1920s, many nurses and their leaders rejected recommendations, such as Stillman's (1910; see chapter 4), to create different levels and types of nurses. Indeed, Reverby recognized that many nurses feared that nursing assistants would legitimize lower-priced competition. Nevertheless, she also stated that there were many nursing and hospital leaders who saw the need for a complex division of labor. It remains unclear just how many nursing leaders supported and rejected these alternatives. Nor is it clear how many nursing administrators simply gave in or compromised because they could see no other pragmatic alternative, given the difficult working conditions of nurses.

How did the status of nurses and their roles compare to those of other women workers? In 1921 Elizabeth K. Adams examined health services other than medicine, in which she acknowledged the impetus given by World War I to effect a public health movement. She recognized that nurses were on the front line in the development of health centers. However, she noted: "Of health workers other than doctors, the hundred thousand odd graduate, or registered nurses are by far the largest, best-known, and oldest group. Nursing, like medicine, is in process of reorganization. But for the present, it is in the main a potential rather than an actual profession, to be compared with teaching more truly than with law or medicine" (p. 86).

Adams recognized the extensive efforts of nurses to deal with the wide variations in the quality and status of hospital training schools, the low standards for admission, the misuse of student nurses for the financial profit of hospitals, and the traditional conception of the nurse as a routine worker. Leaders in nursing clearly recognized these defects and had taken active steps to remedy them. Adams stressed that training and teaching could no longer be confined "within the walls of the hospital" (p. 89). The emphasis on nursing outside the hospital had emerged through the public health nurse, who "becomes an expert field agent . . . rather than the subordinate of a single physician" (p. 90). Adams stated that the problems between nurses and physicians "still remain to be worked out by the two groups" (p. 90). However, she did not state that the basic conflict was between direct control by men in medicine of women in nursing; thus, she considered nurses' salaries favorable to those in other professions when the median was only around $1,200 to $1,300 in the small samples she surveyed, which even included nursing superintendents.

Adams delineated the newly emerging role of social worker from that of the nurse by quoting physician Richard Cabot: "It may be said with truth that the training of a nurse, as we know it in America, at any rate, really unfits a woman in some respects for the work of a social worker, since it accustoms her to habitual obedience and subordination" (p. 96). Small surveys indicate that the median salary for social workers was about $1,800, although it was lower in the psychiatric area. In Adams's book, it is clear that women in nursing were seen as more subordinated and poorly paid than women in social work, who were beginning to extend the original work of nurses begun, for example, by Lillian Wald at the Henry Street Settlement, a center for nurses to serve the poor in their homes in lower Manhattan, New York City. Gender discrimination was very apparent, although not named as such by Adams.

That nurses were well aware of their subordination and fighting for better education is apparent in Josephine Goldmark's (1923) work with the Committee for the Study of Nursing Education (see chapter 4). The Goldmark Report was clear on the differences between nursing and other professions. The excessive hours and free labor of nursing students resulted in economic profit for hospitals but also in shortages of women applicants who did not want to work twelve- to sixteen-hour days all week long for no money. The conditions revealed by the nurses' study of typical hospital training schools included inadequate fundamental science courses, inadequate clinical experience, ward assignments reflecting marked differences in time spent on different services, inadequate supervision of clinical work, excessive time spent in housekeeping work, and inadequate lecture and classroom time.

Goldmark pointed out that these inadequacies were caused by a lack of budget set aside for training the women students. Hospital exigencies took priority. In short, although the Goldmark Report does not state it, men in power were using women in nursing for their own profit. The nurses proposed the obvious: women must control the "training" of students, with a separate budget and separate control of education. In short, the nurses were demanding what Nightingale had previously demanded. To take control, advanced training for nursing leaders was also recommended. To achieve this end, university schools of nursing were needed. Nurses were largely successful in setting minimal standards for registered nurses; however, new categories of women workers continued to be created by physicians and hospital administrators, which undermined these standards.

This New, but "Really Quite Ancient Nurse": How to Control the Public Health Nurse?

While women in nursing were trying to change, improve, and gain control of hospital education, physicians were busy extending their power from hospital nurses to public health nurses. As Adams noted, the potentially more independent public health nurse had become an important part of health care by the 1920s, and predictably, physicians moved quickly to exert control over these women. A 1924 article in the *Journal of the American Medical Association* argued that the scope of the public health nurse now needed "definition" due to "a lack of sympathy" (p. 1339) between the nurses and physicians. Dr. Ira S. Wile (1924) found it strange that the debate by physicians on the public health nurse had continued so long. As he noted, sixty-three years had passed since Nightingale had defined nursing in all its public health dimensions, and thirty years since Wald had used the phrase "public health nursing." Contrasting the obedient hospital nurse with the more independent public health nurse, Wile paradoxically stated, "She is the handmaiden of preventive medicine and her field of service is without limit" (p. 107). Could the nurse's service be without limit if she were also the "helping hand of the public health administrator seeking to reduce morbidity and mortality in his community" (p. 107)?

Wile admitted a "difference of opinion concerning the extent to which her ordinary nursing training should be employed" (p. 107). Should she engage in practice or education or both? (Obviously, competent nursing always involves both.) Should she be paid for a particular specialization or for more generalized service? (Obviously, good nursing incorporates both.) Wile noted that "she no longer is dependent upon the call of a physician to enter a home" (p. 108), but the medical profession still refused to recognize the independence of this newer, but "really quite ancient, nurse."

Wile decided that regardless of differences in training, there must come a recognition that the nurse is not inferior to the physician. He acknowledged that the overlap of actual functions was great and that "obviously it is impossible [for her] to avoid making some diagnoses" (p. 109). In short, the nurse could not help but assess and make judgments. If smallpox, for example, were diagnosed, she must not wait for the physician to confirm her own diagnosis (which, of course, is technically "practicing medicine").

Wile stressed that, whatever her judgment on physicians, the nurse should not show partiality, nor should she contradict the physician in front of a patient's family. Although Wile called for cooperation between physicians and public health nurses, genuine cooperation under the circumstances he outlined was replaced by artificial game playing. The most interesting aspect of the game is Wile's "liberalism," which in reality reinstates patriarchal privilege by the process of "including" nurses in order to continue to control them.

The particular strategy used by Dr. Clemens Pirquet (1927) to control the public health nurse was historical reversal: "In olden times nursing was a part of the art of medicine and it is only since the days of Miss Nightingale that the two have begun to separate" (p. 757). As documented in earlier chapters, history shows that women have always been healers, frequently without the aid of men! Pirquet tried to appear well-intentioned, differentiating himself and his generation from older physicians, who believed that no training for nursing was necessary. In contrast, Pirquet believed the nurse should "learn to think independently and form new conceptions. We must not, however, go to extremes and demand independence of thought in every nurse" (p. 758). Previously excluded from scientific education, some nurses could now be involved in science by observing patients, particularly children. With paternalistic "good will," Pirquet urged nurses to think but not act on what they *already* knew.

In the same year, Elise Van Ness (1927) stressed "teamwork" between nurses and physicians, a team which, under different guises, has appeared in the nursing literature in subsequent decades. Van Ness looked with "gratitude" to a committee on nursing appointed by the Medical Society in Brooklyn, which conducted a survey on nursing. Four men and a woman, a nurse whose time was "loaned," decided to obtain opinions on the "nursing problem." (It is strange how the subordinated always seem to be "the problem"!) They also considered the report of the Erie County Medical Society, which, predictably, expressed fear that nurses were assuming the functions of physicians. Members of the committee acknowledged that with population increases the former personal relationships between nurses and physicians had broken down; however, they concluded that hospital administrators wanted nurses to be "soldiers rather than officers, especially not commissioned officers" (p. 168).

The committee considered the assertion by the *American Journal of Nursing* editor Mary M. Roberts that private-duty nursing had become a blind alley. In discussing nurse registries, the committee concluded: "[T]he subject is so tremendous that no final decision . . . should be outlined or devised . . . without . . . conference between the medical and nursing profession" (p. 169). Nevertheless, the nurses went ahead and set up a registry, and Van Ness concluded: "Endeavor like this on all sides, and the three great professions some day will peer over one of the rocks on the horizon to say, 'Aha! we have the solution'" (p. 170). Clearly, Van Ness used the concept of teamwork in the *hope* of equality, not the reality of actual interaction since state medical societies soon moved to join the AMA and the American Hospital Association in denouncing nurses who did not give evidence of sufficient subservience and humility.

The Politics of Protection: Women Reformers against the AMA in the 1920s

The issue of public health brought opposition, not cooperation, between nursing and medicine on the direction and form of health care. Sheila M. Rothman (1978) in *Woman's Proper Place* presented a history from 1870 to the present of the changing ideals and practices and the actual political struggles between gendered groups. More specifically, Rothman analyzed the politics of protection in the 1920s, focusing on the Sheppard-Towner Act, which was the first federally funded health-care program implemented in the United States. The act, according to Rothman, was "a stunning victory for women reformers, who saw in its passage the first result of female suffrage. Here was compelling evidence that women could translate their political power into a special kind of effort to raise levels of health and welfare. For one, the Act gave women a primary, although not exclusive, role in the field of community health and welfare" (p. 136). The program provided a type of service that presumably would not conflict with the practice of private physicians. Nevertheless, it also became a test of the relative power of gendered groups, particularly of nursing and medicine. And the struggle depicts the politics of medical takeover of women's and specifically nurses' functions and programs.

Preventive care to improve women's and children's health had already been tested in clubs and settlement houses, such as the one established by nurses at Henry Street. It is important to realize that educated women felt confident to lead in the health field because they had, as Rothman stated, led the campaign to create municipal bureaus of child hygiene and baby health stations to educate parents about hygiene. Public health nurses visited homes and created clinics to promote child welfare; these reforms focused on both private and public prevention of illness and were comparable to the public schools, playgrounds, libraries, and other community services promoted and achieved by women. Activists such as Josephine Baker believed that well-baby clinics should be as free as public schools since public health was a birthright, not a special privilege.

The women, particularly nurses, took over preventive health care at a time when there was no rival: "physicians engaged in private practice were generally unwilling and often unable to offer this type of preventive health care to their individual patients" (p. 137). According to Rothman, physicians were trained to cure the sick; they were unable or unaccustomed to conducting preventive health examinations. Separating the role of the private physician from the role of the public clinic, as Rothman stated, seemed reasonable since physicians had already agreed that municipal and state departments of public health should act to control communicable disease and to purify water, milk, and sewage. Such public health campaigns were seen as charitable and humanitarian. Nevertheless, the AMA opposed state involvement and worked to prevent passage of the Sheppard-Towner Act.

According to Rothman, politicians were uncertain of the new female bloc, but understood that many physicians saw the program as belonging to women and the state. Indeed, "To the staff of the Children's Bureau, physicians were a 'reactionary group of medical men who are not progressive and have no public health point of view'" (Rude, 1922; cited in Rothman, 1978, p. 138). Nevertheless, reformers were still careful to avoid conflict with physicians, stressing that the programs would not focus on the symptoms of disease but on the general physical conditions of the well child.

Key staff were public health nurses and female physicians. The latter were already disproportionately located in public health departments, partly because the bias of male-dominated medicine closed many hospital positions to them. Furthermore, women physicians and some nurses saw the act as furthering the goals of all educated women; thus, identification with women reformers was as important as identification with professionals, and "female medical societies were affiliated both with local medical societies and with the General Federation of Women's Clubs" (p. 140). Under the act, women physicians were to be appointed to positions of leadership in the new clinics; however, the public health nurses far outnumbered the physicians and were, therefore, central to the services. Essentially, the act relied on women's skills and female-led campaigns to reduce infant and maternal mortality.

The women had a broader view than obstetricians: their goals included "normal family life, freedom of the mother from industrial labor before and after childbirth, ability to nurse the child, above all, education in standards of care so that women and their husbands will demand good obstetrics and will no longer voluntarily run the risk of unnecessary child bed fever and similar preventable tragedies" (National League of Women Voters, n.d.; cited in Rothman, 1978, p. 142). Clearly, these goals were directly connected to feminist aims.

Unfortunately, this female autonomy and worldview did not sustain over time. As Rothman said, the Sheppard-Towner Act was not destined to be the model for health services because by 1929 the medical profession had mounted a very effective campaign that eliminated the program and the assumptions on which it was based. This was accomplished by private physicians expanding their domain to subsume the role and functions of women and the responsibility of the state: "Women trained in hygiene working in state supported clinics gave way to physicians engaged in private practice" (Rothman, 1978, p. 142).

The Medical Takeover: A Social, Not a Medical, Phenomenon

At a 1923 meeting of the AMA, John M. Dodson advised his colleagues to enter the field of preventive medicine, becoming the family health advisor as well as the family physician. By the end of the decade, periodic health examinations were being given and the physician "now judged both the progress of disease in the sick and the level of health in the normal and gave advice on personal habits as comfortably as dispensing drugs or recommending surgery" (Rothman, 1978, p. 143).

According to Rothman, by 1927 the AMA had persuaded the federal government that "private doctors were the appropriate and the exclusive guardians of *all* matters of health" (p. 143). By 1930 the shift in private practice was from sickroom to office, from emergency calls and bedroom care to advance appointments and routine examinations. According to Rothman, "This shift does not reflect scientific advances . . . [or] new techniques that dramatically increased their diagnostic abilities . . . [or] novel equipment that justified this change" (p. 143). The takeover was "*a social, not a medical, phenomenon*" (p. 143, italics added).

Physicians were able to incorporate women's health care because state agencies would not permit communities to receive funds allocated by the Sheppard-Towner Act without the endorsement of local medical societies; thus, local physicians were forced to take public positions on public health, and they could not afford to oppose a program that saved babies and mothers and promoted children's health. According to Rothman, nurses were edged out when health examinations were conducted by physicians, who then simply transferred these patients to their private practices. To avoid a fight with physicians, nurses had to ask private physicians for permission to examine a woman. But, noted Rothman, physicians were not trained to offer complete health care; thus, the AMA and local societies, ostensibly to remove government control from health care, offered instruction in the techniques of well-child and adult examinations and on routine prenatal care for women.

Some insurance companies and army units had previously recommended health examinations, but the AMA did not endorse these until *after* the passage of the Sheppard-Towner Act. Subsequently, in long articles in the official journal of the AMA, physicians learned how to take lengthy and highly detailed patient histories, already in use by women in public clinics. Hour-long appointments were to be made, but no costly new equipment was necessary. Knowledge of hygiene went beyond their training in serious disease processes, so physicians were encouraged to review physiology, nutrition, and the effects of physical exercise on bodily functions. Rothman concluded: "The view point of the average physician now took precedence over the judgments of educated women and . . . the consequences of this change were far-reaching" (p. 147).

The proliferation of instructions and the sponsorship by medical societies, as Dr. Frank Billings stated at an AMA meeting, relieved "the family physician of any accusation that he is pushing this thing for his own benefit" (Billings, 1924, p. 967; cited in Rothman, 1978, p. 147). Nevertheless, President E. S. Levy of the American Public Health Association stated in 1923 that there had never been a time when people had less confidence in medical practice because doctors were not identified with public health improvement; many did not even offer immunizations against disease.

Some specialists did support the act, but, in the case of obstetricians, gynecologists, and pediatricians, such support made it possible for them to attract sufficient patients to sustain a lucrative practice. The Children's Bureau appointed them as lecturers, consultants, and demonstrators of health examinations. Indeed, the pediatric section of the AMA initially supported the act in opposition to the larger body of the AMA, which subsequently "prohibited sections from making their own recommendations" (p. 149). Soon the specialists moved to capture leadership from women by defining the field of child and maternal health as their own exclusive province.

In 1923 physician L. E. Holt admitted that medicine had been neglectful in the past and deplored the fact that popular health education had been left "too much to the nurse, the social worker and the nutrition teacher and some of these groups largely owing to our neglect, have gotten somewhat out of hand" (Holt, 1923; cited in Rothman, 1978, p. 149). Specialists began to take on the supervision of pregnancy, to manage the significance of general rules of hygiene, and to stress the possibility of the pathological, making "the advice of public health nurses almost irrelevant" (p. 150). Having lost independent authority, the nurse, as physician Robert L. de Normandie (n.d., c. 1927) said, must not assume responsibility for medical supervision, but only carry out physician's instructions.

Eventually, the Children's Bureau gave physicians almost exclusive authority to set standards and relegated the education of mothers to the periphery. Indeed, even college-trained women now presumably lacked the medical knowledge needed to raise their children. Even with these changes, the specialists continued to disapprove the continuation of the Sheppard-Towner Act. Instead, they advised that the correct way to reduce maternal mortality was to provide funding and facilities for training obstetricians. Furthermore, they warned that visiting nurses and social workers should not deal with pathology; by emphasizing this, the physicians not only blocked the extension of Sheppard-Towner in 1929 but, as Rothman noted, also channeled federal funds to suit their own priorities.

For women reformers to be defeated, their skills had to be denigrated and their use of public funds repudiated. As Rothman stated, both women's abilities and politics were discredited. Thus, Florence Kelly, associated with Lillian Wald and the Henry Street Settlement, was labeled a "Communist" and the act a Bolshevik plot. Attacked with vicious smear tactics, women, including public health nurses, were subordinated or eliminated when the act was discontinued. In 1909, at the first White House Conference on the Health and Protection of Children, the emphasis was on educated women helping children and mothers; by the 1930 conference, the problems discussed were ironically and seemingly beyond the power of mothers to handle. Subsequently, most women, regardless of education, would go to male specialists with their problems, rather than consult female nurses.

Educating Women to Follow Orders, Follow Orders, and Follow Orders

After the AMA-induced collapse of the Sheppard-Towner Act and program, the reduction in the number of women organized to help others left a gap that the physicians could now fill. John Dill Robertson (1929), commissioner of health in Chicago, claimed that the most recent influenza outbreak required the training in two-month periods of about a thousand women. His program severely reduced the amount of training required of nurses and placed the education of these women totally under medical control. He admitted that graduates of three-year programs warned that nurses could not be educated in two months, but in his view all that was needed was a woman to follow intelligently the physician's directions and do some housekeeping. Robertson asserted: "Throughout the course we hammered on two main propositions—absolute adherence to the physician's orders and cleanliness" (p. 482). Since it was no part of the nurse's duty to diagnose or prescribe, no attempt was made to teach the women to read the meaning of symptoms. "We made not the least attempt to teach the women to prescribe; on the contrary, we tried to make clear to them the danger of attempting to prescribe even castor oil of their own accord. . . . These women know that they know nothing about materia medica—at least we told them so often enough" (p. 482).

Again, Robertson stated: "Our aim throughout has been to train them to follow the physicians' orders explicitly, but not enough to make them think they can assume any part of the duties of the physician" (p. 482). Robertson thought he could train 10,000 women, some of whom would nurse only their own families, while others would work for $18 to $25 a week. Even though the economic competition would obviously threaten fully trained registered nurses, Robertson claimed he did not oppose them. Nevertheless, housekeepers, practical nurses, or attendants—"[w]hatever you want to call them"—were being trained to be "soldiers to serve under the leadership of the physician in the fight against disease; we are not training subofficers" (p. 483). It is interesting to speculate on how physicians would have reacted if nurses had created lower-level medical men for work in the community and called them doctors, or, as Robertson said, "whatever you want to call them."

An Unwarranted Medical Intrusion: The Proliferation of Medical Committees on Nursing

Following the expiration of the Sheppard-Towner Act, the problems between nurses and physicians were "resolved" by increased efforts to dominate nursing. In Ashley's (1976) words, there occurred "an unprecedented proliferation of committees on nursing appointed by the AMA. . . . Completely ignoring the nurses' professional organizations, the AMA through its own isolated deliberations set itself up as the nominal authority on nursing" (p. 87). In 1927 the AMA's position on nursing was that:

> All surveys, studies and recommendation shall emanate from the AMA and not from any newly constituted independent organization. The problem of nursing education and service is a vital one to the public and to every physician. It is a problem in which we should exert and evidence opinions and recommendations and accomplish their institution. It is a service we owe to the public, to hospitals, to training schools and to fellow members. The AMA should, yea must, undertake its solution and formulate the resultant principles when they are announced. We become negligent and shirk our responsibilities and forfeit guiding direction if we delegate the task to others. (*Journal of the American Medical Association,* 1927; cited in Ashley, 1976, p. 87)

As Ashley noted, only a few men spoke out against "unwarranted medical intrusion" which neither respected the rights of women nor served the ends of social justice.

Various state and national groups of physicians debated what to do with nurses. By 1929 the Committee on Relationships of Nurses and Physicians in Massachusetts was formed by the state medical society to deal with the function of nurses in various settings; it issued several short reports in the *New England Journal of Medicine.* Again, the assumption was that physicians had the right to define and direct nursing education and practice. A 1931 article on "The Doctor and His Patient's Nurse" made it clear that women obtain employment only through men in hospitals or private practice (*New England Journal of Medicine,* 1931b). The majority of physicians were satisfied with the majority of nurses, but what the nurses thought of physicians was not reported. Also in 1931, a review of physicians as teachers of nurses found that the student nurses were fitted into the men's schedules (*New England Journal of Medicine,* 1931d). Indeed, nurse training often had no budget and could, therefore, pay little to physicians for their lectures.

Still another article in the 1931 series reported on "The Doctor and the Bedside Nurse," noting that physicians wanted women "of good breeding and ability to observe and report symptoms well . . . and to carry out the doctor's order" (*New England Journal of Medicine,* 1931a, p. 115). The effects of the Depression were noted in the unemployment figures of nurses. The typical salary was $1,300 for the private-duty nurse. The physicians concluded that "in spite of complaints about irregular employment, uncertain and often small incomes, and the professional loneliness of private duty, nurses love to nurse" (p. 122). The segregation of women in the labor force and the sexist devaluation of women in nursing, though not stated, were amply apparent.

Still another article reported on contagious disease and nursing care: "At least six out of ten nurses . . . who were graduated in 1928, received no practical experience at all in a communicable disease service during their entire training" (*New England Journal of Medicine,* 1931e, p. 980). Physicians complained about a lack of nurses for contagious cases. While giving little support for nursing education beyond minimal "training," the physicians wanted nurses to enter dangerous situations with little if any knowledge. Supported by pitiful and uncertain salaries, the nurses were expected to give genial care, report symptoms, and, as usual, follow orders. It was unclear how they were to do this when, as the committee reported, nursing procedures on contamination and cross-infections were not taught in hospital schools.

Another report was on "Maternity Cases and Nursing Care" (*New England Journal of Medicine,* 1931c). Only a few decades previously, women midwives had given most obstetrical care, but by the 1930s, 18 percent of nurses would not take on such cases and about the same number had *no* obstetrics in their training. The physicians noted that the nurse "is unwilling to nurse a patient to whom she cannot give proper care" (p. 571). Yet 94 out of 100 physicians in obstetrics said they needed nurses. It is ironic that by the early 1930s childbirth was the one area in which women were so unlikely to be adequately educated. The process leading to the demise of women's historical prominence in childbirth is clear: traditional women healers are denigrated and ousted; then, excluded from education, they are allowed very limited and inadequate "training"; then, used as workers rather than educated professionals, they come to be seen as inadequate; losing their old historical knowledge, they then experience further inadequacy and subservience to physicians who use statistics, such as those above, to prove the inadequacy of women to do what they have done for centuries. But the statistics that show women's inadequacy also provide historical proof of the misuse and abuse of nurses and women healers.

The Depression, Nursing in Distress: Educating Nurses beyond Their Sphere of Usefulness?

By the 1930s nursing finally lost the battle to the physicians' monopoly of knowledge and technology and to society's sexist relegation of women to their "proper" roles as aides to men. With the muting of feminism in the Depression came the loss of external support necessary for the empowerment of women as autonomous professionals. During the Depression key changes were made because patients could not afford private-duty nurses or physicians. Conditions for hospital nurses worsened and included twelve- to fourteen-hour days on split shifts, excessively strenuous work in rotations from service to service, inadequate pay, and dismissals as patient loads dropped. According to Reverby (1979), the nurses' use of time-management studies to prove their functions and workloads did not help them, but did help the hospital administrators, who used the data to shunt nursing functions to others. In addition, chronic understaffing forced nurses to accept a variety of "aides" and "subnurses."

To ensure nurses' subordination, the republished Victorian sentiments of Osler, as noted in chapter 4, were redistributed to nurses and physicians in the 1930s. These ideas were sustained in the writings of physicians who, like Lewis A. Sexton in 1931, proclaimed that higher education for nurses was educating "a people beyond their sphere of usefulness" (Ashley, 1976, p. 92). What this physician wanted was women who had "that gentle touch that soothes an aching brow" (p. 92). Such nurses had no need "for a knowledge of the solubility of salicylic acid or the atomic weight of sulphur" (p. 92). In sharp contrast to these views was nurse Mary M. Roberts's article (1932) on fusing the triple viewpoints of physicians, nurses, and hospital administrators. In her paper, which was presented at the American College of Surgeons' conference on hospital standardization, Roberts stated that chronic unemployment, combined with overproduction of poorly prepared nurses and uneven geographic distribution, had produced a grave situation. Even with high unemployment, 33 percent of applicants for general-duty nursing in one instance were ineligible because of poor qualifications caused by inadequate training. Roberts believed that physicians knew extraordinarily little about nursing, which was "infinitely more than medicine's left overs" (p. 34) and following orders. She called for nurses' control of their own curriculum, for the training of more nurse administrators, and for better education of clinical nurses. She demanded that the overuse of young students' free labor be eliminated. The system of free student labor was wrong, even though previously justified because hospitals needed workers.

Because of the Depression, Roberts believed that nursing education could now take priority and the hostility of hospital administrators to graduate nurses could be overcome. To her, clinical service and nursing education were not synonymous parts of hospitals; the system, she stressed, was outworn. Nursing leaders had watched previous studies of the Committee on Grading of Nursing Schools fall on deaf ears; now they were engaging in studies of costs of medical care, the quality of nursing care, and organizing local councils of community nursing service. Yet in response Donald Guthrie, MD, simply emphasized more clinical learning, while applauding the "splendid women in the nursing profession" (p. 37). So much for Roberts's vision of a triple fusion among nurses, physicians, and hospital administrators!

In the 1930s, as in the 1920s, nurses continued their fight for control of adequate and appropriate education. They moved to set standards by registry of hospitals and their accreditation by the state boards of nurse examiners, which would specify the size of hospitals; demand separate training school committees; establish low ratios of students to registered nurse staff; set high school educational admittance levels; require college training for nursing faculty; and require registered nurses as head nurses and supervisors. Nursing leaders further demanded health examinations for student nurses and an end to using students as special-duty nurses in private homes for hospital remuneration; they insisted that students receive preliminary instruction *before* beginning bedside work and work no more than a six-day, forty-eight-hour workweek. They insisted that student records be maintained and diplomas awarded only on passage of state examinations. As this list of demands indicates, nursing was fighting a system of control in which women were overused in clinical settings, given inadequate and poorly funded education in hospitals, and systematically underpaid for their services.

If hospital nursing was in such difficulty under the increasing medical monopoly, public health nursing had not fared much better by the end of the 1930s, a decade after the end of the Sheppard-Towner Act. In 1939 nurse Grace Ross questioned whether the public health officers were fulfilling their responsibilities to women in the nursing program. From national survey results, the number of nurses considered necessary to public health departments varied widely; the percentage of nurses of total staff, although high, differed greatly from place to place. Adherence to the minimum requirements for nurses was met by only 23 percent of the departments; not even a license was required. Indeed, it was not until 1938 that New York State passed laws on licensure for professional and practical nurses, each with different functions, as part of mandatory licensure to restrict the title "nurse" to a particular group of persons: "The older nursing laws merely made it illegal for an unauthorized person to use the title *registered nurse,* but it was not illegal for such a person to practice nursing" (Bullough, 1986, p. 351). To change this, a definition of the scope of practice had to be legislated (see chapter 6). In some cases, a single course was thought adequate preparation and graduates of deficient programs were also acceptable. About half of the departments had public health nurses in charge of the nursing staff. Salaries continued to be abominable, ranging from $1,800 to $3,600 per year with few nurses receiving more income with greater experience. Ross stated: "Most administrators find that nurses on the whole make poor clerks and nurses accept this criticism" (Ross, 1939, p. 309). With biting sarcasm, she remarked: "It is crediting nurses with more altruism than they possess to suppose that salary is not an important matter to them and they are so eager to serve the community well that they will spend hundreds of dollars for additional education on which they expect no financial return" (p. 310). Ross concluded that it was in the hands of the health officers to decide if they wanted "Grade A" nursing. It was clear that medical control of health care had not necessarily improved conditions in public health nursing or in general hospital nursing.

Nursing: Scientific Work or Womanly Ministering?

Physicians' increasing dominance over all aspects of health care and nurses' continuing subordination were interconnected with gender stereotypes that exaggerated physicians' importance and defined nurses' work as womanly ministering rather than scientifically based clinical practice. In reality, nurses' work consisted of a combination of technical knowledge and the skills they needed as the primary providers of direct patient care. Yet their roles, claim a group of Canadian researchers, continued to be perceived, particularly by physicians, as primarily womanly, nurturing, and suited to females and mothers (Keddy, Acker, Hemeon, MacDonald, MacIntyre, Smith, and Vokey, 1987). In the public imagination, nursing, women, and femininity had become firmly linked; thus, nurses in the 1930s were seen as doing "womanly tasks," usually those done by women at home, but now without the control over the full spectrum of functions they had previously provided. Authority over clinical diagnosis and prescriptions by physicians became centrally important, and the nurse was ideologically marginalized and characterized as a nurturant but "unscientific" woman. This process was and still is perpetrated through physicians' paternalistic authority, which is used to devalue the nurse. As one physician put it in 1894, nurses knew no more science than a first-year medical student; variations on this theme are apparent throughout the first three decades of the twentieth century.

Were the physicians' perceptions true or were they simply sexist stereotypes used to bolster medical authority? By analyzing the histories of thirty-five older nurses, Keddy and her colleagues studied the extent to which nurses in the 1920s and 1930s actually used scientific and/or technical knowledge. Analyses of taped responses to a semistructured interview in which the nurses were asked to recall their work experiences produced several themes, one of which was labeled "hands-on nursing," defined as direct-patient contact and the use of health-care knowledge through tasks or skills. The responses were initially analyzed by disease categories; others were developed from the content analysis of the "hands-on-nursing" theme.

To deal with pneumonia and polio, two widespread diseases in the 1920s and 1930s, the nurses, in the absence of sulfa, penicillin, and other modern drugs, directly administered poultices, plasters, fomentations, and dressings and positioned patients to avoid contractures and bedsores. Were these technologies scientific? One can argue that yes, they were the primary type of treatment because bacteriological discoveries between 1878 and 1887 had not been successfully applied, often because many conditions, including pneumonia, could be caused by the action of more than a single bacterium. Until 1935, with the introduction of sulfa and penicillin, and the 1940s, with newer antibiotics, the nurses provided the most and, in many cases, the only rational treatment available for pneumonia and, until much later, for polio. This was confirmed in the extensive use of these technologies by the older nurses interviewed.

The interviews also produced evidence that the nurses often *invented* equipment or procedures to carry out rather difficult tasks, for example, those involving blood transfusions, which in earlier years were very complicated procedures. Although the transfusions themselves were conducted by physicians, nurses carried much of the responsibility for handling the multiple syringes and citrate techniques required. One nurse remembered using a vial of citrate, putting the needle and syringe in the donor, connecting it to a table, then putting it in a sterile beaker with citrate, which was stirred by another nurse using a sterile rod. The two then gave the IV (intravenous therapy) and stirred and poured. From this and other examples, the researchers asserted: "Without much equipment to work with they [the early nurses] turned their workplaces into institutions which functioned primarily because of their ingenuity" (Keddy et al., 1987, p. 38).

Because limited scientific knowledge was available for practical use by any health-care provider in the 1920s and 1930s, Keddy and her co-researchers noted that "the fate of the patient often depended primarily upon the ministerings of the nurse" (p. 38). From this, they concluded that nurses were technically critical to applied science to the extent that it was usable in their work. Ironically, physicians "ordered treatment which was solely nursing care and which was patriarchally devalued as women's work" (p. 38). If the same techniques had been administered by physicians, they would probably have been considered to be "appropriately scientific for the era" (p. 38). In other words, *gender,* not science, determined the degree to which a particular technology was perceived as scientifically based. Keddy and her colleagues concluded that nursing and medical responsibilities in the 1930s, as today, are directly traceable to class and sex roles and only peripherally determined by the actual scientific content of the work itself.

Early Evidence of the Doctor-Nurse Game

In their 1987 article, Keddy and her colleagues focused on nurses' technical work and skills in the 1920s and 1930s. But a year earlier, Keddy and other colleagues had interviewed the same group of older nurses to provide an historical perspective on the evolution of doctor-nurse relationships (Keddy, Gillis, Jacobs, Burton, and Rogers, 1986). Content analysis of the nurses' past experiences produced a main theme—the doctor-nurse relationship—and provided evidence that the doctor-nurse game had been in force many decades before Stein's (1967) classic analysis. (For a comprehensive analysis of the doctor-nurse game, see Roberts and Group, *Gender and the Nurse-Physician Game*, publication pending.)

From their data, the researchers found that these nurses were trained primarily by physicians: "In some schools of nursing the doctors also gave the exams to the nursing students" (p. 747). The nurses said that the physicians thought they knew how much the nurses should or should not know. To them, a nurse's worthiness was "equated with helpfulness to the doctors, much as the wife was considered to be the appendage of the husband since she was his helpmate" (p. 746). The physicians had a great deal of control and power over what the nurses learned: how they were examined, whether they passed or failed, and who would be registered after graduation.

The physicians also controlled the economic situation of early nurses, one of whom noted that she had lost a position in one community because the physician knew the other applicant and her family. Indeed, the nurse also said she knew she would get a job if a physician recommended her; physicians hired the nurses they preferred. The researchers found, too, that "to be a doctor's preferred nurse meant you were a good nurse and occupied a special status with other nurses" (p. 747). However, as Keddy and her coauthors asserted, this system of competition for jobs and favors from physicians kept the nurses from becoming unified. They concluded that, at least from their sample of older nurses, the women had little scope for greater power because "They tried to become 'good' nurses in order to obtain jobs" (p. 747).

What made a woman a "good" nurse? The researchers found that physicians had "very clearly defined expectations of nurses . . . [which] involved doing exactly what the physicians dictated," and to these women they gave as a reward "a certain degree of respect" (p. 748). One older nurse said that the physicians had confidence in and relied on the nurses to carry out all their orders exactly as given. Indeed, the nurse's role was "not described in terms of patient care, but in terms of proficiency with which she carried out the physician's orders" (p. 748). Thus, "obedience" equaled "good nurse," which presumably equaled "good care."

Keddy and her colleagues believed that this attitude extended even to humanitarian men. For example, Jean Ewen, a nurse in China in the 1930s, worked with a famous physician, Norman Bethune, who told her never to call him by his first name—a "sin" she had, in fact, not committed. He told her that beyond the doctor-nurse relationship, they were to have no particular contact. Furthermore, Ewen was not to diagnose or treat patients. In response to this, Ewen wrote: "I was hopping mad. I was a servant, no more, no less. I did not show my anger, at least I hoped I didn't. I resolved to put forth every effort to please the good doctor" (Ewen, 1981; cited in Keddy et al., 1986, p. 748).

Certainly, the results of the interviews with the older nurses dovetail with Ewen's account from the 1930s and give some historical basis for the doctor-nurse game later exposed by a number of researchers. For example, Raisler (1974) stated that a nurse is perceived as "good" if she helps the physician *regardless* of patient outcome; thus, intelligence and judgment are not useful "unless it improves the doctor's self-concept and feeling of authority" (cited in Keddy et al., 1986, p. 748). This calls for gendered game playing, a fact recognized by Keddy and her associates: "In analyzing the data, it becomes apparent that most of the nurses interviewed were involved in the interactive methods of the doctor-nurse game, although none referred to it as such" (p. 748).

The first rule of the game, showing respect to physicians, often involved an expected "form of idolization of the physician" (p. 748). Nurses remembered being told to jump to their feet in military style when a physician appeared. If medical personnel were able, knowledgeable, and devoted to community health, they were respected. However, the nurses' "respect" for physicians was at times "far from genuine"; indeed, nurses were more apt to resent than respect the medical students who thought they were gods and expected idolization. Keddy and her co-researchers found that sometimes the early nurses' feelings were "based on fear of humiliation, developed in the student nurse's mind throughout her training" (p. 749). If physicians controlled nursing education, then it is not surprising that one of the first rules taught was the power of the hospital and medical hierarchy. The researchers asserted that "feelings of inferiority and fear give rise to docility and submission in nurses" (p. 749), making it difficult for them to feel free to contribute to decision making.

The second rule was that "nurses cannot openly diagnose or make recommendations to doctors" (p. 749). As Keddy and her colleagues noted, nurses spend a great deal more time with patients than do physicians; thus, the nurses have information the physicians need. But they found from the interviews evidence of the maladaptive interaction. One early nurse, for example, "referred to two different methods of treating pneumonia that she used in the same ward, depending on which doctor the patient had" (p. 749). Significantly, the nurse noted that one physician's treatment, which involved fresh air, produced better results. Her observation has been subsequently substantiated, but because she could not voice her opinion, the patients of the physician whose treatment was not as effective continued to receive the inadequate treatment. Even if this nurse had stated her opinion, the researchers noted that it could and probably would have been overruled by higher authorities.

The third rule was that no open disagreement or confrontation was allowed. To Keddy and her colleagues, this rule followed the second; if no opinions were allowed, then no disagreement was possible: "In order for the patients to believe and continue to believe that doctors are omniscient and omnipotent, they must not see anyone expressing disagreement with a doctor's judgement" (p. 749). The result was also nebulous communication. One early nurse recalled bathing patients diagnosed with pneumonia; in doing this, she was in opposition to the physician, whose patients were often not allowed even bed baths for days or weeks at a time. She simply did not tell him what she did to keep her patients clean and comfortable. In an understatement, the researchers noted that physicians did not appreciate that nurses' views might differ from their own: "Part of what keeps nurses from asserting themselves is no doubt their stereotypic female role behavior" (p. 750).

Both gender and class discrimination in the hospital hierarchical authority were encountered during training. The researchers recognized that the women in their study were part of a sex-segregated labor force, part of a disciplined corps of subordinated individuals, whose experience with physicians produced the early basis for later problems in the profession: "In a number of interviews, it was strongly reinforced that the medical profession influenced nurses' status in the workplace, their education, and also their actual registration to practice" (p. 750). The gender stereotypes of passivity, subservience, and subordination, based on class and sex discrimination, has been passed on to subsequent generations as the nurse-physician game.

Keddy and her colleagues noted that *some* nurses did express their ideas and acted to improve patient care. These women were unpopular with physicians, the early nurses noted, and often acted "on their ideas furtively" (p. 751). The women's movement has influenced current nurses to be more assertive; however, this recent change has also brought resistance. From the interviews, some change was apparent; one early nurse noted that the nurses eventually stopped standing up for physicians, even though the physicians did not understand or like the women's changed behavior. Even so, it was observed that the doctor-nurse game continued and that ineffective communication had frightening consequences for patients.

To these researchers, change requires honesty about what nurses have actually been doing: "Nurses have been performing duties and roles traditionally intrinsic to that of doctors, especially on night and weekend shifts, for years" (p. 752). Nursing *does* encroach on physicians' presumed territory, which can be perceived as a threat—a loss of power and status. The researchers warned of continued opposition from physicians who, on decision-making committees and boards, can exert influence to limit nurses' roles. The only recourse is to place nurses in these groups. But from their data, the researchers believe that the movement away from the "strictly silent handmaiden image towards the equal team member role will be slow and necessarily involve stress" (p. 752).

The Development of the "Good Doctor and His Loyal Nurse" in the 1930s

Stereotyped images of nurses as subservient, nurturant, and not scientific persons were promulgated early on, not only by physicians but by the male-dominated media in newspapers, magazines, and books. By the late 1920s and early 1930s similar stereotyped images appeared in radio programs and movies; later they would surface in television commercials and programming.

The process by which the public came to perceive physicians and nurses in stereotyped gendered roles was still familiar even at the close of the twentieth century. From the extensive and excellent research by Beatrice J. and Philip A. Kalisch there is more than ample evidence that media gender stereotyping was directly involved in establishing the primacy of physicians. In one historical case study, the Kalisches (1984a) used the massive publicity on the Dionne quintuplets to trace the emergence and establishment of the images of the "Good Doctor and His Loyal Nurse" in both Canadian and American culture. In 1934 five identical baby girls were born prematurely in Canada and survived. The birth of quintuplets had been recorded only twice previously in history, and there was no record of any identical quintuplet surviving beyond a few days. Thus, the birth and survival of the Dionne babies captured the world's attention, particularly since the event happened in the Canadian backwoods.

The government built a private hospital where the girls were raised by a group of nurses. The parents had limited visiting rights and the siblings had none at all. A government committee decided on sterile surroundings and the latest child-rearing procedures. The parents unsuccessfully fought all these arrangements for the first nine years. The newspapers influenced what the public knew, and the press reports, according to the Kalisches, were biased. Indeed, the media view of Dr. Allan Roy Dafoe "approached adulation . . . a rather odd man, [he] had fame thrust upon him, and he thoroughly enjoyed it" (1984a, p. 243).

Shortly after the births, experts rallied around, but "Dr. Dafoe received all of the credit" (p. 243). He was portrayed in the media as a modest and altruistic man of "unlimited medical skills . . . who lovingly treated the families in his neighborhood without regard for money and who remained untouched by sudden fame" (p. 243). In reality, he was "a man of quite ordinary, even mediocre skills—both medical and social" (p. 243), who had purposely gone to a small, remote town to escape comparison to a younger brother, a famous physician in Toronto. Dafoe was reclusive, never becoming part of the community and "never bothering to learn French, the primary language of the area" (p. 243). Although portrayed as giving help without money, he became rich through his association with the quintuplets by giving speeches and writing a syndicated column. He even paid another physician to write articles at which "he scarcely even glanced" (p. 245). Obviously, his actual and public images did not coincide.

The nurses who cared for the quintuplets appeared relaxed, cheerful, and confident and "didn't look capable of the tiredness, indecision, untidiness, or short tempers that ordinary mothers were heir to" (p. 249). The quintuplets' real mother was only a visitor and the five girls said later that their early years with the nurses were their happiest. As the Kalisches noted, four of the girls later chose humanitarian careers, two as nurses and two as nuns. Their real mother "was having a bitter fight with Dr. Dafoe, whom she hated" (p. 250). He never allowed the children to have a nurse as a permanent mother-figure; thus, they had fourteen nurses in six years. The so-called scientific upbringing failed: in adulthood the quintuplets had severe problems about which they were very bitter. This contrasts with their public image as happy children playing with their nurses. What did succeed was "the image of the courageous country doctor and the devoted, happily subservient nurse" (p. 250); these, said the Kalisches, still create a formidable obstacle to changing the current public image of nurses.

Media Stereotypes of the Country Doctor and His Devoted Nurse

According to the Kalisches, in the 1920s "physicians were frequently portrayed negatively, as criminal, avaricious, promiscuous, and/or foolish" (p. 242). But this image changed with a 1930s movie series, beginning with *The Country Doctor* in 1936 and continuing in the next two movies in which Jean Hersholt played Dr. John Luke, a barely disguised but idealized Dr. Dafoe. Hersholt repeated the lovable country doctor in various physician roles for twenty-five years. In the first three films, nurses appeared but "were not idolized as the physician was nor were they shown in any consistent characterization" (p. 245). Nevertheless, the public considered the babies' nurses to be "privileged and wonderful women who were somehow immune to the failings of normal motherhood" (p. 245).

In all three of the original movies, the plot involves good deeds by Dr. Luke, who runs into trouble before succeeding. This theme remains constant, although plots vary: he delivers a small baby, which is quickly followed by four others; he then fights to save the babies; wins the small hospital he wanted over the opposition of the lumber company; saves the town from a diphtheria epidemic; saves a lumber man from having his legs amputated; acts as a role model for a younger man; and finally receives the Order of the British Empire.

As Dr. Luke, Hersholt "exhibited all of the characteristics that later became standard traits for the 'good doctor'" (p. 247). Solid and fatherly, both Hersholt and Defoe had "gray hair and mustache; both wore round, wire-rimmed glasses; and both had a comfortable paunch that rounded out their dark, three-piece suits . . . the eyes shone with sympathy, concern and good humor" (p. 247). Dr. Luke with his "kindly, avuncular figure . . . [had] exceptional medical skill" (p. 247). As a sensitive human being, he treats people holistically, gives them a sense of personal worth, waives his little medical fees even when he is in difficult financial straits. He is "completely trustworthy," with integrity that "transcends all consideration of personal gain" (p. 248).

The Kalisches found that nurse Katherine Kennedy was cast as a loyal assistant to Dr. Luke, concerned primarily with practical matters and with monitoring the physician's finances. However, "the nurse's importance is completely overshadowed by the central role of the doctor. Whatever her talents, however much she works, no matter how much good she does, all goes toward making the doctor a more effective, more beloved, and more altruistic character" (p. 248). If he is not there, the nurse diagnoses and splints a broken arm; however, when he is there "the nurse is reduced to carrying out only simple tasks requiring no special skills or knowledge, such as calling for boiling water" (p. 248).

The nurse is shown working twenty-four-hour days for a week, but the camera focuses on the physician as "he falls wearily asleep in a chair" (p. 248). The nurse goes on working, but "her tireless devotion seems to be taken for granted" (p 248). Taking care of practical matters, receiving no share of the glory, the nurse's image is primarily maternal—for the "nourishment, protection, and comfort of doctor and patient alike" (p. 249). She is liked, but as the physician's adjunct; although capable of replacing him, this fact is not emphasized; she simply helps the man perform modern, "miraculous" medical feats. Actress Dorothy Peterson, as nurse Katherine Kennedy, was chosen because of her blameless character. She looked older than her twenties and played middle-aged mothers as well. The Kalisches quoted Peterson as saying she was chosen to play a nurse because she was not colorful and glamorous.

According to the Kalisches, these images persisted in the *Dr. Christian* radio series from 1937 to 1953, in which "the doctor is very nearly a religious hero" unselfish, dedicated, with integrity emphasized to the point of saintliness, "a repository of all the 'Christian' virtues" (p. 249). The incarnation of love with no hint of sexuality, "He is, like God Himself, the perfectly loving father-figure, the perfectly wise counselor, the perfectly skilled miracle worker" (p. 249). The handful of nurses could not compete in their brief appearances even though they were "pleasant, attractive, clean, neat, and kindly . . . [and] loving, trusted, competent, helpmates . . . they performed almost no duties requiring any expertise, nor did they demonstrate any real importance in health care" (p. 249).

These images have influenced generations of Americans; many older people still remember the movies and the radio series. Those who grew up from the 1960s to the 1980s "take for granted the almost archetypal 'good doctor,' as represented by such men as Drs. Kildare, Welby, Casey, and Gannon and their current television counterparts . . . [who] know all their patients by name, recognize and solve all of the patient's problems—both physical and psychosocial—and charge little or nothing for their services" (p. 242).

A Nurse Who Questioned Medical Authority

While the media fostered the stereotyped image of nurses, what happened to those women who defied gendered perceptions? They were in for some real difficulties, which are obvious in the life of one nurse, Elizabeth Kenny (1886–

1952). The "woman who challenged the doctors," as she was described in one of the biographies of her life, Kenny represents "an interesting case study of a nurse who was willing to question the prerogatives of the physician—even if it meant going her way alone" (Bullough, 1985, p. 4).

After attending St. Ursula's College, Kenny became a visiting nurse in the Australian outback, where, in 1910, she attended a two-year-old girl who lay "with one knee drawn up toward her face, the foot twisted and turned outward, and one arm bent at the elbow across the chest" (p. 4). After a ride on horseback to the closest telegraph office, Kenny received a response to her wire from Dr. Aeneas John McDonnell, who diagnosed infantile paralysis, indicated no known treatment, and recommended that Kenny do her best with the symptoms. Accordingly, Kenny worked on the contractions and muscle spasms, trying several methods until she found that cloths dipped in boiling water, wrung dry, and wrapped around the areas of greatest pain brought relief and sleep to the child. Kenny reported recovery to McDonnell, who said her treatment was contrary to existing medical knowledge but advised continuation of her therapy.

With the advent of the First World War, Kenny served as a nurse in France where she was wounded by shrapnel and then served on a hospital ship. On her return to Australia, she concentrated on patients crippled by polio, reeducating muscles to increase physical activity. Kenny always insisted on an initial examination by a physician. Finally, she was invited to lecture in Queensland, where she spoke to physicians on muscle spasms that, if untreated, created deformity: "When Kenny stated this, the physicians laughed her off the platform" (p. 4). Hospitals refused to admit her patients, but the government health department opened a clinic for her in 1934.

Kenny did not claim a *cure*, but a *treatment* for muscle spasm that reduced or eliminated physical disability; nevertheless, as Bullough notes, "the Australian Royal Commission denounced her treatment in a 120-page tirade" (p. 4). Kenny received better treatment from physicians when she traveled to England and the United States; however, even by 1940, few American physicians listened to her. The Mayo Clinic received her more positively and started to use her form of treatment under her instructions at the Minnesota General Hospital. Although some medical reports found her treatments unsuccessful, her techniques spread, even after her death, until Salk in 1955 and Sabin in 1961 produced efficacious vaccines. To her credit, Kenny "persisted in her treatment in spite of medical opposition and in the process helped establish the importance of physiotherapy" (p. 4). Other nurses have faced similar condemnation from physicians and still persevered in their work. Yet their numbers and names are largely unknown.

In this chapter we have seen the successful efforts by physicians to monopolize health care for their own monetary and social aggrandizement at the expense of nurses and even, at times, of patients. The medical takeover of pre-

ventive health, the defeat of the women's model of state-sponsored health programs, and the subordination of nurses could occur only if socialization for
female subordination was extended from the private to the public arena. This
made it extremely difficult for nurses and women health-care reformers to
succeed. The unequal and gendered struggle, heavily weighted in favor of men,
produced a disease-oriented model of health care that prevailed as the medical
monopoly was consolidated by the end of the 1930s. This eventually produced
the overpriced, complex, and cumbersome health-care system so evident at
the end of the twentieth century.

In the next chapter, some of the forces and events which helped to create
the massive, bureaucratic health system in the United States will be analyzed,
focusing particularly on the period from the 1940s to the 1960s. During these
decades, nurses secured their positions in hospitals and other health agencies,
but physicians capitalized on the new era of medical specialization to gather
more support for their monopoly over health-care provision. At the same
time, a swing toward more conservative gender roles following World War II
caused a temporary cessation of feminism and feminist political action. This
was to make nursing's struggle for increased professional and economic status
even more difficult.

6 | A Growing Unease
Nurse-Physician Interprofessional Relations from the 1940s to the 1960s

With the entrance of the United States into the Second World War, the prestige of physicians and the power of organized medicine were substantially reinforced. Following the war, the rapidly expanding knowledge in the basic sciences; the widespread use of sulfa, penicillin, and eventually antibiotic drugs; and increased technological capacities provided even more support for the medical monopoly. The era of medical specialization began, and the health-care industry grew into a massive, costly, but fragmented business, one that brought substantial financial profits to physicians, whose prestige was augmented by the American Medical Association (AMA), the most heavily funded political lobby in the United States. If the medical monopoly was essentially achieved in the 1920s and substantially consolidated in the 1930s, the next three decades marked the widespread extension of physicians' power. By the 1960s, however, the image of the dedicated, self-sacrificing doctor, although still prominent in the media, began to crumble as consumers became more and more disenchanted with poorly coordinated, expensive, and impersonal medical services. Nevertheless, the AMA, as in previous decades, continued to oppose any national health-care system and fought against Medicare and Medicaid, both of which were supported by organized nursing.

By the 1940s many nurses had shifted from private-duty to hospital nursing; with the proliferation of new health-care workers, largely created or approved by physicians, nurses were increasingly involved in administration. These responsibilities, however, were assumed without the autonomy necessary to coordinate effectively the medical specialists and the new array of technologists, aides, and other auxiliary workers. Like the First World War, the Second World War brought praise for nurses, but it did not produce a parallel increase in their economic status compared to that of physicians. Nor did the war years create greater autonomy or substantially more independent organizational authority for nurses. The struggles of organized nursing with medical and hospital monopolies were made even more difficult during the societal shift following the war toward very conservative gender roles for women.

Although nurses gained more informality in their relations with physicians by the 1960s, organized medicine provided little support for the nurses' move toward full professional status through university-based education. Nevertheless, nurses pushed for greater collegiality with physicians, leading to the first joint national conference of nurses and physicians in 1964. Other conferences followed, eventually culminating in 1967 in the National Joint Practice Commission, which was supported by both the American Nurses' Association and the American Medical Association. Nurses' efforts toward unionization were blocked by federal legislation, specifically the Taft-Hartley Act of 1947, which legally restricted many nurses and other hospital employees from organizing unions and taking strike actions—a restriction strongly endorsed by hospital and medical organizations. Thus, the strategy of unionization available to the vast majority of other workers was largely unavailable to nurses, and the other strategy, professionalization, was very difficult, given administrators' opposition to the closure of hospital schools. Ironically, nurses' successes in achieving greater professional status and in organizing as women workers contradicted the general trend of pushing women back into the home and glorifying their roles as homemakers.

On a Collision Course with the Ideology of Domesticity and the Feminine Mystique

Given the prevailing conservative gender stereotypes, the odds in favor of nurses defining and directing their own area of expertise and gaining the power to establish their own practice and profession separate from medicine were not very high. The nurses' difficulties are very apparent in Barbara Melosh's (1983) research on gender and work in the postwar hospital from the 1940s to the 1960s. Analyzing a variety of sources, Melosh found that "sociological studies, prescriptive literature, and popular fiction all reflected a growing unease with the nurse's expertise and authority" (p. 158). Though subordinated to physicians, nurses had achieved "enough expertise and authority to threaten cultural prescriptions for women" (p. 164). To Melosh, nurses were on a "collision course with the postwar ideology of domesticity, later named the 'feminine mystique'" (p. 165). In diverse sources, there was increased concern about nurses as women and "a new sense of the possible contradictions and conflicts between the demands of work and the claims of gender" (p. 165).

Postwar writers, said Melosh, often depicted nurses as failed women, pathetic or even dangerous. Their distance from traditional women's roles supposedly had a "pernicious" effect on female character. Even nursing manuals covered not only professional and ethical but also gendered behaviors of the nurse as woman. In fiction, nurses were often present simply to round out novels centered on medical themes.

By the 1950s gender and occupation came together in nurse romances, a whole genre by itself and one seldom characterized by any feminist message. Melosh found a few stock plots in the nurse romance, all reflecting the prevalent and stereotyped cultural imagery of women's work and status. Even though more women were employed outside the home, American culture had given only a "reluctant and partial assent to the notion of women in the paid labor force" (p. 167). Even the defense economy of war "did not shatter time-honored conceptions of women's proper place" (p. 167). Women were recruited in the name of their traditional relations with men and only for the duration of the war. Even nurses with rank or those centrally involved on the war front were portrayed as stereotypically feminine, though courageous, and were expected to return home following the war; however, as Melosh noted, women did not stay at home—many remained employed while sustaining their family responsibilities. Nurses "experienced the contradictions of the feminine mystique in an especially acute and hostile form" (p. 167). While other women were urged to return home, nurses, were urged to go to work because of nursing shortages, despite a society that believed that paid "work and womanhood posed conflicting and irreconcilable demands" (p. 168).

The most negative fictional portrayals represented the nurse's position as "anomalous and unnatural, distorting female personality into a new and threatening posture of dominance" (p. 168). Even sociological research sustained the negative gender stereotypes. For example, a study of authoritarianism in nursing by sociologist Richard R. Lanese (1961) failed to support his hypothesis, but he still claimed to find authoritarianism among nurses even though his data did not support this conclusion. As Melosh observed, "More powerful doctors or administrators were surely more prone to abuse of authority than nurses. But as women in some semblance of command, nurses were both more visible and more threatening" (Melosh, 1983, p. 168).

The degree of threat to men from women in power was especially apparent in one short story in the 1950s in which a male patient who had lost his vision and his arms and legs was depicted as experiencing frightening dependence on his nurse. She had become sexually involved with him, not to affirm his humanity but to treat him as an object. After his experience with this fictional "man-hater," the man commits suicide. Melosh concluded, "In a world turned upside down, men lose their power to women, and women with unnatural power abuse it" (p. 169). It is this thread that Melosh followed throughout postwar popular culture about nurses, who, as fictional characters, were seen to "unbalance the proper relationships between men and women, alternately ordering men about and ignoring them; often asserting an unseemly sexual autonomy either by seducing male patients or by abandoning them altogether for celibacy or lesbianism" (p. 169). To Melosh, the "time worn identification of nurses with forbidden sexuality touches deeper cultural sources than postwar social and economic changes alone" (p. 170). Indeed, the views of nurses' presumed sexuality from the 1940s and 1950s simply reflected the stereotyped dichotomy between virgin and whore: "nurses appear either as saintly angels or as degraded creatures of the flesh" (p. 170). To Melosh, the view of nurses as marginal women in earlier literature was altered in postwar fiction to depict "competent nurses as questionable women" (p. 170). The earlier idealized female character changed as nurses were more frequently depicted as involved in work that unsexed or perverted them. By the 1950s nurses were threatening, said Melosh, because they as women had too much control.

All sources researched by Melosh dealt with the conflict between womanhood and work. In fiction, nurses with authority were depicted as battle-axes, or as frustrated, or single, or unloved. Even in sociological research, nursing students were depicted as immature, wanting to be close to people but not ultimately responsible; needing the warmth of the maternal role, but not children; seeking contact with men, but without sexuality (Mauksch, 1963; cited in Melosh, 1983, p. 171). In nurse romances, women in nursing rejected their profession for "feminine" work. Indeed, those who wanted to continue as nurses had to be set straight by male suitors or advisors. As Melosh noted, such novels usually ended with marital bliss ahead, but little was said about the heroine continuing her nursing work. Some nurse characters, however, insisted that the men accept them as they were and these nurses did continue their careers.

Even nursing manuals asserted the need to be "feminine." A 1959 column in *Nursing World* directed readers "to seek the delicate balance of 'the feminine principle of feeling' versus 'the thinking characteristics associated with the masculine principle'" (Muller, 1959, pp. 28–29; cited in Melosh, 1983, p. 174). If the "masculine" were overemphasized, the nurse would presumably become depressed, lack zest, and feel dissatisfied. Some nurses emphasized the female fitness for nursing, asserting that nurses made the best mothers and wives: "Nurses trained in the 1940s and 1950s remembered hearing this justification again and again" (p. 174). This was happening at a time when nurses were increasingly involved in more technical work that removed them even further from their domestic origins. Given the societal attack on women workers, Melosh concluded that "without the defense of an articulate feminist ideology or the support of an active women's movement, nurses often met this attack with rhetorical efforts to accommodate their work to the demands of the feminine mystique" (p. 175).

The pervasive sex discrimination basic to medical, hospital, and agency practices was seldom overtly named, analyzed, or attacked. Even with clear evidence of unfair, gendered treatment of women nurses in salaries and work conditions, sexism was very infrequently noted or discussed by nurses or even by social scientists studying nursing. Yet as Lovell (1980) concluded in her historical study, organized medicine continued to function as a business from the 1940s to the 1960s, and relied on paternalism to sustain its monopoly. Few other historians have focused as clearly as Lovell on nurse-physician relations. Indeed, Melosh charges that nursing history has yet to be incorporated into medical, social, labor, or even women's history or sociology. This is particularly obvious when military historians studying World War II or the Korean or Vietnam Wars—all major conflicts during the decades covered in this chapter—have demonstrated only a peripheral interest in nursing, despite the obvious importance of nurses in wartime.

Indispensable in Wartime, Subservient in Peacetime

During the Second World War, the tremendous need for women workers, and especially for nurses, changed priorities and caused a temporary emphasis on the value of women in the workforce. However, the patriotic appeals to nurses were based on traditional gender images which were mixed with contradictory messages. To recruit more women nurses, the media, for example, produced a number of movies with nurse heroines, all positively portrayed, but all clearly sex-stereotyped.

Physicians in the military had, at best, a mixed record on accepting nurses in the armed forces. (For a fuller discussion, see Roberts and Group, 1995.) Even before World War II, nursing leaders requested that the surgeon general reopen the Army School of Nursing, but he refused, despite clear evidence that a very large number of nurses would be needed if war was declared. With the outbreak of hostilities, nursing organizations had a very short time to create nursing programs and train thousands of women, as they had during World War I. Beginning in 1941, Congress provided funds to increase the numbers of nursing students, augment nursing services at some eight hundred nursing schools, supplement public health nurses to care for defense workers, and help agencies, including nursing organizations, to provide services for communities. Nursing leaders and nursing organizations subsequently created national recruitment and training programs, such as the Nurse Cadet Corps, which located and educated some 125,000 students. In addition, 100,000 women hospital volunteers were recruited and trained as unpaid aides, presumably to supplement but not replace nurses. By 1944–1945, one-half of the 240,000 active nurses had volunteered for military service, leaving civilian facilities in dire need of more nurses. Still the need for military nurses was so great that President Franklin D. Roosevelt finally requested the draft of nurses; only the end of the war stopped the proposed conscription of women.

As in past wars, the much-needed nurses who entered the military continued to be subjected to sexist treatment. Assigned relative, not permanent, rank, they earned about 60 percent of the pay of men at the same rank and had no retirement, dependents' allowances, or other usual benefits. The women wore officers' uniforms and held officers' titles, excluding the highest rank of general, but received no commissions. Even with intense struggle, it was not until 1944 that nurses received permanent rank, but only for the duration of the war and six months after the cessation of fighting. This, despite the fact that the women dealt with the worst product of war, the wounded and dying, and often served in extremely dangerous situations. It was not until the late 1950s that *both* women and men nurses would be free from some of the worst practices of sex stereotyping and discrimination.

World War II also fostered the rapid development of industrial and public health nursing, fields in which the number of nurses doubled. The severe shortage of nurses and physicians in civilian hospitals forced many nurses to take on medical tasks for which they received no increased pay and no formal recognition. As congressional funds became available by the 1950s, more psychiatric nurses were recruited and educated to deal with the aftermath of wartime experiences and other psychological problems. These changes, along with the sharp reduction of private-duty nurses as these women shifted to hospital employment, did not, as Melosh (1983) observes, "overturn the ironclad rule of medical dominance: by law and custom doctors were nurses' supervisors" (p. 160).

In theory, the nurses' move from private homes to hospitals and public health agencies lessened physicians' direct control over the hiring and firing of individual nurses. The massing of nurses in organizations also provided the possibility of unified work actions and female support in confronting male physicians and administrators. Theoretically, the option of creating and using formal institutional channels for complaints was also possible. In reality, health-care institutions, hospitals, and medical organizations repeatedly blocked the closure of hospital training schools and the opening of university nursing departments, and successfully lobbied Congress to close unionization to the majority of nurses. Furthermore, complaints by nurses about their treatment as women workers were not possible until the passage of the 1964 Civil Rights Act and subsequent acts and executive orders outlawing sex discrimination and harassment in education and employment.

The one clear recourse for nurses following the war, and one fostered and sanctioned by the return-home rhetoric, was to refuse to return to their prewar nursing jobs. Among nurses who had carried significant responsibilities during wartime, there was, as Melosh noted, clear dissatisfaction with returning to rigid and subordinated roles and to poor salaries; thus, in one survey of army nurses, only one in six expected to return to their civilian nursing jobs. In 1946 hospital nurses averaged 74 cents an hour for forty-eight-hour workweeks, compared to typists, who averaged 97 cents an hour, and seamstresses, who averaged $1.33. Rejecting these salaries, *and* blind obedience, *and* unbending discipline, *and* peripheral status, up to 75 percent of nurses in one survey saw themselves leaving nursing or working only to supplement their husbands' incomes, again reflecting the postwar propaganda designed to push women out of the public workplace. Dissatisfaction among hospital nurses was especially high because of long working hours and split shifts that made combining work and family tasks particularly difficult. Nevertheless, a substantial number of nurses did continue their work, many responding to the needs of patients and to the calls for help from nursing organizations.

Ironically, nursing had even greater difficulty in organizing and unifying its ranks after the Second World War because wartime emergencies had provided the rationale for a growing division of labor and the proliferation of new roles. Thus, registered nurses' attempts to unify women into a relatively independent profession were undermined by the swelling numbers of subsidiary, mostly female workers in roles often created by physicians and hospital administrators. Gradually, nursing leaders were forced to yield to pressures for the formal definition and preparation of subsidiary nurses. As in previous decades, nurses understood that medical and hospital men could keep creating new classes of cheaply paid women workers rather than meet registered nurses' demands for sufficient education, decent working conditions, adequate salaries, and control of nursing practice to ensure quality patient care.

With increasingly large bureaucracies, registered nurses became more and more involved in supervision and administration, but Melosh observed, they "were still far from claiming real control over their work . . . [and] were bitterly aware of these constraints of their new relationship to administrators" (p. 164). Some private nurses felt "a loss of personal independence . . . [and] many disliked the new division of labor" (p. 164). Others resisted demands to streamline and speed up patient care and decried new definitions of "efficiency." Charge and head nurses "chafed under new mountains of paperwork and complained of the frustrations of heavy medical and administrative demands, overcrowded wards, and understaffing" (p. 164). Nurses questioned whether they had "stopped being the servants of private duty patients merely to become the slaves of administrators" (p. 164).

Even during the war physicians continued to stress the "rightness" of nurses' subordination. For example, in 1943 one physician cautioned a graduating class of young women not to get out of line and warned them "to be good little girls and obey the physicians and the medical profession would not desert them" (Lovell, 1982, p. 218). Although nurses were much praised for their work in the Second World War, physicians' efforts to control nursing were sufficient to suppress any noticeable increase in nurses' formal power. By the late 1940s the nurse as supplementary handmaiden to the physician was still very much evident. This is obvious in one example of the legal cases of that period. In this proceeding, reported in the *New England Journal of Medicine* (1948), a nurse brought action against a physician who claimed she had made derogatory remarks about him. Despite the proven competence of the nurse, she had been removed from the nursing registry, effectively eliminating most of her employment possibilities. Although the jury decided in favor of the nurse, the court stated that in a "privileged" situation involving medical professionals, the physician had the right to take action; thus, the legal system supported further subordination of nurses, and therefore of women in general.

Freedom of speech was not directly tested, since the jury believed the nurse, who asserted that she had not made the derogatory comments.

Gender stereotypes continued to be used by physicians to reinforce their monopoly. For example, in 1946, another physician relied on the myth of "man the mighty hunter" to reaffirm patriarchal authority. Thus, he said, in the beginning, the first mother in the first primitive forest was the first nurse, not the first physician. She remained behind in the cave while the male, the hunter of all living things, stepped out of the cave and began to create specialized work and eventually, in Lovell's term, businesses, such as the medical profession. The moral of his tale? Women were "born nurses," but evidently not "born physicians." Despite flagrant disregard for both historical and anthropological fact, such sentiments were hard to attack without the support of a strong feminist movement.

The Repetitious Litany of Nursing Obedience and Peripherality

As noted previously, World War II led to the increased importance of public health nurses, whose qualifications eventually included college or university degrees. Following the war, more highly qualified nurses entered the public health field, in part to avoid direct medical control in hospitals. As in previous decades, this led to more published pronouncements by physicians, again emphasizing obedience, but now connected with the ideology of domesticity. For example, in 1948 physician Albert D. Kaiser called the public health nurse the "physician's ally," evidently assuming, as prewar physicians did, that the physician was central to the "battle." To Kaiser, maternity service was one of the public health nurse's most important functions. Ironically, he seemed unaware that nurses and other women had tried to create, through the Sheppard-Towner Act, a national system of maternal and child care in the 1920s (see chapter 5). Nor did he acknowledge that the AMA had successfully destroyed the system.

Given Kaiser's own ignorance or intentional dismissal of nurses' history, there is a peculiar contradiction in his charge that "Relatively few physicians appreciate the scope of the public health nurse in maternal services" (p. 24). Evidently, the subordination of women health reformers and the elimination of midwives by organized medicine in the 1920s and 1930s were so complete that physicians were unaware of the maternal and child care provided by nurses less than two decades earlier! Indeed, Kaiser felt it was necessary to explain to physicians the "woman's" role in the fields of child and school health. In the process, he, like his predecessors, emphasized that the female was to "assist," not "direct," others. It is the physician who "directs" the nurse in preventive service or follow-up care; she then becomes of "maximal benefit." According to Kaiser, the physician still did not understand the nurse's work and continued to object to the women because of their "interference with the management of his patients" (p. 26). Kaiser concluded: "The real function of the public health nurse is to supplement the physician's services" (p. 27). Clearly, a subordinated, peripheral female assistant, who was also minimally educated, would represent no threat to male medical authority.

You Don't Need a PhD to Carry a Bedpan

Many physicians feared that with increased education, nurses would pose a threat to the medical monopoly. As already discussed, in earlier decades nursing leaders had pushed for collegiate education to eliminate the worst abuses of hospital-based training of nurses and to achieve higher professional status. However, after World War II, this strategy was severely tested as the American Nurses' Association (ANA) noted a decline in the number of nursing students and a nursing shortage that was partially offset by the success of organized nursing in obtaining federal support for nursing education and services in the 1960s. Nevertheless, hospital and medical organizations, as in previous decades, blamed such shortages on the "minority" of "political" nurses who pressed for collegiate-based education and created an economic package that authorized state nursing associations to act as bargaining agents for their members. Former AMA president Frank Lahey claimed that nurses were "legislating and educating themselves out of jobs" (Brent, 1949, p. 68). Physician A. M. Frank said "one definitely does not need a PhD degree to carry a bedpan" (p. 70) and claimed that nurses were spending too much time in lecture halls. The American College of Surgeons issued a statement that the postwar development of nursing education was incompatible with the finding that 84 percent of illness needs could be handled by auxiliary personnel; therefore, they unilaterally called for immediate action and passed a resolution for training "vocational" nurses in short courses without bothering to consult nursing leaders and organizations.

By the early 1950s licensed practical nurses and schools for practical nurses had increased substantially. They represented a significant proportion of caregivers, but even by the late 1940s, student nurses were still providing most of the care in hospitals with nursing schools. In addition, the Red Cross recruited and trained women for jobs that paid salaries close to those of experienced, professional nurses.

Clearly, medical and hospital organizations were hardly supportive of nursing's professional and economic goals. This was most evident in the attack on Lucille Brown's 1948 research report, *Nursing for the Future,* which supported nursing's move to collegiate settings, deplored medical and hospital authoritarianism, called for more freedom for nurses and more involvement in setting health-care policies, and recommended the closure of many of the 602 hospital nursing schools, particularly those with fewer than 100 students. Of these schools, 46 percent were rated as poor or very poor. Although

Dr. Brown's work was strongly supported by nurses, her research and book were attacked at the 1948 AMA convention, and she was dismissed because she was not a nurse. Nevertheless, nursing organizations such as the National League for Nursing Education (later the NLN), the American Nurses' Association, and the National Organization for Public Health Nursing joined forces in the late 1940s and moved quickly to establish accreditation procedures for all nursing programs in the United States. The newly formed National Committee for the Improvement of Nursing Services (NCINS), which surveyed 1,150 state-accredited schools, found some two hundred substandard hospital schools of nursing and excluded them from the "accredited" list. In retaliation, the National Organization of Hospital Schools of Nursing was formed to defend such schools and attacked the NCINS as an enemy of freedom and even of free enterprise (Kalisch & Kalisch, 1978). Nevertheless, by 1957 about 75 percent of nursing schools were accredited and the smaller hospital schools were on the decline.

Eliminating Nurses' Right to Bargain Collectively

If the professionalization strategy of shifting nursing into higher education was considered unacceptable to many hospital administrators and physicians, even more potentially threatening was the possibility of nurses' unionization and collective bargaining, which Congress legalized for most workers in 1935, though they were discouraged during the war. In 1946 the ANA passed an economic security program and authorized state associations to act as exclusive bargaining agents for nurses on such issues as the forty-hour workweek and a minimum wage for nurses. Many nurses feared the possible negative effects on patients if nurses took collective action, and others were concerned about losing professional status if they were identified with union workers. Nevertheless, some nursing leaders, such as Shirley Titus, executive director of the California State Nurses Association, approved of this strategy. After the passage of the ANA economic security resolution, she said:

> Both organized medicine and the hospital have always sought to assume active and positive direction of nursing affairs in order that both nurses and nursing should function in a way that would best serve their special interests. These controls have prevented nurses from securing that background and experience which would have prepared them to live more fully and function more effectively ... [and] have also seriously retarded and deflected the normal evolution of nursing from the status of a craft to that of a profession. (Titus, 1952, p. 1110)

In an environment dominated by hospital management and physicians, the nurse, said Titus, had remained more docile and subservient than any other American worker and had even come to accept the thinking of the dominant groups that had encouraged nurses' fears of jeopardizing patient care and losing professional status. Consequently, the nurse "has been like a sleeper who has slept serenely on when a great battle—a battle for human freedom and the rights of the common man—was being waged. But eventually the sleeper awakens" (p. 1110).

Titus and other nurse leaders led the struggle for collective bargaining for nurses, but the nurses' awakening proved too threatening for physicians and hospital administrators, whose lobbies pressured Congress to exclude from collective bargaining nurses and other predominantly female health-care workers in nonprofit institutions that qualified as charities. When the Taft-Hartley Act was passed in 1947, collective bargaining, a right of most other workers, was denied to many nurses because of their location in such institutions. Since most of the workers affected were women, the Taft-Hartley Act is a textbook example of gender discriminatory legislation that effectively stalled women's unification against sexist treatment in salaries and work conditions. It also served to strengthen the medical monopoly and the monopolistic practices of hospitals. Nurses who could not unify in their own behalf or that of their patients could hardly mount a successful threat to male-dominated practices and procedures.

It is not surprising, therefore, that by 1955 nurses' salaries had fallen behind those of teachers, recreation workers, librarians, and even women factory workers. Other women workers, even with average salaries only two-thirds of their male counterparts, were doing better than nurses, despite the fact that nurses worked longer hours and had fewer benefits than most other male and female workers. Nevertheless, the American Hospital Association (AHA) in 1956 and again in 1959 reaffirmed the Taft-Hartley exemption. By 1960 university-educated nurses were earning little more than hospital-trained nurses; this limited incentives for nurses to acquire more education and thus jeopardized the goal of professionalization emphasized by organized nursing.

A Sociological Critique: The "Ambiguous Status" of Nursing

Just in case the nurses did not get the message, sociological researchers and commentators in the 1950s began to question whether nurses were really professionals or merely skilled workers. For example, Lyle Saunders (1954), targeting a nursing audience, characterized nursing as highly diversified and marked by a wide variation in training. In short, it was an occupation of "somewhat ambiguous status" (p. 119) with a discrepancy between status and responsibilities. Barely alluding to gender discrimination, Saunders commented: "It is not without significance, that even in a time of great demand for their services, the salaries of nurses remain relatively low. A part of the discrepancy between requirements and rewards may lie in lingering notions we all have about the relative capabilities of men and women" (p. 118). Following this cautious assertion, Saunders observed similarities that nursing shared with teaching and social work, two other traditional women's professions. Without overtly carrying the analysis of sexism further, Saunders stated that nursing was almost the only profession in which decisions about what work is done and how it is done are made by people outside the profession. He did not describe how these "people" came to achieve such control and monopoly. That these people were historically and currently predominantly male is a point also not made. Saunders noted the social isolation of nurses, without commenting on the gender-segregated character of nursing: "It is very striking to an outsider to see doctors and their student flocks proceeding through a ward, discussing cases and a nurse instructor and her students working on the same ward, with no indication that either group has any awareness of the other's existence" (p. 121). Another characteristic of nursing, claimed Saunders, was its location in organizational bureaucracies, where nurses are "drawn into the machinery . . . and tumbled about by it" (p. 123). He predicted an increasing distance between patients and nurses, caused by complex organizational structures. Again, Saunders ignored the fact that men controlled and monopolized the machine in which the women were tumbling.

Emancipation from "Feudalism" or Retracting Errors?

Still another commentator, Daniel S. Schechter (1954), gave his somewhat more positive impressions of nurses who, he claimed, "are pleased with the improvement in their relations with physicians" (p. 192). To him, a "new note" of informality reflected the change from the handmaiden image of nursing to one of partnership with medicine. This was caused, first, by university-based education, which promoted democratic principles of organization, and, second, by the wartime experience of younger physicians with nurses as commissioned officers, both working under adverse conditions. From interviews with nurses, many of them "spoke in the strongest terms of their emancipation from 'feudalism,' [and] 'a military regime'" (p. 192).

Nurses were now more likely to use physicians' first names and less likely to rise when a physician approached the nurses' station, to step aside and wait until a physician had exited an elevator first, or to hold doors open for physicians. Schechter also claimed that nurses were also more likely to meet with physicians in informal and social situations. There were more joint committees, particularly those pertaining to operating room management. The use of some nurse educators in medical schools to teach medical students about nursing was also noted. However "not all physicians are happy about the results of nurses' increased education" (p. 192), which presumably led nurses to be more openly critical and to act as "pseudo doctors." As one nurse stated: "Some doctors seem quite threatened by the fact that nurses are getting more education. Nurses are asking more questions and are not so willing to blindly follow doctors orders" (p. 193). As nursing shortages continued and more non-nurse technicians or subnurses were created and hired, physicians complained that they could not distinguish between professionals and auxiliary workers. Ironically, it was the medical profession itself that had for decades demanded these workers! Nurses were "cheered by their increased economic and social status, but they recognize that . . . their struggle for recognition is not yet completely won" (p. 193). The physicians did not like the women's "aggressiveness," but, said Schechter, the nurses acknowledged they "have been at fault . . . and forged ahead without taking the time or the effort to acquaint the medical profession" (p. 193) with the goals and objectives of nursing, a "mistake" the nurses were now trying to correct.

It is important to recognize that some changes did occur in the late 1940s and 1950s. These were created by nurses in an era of "ultra femininity," of the return of some women workers to their homes and of an extreme emphasis on motherhood and marriage. At a time when the highest marriage rate in the Western world was recorded, some nurses were capitalizing on their gains from university education and the war. However, according to Schechter, they were also beginning to retreat from their "aggressiveness" and to retract their "errors" (p. 193).

One way to retreat was to use the conservative cultural gender templates as a way to organize the perceptions of nurses' and physicians' work. For example, nurses who were influenced by the widely recognized sociologist Talcott Parsons began to consider nursing as expressive, focused on subjective, often psychological aspects and on caring. Medicine on the other hand, was task-oriented, centered on curing and objective, goal-oriented work. Such a reconstitution of the actual work of nurses was a compromise that could not stand real analysis, but it was acceptable to many physicians whose monopoly of health care could hardly be threatened by such emotion-oriented women workers. Over time, Parsons's dichotomized theoretical constructs would collapse under feminist analyses. Similarly, such sociological theories applied to nursing would eventually give way to more accurate portrayals of nurses' work that would be more threatening to the medical monopoly. Nevertheless, in 1955, the nurses themselves, under the pressure of increasingly successful medical innovations and powerful national medical organizations, gave part of their power away by amending their own practice acts to include a phrase about obedience and loyalty to physicians.

In fact, the ANA adopted a "model" definition of nursing practice, which excluded any "acts of diagnosis or prescription of therapeutic or corrective measures" (Bullough, 1986, p. 352). According to Bullough, the women themselves enshrined their subservience in their own nursing model for state licensure. Sadly, it is not uncommon to find this form of "self-policing" in behaviors of oppressed groups, particularly those that fear retaliation by the powerful.

Nevertheless, while enshrining their subservience in legislative acts, nurses embraced the rhetoric of "teamwork," a code word that expressed their hopes for equality with medicine. In reality it usually covered up the widening disparities in income, authority, and prestige between the two occupations. Indeed, physicians, such as Hugh R. Leavell (1955), continued to discuss the "independence" of the public health nurse in very traditional and sex-stereotyped ways: "The nurse can be the heart of the team. With her feminine intuition and human sympathy, she compliments [*sic*] the physician's personal attributes and supplies elements that are so essential to the completeness of the team" (p. 15). He even suggested that the nurse overcome her "very natural timidity," while paradoxically stating, "Any experienced public health physician should be willing to admit that he has learned a tremendous amount from the nurses with whom he has worked. But he may not know how this learning took place. The process probably occurred so quietly and unobtrusively that he was hardly aware of what was going on" (p. 15). The "timid" woman, whose feminine sympathy allows her to be the "heart" but not the "head" of the team, was actually teaching physicians, but they evidently did not know how this occurred!

Ironically, the "expressive," even naturally "timid," nurse had to deal with rapidly changing and increasingly complex technology, instrumentation, and treatments, often requiring more "head" than "heart." Indeed, a major challenge was to retain her humanity, her concern with patients as whole people in real families and communities. This became increasingly difficult both for the individual nurse and for the profession as a whole, which once again was forced to oppose the AMA and AHA on how health care should be organized.

Nurses Oppose the AMA and AHA on National Health Insurance

From the 1940s to the 1960s, as in the 1920s, organized medicine opposed *any* form of national health insurance as socialist or communistic. Early efforts by President Harry S. Truman and Congress to pass a national health-insurance bill were fought by both the AHA and the AMA, the latter spending millions of dollars to distribute fifty-four million pamphlets to the public depicting a physician at the home bedside of a sick child; this imagery was an obvious throwback to the 1930s country doctor. The National League for Nursing Education consistently backed a nationwide health program, and the ANA, after initial uncertainty, also backed the legislation; thus, nurses were again, as in the 1920s, in direct opposition to physicians who pushed private insurance primarily focused on payments to themselves and hospitals. The nurses were under heavy pressure from physicians to oppose the legislation. But the ANA in 1950 tabled a resolution sent by the AMA, which expected the nurses to also pass the statement opposing compulsory health insurance. The nurses had their own views, and they rejected the AMA proposal. Thus, even during a very conservative, highly traditional period for women, the nurses maintained their own value system. As in the past, the physicians and hospital administrators won their campaign, but they did so without the approval of organized nursing. Increasingly, medicine and nursing were going in different directions and the sex segregation of health care was to become even more obvious.

"Mother Surrogate" without the Power to Coordinate Multiple Pressure Groups

Despite the nurses' efforts toward independence, the metaphoric hospital as "household" was still analyzed, sustaining an updated version of the traditional view of nurse as woman. For example, Sam Schulman (1958) differentiated the roles of mother surrogate and healer and claimed that the nurse as mother surrogate enacted a "feminine" role characterized by affection, intimacy, and physical proximity and identified with the protection of her patient. But as healer, skilled technical care was required, and this was centered on curative and therapeutic practices: "The healer stands in sharp contradiction to the mother surrogate . . . which not only stands as contrasting but possibly as antagonistic to one another" (p. 33). Presumably, the mother surrogate expressed feeling; the healer did not. To meet a host of needs, the healer, a single great authority, must be recognized. It is strange that early women healers, whose mothercraft included *both* domestic nursing and medicine, were now divorced from cure, ironically the one important reason for their survival over the centuries. Nevertheless, to Schulman, the mother surrogate equaled feeling and the healer provided cure that equaled "objective" treatment.

Sociologist Hans O. Mauksch (1957) drew a more convincing analysis of nursing dilemmas in the organization of patient care, recognizing *multiple* pressures from *diverse* groups: patients, nursing service, hospital personnel, paramedical and physician groups. The nurse was held accountable for the effects of all these groups, for the functioning of every person coming into contact with the patient. The hospital unit was her unit, yet few of the members of other groups overtly recognized her authority over her unit. This situation was often complicated by as many as fifteen physicians, all writing orders for a large number of patients over whom they retained clinical control, often in absentia. Mauksch stated: "Without the normal power to do so, but informally expected to, the nurse assumes responsibility to mediate, coordinate and safeguard the continuity, compatibility and even propriety of the medical care prescribed" (p. 31). He concluded: "The disappearance of the older, motherly head nurse . . . has given way to a younger, but better prepared, woman. They may handle the formal aspects of the job superbly, but . . . they do not present symbols of authority to men in our society" (p. 132). Whether any woman, young or old, would be accepted as an authority figure is questionable, particularly given Melosh's analysis of the increasingly negative cultural images of nurses in the 1950s.

A Feminist Perspective on Nurses' History and Needs in the Conservative 1950s

Amid the spate of sociologically oriented publications in the 1950s, it is difficult to find nurses' own views on gender and nurse-physician relations. However in 1957, Florence Flores, then nursing director at Massachusetts Memorial Hospitals, published a historical view of the current status of nurses. Although softened by humor, it laid out the problems quite openly. This work, atypical at the time, is considered at length because it is important to see what remained of feminism and what interpretation of early nursing history survived in the very conservative decade of the 1950s.

To Flores, women from Eve onward were nurses, responsible for binding the everyday bruises of living and strife, and nurturing mankind. Over time wise women emerged from among those who showed more aptitude in their knowledge of herbs, simple treatments, and midwifery. Satirically and pointedly, Flores defended these wise women: "They were not the counterpart of the medicine men and magicians who developed trephining, pummeling and sweating accompanied by loud noises, dancing, and the use of hideous masks to drive out evil spirits" (p. 52). According to Flores, there was little subordination of women since the practitioners usually functioned independently. Over the centuries, wise women could be found among pagan priestesses, or highborn Roman matrons, who founded hospitals, or Christian abbesses, who lived in the great medieval religious orders of women. To Flores, the severest blow to nurses was the elimination of women's orders during the Protestant Reformation, which left nursing "shattered and lying in the dust . . . [of] hopelessness and despair" (p. 52).

The Deaconesses, who emerged in Germany, the Flemish countries, and later in England, were constrained to work with medical men; thus, nurses were no longer independent in their action, but were required to function wholly under the jurisdiction of physicians. With tongue in cheek Flores claimed: "Man, the lord and master of his household and his institutions, was busily preparing the ground for great social, scientific and cultural changes; but for the most part he was ignoring his women, who in his opinion lacked the strength or the wit to participate in what was going on" (pp. 52–53). Although resentful, many women did not know how or did not dare to enter into conflict with men, but, said Flores, a few women, such as Florence Nightingale, Dorothea Dix, and Clara Barton, were made of "sterner stuff." They didn't like what they saw and started the revolution which led to their emancipation. No feminist leaders external to nursing were mentioned by Flores.

By the turn of the century, hospitals were perceived as extensions of the household in which women's "main responsibility was the custody of the patient between the doctor's visits, their chief concern his comfort and safety" (p. 53). The hospital "household" was an extension of the Victorian family: "the doctors gave the orders, the nurses carried them out without question, and the patients—in the role of the child—got what was 'good' for them" (p. 53). Nurses ran the hospital household, "handled its accounts, kept it in repair, clean and orderly, purchased its supplies, did the laundry, prepared the food, hired and supervised the personnel and of course, nursed the patients" (p. 53).

Women's move out of the home "provided them with an opportunity to express their need for emancipation . . . Little did they know that they were subjecting themselves to a lifetime of servitude and restriction the like of which most of them had never known. Nor could they have been expected to foresee the headaches they were developing for their sisters at the coming mid-century" (p. 53). Physicians delegated more responsibility, nurses' activities became more complex, and their training increased in order to work in a complicated institution, which, however, was "still being administrated as a household" (p. 53). To Flores, the student apprentice "worked where and when she was told," lived "a life of monastic subservience," and received a "low grade subsistence and an education of sorts" (p. 53).

Out of this gendered situation an off-balance triad developed. Eventually, patients' needs and physicians' desires exceeded the nurses' abilities to meet all of them. Thus, said Flores, other workers took on nurses' functions; first the dietitian, next the social worker, then the executive housekeeper, X-ray technician, physical therapist, occupational therapist, and even the records librarian. In all cases, the majority were women, and they all saw the need for academic degrees. The complexity of scientific discoveries, plus the unequal demands, forced nurses to take on more procedures and to coordinate and supervise; however, prohibited from diagnosing, treating, or prescribing, they ended up providing the care. Given the galaxy of specialists over whom the nurse had no control, she still remained the chief link between physician and patient. The physician saw her as alter ego, but only up to a point. The patient saw her as mother, someone "to love him in spite of his infirmities . . . and to sustain him when his spirit needs sustenance," but neither patient nor physician was "interested in having a woman who thinks she is a specialist" (p. 55).

What did the *nurse* want? Education, economic security, leisure, status, prestige, "the right to choose where and how and when she will work . . . above all, she wants her area of independent action defined" (p. 55). To Flores, the fractionating of patient care had left so many "holes in the dike" that the nurse did not have enough fingers to plug them. How could this web of circumstances be untangled? How could a nurse achieve education and prestige "without making her feel that she has aspirations beyond her station" (p. 55)? Flores recognized that nurses were fighting against difficult odds, but warned that, though they may confuse the men, the women themselves were not at all confused about what they wanted.

Despite Increased Pressures, Nursing Records Some Gains

Whether nurses would get what they wanted was questionable. Despite their efforts to upgrade the profession, by 1959 nurses were still the lowest paid of all professional women. For example, nurses had a median annual salary of $3,200, compared to $4,900 for secondary school teachers. This was in spite of the increase in collegiate programs and in the larger numbers of nurses with BS and MS degrees. The political actions of organized nursing had produced federal educational funds through the Nurse Training Act of 1964, a five-year legislative package that nurses had to fight to extend to 1971, when the act was renewed.

The ANA pushed for repeal of the nurses' exemption under the Taft-Hartley Act. Although the act was not repealed, at least federally employed nurses were given bargaining rights in 1962. As an alternative to direct strike actions, in 1966, 2,000 nurses from thirty-three San Francisco Bay Area hospitals handed in their resignations, protesting low salaries, difficult working conditions, and inadequate provisions for patient care. However, even with this and subsequent alternatives to strikes, it would not be until the mid-1970s, with the reemergence of feminism, that nurses in 3,500 nonprofit hospitals would be successful in their fight to repeal the act and become free to engage in collective bargaining. But this freedom would again be jeopardized in a subsequent 1994 Supreme Court ruling that reclassified many nurses as managers (see chapter 10).

Although the number of nurses had substantially increased by the 1950s, nursing leaders continued to be accused of causing shortages because of their insistence on high educational standards. It was more likely that nurses' restrictive roles, inadequate salaries, and difficult working conditions were causing shortages. These factors, combined with the back-to-home rhetoric and expectations of traditional female roles, led to an increase in the national birth rate of 45 percent from 1940 to 1947, continuing at a very high level throughout the 1950s. The back-to-home rhetoric also led to earlier ages at marriage, which, combined with high birth rates, contributed to the larger numbers of potential and actual patients and a lower number of women available to nursing as a predominantly female profession. This situation was exacerbated in the early 1950s when the Korean War put even more pressure on organized nursing to provide more nurses for military duty. Shortages were used by hospital administrators and physicians to justify shifting responsibilities in and out of nursing departments and to create more auxiliary workers and aides. Eventually, in 1952, nursing countered the proliferation of new roles by developing the highly successful associate degree program, based in two-year community colleges.

As specialization increased among physicians, they tended to transfer more medical tasks to nurses, despite the nursing shortages. This created problems, given the increasingly restrictive state nurse practice acts, most of which incorporated the 1955 ANA disclaimer in its "model" definition of nursing practice: "The foregoing shall not be deemed to include any acts of diagnosis or prescription of therapeutic or corrective measures" (Bullough, 1975, p. 232). Difficult restrictions to follow indeed, since nurses were already involved in countless diagnostic and prescriptive acts! For example, in 1957, the right to start intravenous fluids, which nurses had actually been doing for years, required joint resolutions by nursing and medical associations because laws technically allowed only physicians to pierce the skin. Over the centuries, as medicine monopolized more and more of the traditional functions of women healers, the overlap between functions among caregivers became larger. Although physicians had achieved legal rights to practice that made it illegal for nurses to engage in many healing functions, in reality, nurses actually performed as needed many of what were now called medical tasks. This was proved in ANA-sponsored research in the early 1950s (Kalisch & Kalisch, 1978, p. 597), which reported that registered nurses performed more than four hundred functions, many of these tasks previously in the province of physicians, who had sloughed them onto nurses. Indeed, nurses had for decades provided relatively independent care in schools, camps, and industry, and in the 1960s established, often with colleges and universities, nurse clinics in demonstration projects involving pregnant women, the elderly, the chronically ill, and children. In all these projects, nurses were highly evaluated. Typical of the positive findings is a University of Kansas study which compared patient care in the general medical clinic and the nurse clinic. The nurses reduced waiting time from 58 to 5.5 minutes; increased consultation time from 35 to 49 minutes; produced fewer hospitalizations; and reduced cost per patient. More importantly, the women provided care that "focused on the person and his family rather than on the disease" (Adamson, 1971, p. 1767).

The most famous early experiment and demonstration project involved pediatric nurse practitioners in Colorado, who at various field stations provided total care to approximately 75 percent of the children in these localities and produced well-documented positive results. Begun in 1965, this successful program was initiated by Loretta C. Ford, RN, and Henry K. Silver, MD at the University of Colorado, who pioneered the formalized shift of functions many nurses were performing anyway. Their program was the first to use the title "nurse practitioner" (NP) and the primary rationale was "to prepare graduate students for clinical specialization and to reclaim a role that pediatric health nurses had historically held" (Ford, 1995, p. 12). Although the Ford-Silver model emphasized nurse accountability, clinical judgment, direct patient care, illness prevention, consumer education, collegiality with physicians, and clinical research, many nurses—leaders and educators primarily—attacked the pediatric nurse practitioner program as medically based and were, regrettably, "destructive critics . . . fearful of takeovers of nursing education by physicians, their control of nursing legislation and practice, and so forth" (p. 12). Ford remembers the abuse she suffered from her own professional nursing colleagues: "It was terrible. . . . They did not believe that it (the NP program) was nursing since the nurses, they said, were learning medical skills, using instruments like an otoscope or ophthalmoscope, and they would appear to be doctors!" (Fondiller, 1995, p. 9).

Such criticisms led some to believe that state nurse practice laws needed to be changed or amended to accommodate the new expanded nursing role. Ford opposed this move, emphasizing that the Colorado pediatric NP program was within current nursing practice laws: "Academic and practice standards were maintained. . . . The nurse practitioner was a professional nurse who functioned within the nursing practice statute [of Colorado]" (Ford, 1995, p. 12). Additionally, even though the Ford-Silver model stressed nurse-physician collegiality and teamwork, critics claimed that the Colorado NPs were practicing under physician supervision. But Ford notes: "It was only when the bastardization of the original model occurred (lack of academic entry standards, sponsoring agencies other than nursing, confusion with the physician assistant, etc.) that medical control became an issue" (p. 12). Duke University, for example, announced the opening of the first physician's assistant program in the United States around the same time that Ford and Silver initiated their nurse practitioner project in Colorado. Unfortunately, Ford's vision and initial intent to prepare nurse practitioners at the graduate level was derailed by others and took a different direction. Indeed, in the late 1960s and early 1970s, there followed a proliferation of more than five hundred programs in the United States which claimed to prepare nurses for expanded roles—as physician's assistants/associates, nurse practitioners, or nurse clinicians. By the end of the 1960s the trend that Ford and Silver initiated would eventually lead to public debate, dissension, and conflict between organized nursing and medicine in the 1970s. (For a fuller discussion, see chapter 7.)

Feel like a Girl, Act like a Lady, Think like a Man, Work like a Dog

The largely informal transfer of functions from physicians to nurses led Henry Pratt, MD, (1965), to publish "The Doctor's View of the Changing Nurse-Physician Relationship." (Note that the historical trend to use "doctor" as a generic term for "physician" was making it confusing and difficult for others with doctorates and more specifically for the small number of nurses who had achieved their doctorates by the 1960s.) Pratt admitted: "The physician's concept of the perfect nurse has been: She must feel like a girl, act like a lady, think like a man and work like a dog" (p. 767). But, to him, these attitudes were changing because "the scientific, economic, and legal aspects of medicine have changed profoundly" (p. 767). What happened to all the women's efforts to create and change nursing? They were ignored and thus eliminated as causative. Instead, Pratt reviewed changes in medicine and, from this one-sided view, considered factors "favoring" change.

The demands of war on physicians and their work in military teams, as well as technological improvements, required sophisticated clinical skills; however, "there is a large grey area where there is constant overlapping of functions, duties and responsibilities" (p. 769). Again, looking to an inaccurate "golden" past when "[t]here was little, if any, overlap" (p. 769), the rapid changes in medicine were used as an explanation for the "current" blurring of roles.

To Pratt, "The nurse has become a Partner" (p. 769). He conveniently overlooked the increasingly large economic inequities in the "partnership" and believed that nurses would become "second class" physicians because of increasing medical complexity and physician shortages. As to his predecessors, things were simple to this physician: nurses made beds and gave backrubs. But by the 1960s, "The head nurse is in essence the superintendent of a 35-bed hospital" (p. 770). Pratt failed to note what Mauksch had earlier, that the head nurse was not given full authority to act in this role, but he did admit that for legal reasons the nurse must "police the activities of her partner, the physician" (p. 770). Caught between administration and medicine, "It takes a special kind of women to resolve these conflicts" (p. 770). Fortunately, said Pratt, such women were entering nursing. Women in nursing, however, had less optimistic and more realistic views of such "superwomen."

How the nurse was to provide care, act as a hospital superintendent, and police her physician "partners" without any increase in authority remained a problem. Indeed, Robert C. Leonard (1966) noted that the physician, administrator, and patient all defined the nurse in different ways, causing role conflict for the nurse, a fact that even in the mid-1960s was considered "well-documented." Although Leonard did not target nurses' roles as women, he did assert that the "expressive," nurturing function was one to which nurses have a historic claim. After eliminating cure, Leonard then questioned whether nurses, caught in bureaucratic, technological, and professional changes, could actually provide nurturing care. Using Talcott Parsons's sociological terms and theory, Leonard continued the stereotyping of the previous decade; the physician was task-oriented and instrumental; the nurse was emotion-oriented and expressive. Presenting four short experiments, Leonard showed the physical effects of the expressive style on patients. What seems forgotten is that instrumental and objective information, goals, and actions are always connected to those that are expressive and subjective. The feminist critique of the Parsonian model shows that it did not work for women and men in families, and it did not work when transferred to women nurses and medical men. In both situations, the division of instrumental and expressive simply continued sex stereotypes in different but really quite old terms.

Bonnie Bullough (1975) claimed that the continuation in the 1960s of these stereotyped attitudes even in research, could be traced to the "weight of past tradition, the subordination of nurses, the sex segregation, and the apprenticeship model in nursing education" (p. 229). All these were reinforced by nurses' emphasis on social and emotional aspects of care and not cure. The division between the rational male who diagnosed and treated and the emotional female who gave care followed gendered lines and was justified because women were "more naturally maternal and expressive" (p. 230). Thus, gender-based stereotypes deterred acceptance of the nurse practitioner, who both cured *and* cared. Indeed, many nurses came to believe they should take no independent action or responsibility: "They are able to believe this in spite of the fact that much of the time the patient's life depends on the nurse's ability to assess his condition and act intelligently on that assessment. Of course, nurses do not actually avoid all decision making. They merely pretend to avoid it" (p. 230).

This pretense was highly correlated with gender expectations that women in general should act dumb in order to not threaten the male ego. Unfortunately, such gender-stereotyped behaviors in health care were and still are deleterious and even dangerous to people's health. The imbalanced division of labor and the excessive authority of physicians had produced, as physician Leonard I. Stein (1967) called it in his now classic work, "the doctor-nurse game," which was a "neurotic transaction" in which nurses could not make a direct statement, but must address physicians in such a way as to make their recommendations sound like nonrecommendations. It is really not helpful to patients when nurses have to act stupid, or constrain intellect, or restrain action in order to prop up medical authority. As Stein noted, the consequences to nurses who refuse to engage in this neurotic transaction were at least "uncomfortable" and at most severe, including job loss (see Roberts and Group, *Gender and the Nurse-Physician Game*, publication pending). An ever-increasing number of nurses were tired of the pretense and game-playing.

We Have Become "Takers" of Doctors' Orders

In 1964, at the insistence of nurses, the first national conference for professional nurses and physicians convened in Virginia to discuss changing patterns of practice, ethical considerations in practice, and legal implications of changing practice. In 1965 (Colorado) and 1967 (California), two more conferences were held that were jointly supported by the American Nurses' Association and the American Medical Association.

At the first conference, Katherine K. Nelson (1964) noted that nurses in the mid nineteenth century collaborated with physicians, but had "little dependence on them" until "Pasteur's notable observations" that opened the "Golden Age of Medicine" (p. 25). This led to a spectacular momentum in medical developments but left the mundane for nurses, whose work of sitting by the ill at night "in the silence of a darkened ward is not nearly as dramatic as the invention and use of the cardiac pacemaker" (p. 25). To Nelson, there is something hidden about nursing practice. The overshadowing of nursing has simultaneously increased nurses' dependence on medicine and constricted the women's sphere of influence: "we seem to have moved to the viewpoint that we are 'takers' of doctor's orders" (p. 25). The emergence of large hospitals in this century exaggerated difficulties for nursing, which as a profession needed an environment in which it could "truly *nurse* its clientele" (p. 26), without simply doing the work of the hospital and meeting all the demands of other professionals.

Nelson claimed that medical treatment and therapy took priority over the promotion of health, prevention of illness, and rehabilitation. She warned physicians that they "violate this principle of economy when they waste so much of their time in the practice of medicine in trying to run the nursing profession's business" (p. 30). Nurses also wasted their time "running around after doctor's orders on how to carry out the simplest of their professional tasks" (p. 30). Since nursing had been placed under the domination of more powerful forces, it had lost the right to make its own independent judgments. Nelson called for research, but not on collaboration, since there had already been a hundred years of "togetherness." Instead, research was needed to study "how far apart can you pull the circles of responsibility and still give safe care to the patient" (p. 30).

At no point in the conference papers or in the printed proceedings of the ensuing panel discussion did the issue of sex-segregated groups arise. Although the gender of the conference members was clearly apparent, no one commented on the all-male physicians' or all-female nurses' groups. Instead, one panel member, nurse Sister Charles Marie Frank, believed that men in medicine were the best listeners, "more so than nurses" (p. 60). Ironically, the men talked a great deal, taking up much of the panel's discussion time, at least as recorded in the proceedings. Nevertheless, Eleanor C. Lambertson stated and restated the problem of dependence and independence of nurses in hospital contexts. One physician, Robin Anderson, believed "doctors talk to each other much better than you nurses do" (p. 67). To this, Lambertson replied, "You are confusing the issue" (p. 67). Anderson saw the issue as "your problem." Lambertson responded, "Yours too." Finally, one physician admitted to confusion, claiming that until nurses specialized they would remain all things to all people. Mary S. Harper spoke of role clarification, concluding that the patient and family "are the victims of our rigid hierarchical structure . . . 'everybody tells us what to do and no one agrees on anything'" (p. 70). To which surgeon Alfred Hurwitz responded that nurses needed factual knowledge: "Therefore I throw the ball back to the nursing profession" (p. 70). Frances Reiter also spoke on this issue, stressing clinical services and concluding, "I would want the chief of professional services to be the doctor as the father is head of the family" (p. 72). But she also wanted a collaborative relationship. How an adult woman was to be subordinated to "Dad" and at the same time collaborate with him as an equal remained unclear. And so the discussion continued, with no overt recognition of the sex-segregated system in which all the participants were located.

Following the conferences on nurse-physician relationships, several articles appeared. For example, Cecil G. Sheps and Miriam E. Bachar (1964), specialists in hospital administration, traced the shift from individual, "custodial nursing care" to institutional contexts and from simple to complex scientific procedures in care. These, they said, created a need for professional interdependence, with an increased number of tasks that could be performed by *both* nurses and physicians. Lacking an understanding of the historical importance of so-called custodial care and the long-term overlap of functions, they asserted: "Until a few decades ago, it would have been quite easy to define the scope and range of the physician's functions and of those of the nurse and there would have been very little overlapping. Today this is impossible" (p. 188). (It was obviously also impossible in the past.) They advocated greater education for nurses, which historically had not provided commensurate increases in rewards and status. "The nurse is no longer the handmaiden of the physician" (p. 189)—but how, they ask, is one to decide which function belongs to which professional? Their answer? Arrange and assign tasks on the minimum required skill and training. For more complex functions, time must be added as a factor. But what happens in areas involving attitudes, roles, and values? Presumably, these are inherent in all situations, but the authors seem unable to separate these; instead they ask whether a nurse should accompany a physician when *he* sees *his* patient on the floor. (Note that shared interdependence quickly breaks down when the "ownership" of the patient and the sex of the "owner" are specified.)

What happens to factors that are not easily specified? The authors suggested that judgment must be used. Whose judgment? The obvious but unstated answer: the physician's. Why? Again, because "he" and "his" group control the system. Again, as in previous writings during this period, the well-intentioned analysis avoided any recognition of the sex-stratified system and the medical monopoly; thus, the analyses were often incomplete.

By the late 1960s organized nursing and organized medicine admitted *publicly* that their relations were marked by hostilities and poor communications. In 1967 the report of the National Advisory Commission on Health Manpower concluded that close cooperation between nurses and physicians was rare and actual conflicts were common, exacerbated by the independent practice of medical practitioners. The need for role alignment was obvious, but physicians had little interest in helping nurses to achieve their full capabilities, preferring instead to retain them as obedient, nonthreatening assistants. Yet the health-care "system" needed massive reorganization to improve efficiency and reduce rapidly escalating costs, which by the late 1960s represented approximately 6 percent of the gross national product.

The trend to medical specialization was very clear. In 1934, 85 percent of physicians were general practitioners, but by 1960 the figure was only 45 percent and by 1964 it had dipped to 37 percent. The majority (63 percent) were located in forty specialties. Increased specialization had produced even larger incomes for the physicians, but no equivalent increases for the more highly educated nurses, even after they had assumed more medical tasks. Just after the Second World War, nurses' average income was a third of physicians', but that had decreased to a fifth by the 1970s.

Exposing women's dissatisfaction with their traditional roles, *The Feminine Mystique,* authored by feminist Betty Friedan (1963), marks the point of transition to a reemergence of feminism. The female labor force doubled from 16.7 million in 1947 to over 32 million by the early 1970s. Many more women, including nurses under 25 and those between 45 and 54 years of age, entered the workforce, despite discriminatory salaries, difficult hours, and grossly inadequate and insufficient child-care facilities. Organized nursing continued to take the controversial position that hospital schools should be phased out. Organized medicine continued to question collegiate education for nurses.

Given the growing number of nurse practitioner and physician's assistant programs, in 1967 the National Commission for the Study of Nursing and Nursing Education supported expanded roles for nurses and recommended that a National Joint Practice Commission be formed to work on changing nurse-physician roles and relations. The governing boards of the ANA and AMA each appointed eight members to the newly created commission, which subsequently, over a decade and a half, published a book and a monograph on legal issues, and started demonstration projects at selected institutions to assess the effects of initiating more egalitarian interprofessional relations. Unfortunately, as we shall see in chapter 8, these early efforts toward cooperation and collaboration were not sustained; the AMA pulled its delegates in 1983 and the commission was dissolved.

Research Proves Nurses' Abilities, but Physicians' Negative Perceptions Continue

Increasingly, research was conducted that proved, for example, that nurses could handle over 50 percent of patients' visits. In particular specialties, other research proved that pediatricians, for example, spent only 2 percent of their work week on cases that had made up the vast majority of those seen during their residency training. Obviously, many physicians were overtrained for the actual needs of many patients, retaining authority over tasks that nurses could and often actually did without formal or legal authorization.

Unfortunately, other research findings proved that physicians' perceptions of nurses were generally not very positive and frequently underrated the women's capabilities (see also Roberts and Group, *Gender and the Nurse-Physician Game*, publication pending). Indeed, medical researchers continued the gender-stereotyped tradition so apparent in earlier investigations: For example, Marshall O. Zaslove, J. Thomas Ungerleider, and Marielle Fuller (1968) described the "somewhat unexpected" results of a brief questionnaire completed by psychiatric residents, nurses, and patients. To the authors' surprise, the nurses were frequently mentioned by patients as being helpful to them. In contrast, the male medical residents seldom reported that nurses were helpful to patients. The differences were sharply drawn, a finding typical of several similar studies, which found physicians often underestimated nurse competence.

Physicians saw nurses as the least helpful of all treatment agents; the nurses were more generous, rating the residents as, at least, quite helpful. Patients saw both as equally helpful. Using the stereotyped family analogy, the researchers equated nurse with mother and resident with father and concluded: "If it is equally important that father in such a family see himself and his tools (i.e., medications) as powerful and his professional wife as relatively ineffectual, then again the family picture fits the data well" (p. 77). This professional "family," according to Zaslove and his colleagues, results from "unconscious transference," not a sex-stratified medical monopoly. The researchers further concluded that the nurse saw herself as a child to the physician; this "transference is, however, seemingly fraught with ambivalence" (p. 77). While overtly compliant, the nurse might sabotage the physician's work behind his back. Indeed, the physician might recognize the nurse as more powerful, but hide this fact. Obviously, without a systematic analysis of the effects of a sex-stratified monopoly, the continued use of family and marriage as a model for nurse-physician relations simply sustained an inaccurate and stereotyped picture of patient care and of caregivers.

The Sex Segregation of Bodies of Research

The sex-segregated character of practice and the separation of nursing and medicine were clearly apparent by the 1960s, but some nurses, such as Ruth Fine (1969), like many nurses before her, still hoped for improved nurse-physician relationships: "One of the dreams of my life is for nursing care—kind and quality—to be decided upon by nurses" (p. 12). Unlike others before her, Fine stated flatly that physicians were "practicing nursing without a license" (p. 13) when they inappropriately intruded into the decisions about the nursing care of patients. Although she believed that physicians and nurses should work together, as in the Ford-Silver model, she questioned whether they were actually doing so. To determine the extent of interprofessional collaboration, Fine conducted a content analysis of all studies published in *Nursing Research* from 1952 to 1967, finding *no* joint study by a physician and nurse in the 270 studies surveyed. Though a few jointly conducted studies were reported in other professional journals (e.g., Andreoli and Stead, 1967; Ford and Silver, 1967), combined research efforts were very scarce. Nevertheless, physicians continued independently to define nursing practices and engaged in stereotyped research, which, as in the study by Zaslove and his associates, produced surprise that patients actually thought nurses' care was equivalent to that given by medical residents, who were still in training. Obviously, the sex segregation of research contributed to the shock and to the residents' denigration of the nurses. Evidently, underestimation and denigration were needed to sustain the medical monopoly, even if maintained on spurious grounds.

Conflicting Views of Nurses Continue: Autonomous Professional? Or Legal Subordinate in the Bureaucratic Hierarchy?

By the end of the 1960s, the disparity between the views of physicians and nurses is amply apparent in a comparison of only two of many publications. Nursing leader Eleanor C. Lambertson (1969) faced squarely the conflict between professional autonomy and the bureaucratic hierarchy. She pointed to the central paradox: "the physician expects the nurse to initiate, coordinate and facilitate institutional and therapeutic services, . . . but deplores any action on the part of the nurse, in support of medical policy or established institutional practice, that appears to curtail his perception of his individual rights and privileges" (p. 75). Lambertson believed that the physician could not continue "to insulate himself from organizational stress and interpersonal conflict," but rather must realize that "his concept of his role may well be a causative factor" (p. 77).

In contrast, physician Charles V. Letourneau (1969), who wrote on hospital authority, claimed that "A man's authority is determined by his subordinates . . . [but] the relationship between physician and nurse is not based upon a willingness to be governed on the part of the nurse, but upon the imperatives of the law" (p. 36). Only the law permits physicians to diagnose and prescribe treatment; thus, "unlicensed persons are guilty of the illegal practice of medicine" (p. 36) if they engage in such activities. The physician must be sure that nurses carry out his orders "to the letter"; the nurse must not "second-guess" the physician. To Letourneau, the nurse might "work alongside" the physician, but the "law provides that she is to exercise no independent judgement" (p. 37).

A comparison of these two articles provides little evidence that better communication had occurred over the previous decade or even the previous century. Clearly, the physician reestablished his authority by resorting to the law, which ironically was created by pressures from his own medical group. He did not recognize that pressure from nursing groups could force such laws to change. Equally clear is Letourneau's lack of understanding that he was, without overtly recognizing it, stating that a group composed predominantly of men has authority to keep an entire profession of women from making any independent, individual judgments at all, except under serious emergencies.

The distance between views of individual nurses and physicians was equaled in the expressions and actions of their professional organizations. When nurses began to reject taking on more medical functions without increased authority, the National Academy of Science Board of Medicine issued a report that advocated that military corpsmen be recruited and trained in the new role of physician's assistant (PA)—a role that would force nurses to accept the authority of men who were usually unequal to the women in years of education or expertise. As in the past, physicians expected nurses to accept this new role, as they had been forced to accept the many previous roles created out of nursing and medical functions. This time organized nursing refused to go along with the men's unilateral action. Though there was substantial deviation from the original Ford-Silver model, the 1970s saw the further development by organized nursing of the nurse practitioner as an alternative to the physician's assistant. As we shall see in the next chapter, the conflict between medicine and nursing would become a public issue in the coming decade.

Reconciling Practice with Protest and
Confrontation with Cooperation
Nurse-Physician Relations in the 1970s

By the 1970s the medical monopoly had been strongly buttressed by the rapid
expansion of knowledge from the physical and biological sciences and by increased technological capacities. The health-care industry had become the
third largest in the nation; indeed, there was an 80 percent increase in the
number of health workers from 1960 to 1970. The greater complexity of work,
the creation of new technologists, and the development of nurse clinicians
and specialist roles in intensive and coronary care units were associated with
diagnostic and therapeutic advances, for example, in the use of radioactive
isotopes and ultrasound and infrared technologies.

The failure to achieve some form of a national health-care system, which
had been opposed by the American Medical Association (AMA) from the
1920s, or even to provide adequate health care for the poor and the elderly,
finally led in the 1960s, despite continuing AMA opposition, to the Medicare
and Medicaid programs. However, private health insurance remained the
dominant mode of reimbursement, one that covered physicians and hospitals
but often left preventive, nursing, home, and long-term care in peripheral positions. Because most physicians were in private practice, there was little direct
control of them by hospitals, nurses, or the public. Indeed, the medical monopoly over patient admissions gave physicians power over the use, even overuse, of hospital beds, thus determining the level of hospital usage. By the 1970s
it was clear from research that physicians conducted many unnecessary procedures and surgeries, particularly those involving women patients, such as hysterectomies. The medical monopoly had not solved fundamental problems
and, indeed, had helped to create a fragmented and expensive "system" of care.

The public became increasingly vocal in their criticisms of medicine and
the health-care industry. Feminists were particularly incisive in detailing the
poor and prejudicial treatment of women by male physicians. With the reemergence of feminism, nurses were more aware of and vocal about their subordination and unwilling to allow sex discrimination to limit nursing and to
prop up the medical monopoly. The number of articles written by nurses on
nurse-physician relations increased dramatically. In these publications, femi
nist analyses and interpretations of interprofessional relationships were often
very apparent, reflecting nurses' renewed connectedness to issues involving
gender equity (see Roberts and Group, 1995). If the decade of the 1920s was
the turning point for the consolidation of medical power, the decade of the

1970s was the turning point for challenges to the medical monopoly by consumers, nurses, and other health-care professionals.

Despite greater clarity on political issues, organized nursing was still forced to fight for federal funds, particularly for nursing education, even though the Nurse Training Acts of 1964 and 1971 had produced a 200 percent increase in active registered nurses between 1950 and 1978. Nurses' efforts to shift from hospital-based programs to college- or university-based education continued without any substantial support from and sometimes even the opposition of organized medicine. From 1963 to 1972, nurses with associate degrees had increased by more than 1,000 percent, those with bachelor's degrees by 90 percent and those with master's degrees by 70 percent, while the number holding doctorates doubled to more than 700. These upward trends would continue throughout the decade.

The struggle for gender and professional equity in the military continued, leading to the promotion of the chief of the Army Nurse Corps to the rank of brigadier general, one of only two women in over two centuries of American history to attain that status. The Navy and Air Force followed the lead of the Army. Nevertheless, sex discrimination and harassment continued in the military, and was particularly evident during and following the Vietnam War (see Roberts and Group, 1995).

The fight for equitable salaries and better working conditions was substantially supported by feminist successes in achieving federal legislation outlawing inequities in the workplace. Non-nurse unions were very successful in organizing nurses, particularly in large urban areas. Believing that nurses were best represented by their professional association, the American Nurses Association (ANA) in 1973 began a campaign to organize all of the registered nurses in the nation. In June 1974 over 4,000 nurses, all members of the California Nurses' Association, walked off their units at forty-three hospitals in and around San Francisco, protesting low salaries, poor working conditions, and inadequate resources for quality patient care. Finally in 1974, the sexist and restrictive Taft-Hartley Act, which had excluded or severely limited many nurses from legally organizing and taking strike actions, was finally amended, allowing nurses to bargain collectively in over 3,500 nonprofit hospitals. By 1975, 200,000 nurses were represented by the ANA in state associations and 515 bargaining contracts had been negotiated. Clearly, organized nursing was more militant and nurses were more aware that political activity at all levels was needed to achieve greater autonomy and to eliminate sex discrimination against them. Nevertheless, according to some sociologists the medical monopoly remained substantially intact.

In this chapter, we consider medical sociologists' views of medicine and nursing, the struggle over physician's assistants (PAs) and nurse clinicians or practitioners, and the continued unilateral actions by organized medicine to define and control nurses. As detailed in this chapter, the refusal to allow more autonomous roles for nurses continued, as did the manipulation of nursing by medicine through the introduction of PAs and of "new" lower-paid occupations, to be filled primarily by women. These roles were hotly debated. To some nurses, the definition and extension of nurses' roles involved the central issues of male independence, dominance, and cure versus female dependence, submission, and care. As will become obvious in this chapter, the primary question was who decides what nurses can do. This issue was especially critical to the nurse practitioners, whose expanded roles and responsibilities were encouraged by organized nursing as an alternative to those of the medically controlled PAs.

We turn next to the issue of nurses' autonomy, particularly in relation to licensure and the nurses' shift from physicians' handmaidens to patients' advocates. The efforts to obtain the legal right to make nursing diagnoses and the gender barriers to autonomy are detailed. The consequences of gendered interaction are apparent in the nurse-physician game, a neurotic interaction pattern based on traditional male-female patterns. A typical conference discussion in the mid-1970s gives a snapshot of the problems involved in changing nurses' roles. The struggle for autonomy is also exemplified at one hospital where the nurses tried to gain greater independence, only to suffer negative consequences mostly caused by physicians.

By the mid-1970s, sufficient research evidence on physicians' acceptance or rejection of nurses' expanded roles had accumulated, and the trends from the data clearly indicate physicians' preferences for PAs and underutilization of nurse practitioners. There was also evidence proving physicians' reluctance to delegate authority, their lagging acceptance of nurse practitioners, and differences between reported attitudes and actual behaviors in hiring and other practices. These generally negative trends continued despite evidence of patients' acceptance of and satisfaction with nurse practitioners. It was also clear that the nurses' own satisfaction grew as their independence increased, as did their dissatisfaction with the status quo. In addition, there was increasing evidence that the nurses' treatments produced a quality of care that equaled or exceeded physicians' primary care. Indeed, some nurse researchers were rejecting physician care as a standard of comparison and demanding that future research incorporate nurses' own perceptions of what constituted high-quality care. By the end of the 1970s, some sociological researchers were recommending that nurses become the primary caregivers and physicians become consultants—a logical solution, but one obviously unacceptable to physicians both past and present.

Medical Control: Unparalleled in Any Other Industry

Ironically, the new militancy of nurses in the 1970s emerged at the same time that medical sociologists were confirming physicians' monopoly and questioning whether nursing as a "paramedical" group could *ever* achieve autonomy. In 1970 Eliot Friedson published the *Profession of Medicine*, which, although it lacked a systematic analysis of the sex-segregated marketplace, detailed the monopolistic control by physicians and proved that they were still working to maintain and extend their exclusive right over healing. Although other occupational groups were useful to physicians, they endangered the medical monopoly, so medicine gained state control over these occupations in order to limit and supervise their activities, thus excluding the possibility of competition. According to Dale Hiestand, "In a way unparalleled in any other industry, the physician controls and influences his field and all who venture near it" (Hiestand, 1966; cited in Friedson, 1970, p. 48). In other fields, the division of labor is ordered by historical accident, or economic and political power, or competition, or purely functional interdependence; however, "the division of labor surrounding the highly professionalized activity of healing is ordered by the politically supported dominant profession" (Friedson, 1970, p. 48). Historically, predominantly male control of economic and political power over mostly women nurses had made them subject to a control not evident in any other industry.

Ironically, medical sociologists such as Friedson found there were few traditional tasks performed by physicians that were not also performed by nonphysicians. Indeed, many of the tasks now performed by nurses were once considered the prerogative of the physician or, from a longer and gendered perspective, of earlier community women healers, empirics, and midwives. In purely technical terms, there is, said Friedson, no way to consider physicians' tasks as distinctly different from those of others around them: "What the physician does is a part of a larger technical division of labor and sometimes not a very distinct or generic part. It is the physician's *control* of the division of labor that is distinct" (p. 48). Thus, said Friedson, a "quack" is determined by physician control, not necessarily by the body of knowledge that the individual uses. The term "paramedical" primarily denotes medical control, not specific tasks.

Physician control is manifested first by the approval or at least supervision of training; second, by using workers to assist with rather than perform the tasks of diagnosis and treatment; third, by the subordination of "paramedical" workers, who perform at the request or order of and under the supervision of physicians; and fourth, by the unequal distribution of prestige allocated to physicians by the public who themselves are under the control of the physician in critical matters of life and death. Thus, Friedson characterized nursing as a "paramedical" occupation, since it was marked by a lack of autonomy, responsibility, and prestige. Although lacking autonomy and prestige compared to physicians, nurses have certainly not lacked responsibility, even if they have, as in Friedson's analysis, received little credit for their *informal* assumption of such responsibilities.

According to Friedson, only in the United States had physicians been able to achieve such widespread control over nursing and other health occupations. Thus, by the 1970s, American nurses were in a decidedly difficult situation. Since the majority of nurses and other "paramedicals" are women, it is clear that the patriarchal culture has made it easy for physicians to impose control to a degree unparalleled throughout the occupational world. According to Friedson, the historical origins of occupational control emerged from guilds or universities; thus, university-trained physicians have been in a stronger position to pressure the state to subordinate their competitors. As noted in earlier chapters, this strength could be monopolistic precisely because of the historical exclusion of women (and thus of nursing) from higher education and, in turn, from professional credentialing. For centuries the organization of workers around physicians was highly unstable, with considerable competition from "irregular" practitioners. Only in cities with a stable wealthy population were physicians able to solidify their power. Friedson did not note that many of those "irregulars" were women; however, he was clear that an extensive and rigid division of labor did not emerge until the twentieth century, a fact stressed in earlier chapters. Ironically, increased male domination based on university credentials led to prolonged female resistance, most obvious in nurses' demand for locating nursing in institutions of higher education.

Nevertheless, medical control over the central functions of diagnosis, prescription, and surgery has sustained nurses' subordination. Excluding gender in his analysis, Friedson noted that the differences in personal backgrounds of health-care providers were broadly distributed throughout the "medical" system. To him, the critical issue was autonomy, the degree to which work could be carried out independently; however, where there is the greatest amount of overlap, there is the greatest amount of attempted control. Friedson noted that chiropractors, dentists, pharmacists, homeopaths, and clinical psychologists have achieved some autonomy, but he failed to observe the historical male predominance in these groups.

A second aspect of control is related to recruitment and training: longer periods of university-based education bring increased prestige and control. Restating the stereotype that nursing is composed of "trained" women who are "unlikely" to remain in the profession, Friedson believed that nursing would be unable to compete for autonomy with medicine. With this pronouncement, he asserted that nursing was supposed to be reorganized to meet the demands of marriage and family. Ironically, the feminist literature published at the same time, the early 1970s, reversed this recommendation, asking whether women should simply leave nursing, not because of marriage and family but because of male control of women and their work, which often led to severe dissatisfaction and, ultimately, departure from the field.

Nursing leaders, said Friedson, had energetically sought to establish full professional status; nevertheless, he doubted that equal status would be achieved as long as women remained subject to orders from physicians within hospital structures. Paradoxically, to obtain professional status, the nurse has had to become part of the institutional "paramedical" structure where, Friedson noted, the physician's stereotypical conception of the nurse has been sustained: she is still considered to be a woman who remains by the patient's bedside following the orders given, most frequently, by men.

Although upward mobility to mid-level administration was possible as an escape route from subordination, Friedson concluded that even with their own nursing schools, licensure boards, and service, nursing would maintain only the appearance of formal professional autonomy if nurses' work remained subject to the orders of another profession. As long as medicine retained the right to diagnose, cure, and prescribe, nursing would retain a "paramedical" status. To Friedson, physicians were autonomous, nurses were not. Physicians gave orders. Nurses gave orders to some, but primarily took orders from physicians. Professionalism as a set of personal attitudes was distinguished from structural professional status, based on the domination of one group by another. Because Friedson's analysis substantially excluded gender, he could not predict the feminist rebellion of nursing leaders and many practicing nurses in the 1970s—a rebellion triggered by the continuous shunting of medical tasks to nurses without an accompanying increase in authority and by the unilateral decision by organized medicine to create still another new category of health caregivers, the physician's assistant.

The Battle for Domination: Enter the Physician's Assistant

Many nurses strongly objected to picking up the physicians' leftover tasks; they asserted their right to their own emphasis on holistic wellness, rejected more responsibility without increased authority, and refused to allow physicians, once again, to dictate to nurses what they should do. There was no question, as T. Elaine Adamson, public health specialist, said in 1971, that productivity could be improved by realigning overlapping duties. Research results indicated that non-physicians could safely handle a substantial proportion of patients' problems and that physicians were therefore monopolizing tasks that nurses could do. Furthermore, research studies also proved that nurses could and already had been doing medical work effectively. By the end of the 1960s nurse practitioners and clinical nurse specialists had emerged (see chapter 6), but hospitals and physicians were not willing to pay more for these highly trained nurses, who were instead often put into administrative positions rather than assigned to jobs where they could use their advanced clinical skills with patients. Physicians, experiencing a self-imposed shortage because of their own restrictions on medical school admissions and facing increased technological demands and excessive specialization, decided to get rid of the "scut" work, not by giving nurses more independent authority but by creating the physician's assistant (PA), who would be responsible not to nursing but to medicine. To counter this move, organized nursing encouraged the development of a different health-care specialist, the nurse practitioner.

Initially, physicians turned from predominantly women nurses to men in creating PAs, who were recruited from military corpsmen. In the 1969 National Academy of Science Board of Medicine report, these men were recommended for such nonmilitary occupations as electroencephalogram or operating room technicians, or as PAs in highly independent positions in which their skills might go beyond those of physicians not practicing in the particular specialty in which the assistant was employed. The AMA's Council on Medical Education listed the responsibilities of PAs: taking histories and conducting physical examinations; doing routine laboratory studies, including EKG tracings; providing injections, immunizations, and care of wounds; instructing and counseling patients about physical and mental health topics; executing physicians' standing orders; delivering continuing care and monitoring treatment and therapy plans; independently performing evaluation and treatment procedures needed in life-threatening situations; and facilitating physicians' referrals to community facilities, agencies, and resources. It is indeed difficult to differentiate these responsibilities from those of physicians, and diagnosis is clearly involved. Not only did physicians welcome other men to their field, but they purposely excluded women nurses, many of whom had more years of education and experience than the medical corpsmen. The economic rewards for physicians who hired PAs could be very substantial. The rewards for nurses who took on more medical functions were questionable at best.

The legal control of PAs was "resolved" by allowing physicians to delegate functions under "standing orders," which enabled them to retain supervisory control and, even when they were not actually involved in the work, to continue to receive economic returns. To get rid of licensure problems, it was even proposed that nurses should be licensed by institutions, not state boards of nursing. For nurses, the legal problems, other than diagnosing and prescribing, could be dealt with by essentially renaming these processes, thus cloaking what might continue to be seen as "medical" functions.

As noted in chapter 6, the first PA training program opened at Duke University; its goal was to prepare the PA "to do anything which the doctor can program him to do" (Adamson, 1971, p. 1771) and hinged on the match of corpsman to physician, analogized by one physician as guide dog and blind person, a highly derogatory image and a dangerous one for patients. The University of Washington's Medex program, also under AMA sponsorship, was another early program that was eventually extended to other states. By 1972, through the 1971 Comprehensive Health Manpower Act, accreditation mechanisms for the PA programs had been established in coordination with the AMA, the Association of Physicians' Assistant Programs, and the National Board of Medical Examiners. At the same time, the National Commission on

Nursing and Nursing Education recommended role expansion, the nurse practitioner, and primary-care nursing.

As usual, the physicians thought they had the right to define for their own benefit the profession of nursing. In 1970, the AMA called for 50,000 to 75,000 nurses to be prepared as PAs, working under physician direction (*American Medical News,* 1970). After nursing's immediate rejection of this unilateral action, the AMA later published a formal position paper supporting the expansion of the nurse's role "in the direction of extending the hands of the physician" (Adamson, 1971, p. 1772) but making no reference to nurses as physician's assistants. In addition, no mention was made of the unique contribution of nursing care to the benefit of the patient. The physicians also continued their support of hospital nursing schools in direct opposition to the nurses' own efforts to move nursing education into colleges and universities. To the extent that it succeeded, this change would further remove nursing education from the control of physicians and hospital administrators and place expanding nurse roles under the control of nursing's own leaders. After many nurses refused to be PAs, nursing leaders established their own nurse clinician and practitioner programs to prepare nurses for expanded roles, and, in 1972, they obtained federal funding for these programs. Given the success of these programs, Adamson could only conclude: "The emphasis in the AMA position statement on diploma graduates and non-clinical degree graduates, the antithesis of current trends, seems to be based on a desire to have minimally trained nurse assistants who will be more willing to work under authoritarian physician leadership instead of highly educated nurses who are capable of independent judgment" (p. 1773).

The main factor affecting productivity, said Adamson, was physicians' reluctance to give up their functions and their need to retain control over the health-care system. Unfortunately, Adamson did not adequately differentiate the PA from the nurse practitioner, simply seeing them as equivalent. Nor did she openly discuss the sex-stratification system that would allow men, some with only a few months of training and often no more than a year of military experience, to function as PAs and conduct minor surgery, diagnose, and prescribe medications, while women with three to twelve years of higher education, some with a lifetime of professional experience, could not do these things and, in fact, must presumably take orders, not only from physicians, but now from the predominantly male PAs.

Adamson understood that physicians viewed delegation of tasks as a potential surrender of power. It could also mean loss of income since "costs of various tasks [delegated to others] could be assessed," which could lead to "reassembling of the professional decision-making structure" (p. 1774). Nursing costs are usually assessed as part of hospital room charges. In this way, the actual cost of expanded roles—particularly if the tasks are performed under a physician's "standing orders"—is blurred, allowing no costing-out of the actual functions and tasks and making, for example, "obstetricians in the United States . . . the highest paid midwives in the world" (p. 1774). By the end of the 1960s, the only specialty groups that had set guidelines for the advanced training of nurses were pediatricians, who alone endorsed a collaborative nurse-physician relationship, though not an independent one.

What was the future of the physician's assistant? The men were largely recruited from the military, which in peacetime would produce fewer corpsmen with less battlefield experience; thus, their supply could not be infinitely expanded. By 1971, sixty-one PA training programs existed, and though some nurses became PAs in the 1970s, the majority were not RNs. Physicians initially expected nurses to become PAs, but forty-seven of the PA programs did not require a degree in nursing at all. Nevertheless, physicians still had to rely on nurses, who had historically been legally restrained from doing anything other than lower-level tasks, regardless of their informal assumption of medical functions.

Adamson's view of overcontrolling physicians as the major impediment to change was sustained in subsequent research by nurse scholars, such as Mariann C. Lovell (1982), who criticized the AMA's Committee on Nursing's "Position Statement" as patronizing because it encouraged nursing to become a primary component of *medical* care, assuming *medical* tasks under *physicians' direction.* Nurses were to receive further training under *medical* supervision and control, thus extending the "hands of the physician" (AMA, Committee on Nursing, 1970; p. 1881). In a perfect example of paternalism, medical "fathers," said Lovell, told women what nursing needed, without input from the profession itself.

Attempting to meet the physician shortage by creating a nursing shortage was hardly appropriate, said Dorothy Cornelius, then president of the ANA. She added, "It is not the prerogative of one profession to speak for another. We strongly object to this unilateral action by the AMA" (*American Journal of Nursing,* 1970, p. 691). In addition, the press and public had responded to the report before the ANA even had the details of it.

Reconfiguring Physician Dominance: Derivative Authority in "Teams"

Regardless of nurses' indignation, in 1970 the Position Statement of the AMA's Committee on Nursing received approval by the AMA membership; thus, the physician delegates supported efforts to increase the number of nurses and to expand nurses' roles—but only under physician supervision—and agreed that licensure was not a problem since the nurse was already required to carry out physicians' orders and because the specific functions of nursing were not legally defined. The AMA membership supported *all* levels of nursing education, rather than backing nurses' drive for college- and university-based education. Physicians also called for nurses' return to patient care and away from administration, which had "interrupted the primary physician-nurse relationship" (AMA Committee on Nursing, 1970, p. 1882). The AMA supported nurses' participation on committees, thus backing the teamwork concept; however, this cost nothing since few teams formally existed and wherever they did exist the physician was to be the captain. Thus, authority continued to be *derived* for the nurse, who would take her place *beside* the physician. Better communication between the nurse and physician as side-by-side partners was necessary, but how, where, and when the nurse was to achieve adequate reimbursement as a "partner" in a "team," or attain the institutional authority needed to act independently, or to receive third-party payment for independent practice—none of these questions were addressed or answered by the AMA Committee on Nursing or by the convention delegates.

Some nurses were clearly aware that becoming a PA would tighten medical authority by making nurses responsible to physicians, not to other nurses. Since physicians and administrators had for decades been demanding and obtaining cheaper women "subnurses" and had for years been creating new categories of health workers, often spinning these off from nurses' or physicians' functions, they evidently believed that their unilateral action in creating PAs would not be blocked by nurses. But nurses such as Margaret L. Shetland (1971) recognized that physicians were simply giving away the functions that were no longer profitable to them. Shetland warned nurses against ignoring the real changes at work, the political and manipulative actions taken by medicine. She insisted that nursing must be perceived as a "responsible, mature profession" and said that "no one profession, no matter how well-meaning, has the right to make unilateral judgments out of its own area of competency" (pp. 1961–1962). It is fascinating to replace professional terms with those related to gender in Shetland's article because this makes the basic problem glaringly apparent. For example: "Until nurses [women] can learn to view themselves as responsible, mature professionals . . . others [men] will not view them as such" (p. 1963).

"Neither Role Is an Exclusive Domain": Recognizing Overlapping Functions in Cure and Care

Some well-intentioned physicians, such as Barbara Bates (1970), tried to explain nurses' role expansion to other physicians. Bates candidly stated that the nurse-physician interprofessional relation is characterized by medical authoritarianism and nursing dependence, which makes full realization of adequate patient care impossible. Following on the three earlier national conferences on nurse-physician relations (see chapter 6)—Virginia in 1964, Colorado in 1965, and California in 1967—Bates's work was one of the few published defenses of women in nursing by a woman in medicine. She visualized overlapping circles of cure by physicians and care by nurses: "Neither role is an exclusive domain" (p. 129). Indeed, with more sophisticated technology, tasks instrumental to diagnosis were increasingly done by nurses. Could the disease-focused physicians work with the psychosocial-focused nurses? "Unfortunately, the physician does not enjoy good reputation in his relations with his co-workers" (p. 130). In Bates's view, the physician thinks of the nurse as his technical assistant, thus constricting the psychosocial characteristics of his own professional viewpoint. The constriction is enforced by authoritarian behavior against which, "except perhaps for an articulate minority, nurses have not rebelled" (p. 131). In addition, "Physicians are usually men, most nurses are women, and the pattern of male dominance prevails" (p. 131). Physicians are older, are more likely to come from a higher social class, and have a stronger knowledge base, receive greater rewards, and achieve higher prestige.

Using the psychosocial focus of nurses as the rationale, Bates described new approaches to patient care, explaining to other physicians the changes nurses had begun to make. It is clear that such a translation was, and still is, necessary because of the obvious sex segregation of the professions. The clinical specialist who focuses on complete patient care is, according to Bates, trapped in bureaucratic schedules, and the role cannot be easily enacted unless she is relieved of technical tasks. In a second approach, the nurse with an expanded role takes on responsibilities usually restricted to the physician, seeing patients independently and referring them to physicians as needed. Despite the documented improvements in patient care, Bates said, "The concept of the expanded nurse role has set off ripples of apprehension within nursing circles lest by a process of professional cannibalism, the extended nurse role be consumed by medicine and deteriorate into an expanded set of delegated tasks" (p. 132). There may be some bases for nurses' concern, said Bates, in the expanded role in specialty areas, such as coronary or intensive care.

A third approach, the physician's assistant, involved doing some tasks previously assigned to nurses and some previously assigned to physicians, as needed by the latter: "The basic approach to the patient and the perception of patient needs appear to be those of the doctor, not of the nurse" (p. 132). Bates admitted that nurses may see the PA not as relief from labor but as "an unwanted replacement or economic threat" (p. 133), or a further complication in the already unwieldy number of roles in massive bureaucracies. Surprisingly, Bates did not describe the anger of nurses who saw sex discrimination in the unequal treatment of male corpsmen as opposed to women nurses.

Bates concluded that nurses were better equipped to meet a "wider spectrum of patient needs" (p. 133), but implementation of the needed complementary nurse-physician relationship might meet several obstacles. Joint communication and decision making are *not* characteristic of the physicians' directive approach. Additionally, physicians may believe that nurses are usurping their responsibility and authority; this is more likely with nurses who can provide comprehensive, not simply technical, care. Bates stated that decisions must be based on "experimentation, reasoned judgment and joint planning," not on "traditionalism, self-protectiveness and professional prestige" (p. 133).

In 1972, Bates again attempted to bridge the gap between the professions, presenting earlier research conducted on nurses' compliance and dependency (Hofling, Brotzman, Dalrymple, Graves, and Pierce, 1966). A physician's telephone call was staged and the nurse was ordered to administer a nonexistent drug at unsafe levels. Finding a bottle of the pseudo-drug in the medicine cabinet, twenty-one of twenty-two nurses set out to administer a drug they did not know, at an unsafe dosage level as indicated on the bottle, ordered by a physician they had never met. These actions were taken despite the fact that the majority had said in a previous test that they would resist or challenge such an order. Given this dangerous result, Bates asked, "What phenomenon in interprofessional relationships is at work in this kind of reaction to the mysterious phone call? I believe it is the highly autocratic tradition that we have inherited and that is still generally accepted today by both of our professions" (Bates, 1972, p. 3).

Hoping that such blind obedience might be giving way to more assertive behavior, Bates provided examples of new nursing roles. The first was a master's-level nurse faculty member who volunteered her services to a hospital clinic, where she and the resident worked out a role that excluded administration or performance of technical tasks for others. Working only on patient care, the nurse took on increased decision making and felt that she was "doing 'real nursing'" (p. 4). A second nurse, with a diploma and several years' experience, took a four-month preceptorship with two physicians for training as a nurse practitioner. In her first two weeks in practice, she saw 175 patients, delivered three babies, did four surgical closures, and performed many physical examinations. A third nurse in a physician's assistant program, taking classes with medical students, now works essentially as an intern.

Bates tried to create models of care, basing them on multiple overlapping functions in nurse-physician roles, for example, in meeting patients' psychological needs and fulfilling tasks basic to diagnosis and treatment. Patient care, according to her, did not reflect the full realization of either nurse or physician roles. Bates seemed to take the view that nurses provided psychosocial care, the usual maintenance role of women, while physicians took on the "masculine" task roles of diagnosis and treatment. Bates returned to the example of the three nurses, indicating that freedom to work with physicians, instead of being stuck in tasks delegated by hospital administration, frees the nurse to practice fully: "it would be fascinating to find out what proportion of patients they could handle on their own" (p. 6). Interestingly, midwives in rural areas and public-health nurses have worked on their own for decades; thus, evidence of independent practice was available, but perhaps unknown to Bates.

Nevertheless, Bates did present research that showed that only 22 percent of patients needed medical expertise after their first visit; thus, nurses could handle most client situations. Similarly, other research on internists showed that of every ten patients, one comes for a physical examination, two for new complaints, and seven for care of a continuing clinical condition. Many of these patients could be cared for by nurse practitioners; indeed, Bates claimed such nurses "may be able to meet most needs of most patients most of the time" (p. 6). If the health-care system could be reorganized around patients' needs, better care of patients and utilization of personnel would occur, as demonstrated in research on patients who were cared for in a nursing clinic and who subsequently exhibited fewer symptoms and less disability, and expressed fewer criticisms of their care. Bates believed the PA role was too often subsumed in the circle of medicine, rather than in overlapping circles of the two professions. Whether nurses were forsaking nursing to become PAs was not as critical to Bates as their satisfaction in using their intellectual skills and increasing their capacity for decision making.

Bates admitted that medicine has acquired a reputation not just for leadership, but for being a "bit of a bully" (p. 7), and that "nursing for the most part has followed in medicine's footsteps" (p. 7), though a portion of the ranks have rebelled, evicting physicians as teachers from nursing programs and declaring nursing's independence. With this "healthy revolt" (p. 7) now presumably over, Bates noted that it was time for individual change from the feminine self-image to one that requires brains, guts, broad shoulders, and a thick skin—all presumably traditional male attributes! Increasing levels of knowledge would be required in expanded roles; this would probably threaten some nurses, who might become hostile. But Bates viewed such nurses not as junior doctors, or technicians, or deserters from their profession, but as innovators who must carry responsibility for new clinical decisions.

To her credit, Bates insisted that physicians needed a wider perception of patient needs. She admitted that physicians constrict the scope of patient care by seeing other professionals as helpers, not as independent professionals with their own perspectives. Bates further argued that physicians must share the rewards of their profession, not only the economic ones but the relationships with patients as well: "We can delegate tasks to others and reallocate some of our functions, but we have much more trouble allowing another person to enter importantly into what we have treasured as a one to one physician-patient relationship" (p. 8).

According to Bates, individual changes would be insufficient; imaginative organizational improvements were needed because there was no long-term continuity of patient care by nurses and physicians in hospitals or public-health agencies. Very accurately she asserted: "We operate in different organizational systems, are responsive to different authorities and belong to few if any groups in which we collaborate together" (p. 8). Individual and organizational change would not suffice; the social—specifically, the economic and legal—

milieu must also change. If nurses take on more responsibilities, they must receive salaries commensurate with effort, education, and responsibilities. Clearly, Bates still perceived nurses as working for physicians and institutions, and not in independent practice. Further, she did not see legal problems as critical if physicians and nurses planned together. Her well-intentioned optimism may, however, have been misplaced; since the AMA has traditionally lobbied for restrictive laws against nurses and other professionals, it is questionable how quickly physicians would be willing to share their power and economic rewards. Similarly, hospital administrators have fought affirmative action measures and nursing professional associations and unions. Unless the monopolistic systems are changed, Bates's hopes may have been premature.

The reactions of nurses to new expanded roles and the resulting confusion surrounding expected tasks and responsibilities varied considerably; some blamed nursing, not medicine, for the confusion. For example, Bess M. Piggott (1971) believed that respect between professionals *was* possible; but to her, respect existed in the operating room, not nursing in general. She asked, "[C]an we continue in this state of disarray and survive?" (p. 57). There were 200,000 nurses not currently employed, an alarming decrease of students, a 70 to 150 percent annual turnover of nurses in hospitals in large metropolitan areas, and a twenty-one-year average working life for nurses. And now the AMA had called for up to 75,000 nurses to practice medicine as PAs under physicians' direction. Although Piggott acknowledged nurses who deplored the unilateral action by another profession to create PAs, she did not think this issue was important. She admitted that nurses still had to make suggestions in a way that made physicians think the ideas were their own. But, she asked, "What difference does it make?" (p. 58).

Criticizing the efforts to shift nursing education out of hospitals and into university programs, Piggott said that when the question is asked, "Where have all the nurses gone?" the answer will be "They are on the outside of the patient care capsule watching the electronic equipment" (p. 64). As far as she was concerned, the major problems were to be found within the primarily female group of nurses. Physicians were evidently not intruding into another profession. There was presumably no sex-discriminatory system against which women were struggling; there were only ill-advised women who were destroying nursing. Piggott seemed completely unaware of the long history of medical efforts to introduce and modify types of nurses and to reject the expansion of nurses' education in order to sustain a medical monopoly.

"No New Dilemma for Nurses": Reconciling Practice with Protest

Claire Fagin and Herbert Lehman (1971) offered a sharply different perspective: professional nursing represented the problems of women in microcosm. Deploring the negative image of nursing in a letter written by a man to the *New York Times Magazine*, the authors stressed that nursing has historically offered one of the few opportunities for women to travel, to obtain leadership, and to provide powerful models for other women. Despite the "variety, mobility, relevance and satisfaction" (p. 8) in nursing, two major problems did exist: status and power.

To escape the inhibiting forces in hospitals, nurses moved to community or school nursing, only to find they must again prove themselves. The authors clearly understood the public confusion about the various kinds of nurse preparation, and realized that physicians had created and pushed practical nurses who "overextend themselves beyond their [level of] preparation" (p. 9). Why had medicine got away with exerting such pressures? Because patriarchal society "does not place a high value on the 'caring for' role" (p. 9). Indeed, medical control of "caring" was now so complete that some nurses were even afraid to wash a patient's hair without a physician's order: thus, an intelligent woman was "behaving like a nincompoop in her work situation" (p. 11). Consequently, nursing shortages were common because physicians manipulated nurses, who are "rarely used at the level of their preparation" (p. 12). The result? Many leave. Thus, men in power create spurious shortages, which in turn free the AMA to introduce lower-paid occupations for women and to manipulate levels of training, which are then used to exclude honest competition. With each new level and type of nurse, women nurses then turn on each other to prove the validity of their own backgrounds. To Fagin and Lehman, this was the wrong way for nurses to gain status and power. The impact of feminism was obvious in this analysis.

With the reemergence of feminism, nurses began to recognize systemic manipulation and to revolt against it. To Ruth B. Freeman (1971), nurses were "reconciling practice with protest, confrontation with cooperation . . . the revolutionary with the . . . professional. This is no new dilemma for nurses" (p. 918). Freeman claimed historical precedent. Florence Nightingale championed the British soldier in an "aggressive, articulate, and sustained interchange" (p. 918). Her *Notes on Nursing* represented a protest about conditions "in medicine and administration and in public policy" (p. 918). Careful strategy, workable solutions, and practical hard work, all based on "getting the facts": these were Nightingale's approach to creating often scathing exposés: "She not only described and deplored the conditions she protested, but was able to suggest possible remedies" (p. 918). In the twentieth century, nursing had turned inward, but it was time, Freeman argued, to share "the cause of the aggrieved," to act as advocates, to build the capabilities of others so they could fend for themselves. Nurses could and should advocate once again for their patients and their rights. Warning against a passive or meek approach, Freeman called for social action, but did not elaborate on the monopolistic and bureaucratic systems that make protest for nurses so difficult.

"A Marriage between Physicians and Nurses? Thanks—but No Thanks!"

Indeed, some nurses were still using the sex stereotypes common in earlier periods. When the ANA refused to sanction PAs and countered with nurse practitioners, some nurses, such as Ludmila Davis (1971), sided with the physicians, still using the metaphor of the "interprofessional marriage." The rejection of such a stereotype is more than apparent in Shirley A. Smoyak's (1971) rebuttal of Davis' article in a letter headed "'A Marriage between Physicians and Nurses.' Thanks—but NO Thanks!" Clearly, the traditional gender roles suggested by marital parallels were acceptable to Davis, but not to Smoyak. There was a clear division between these women on the propriety of gender roles as a model for professional roles. Smoyak attacked Davis's article as a "throwback to a pre-Nightingale era" (p. 53) and said Davis should obtain a salary raise, since she was so sweeping in her praise and so uncritical of the physician's assistant, which "can only reflect the author's enormous need for approval from—and fear of disagreeing with—physicians" (p. 53).

What arguments, asked Smoyak, does Davis present that justify unilateral action by the AMA, without consulting the nursing profession? Absolutely none. Unambiguously, Smoyak stated: "Nursing as a profession speaks for nursing. Physicians speak for physicians" (p. 53). Though Davis asserted that using the word "subordination" is not hostile, Smoyak countered, "The title 'physician's assistant' deletes the title 'nurse' and gives the nurse full status as a subordinate rather than a colleague" (p. 53). Indeed, she argued, the word "subordination" *is* demeaning and derogatory.

The interesting issue in this exchange is that both women were positioning themselves in relation to men: Davis as subordinate and Smoyak as equal. But what of their relationship to the patient? Like a good wife, it is impossible, said Davis, to make a commitment directly to the patient, so make it to the physician. To this, Smoyak said that "it is indeed a sad day" (p. 53) when nursing loses sight of the patient as its reason for being. The old gender-typed metaphor of patients as children, physician as father, and nurse as mother, was no longer acceptable. Smoyak clearly and unambiguously represents the change: "I prefer to keep my social and professional roles distinct" (p. 53).

Other nurses, such as Rheba de Tornyay (1971), believed that expanding the nurse's role did not necessarily make the nurse a physician's assistant. To her, expanded roles grew out of need, just as nursing aides and vocational or practical nurses evolved out of need. At no point did she acknowledge that these roles also saved hospital administrators money and allowed physicians to increase their own income at the expense of nurses, whose competition for decent salaries was consistently undercut by the simple expedient of hiring other, more poorly paid women and then redefining nurses' roles accordingly.

The development of new roles, noted de Tornyay, had historically been handled by nurses in reaction to the initiatives of non-nurses. This time was no different, but it was time to reconsider the preparation of the nurse-as-generalist and to focus on specialization. However, given the tremendous technical advances, could more and still more be added to nursing curricula? De Tornyay recommended giving stronger clinical training and demanded a different approach to educating women: "We have socialized nursing students to the submissive role . . . to be tactful and diplomatic to the point of obscuring their collaborative role . . . [and] so filled nursing students with the fear of making a mistake that they are low risk takers" (de Tornyay p. 976). Thus, female students learn to be dependent on physicians and become "reluctant to accept responsibility and accountability for their own actions" (p. 976). Nurses did not want to take orders from PAs, said de Tornyay, and she speculated that in the future nurses might actually take orders from other nurses. Nurses had to "clean up" their language and get away from the caste-oriented terminology. How this change in communication would change actual institutional authority structures remained unclear.

In the same issue of the *American Journal of Nursing,* Abraham B. Bergman (1971) claimed that the nursing profession should accept and incorporate the wider functions of the PAs: "I work with large numbers of nurses and I sense that they have greater unease and dissatisfaction with the fate of their profession than any other group in the health field" (p. 975). To him, endless charting of trivia and a degrading supervisory system led "women with brains and spirit to chuck it all to become airline stewardesses" (p. 975). Public health nurses were bogged down with fossilized department leadership and financial eligibility forms while office nurses working with physicians were seldom involved in "any meaningful patient care activities" (p. 975).

Bergman attacked nursing education for not dealing with shortages, instead issuing "narcissistic pronouncements on the image of the nurse" (p. 975). After criticizing nurses, Bergman concluded: "The cold, harsh truth is that physicians control the delivery system, and despite changing political winds, are likely to do so for some time" (p. 975). Whether this was right or wrong, Bergman did not profess to know. He did admit the frustration of other health professionals with medicine's "undistinguished track record for innovation," but called on the nurses to accept being PAs, because, after all, "it pays to view the world as it really exists" (p. 975). Since men were in control, then women must recognize that they could do nothing without male support. Some nurses had other views, however.

Nursing Exists to Serve Society, Not the Ends of Other Professions

Martha Rogers (1972) protested the imposition of PAs by organized medicine. To her, nurses could either support independence or leave the ranks and join physicians as their subordinates. Medical efforts to stop nurses' march to an independent identity have been, Rogers said, "continuous and diligent" since Florence Nightingale; the most recent effort was cloaked in a "nonsensical nomenclature" to gull women into leaving nursing to "play handmaiden to medical mythology and machines" (p. 42). Tinkering with traditional sick services, making shamanistic claims to medical omnipotence, frightening people into compliance with "authoritative" magical threats—these will not prevail against the "embryonic concern for human rights and the dignity of people" (p. 42).

In sharp contrast to de Tornyay, Rogers charged that categories of health workers had multiplied *without regard for human safety.* Vested interests try to do away with nurse licensure and still subject it to the "control of some medical priesthood" (p. 42). The struggle for control had even forced the government to recommend a two-year moratorium on establishing new categories of health workers. To Rogers, "the battle for domination" became explicit in those anomalous phrases "physicians' assistant" and "pediatric associate" (p. 43).

Uncompromising, Rogers stated that professionally educated graduates of baccalaureate programs are the peers of physicians, and to recruit them as subordinates to function at a lower level in medicine represents a human and intellectual waste. Nurses may swallow the proclamations of "new functions" that have been "integral to nursing practice for many decades" (p. 43) but are now limited to the confines of medical knowledge, concerned with physiological pathology, not human unity. Medical practitioners are "not competent to practice in or exercise control over any other professional field" (p. 43). Medicine is only one of several disciplines required for comprehensive health care. Nursing exists to serve society and is directly responsible to the people served: "The nursing profession does not exist to serve the ends of any other profession, nor does one profession delegate anything to another profession" (p. 44). Here the boundaries are clearly set. Men may rule their profession, but women will rule their own.

Nursing emphasizes wellness, for example, in community health services, and this orientation is needed to transcend "sick services." Aggressive leadership is needed to transmit the nurses' model in health maintenance and promotion centers. The nature and delivery of present services are "critically inadequate and unsafe and notably obsolete" (p. 44). The physicians present "short-sighted, narrowly conceived modifications of long existing practices" as "innovations" (p. 44). Home-care services, for example, were started over a century ago by nurses, but were now claimed as the physicians' "creation."

Monitoring new machines is a needed skill. For this, a college or graduate education is not necessary, but the assessments made of data collected from machines *do* require the scientific basis founded in higher education. The medical divide-and-conquer attack on nurses had ranged from preventing nurses from joining professional associations (by threatening loss of employment) to setting up competing occupational groups under a paternal control. Nurses had too long adhered to a "sad state of dependency," frightened of confrontation with the status quo, a confrontation which requires "commitment and courage" (p. 45). If women are socialized to be passive and dependent, then confrontation with men, particularly those at the pinnacle of the occupational prestige pyramid, is indeed threatening. But, said Rogers, this confrontation was necessary if proliferation of bureaucratized roles was to be halted, if nurses' emphasis on health, not disease, was to be sustained, and if the medical monopoly was to be challenged.

The situation was so bad that in the 1972 report, *Extending the Scope of Nursing Practice,* to the Department of Health, Education, and Welfare, the AMA's Committee to Study Extended Roles for Nurses—which was composed almost equally of physicians (only one of whom was a woman) and nurses— recognized that wider professional responsibilities made "both nurse and physician feel threatened and . . . troubled by ambiguities, uncertainties, and misconceptions of their symbiotic roles" (American Medical Association, 1972, p. 1231). The "enormously wide range of tasks [were] often under close supervision by a physician" (p. 1231), but sometimes they were not. The committee claimed there was inadequate preparation of nurses and recommended curricular innovations involving physician-nurse teams. The issue in the orderly transfer of skills was role definition, not licensure or other legal problems. Increased salaries for the women in advanced roles would be offset by greater freedom for physicians and others in the system. Primary-care functions were then delineated, including those shared by both professionals. All these were spelled out without consistent reference to the gender role inequities upon which they were, in part, based. Indeed, the HEW-sponsored report recommended the orderly transfer of medical functions to nurses but did not define the nature and scope of the roles. In reality, the transfer of functions had been proceeding for many years and nurses were already performing many "medical" functions. Although admitting that relations were far from ideal, the report did not clearly implicate a sex-stratified system as a basic factor in the physicians' monopoly and the nurses' subordination.

The Imposition of the Physician's Assistant: A Gendered Struggle over Dominance and Submission?

In contrast to other analysts, June S. Rothberg (1973) directly confronted the gendered nature of the battle over PAs. The surface problems—citizen discontent with health care, shortage or maldistribution of personnel, lack of access to care, exponential expansion of knowledge, pressures for updating skills, public and peer demands for closer evaluation of science—were all based on deeper issues: "independence versus dependence, male versus female, dominance versus submission, medical cure as differentiated from health care, control in contrast to freedom, and—underlying all—economics" (p. 154).

A deceptively simple but important issue is that of title and identification. What is nursing? Is it a part of medical care with no independent functions? Is it an independent practice with no dependent functions? "A state health department official goes on record in an open meeting . . . that in ten years nurses and physicians' assistants will be doing the same thing and that, in fact, 'there will be no nurses by that name in practice'" (p. 155). The future for nursing was clear: women would be subsumed as "totally dependent practitioners" (p. 155).

The move by physicians to force nurses into this position occurred in the context of the physicians' perceptions that their monopoly and control were being eroded by "unwarranted attempts to obtain privileges rightfully delegated to the medical profession" by a wide variety of professional groups (p. 155). Physical therapists, chiropractors, psychotherapists, psychologists, and even nurses, the "handmaidens," were rebelling. Physicians still controlled the health-delivery system: "Yet there is not a discipline in the field of health services today that is not trying to attain greater control over its own practice" (p. 155). According to Rothberg, the physicians' move to turn nurses into PAs could symbolically represent medicine's reaction to the movement toward independence by all health workers.

As a predominantly women's profession, nursing requires liberation, since it has, as Rothberg stated, "inequality forced upon us from sources external to our occupational group" (p. 156). In agreement with Fagin and Lehman (1971), Rothberg believed that nursing "epitomize[s] the inequitable sex role that women's rights groups are rebelling against" (Rothberg, 1973, p. 156). Although predominantly a woman's discipline, it was not dominated by women. The classic signs of second-class citizenship included persistent low pay despite advanced preparation, a sense of powerlessness and frustration, and lack of advancement to the highest levels of policy-making positions. Rothberg contended that "nursing is going through its own process of 'consciousness raising' in precisely the same sense that the women's rights movement advocates for individual women" (p. 156). The extension of the roles of wife and mother into the workplace makes rebellion for nurses an act against not only occupational subordination but traditional "femininity."

The question of extended roles must be seen in the broader context of dependence versus independence. The PA is delegated a defined set of tasks to be carried out *only* under medical supervision; thus, by name, definition, and practice, the PA is dependent on physicians. Although there are overlapping areas with medicine, nursing, in contrast, has a distinctive field of practice and a separate legal professional identity. Though the nurse may be dependent on an MD's orders in some situations, she is also able to function legally in independent ways. To Rothberg, interdependence is the highest state of development and "to expect that mature adults . . . will complacently accept a dependent role for all time is to defy what is known about psychological development" (p. 157). The PA is denied this interdependence because his or her occupational identity is completely defined by subordination to a member of another profession. For female nurses to accept PA status is also to accept stereotyped sex roles (male equals dominant-aggressive independent, and female equals the opposite); "the mind boggles at what the predominantly male physician's assistants will be expected to accept" (p. 157).

Eventually, warned Rothberg, physicians might upgrade PAs to replace house medical staff, especially as the flow of foreign physicians decreases. If this occurs, then women in nursing will acquire another layer of male authority, this one with credentials of a lower level than the women themselves may possess. If PAs are physician surrogates, nurses may be forced to accept their orders. Nevertheless, physicians assert that PAs would not disrupt the physician-nurse relationship because the nurses could now consult the PA without disturbing the physician. "Upon occasion a nurse will be called upon to carry out the instructions of a P. A. This should not pose a professional problem since the instructions are for the good of the patient" (*Physician Associate Program*, 1972; cited in Rothberg, 1973, p. 157). Rothberg countered, "This incredibly naïve statement overlooks the fact that the nurse alone is legally responsible for her actions" (p. 157). Kansas nurses, in fact, had found that following a PA's orders placed them at risk as far as liability was concerned (*Kansas Nurse*, 1972). The writings of PAs clearly show that they avoid the drive for status afforded by education and independent professionalization, accepting instead an employee relationship with the physician, whom they can expect to mention their names "with respect and admiration to the administration" (p. 158).

Rothberg decried nurses who were caught up in this mentality and noted a "rising tide of concern and caution . . . to say nothing of the furor among nurses" (p. 158). An AMA report advised sound thought and action "to prevent the chaos on which the situation is bordering" (American Medical Association, 1972, June; cited in Rothberg, 1973, p. 158). To Rothberg, the root problem was that neither medicine nor nursing had been able to define its separate role or deliver an acceptable level of care; thus, the PA was a symptom of a dishonest sex-segregated system that could not admit or deal with the overlapping functions of the professions, insisting instead on nurses' pseudo-independence and PA's excessive dependence.

Maintaining the Status Quo While Expanding Roles?

This confused state of affairs led nurse Nancy S. Keller (1973) to conclude that "we are apparently going to attempt both to maintain a status quo *and* to move into contexts of practice as yet unexplored. Nursing functions, like it or not, are predominantly medical orders translated into action; only very indirectly do they evolve from the needs of patients" (pp. 236, 237). Influenced by medical sociologists, Keller further concluded: "We have sought valiantly to professionalize the work of nursing, but the most that we have accomplished is to professionalize the viewpoint of the worker" (p. 237).

In the attempt to professionalize the work of nursing, Keller claimed that a "supernurse" was envisioned: a person who would devise effective nursing care plans, teach her staff, implement procedures for early rehabilitation, see to her patient's comfort, and individualize patient care. But these goals were incompatible with routinization in complex organizations. Such a nurse was an impossible fantasy. "Neither," said Keller, "have we reckoned on the pervasiveness of the 'feminine' ideal as the basis for nurseliness" (p. 239). Medicine, hospitals, government, and communities exerted more influence on nursing than nurses did. Given the very large number of nurses, why did women en masse accept the decisions of a small number of men in medicine and hospital administration? If nurses were socialized for subordination, sex-segregated in the marketplace, and subject to patriarchal control in all cultural systems, the explanation for their disunity in political actions becomes clearer.

What Can Nurses Do and Who Decides?

The need for political unity among nurses was increasingly apparent to answer the question, who decides what the nurse can do? Katherine B. Nuckolls (1974) tried to answer this question by tracing some historical events which influenced nurse-physician relations. Citing the initiation of the Ford-Silver pediatric nurse practitioner program in Colorado and Duke's training program for PAs (see chapter 6), Nuckolls acknowledged that these programs were seen by many as "efforts by doctors to foist unwanted tasks off on to nurses and to control nursing for their own benefit" (p. 626). Thus, when the AMA in 1970 announced its plan to turn thousands of nurses into PAs, Veronica Driscoll, then executive director of the New York State Nurses Association, responded: "It is incongruous to believe that one profession could or should 'expand' or 'extend' or otherwise transform itself into another. Nursing is nursing and medicine is medicine" (p. 626).

What, asked Nuckolls, has led to this schism? Relying primarily on a technological explanation and ignoring the purposeful development of a medical monopoly, Nuckolls noted that, until sulfa was introduced in the mid-1930s, medical interventions were limited and nursing care was frequently the critical determinant of "medical cure," particularly given the absence of auxiliary specialists and the small number of physicians serving full-time in hospitals. In addition, most nurses were engaged in private-duty or public-health nursing, where they often made decisions about medical care on their own. Nuckolls did not see the shift to increased medical control in the 1940s as an intentional political and economic maneuver but as a development caused by new antibiotics and improved technology, which reduced the central and critical importance of nursing care and, at the same time, reduced mortality, thus increasing population growth. The larger number of potential patients created nurse shortages, which were exacerbated by unsatisfactory nursing roles, since nurses were reduced to "routine" tasks. Why and by whom they were reduced and the reasons for their reduction remained unclear in Nuckolls's analysis.

At the same time, collegiate preparation shifted the teaching of nursing away from physicians to nurses, who were prepared at advanced levels to teach their own; thus, by the 1960s, physicians as preceptors were largely excluded from nursing, and the two professional groups "were barely able to carry on a civil conversation. Independently, each profession began to develop new types of educational programs" (p. 628). The women developed master's degree programs for clinical specialties, creating the clinical nurse specialist, while the men sponsored techniques of physical assessment and the management of minor illnesses, euphemistically dubbed "expanded role functions." Since 1969 the programs have proliferated, but with no consensus as to "who should be trained and for how long, or who should be responsible for the training" (p. 628). In addition, licensure laws "often present obstacles to educational advances, new techniques, and effective delegation of tasks" (p. 628). As noted previously, in 1972, the AMA, at the request of the Department of Health, Education, and Welfare, prepared a major paper on licensure, recommending that the states expand the functional scope of health-practice acts and extend broader delegational authority. Meanwhile, the transfer of responsibility proceeded, with nurses diagnosing, treating, and even prescribing, all functions previously carried out by physicians.

Nevertheless, what nurses could do was still controlled by physicians in employing agencies and institutions. Furthermore, nurses, who are "well-trained to obey orders, are also unlikely to rock the boat by trying to change organizational policies" (p. 629), even though failure to question irrational or outdated policies produces poor patient care. Organizations further restricted nursing by failing to provide space, equipment, or backup services, which forced the nurses to perform secretarial or housekeeping functions. However, organizational limitations were still not as critical as physicians' expectations, and these would not change unless students in both professions were educated together. If this did not occur, "mutual misperceptions of roles" would continue: "The physician may be reluctant to share the close personal relationship he has developed with his patients, or he may feel threatened by the nurse's competence . . . [or] may be concerned that his patients will not accept a nurse in the new role. . . . Yet when patients respond favorably . . . he may feel threatened by her success" (p. 629). Still, Nuckolls expected that the "nurse practitioner should see herself, and be regarded by the physician, as a professional colleague with a legitimate voice" (p. 630).

How she could accomplish this without joining with other nurses in a direct attack on the medical monopoly is unclear. Indeed, the ultimate determinant of what the nurse can do is the nurse herself: "In this context, since most nurses are women and most doctors are men, the role expectations for each are highly sex-linked, and gender behavior enters into the picture. As a woman, the nurse has most likely been socialized toward compliance," with the central concepts of security in interpersonal relations and social acceptance "valued more highly than social achievement" (p. 630). This socialization is reinforced by the physician, whose ego is bolstered by the presence of a compliant handmaiden and whose identity may be threatened by a competent woman.

Nuckolls found no one answer to the question of who decides what a nurse should do; however, she recommended interdependence between professions that clearly had jurisdiction over these functions. How these came to overlap and how medicine achieved a monopoly over them remained unclear. How interdependence would help nurses deal with the medical monopoly was equally unclear. Lacking a system-wide analysis of monopolistic medical practices, Nuckolls was left with the effects of a changing technology—an inadequate historical explanation, as Gamarnikow would later claim (see chapter 2). Even with attention to gender, recommendations for interprofessional education and interdependence were unlikely to find much support from physicians if these threatened their monopoly.

The Word "Autonomy": Producing Fear, Perplexity, and Paranoia

The extent to which nurse autonomy threatened medical and hospital men was exemplified at the 1976 ANA convention in the discussion by panelists Genrose J. Alfano, nursing director; Karren Kowalski, nursing professor; LeRoy R. Levin, surgeon; George Bruce McFadden, hospital administrator; and others. The session was sponsored by the National Joint Practice Commission, which was then still viable, and the entire proceedings were subsequently published (Alfano, Kowalski, Levin, and McFadden, 1976).

Panelist Levin deplored the loss of medical, not nursing, autonomy, particularly to government organizations, and believed physicians were being pushed to "cookbook ideas. All hernias should have so many days in the hospital. All patients with such and such problems are expected to have such and such tests" (p. 46). Given the increased need for justification to government for types of patient care, Levin warned nurses that autonomy meant increased responsibility and accountability and questioned how registered nurses could provide these if they could not be differentiated from practical nurses. Dr. Barbara Brown, a nurse, responded that there were extremely competent nurses at all levels who were already held accountable, but that nurses must work out their lack of differentiation by requiring of all nurses college- or university-based education, advanced clinical training, and doctoral education for nurses at the upper levels of practice. Nurses were *already* involved in governmental processes, for example, as utilization review coordinators in hospitals; therefore, "It isn't the physician; it's a nurse who is doing the physician's work, so we are accountable" (p. 46). At one hospital, said Brown, her own research showed that with an increased RN staff, primary nursing care cost $3 less per day, produced more hours devoted to direct patient care, and decreased patients' length of hospitalization by a day and a half.

George McFadden said that the hospital administrator was in the center of controversy and "caught in the middle over the allocation of resources" (p. 47). He admitted that many administrators "do not have a particular interest in nursing arts or the promotion of collaboration between nursing and physicians," and further questioned "whether 10 percent, more than 10 percent possibly, fully understand what you [nurses] are talking about" (p. 47). He anticipated that health-care costs would soon exceed the current $135 billion a year and stressed that someone had to make decisions on allocation of resources. He admitted that there was a loss of confidence in the government, in politicians, in hospitals, and in physicians, and "obviously nursing is identified with physicians and with hospitals" (pp. 47–48). A congressional committee had recently reported more than two million unnecessary surgeries and "some 11,000 unnecessary surgical deaths" (p. 48). Although the AMA challenged the committee's report, McFadden doubted medicine would be fully vindicated and said, "I'm not certain it should be fully vindicated" (p. 48).

McFadden warned nurses that administrators may have no resources to give them. Even though he did not disagree with Dr. Brown's data, he did not seem to grasp their implication for cost savings. At least he admitted that "nursing is at the point of becoming autonomous" though it had yet to be "legitimized" (p. 48). How nurses would be legitimized without resources was unclear. Nevertheless, he advocated nurse-physician collaboration, but noted that the hospital may not be the central locus of such interaction. Nurses must go beyond institutions: "I'm not certain, for example, whether the nurse could not fulfill the role of a family practice physician" (p. 48). He immediately backed off from this speculation and questioned whether nurses could be autonomous in service organizations such as hospitals, in contrast to educational institutions, because, although medicine was losing some of its autonomy, it was still in control of professional activity within the hospitals, such as the credentials committees.

Dr. Brown agreed that the medical staff had responsibility for its own credentialing committee, but insisted that nurses should assume responsibility for allied health credentialing committees: "It's time nursing protects the rights of patients by looking at credentials of physicians' assistants, practitioner associates and others. . . . We have all kinds of sporadic Allied Health professionals springing up that a doctor wants to bring in. So I'm talking about the Allied Health credentialing of employees of physicians" (p. 49).

Karren Kowalski was equally committed to autonomous primary-care nursing. Consumers want personalized and individualized care, which was obvious, for example, in the popular women's magazines that patients read for coverage of health issues. Now, women patients in labor and delivery have nurses who followed them through ante- to postpartum care. Speaking directly to Levin, Kowalski pointedly said that creating the changes that women consumers wanted was not easy. She continued, "I think nurses should nurse patients; they should not nurse physicians and nurse systems, bureaucratic systems" (p. 51). However, she admitted that nurses have usually received their "strokes from physicians. We are women; they are men" (p. 51). She asked Dr. Luther Christman, a male nurse, what was the difference in getting what you wanted as a man. He responded that there was no difference. Brown disagreed: "[T]he first medical executive committee that I sat in on, the boys looked at me, like who are you and what are you doing here? I stayed and I went to every staff committee meeting I could and then worked in the appropriate nursing staff to take my place" (p. 51).

Moderator Alfano half-jokingly asked Levin if he would like to comment, now that he had discovered the failure of the medical profession to identify nurses as vibrant people. Levin responded that he felt like a whipping boy and stated that he had never been comfortable with the idea of the physician's assistant or associate: "it was something that politically became a fact not on the basis, really, of reality" (p. 51). Indeed, Levin contended that few physicians would choose a PA over an "autonomous thinking nurse, a responsible nurse" (p. 51). Why then had physicians forced PAs on themselves and on nurses?

To Alfano, a major problem was one of access to patients: "Perhaps, when it truly becomes 'our patients' between nurse and physician rather than 'their patients,' then we will have an even better base for our communication because we will have a better goal" (p. 53). McFadden agreed and stated that communication was "our strongest potential power base . . . [but] the weakest link that's been in the system" (p. 53). In reviewing medical staff committees, he could always "identify the nurses, and not because they were female, (they all were, incidentally) but because they all had R. N. beside their names. But . . . it was R. N., ex officio" (p. 53).

One nurse in the audience understood that better communication would not solve structural problems. She asked Brown how she had obtained hospital privileges for nurses who were external to the hospital. Brown responded that these nurse practitioners went through not the medical, but the *nursing* credentialing committee, which reviews their credentials and states what they may or may not do in the hospital. Another audience member questioned Brown on patients' charting of their feelings, concerns, and needs. Brown responded that this change had forced physicians to read the notes, thus creating better communication among patients, nurses, and physicians.

Christman focused on structural changes; in his hospital all services were coequals; they did not report to each other, but reported upward in the structure. However, an audience member said, "The power structure does not always permit all three powers to function equally . . . the hospital administrator . . . is sometimes the key and can be swayed more strongly by the medical end of this structure, than he can by the RN end" (p. 54). Christman claimed that only happens when nurses are dependent, not when they assert their competence. The moderator laughingly commented that Christman kept saying nurses should be strong, but everyone continued to ask *how* to be strong. Clearly, this male nurse saw achieving power through strength as an easier proposition than did the women nurses who questioned him.

Levin's honesty in saying he did not fully understand autonomous nursing and McFadden's assertion that most hospital administrators were unaware of changes by nurses led another nurse in the audience to ask what nurses could do to create awareness. Levin responded that it was all individual and personality. His own reaction to the word "autonomy" was that "it meant independent and that I would fear it or be concerned about it" (p. 54). He advised nurses to define autonomy succinctly and to communicate with a physician by grabbing him and talking to him: "Make him know that you exist. . . . You've got to push" (p. 54). Once again, the onus for change rested on the nurses. Clearly, as long as physicians controlled access to patients, this form of forced communication would continue to be expected of nurses.

To McFadden, the word "autonomy" in nursing was considered by some administrators to be the foundation for collective bargaining. When the audience laughed, McFadden warned them not to, because some "people do have paranoia, even hospital administrators, and that's their immediate reaction to this" (p. 54). He advised nurses to think politically outside their "own little world" in order to deal with the possible lawsuits that might emerge from nurses' autonomy. But a nurse from the audience seemed more concerned that highly educated nurses were exiting the profession, making such political action more difficult, to say nothing of patient care.

Another member of the audience, a head nurse on a twenty-four-bed surgical unit, asked how to convince physicians to stop "unnecessary orders such as vital signs, intake and output, ambulate" (p. 56). When she talked with them about unnecessary orders, they said they wanted to be sure they are covered. Christman said he had presented physicians with data on "all kinds of unnecessary, fruitless kinds of activities in which they ask nurses to scurry around" (p. 57), and he had placed the burden of finding more time for nurses on the physicians, not the nurses.

Alfano targeted the issue of how nursing autonomy would change the physician's role. Brown said her institution conducted a "humanizing medicine" symposium in which, for example, physicians learned that by sitting rather than standing with patients, physicians were perceived as spending more time with patients. Some change in physicians' attitudes was accomplished, but Brown admonished nurses to get over their hang-up over "whether we are female or male nurses and get on with demonstrating competence in practice" (p. 60). She advised nurses to stop reacting to physicians who get upset over something that is wrong. Nurses should accept the fact that they are going to make mistakes in integrating a new system of care into the organization: "Stop becoming defensive about it" (p. 60). She continued, "Physicians have to learn to do the same thing instead of shouting at each other over human error" (p. 60). She advised establishing the superordinate goal, improvement of patient care: "We try to teach every nurse not to react, but to deal with the problem rather than the behavior" (p. 60).

Christman strongly advised a shift from changing individuals to altering organizational structure: "You have got to work on means and one of the means is joint practice" (p. 60). To him, the problem was to create organizational designs in which nurses and physicians could "relate differently instead of antagonistically" (p. 60). The current design was set up for failure. One nurse from the audience, however, did not entirely agree, saying she was a pediatric nurse practitioner in practice with a pediatrician: "I have been very successful in implementing the role and I think you have to jump in somewhere, whether they are hostile or not and if you can demonstrate a personal competence, nobody can argue with success" (p. 60). In her view, nurses had waited too long and had not valued themselves as individuals. Even though she was initially suspected of being a physician's assistant, she had created changes in attitudes.

Where, asked another nurse in the audience, was the bulk of monetary savings realized by instituting primary-care nursing? In the reduction of costs, said Brown, from fewer days in the hospital, but she observed that all institutional components had to be analyzed, including reduced turnover rates. Still another nurse asked whether nursing schools ought to produce a new type of nurse, and Brown firmly agreed. But Christman again stressed that different socialization would not work unless both the structures in which nurses practice and the ways they learn to practice are changed: "We have to change the milieu before the student being inducted into it can understand what it's all about" (p. 61).

However, another nurse from the audience said that at her school the more autonomous primary nurse had been emphasized, but when she went into a work setting and enacted the new role, "I was put down by all the . . . nursing staff, because this is totally new to them. They didn't understand it; they did not condone it; they thought it was out of line. The doctors loved it. They really appreciated it. It helped them a lot. We had good communication going, so I disagree. There are things you should start with your student nurses. You should start the change there" (p. 61). Christman disagreed, saying that the autonomous nurse, entering as a stranger on a unit, would be co-opted and thus unable to change the system. He agreed that new socialization was needed, "but you can't socialize people into something that isn't there" (p. 62).

McFadden, although admitting problems with hospital administrators and with communication and rapport with physicians, concluded that the biggest challenge for nursing was to change nursing itself: "It's you and your group" (p. 62). How did nurses, the subordinates in systems headed by men such as McFadden, come to be the group responsible for organizational change? Clearly, nurses such as Christman and Brown *were* trying to change systems, but these were predominately controlled by men who, as both McFadden and Levin had noted, were often unaware or hostile or simply unwilling to change professional and organizational structures to accommodate more autonomous roles. What was the responsibility of these men to change their *own* attitudes, behaviors, organizations, and professions?

New Nurse Practice Acts: Legal Freedom or Entrapment?

By the 1970s it was very clear that system-wide changes would be required if nurses were to take on more medical functions legally. But nurses were still trapped in the legalities of practice and caught in a legal system heavily influenced by pressures from the AMA earlier in the century. Whether the nurse protested her role or changed it according to new definitions or simply followed orders, she might be in real trouble. Ironically, the traditional nurse who followed orders which led to a patient's death was, according to attorney Michel Lipman (1972), likely to be arrested for manslaughter. Peculiarly, sociologists such as Friedson considered nurses paramedical, but the law, at least in the area of liability, treated nurses as professionals, capable of exercising independent judgment. Of course, if the nurse did *not* follow orders and "wrongly substitutes her own judgment" (p. 55), she was also liable. The nurse was caught in a double bind: if she wrongly followed orders, she was liable; if she refused to follow orders, Lipman warned, the "nurse will have to face the fact that her action won't endear her to the physician, whether she is right or wrong" (p. 86). Thus, the nurse, hemmed in by monopolistic restrictions, was still legally responsible even for carrying out a physician's improper orders. If this was the situation for traditional nurses, how much more difficult was it for nurses in expanded roles? The need for new nurse practice acts in all the states was obvious, particularly in the areas of diagnosis, treatment, and prescriptive authority.

By 1970 every state licensed professional nurses, but in twenty states licensure was optional or more permissive, rather than mandatory. With permissive statutes that did not require licensure, unlicensed nurses could not use the title

RN or claim to be licensed; however, mandatory licensure involved a definition of nurse and banned all unlicensed persons from nursing practice. Even in states with mandatory licensure, the nurse practice acts were riddled with exemptions from the requirements. At least thirteen different exemptions existed, including one for *any* persons providing nursing care under physicians' orders. At the insistence of organized nursing, twenty-one states were forced by 1971 to change their nurse practice acts, and in twenty-nine more, nurses were steadily involved in efforts to convince the legislatures to amend the nurse practice acts.

The most recent changes in licensure started with the 1971 Idaho revision of the nurse practice act, which authorized particular nurses to diagnose and treat patients; then in 1972 New York revised its nurse practice acts. In 1903 New York had been the second state to establish a registration act, and in 1938 the first state to establish a nurse practice act; following Idaho, it was the second state to allow nurses to diagnose and treat "human response to disease and illness." This action was quickly followed by many other states.

The success of organized nursing in New York was achieved only after a protracted struggle caused by the bitter opposition of the medical society and the hospital association. The latter even distributed a memorandum to state legislators that accused the nurses of improperly seeking authority to practice medicine. This delayed the revised definition of nursing, but eventually nurses obtained statutory independence, only to have to defend the new statute continually throughout the next two decades.

In 1975 Carol Ann Mitchell reviewed the efforts by New York nurses to change the legal restraints on professional autonomy through political pressures leading to the enactment of the new nurse practice act. But, she asked, had legal freedom led to changes in actual practice for the majority of nurses? Mitchell claimed that institutional constraints still defined nursing: "nurses generally are not—and cannot be—person-oriented in the environment as it now exists. This particular milieu forces a relationship that is managerial, technical and task oriented" (p. 15). As long as roles are defined by the employing agency, "without either the consent or counsel of nurses ... [they] cannot practice professionally within the walls of hospitals" (p. 15).

To Mitchell, the foundation for impediments to professional practice was "basically one of societal expectations and sexist struggles. Most physicians and hospital administrators are men: nurses are generally women" (p. 15). Women were forced to depend on men for "permission to perform our independent professional functions" (p. 15), and then left to rage about the medical chauvinists. The movement of nurses into private practice may help to destroy the idea that their sisters who remain in hospitals are incapable of independent practice. This was Mitchell's hope for channeling energy into constructive action.

Sexist Barriers to Autonomy: The Physician-Nurse Game

Bonnie Bullough (1975) agreed that the worst barriers to the nurse prac-titioner movement were basically the problems of women in a woman's field. Nursing had always lived with sexist barriers, "learned to cope with them, and now finds that those very coping mechanisms are blocking progress" (p. 225). Why, she asked, did nurses stand by and allow a new occupation, the physi-cian's assistant, to develop to meet a need that nurses, with only a minimal amount of added training, could fill? Why did the women not preempt the field from the beginning? To Bullough, the answer is found in the fact that, with the possible exceptions of housewifery and prostitution, nursing more clearly embodies the female stereotype than any other occupation. Therefore, nurse-physician relations reflect extreme female subordination, which nursing education had reinforced by creating "ladylike" and subservient nurses.

The early Nightingale reforms emphasized that women be clean, chaste, quiet, and religious workers who toiled long hours, never complained, and obeyed their superiors and physicians, valuing good character even more than education. All these presumably reinforced their gender-stereotyped behavior. Nevertheless, Bullough lauded the nineteenth-century women and placed re-sponsibility elsewhere: "The real culprits are their twentieth century followers, who have uncritically accepted the more repressive assumptions along with the positive contributions" (p. 228). To her, sexism was institutionalized in hospital training schools, where service to physicians and patients, not educa-tion, was the primary goal for women, whose work produced profits for oth-ers. Nurses' intellectual subordination was validated by the "belief that the physician was always right and even when he was wrong he must be made to appear right" (p. 229). These sexist traditions, said Bullough, slowed educa-tional reform so that a half century passed between the opening of the first collegiate nursing program and the time when even 16 percent of nurses were graduated from a program operated by an educational institution. Not until 1972 were more nurses graduated from collegiate institutions, both two- and four-year, than from hospital diploma programs.

The force of tradition, nurses' subordination, their sex segregation, and their history of apprenticeship training were reinforced by nurses' subsequent emphasis in the 1950s on social and emotional support for care, not cure. This division, the rational male diagnosing and treating, and the emotional female giving care, followed gendered lines and was justified because women were "more naturally maternal and expressive" (p. 230). Thus, gender deterred the emergence of a nurse practitioner who cured *and* cared. Bullough noted that there were still nurses who thought they should take no independent responsi-bility: "They are able to believe this in spite of the fact that much of the time the patient's life depends on the nurse's ability to assess his [sic] condition and act intelligently on that assessment. Of course, nurses do not actually avoid all decision making. They merely pretend to avoid it" (p. 230).

This pretense is best exemplified in the doctor-nurse game (Stein, 1967; also see Roberts and Group, *Gender and the Nurse-Physician Game,* publication pending). Bullough reported the results of research conducted by her and graduate students, finding that the types of these games varied by situation; however, in the questioning of orders, *none* of the 103 nurses surveyed would state, "Doctor, you have made an error" (Chaffee, Kingstedt, Reiss, Baron, Brady, Lee, Kyung, Stuart, and Bullough, 1974, p. 231). Of the 40 physicians, 86 percent preferred "Doctor, would you like to check this order?" (p. 231). The most worrying finding was that nurses chose the indirect approach *regardless of age.* Older physicians also preferred this approach, but younger men were more likely to accept a direct communication from the nurses. Clearly, the nurses were still playing the game of making recommendations without appearing to do so: "Similar patterns of anticipatory withdrawal are fairly common among minority groups; the ghetto walls are often as well policed from the inside as the outside" (p. 231).

Despite game playing and legal restrictions, Bullough quite rightly pointed out that nurses' acts of diagnosis and therapy had been happening continuously. Nevertheless, the extreme superordination-subordination of physician-nurse roles had led physicians to conclude that nurses were simply not "capable of independent or even cooperative decision making" (Bullough, 1976, p. 1478). But to Bullough the most important barrier to change was the nurses' own perceptions:

> Many could not conceptualize themselves as able to make diagnostic decisions. They had, of course, been making them for years, but they had protected themselves with elaborate games which cast the physician, captain of the team, as the only legitimate decision maker. . . . [T]he women's liberation movement came at a most fortunate juncture to combat some of these ideas. The care-cure dichotomy was to a certain extent based on a sexist argument that nursing should pursue the care element because it is feminine, maternal, expressive, and natural for nurses, while the cure element is masculine, paternal, instrumental, and natural for doctors. (p. 1478)

With the reemergence of feminism, nurses were encouraged to gain autonomy in decision making; they began to feel increasingly foolish about the blatant game playing and a "long-needed honesty [was] creeping into the interaction between physicians and nurses" (p. 1478). In addition, the technological developments that led to intensive care units also caused "significant incursions of nursing into what was formerly considered medical territory" (p. 1477). By the 1970s nursing had largely eliminated the "virtual monopoly of the hospital apprenticeship" programs (p. 1477) and moved into institutions of higher education. To Bullough, these trends converged to force role expansion, which led to nurses' attack on the power of medicine to write unlimited statutes through professional regulatory boards that advised legislators. Not only had a number of states modified their nurse practice acts, although only after struggles with many physicians and health administrators, but by 1975, approximately 10,000 nurse practitioners were active and 1,500 midwives had been certified, compared to an estimated 900 PAs. Clearly, the nurses had been very active. Despite the support of PAs by medical societies and some hospital administrators, by 1977 there were over 150 nurse practitioner programs in existence.

The Anatomy of a Conflict: The Struggle for Autonomy at One Hospital

What actually happened when nurses assertively moved to achieve greater autonomy and rejected vulnerability by uniting in joint efforts to enact the new state practice acts and to introduce independent, advanced nurse specialists? Gloria Donnelly, Andrea Mengel, and Eunice King (1975) described events that occurred at St. Agnes Hospital in Philadelphia that eventually resulted in the dismissal of the director and associate director of nursing, which was followed by a protest by many nurses. Based strictly on the principle of the nurse's right to practice under the new Professional Nursing Law in Pennsylvania, the nurses claimed that medicine and hospital administration had repeatedly interfered with nursing care. Nurses picketed with signs proclaiming "Medical Imperialism Wins Again" and "Doctors Are Not Gods." Student nurses and those who had been on the staff for many years joined the pickets. Nevertheless, of the 140 nurses who committed themselves to this political action, 33 eventually resigned. What were the events that led to these results? The nurses insisted on greater autonomy and independence and introduced advanced nurse specialists into the hospital. As the authors noted, the primary product hospitals provide is nursing care, yet an "organized, intelligent progressive, assertive nursing department" was termed by a board member as a "'monster'—too bright, too well educated, and too well functioning for a community general hospital" (p. 30).

A small group of physicians charged the nurses with inaccurate and negligent care; to this the nurses responded by conducting three research studies. One investigation, a one-month survey of incident reports and medication errors, discovered only 15 errors (9 of these by foreign nurses) in some 50,000 doses, and 67 incident reports, of which 37 involved patients, including 5 injuries and 19 falls from beds (side rails were up in 13 cases). These data temporarily quieted the physicians, but the arrival of the first clinical psychiatric nurse specialist produced more resistance. Although her role had been discussed and approved by physicians, after two months the physicians began to ask their own department head if she should be reporting to them and if she should have a physician's order before seeing a patient. Reporting to the director of nursing was not deemed appropriate by some of the physicians.

A small group of men, many holding administrative posts, repeatedly interfered and seemed "baffled" by independent, thinking women and uncertain of their relationships with them. The relationships with the male nurses were even more cumbersome. According to Donnelly and her colleagues, the physicians frequently invoked the "Captain of the Ship" theory to defend their interferences. To this, the nurses replied that the captaincy had been successfully challenged in court. Physicians then moved to pressure administration to place their own chosen women in nursing administration; however, when this was accomplished, it did not lead to a reduction in tensions. There followed a meeting to request the dismissal of the director and associate director of nursing; a campaign of intimidation ensued, threatening nurses at all levels. Finally, after the nurses picketed, a committee was formed by hospital administrators, but it supported the original administrative decision to dismiss the nurse leaders.

Donnelly and her colleagues noted that many nurses protested with great reluctance because they were afraid of being fired and were concerned about adverse effects on future employment; they also feared lack of support and experienced anxiety "about acting so out of character with the traditional image of the nurse as a passive, submissive person" (p. 36). The nurses eventually split into two groups, the larger actively protested but the smaller group interpreted the problem as a personality issue; thus, "Trust among peers was constantly threatened" (p. 36), particularly as supporters withdrew out of fear of reprisal or removal of opportunities for advancement.

As the authors noted: "The violation of a nurse's rights can be a subtle process, particularly if the nurse had been educated in a regimented, traditional system where she is socialized to 'know her place'" (p. 37). However, the nurses learned that to remain silent to appease physicians was nonproductive. For example, one physician during the struggle accused a nurse of causing the death of a patient, and, after the nurse's initial silence, an investigation instigated by the nurses found the charge unsupported. The initial failure to counter the physician's accusation, however, had simply contributed to the MD's refusal to accept nurses' new roles. Although the nurses won the case involving the one nurse cited above, they lost their fight to achieve greater nursing autonomy and to reinstate the nursing administrators who had been dismissed. Nevertheless, the media coverage was extensive. A few physicians were supportive, trying to understand better the Pennsylvania Nurse Practice Act, and nurses in the city, and across the state and nation, provided welcome support. In the final analysis, "In the choice between our consciences and our careers we chose the former" (p. 38).

The "Captain of the Ship" theory, so fondly embraced by most physicians for decades, supported the belief that the medical system was untouchable. Indeed, both medical and hospital systems were exempt from federal antitrust laws until 1975, when the United States Supreme Court ruled that the Sherman Act applied to professional workers as well as to those in other industries. This ruling opened the door for nurses, especially nurse practitioners, to seek greater opportunities for independent practice and autonomy (for a more detailed discussion see chapter 9).

A Common Vulnerability: A Strategy to Unite Splintered Nurses

Given the negative reactions of physicians to nurses' efforts to change their roles at only one institution, could nursing actually control or direct change in the hundreds of educational institutions and health organizations across the nation? Margretta Styles and Mildred Gottdank (1976) spoke of vulnerability, which by definition means assailability—being susceptible to threat, attack, and assault. Admitting that nurses are vulnerable, the authors asserted that this vulnerability could be used to *unite* the separate factions in nursing: "The notion that we, in nursing, might be most available to and successful in achieving unity with the stench of our own fear in our nostrils is repulsive" (p. 1978). To the degree that nurses are vulnerable, so is the public. What is the best strategic position to help the public and nursing? "Our numbers are one obvious strength" (p. 1979). Yet these numbers reflect disunity, which is a negative factor: "we have subdivided ourselves until there no longer seems to be a community of interest with which we all identify. . . . We engage in territorial conflicts among our organizations while a vast and potentially most valuable segment of our world—those who belong to none—goes unmapped and untapped and periodically bursts forth in opposition to our positions and platforms" (p. 1979).

To Styles and Gottdank, "We are splintered, and many of the splinters do not belong to us" (p. 1979). The perception of powerlessness, if not the actuality, is a paradox given the nurses' tremendous potential for power. The actual threats, though numerous, can be lumped together, claimed the authors, under the headings of "loss of autonomy" and "separate identity." These could only be attained through a unity based on mutual recognition of a common vulnerability.

Unity could also be based on more than common vulnerability. From the mid-1960s through the 1970s, research accumulated that proved nurses' competence, providing a more positive base for a unity grounded in self-worth. Unfortunately, the research also provided evidence of physicians' often negative attitudes, their underutilization of nurse practitioners, and their preference for PAs, directly under medical control. In the next section, we consider several research studies that describe physicians' reactions to nurse practitioners and PAs.

Research Proves MDs Prefer Physician's Assistants, Resist Nurse Practitioners

The disparity between the early growth rates of the PA, certified nurse midwife, and pediatric nurse practitioner programs was evidently directly related to role challenges to physicians. Jane Cassels Record and Merwyn R. Greenlick (1976) studied the Kaiser Foundation Hospitals in Portland, Oregon, and reported that over a three-year period, the PA program had expanded but the nursing programs had not. The researchers found that the disparity was related to the differential implications for the role and status of physicians. The new programs "evoked substantial negative response from some department chiefs in the form of open opposition or passive resistance" (p. 7). The three types of departments studied, medicine, pediatrics, and obstetrics-gynecology, had different recruitment problems: internists were in short supply; pediatricians relatively plentiful; obstetricians and gynecologists in heavy demand. Thus, market conditions should have produced greater receptivity among different specialties according to varied needs. In fact, this did not occur. Instead, the attitudes of the department chiefs were the critical determinant.

Although the female nurses' education often exceeded that of the predominantly male corpsmen serving as PAs, gender was a significant determinant of the success of the different programs. The nurses were at an advantage in obstetrics and gynecology. The physicians believed that the female nurses would "know what the proper relationship between a physician and an assistant ought to be; . . . [they] would have an inculcated 'sense of their own limitations'" (pp. 8–9). Indeed, gender segregation was evident, even in social situations: at cafeteria tables, the nurse practitioners sat with nurses and the PAs sat with physicians. The researchers concluded that the ease of role definition and the breadth of roles allowed the male PAs were concessions of medical rank and privilege, which were easier for a physician to share with other men, "thereby avoiding an implicit threat to his maleness" (p. 9).

The physician's assistant relieved the internist of general practitioner functions, thus enhancing the physician's functions at "higher" levels. In contrast, the certified nurse midwife and pediatric nurse practitioner threatened the status of physicians in their areas because nurses' training encompassed the entire maternity cycle, "thus paralleling rather than buttressing the obstetrician's specialty" (p. 9). Although the nurse midwife was limited to "normal pregnancies" (p. 9), these constituted the majority of cases; thus, the total number of obstetricians could be substantially reduced if they only had to care for the few abnormal cases. In short, the nurses with lower-level degrees could do what the physicians usually do. However, when asked what the midwives *should* do, only three of ten physicians indicated delivery and labor. After three years, only one midwife remained; she performed no deliveries, despite the fact that women had historically preceded men in this field.

Among the pediatric nurse practitioners, 62 percent of the babies referred came from only 4 of 14 pediatricians; indeed, a large proportion of the pediatricians thought they were better even at well-baby care than were the nurses. These opinions probably reflect the fact that a substantial proportion of the physicians' practice involved well babies; thus, the researchers observed more physician interventions and explained these as physicians' defensive actions to preserve their economic status, which was derived from "the continued exclusive performance of at least one set of functions which define the desired higher role" (p. 11). The authors postulated the same behaviors would occur in departments of medicine with PAs, but only if the physicians were general practitioners, not if they were internists, whose elevated status allowed them to disperse less complex tasks, given their higher degree of specialization. Since the male PAs had higher patient loads from the start, obvious and unnecessary physician interventions were probably lessened, compared to those with nurses, who had only gradually built up their caseloads.

Although the researchers noted gender as contributory, they did not explicate the general research finding that male affiliation with females is not traditionally seen as providing status, nor did they refer to the equally sound research generalization that males feel they have the right to use females as subordinates and therefore are more intrusive with them. Nevertheless, Record and Greenlick established that both gender and professional role challenge were evidenced in physicians' attitudes and behaviors, which are critical to the extent and manner in which women professionals are used in new roles. Furthermore, there seemed to be a differential usage in specialties according to status threat.

Autonomy: Only under Physician Surveillance?

One of the earliest specialties to be researched involved pediatric nurse practitioners. In 1973 Edgar J. Schoen, Russell J. Erickson, George Barr, and Harvey Allen conducted a survey of 568, or 53 percent, of the members of the American Academy of Pediatrics. Since 1965, eighteen "training" programs had produced 350 pediatric nurse practitioners, and by 1971, a joint statement of the American Academy of Pediatricians and the American Nurses' Association (ANA) set practice guidelines. By 1973 the results essentially proved patient acceptance and established the professional and economic advantages of pediatric nurse practitioners to physicians' practices under particular conditions. The results supported an explanation of changing gender expectations: those physicians most favorable to pediatric nurse practitioners were the youngest and in group practice; the least favorable were solo practitioners who were older than sixty. The majority of physicians thought a nurse-physician team would enrich both professions, that parental acceptance was likely, but that the pediatric nurse practitioner would not reduce costs.

Of critical importance was the extent to which physicians approved autonomy for nurses; the majority favored nurse practitioners, but only under constant pediatrician surveillance. Control would be exerted, for example, by allowing the patient to be seen for only part of a visit. This, of course, excluded the possibility that the nurse might be preferred by some patients or that she could build up her own independent practice. Similarly, the physicians approved the nurse's care, under supervision, of minor illness; however, she would not replace the pediatrician even in well-child care. Since the pediatric nurse practitioner hoped for a more independent role, the researchers believed that some modification of attitudes would be necessary.

Schoen and his colleagues found several discrepancies. Of the respondents, 96 percent still believed that the nurses could not function successfully unless the physicians fully accepted them. As in previous research, pediatric nurse practitioners were perceived by 86 percent of the physicians as supplementing their own work, *never* as replacing it. In general, the physicians agreed that nurses could work where the physicians did not want to—rural areas for example, where only 3 percent of the respondents were located. The physicians agreed that nurse practitioners would be acceptable to parents, and 64 percent said that "many mothers would rather talk to a PNP . . . about certain problems" (p. 65). However, 58 percent felt that given a choice, the mothers would rather see a pediatrician, even if the child was healthy. Illogicalities are obvious and fears of competition are inherent in these responses.

The physicians did not believe expanded roles were a fad that would go away, but the vast majority did not expect that using nurse practitioners would reduce health-care costs. Strong support came from some physicians who had worked with pediatric nurse practitioners; but strong disagreement was expressed by many physicians who feared the nurses would be "second-class MDs" (p. 66). Furthermore, many did not want to take on more sick patients as a result of the nurses assuming responsibility for essentially healthy children. Schoen and his colleagues, still viewing the role as defined by delegated tasks, asked why, if there were generally positive attitudes, only 12 of 88 women educated as pediatric nurse practitioners since 1965 at one medical center were, as of 1972, employed with physicians. Perhaps the delegated task expectations were different from the nurses' ideas of independent and parallel professions, or maybe this difference was recognized but rejected by many physicians in the early 1970s.

Reluctance to Delegate Responsibility

By mid-decade, research on physicians and family nurse clinicians was reported by Edith Wright (1975), who, in preparation for starting a collegiate graduate program, assessed factors that would hinder or help nurses to assume the expanded role as primary caregivers in the community. Acknowledging the problem of subordination, Wright questioned whether family practice physicians would "allow" nurse clinicians to extend their work in other practice settings. Where did the physicians see nurses' positive influence, and where did they see problems? Would they support or hire a family nurse clinician? Interestingly, no questions pertained to *independent* practice by nurses. Of the 194 questionnaires distributed, only 49, or 20 percent, were returned, an indication of the physicians' interest. The low response rate, which could have been biased toward those who were supportive, indicated just over 50 percent were favorable to the expanded role. About half (53 percent) thought the family nurse clinician would enhance the delivery of health care, while 47 percent did not. Only 35 percent were willing to employ or to help educate a family nurse clinician, and 65 percent would do neither.

As Wright stated, the physicians' opinions varied greatly on nurses' responsibilities, but a large number were reluctant to give the nurses any new responsibility, and if they would "allow" any, it was not a great deal. Some physicians held definite and extreme opinions, called by Wright the all-or-nothing views: some would delegate a great deal of responsibility and others none at all. Great resistance was expressed to nurses conducting physical assessments and managing common illnesses. Surprisingly, Wright felt the results of the survey were encouraging, presumably since *some* areas of responsibility were allowed. Wright and her nursing colleagues intended to go forward with their program, regardless of the physicians' low response rate, their mixed approval of only limited functions for nurse clinicians, and the very hostile reactions by some respondents.

Independent versus Dependent Styles of Nursing Practice: Patient and Physician Perceptions

In 1976 Charles E. Lewis, physician, and Theresa K. Cheyovich, nurse, replicated a previous study conducted by Lewis and Resnick (1967) on extended roles for nurses, which had been followed by several research articles by Lewis and other colleagues from 1969 to 1975. Previous research had usually categorized nurse practitioners according to the age, sex, or health problems of patients, or to the specialty orientations of the nurses themselves. Lewis and Cheyovich observed that classification would be more functional if it were based on health-care *actions and processes* and the extent to which nurses function independently, interdependently, or dependently with physicians. More information was needed than simply the symptoms or diagnoses of patients. Indeed, the researchers wanted more detailed data on the *processes* of care. For example, what functions do nurse practitioners perform? What tests do they order? What drugs do they use? What nursing services or interventions do they provide in addition "to those activities formerly performed (officially) only by physicians" (Lewis and Cheyovich, 1976, p. 366). Lewis and Cheyovich were

particularly interested in the degree to which care allowed patients "to participate in the decision-making process related to his or her care" (p. 366). Beyond
the necessary high quality of technical performance, research was needed on
interpersonal strategies to improve client attitudes and behaviors, including
compliance in dealing with their illness and health.

Recognizing the proliferation of nurse practitioner programs throughout
the United States, Lewis and Cheyovich asked who was a nurse practitioner
and what were her functions, scope, and competence, according to specialization. Importantly, they asked, "Who should decide what that scope of functions should be?" (p. 366). Formal certification examinations and accreditation mechanisms had not yet been clearly established; although some state
laws had, as noted previously, changed to redefine nursing, what was their
actual practice to be? What, asked the researchers, differentiates a nurse practitioner from a physician's assistant, a registered nurse, or a physician?

In the process of partially replicating the earlier 1967 study, Lewis and
Cheyovich were able to compare the care given by two nurse practitioners with
similar backgrounds and training, working in the same setting and caring for
patients randomly assigned as part of the larger study. The previous research
had proven that patients receiving care from nurse practitioners, in comparison to those in a control group, had a significant reduction in their levels of disability; were significantly more satisfied with their care; were less likely to experience hospitalization and had, therefore, lower costs; were less likely to seek
care for minor problems; and experienced no greater mortality or morbidity.

The two nurse practitioners studied for the 1976 report both held master's
degrees, and both had fifteen years of experience in public health nursing and
in ambulatory care. Despite similarities in past work history, participation in
the same short training program, and practice in the same environment with
the same physicians, the two nurses provided care quite differently: "Nurse A
worked more independently, used physician consultations less frequently,
more often ordered tests and x-rays for follow-up, and more often ordered
medications for patients. Nurse B more often used laboratory tests for screening or diagnostic reasons, was more dependent on physicians, and described
the results of her care in a less optimistic fashion" (p. 368).

How did these differences in interpersonal style, characterized as differing
in independence, affect other processes of care? Cheyovich and Lewis asserted
that on the pretest, both nurses were considered a relatively infrequent source
of information, but this perception was significantly altered in the retest by
patients in the experimental group. However, changes in rankings were not so
striking for the more dependent Nurse B. On pre- and retests of ten particular
functions—some of which were traditionally nursing, e.g., changing a dressing, and others traditionally medical, e.g., deciding on medications—there
were also statistically significant shifts in patients' increased preferences for
nurses, particularly by those treated by Nurse A.

One of the most important findings: "doctors significantly increased their willingness to refer patients to both these practitioners. The physicians did not differentiate between the two practitioners in terms of their referral patterns. Also, no anecdotal evidence that the physicians perceived the nurses to be providing care differently within the Clinic was found" (p. 370). Yet the data on processes showed that Nurse A was far more independent, had more successfully integrated physician and nursing activities, and produced a greater effect than Nurse B on patients' perceptions of nurses as sources of information and as preferred caregivers.

Unfortunately, no data were collected to show differences between these nurses on attitudes toward gendered roles in general or on their perceptions of themselves as women. That gender was important is clear and obvious from the researchers' speculation that differences in findings between the 1967 and 1976 studies might be attributed to the differences in gender of patients, who in the first study were female and in the second male. If gender of patients had some bearing on the processes and outcomes of care, then logically gender roles must also have an impact on nurses (primarily women) and physicians (primarily men), including the individual perceptions and care given by two women: Nurse A, who provided, from a gendered point of view, more "androgynous" care, blending traditionally defined male and female functions and tasks more successfully and independently; and Nurse B, who continued to behave in a more dependent fashion, typical of the traditional female role. The perceptions and interactions involved in care intersect both professional and gendered roles. Yet these may go formally unstated. Indeed, the predominantly male group of physicians, initially unenthusiastic about working with the nurse practitioners, "eventually worked with them in a relatively distant fashion, [and] were unaware of any differences in the processes of care they provided" (p. 371).

A Waste of a Valuable Resource

Apparently, nurses have something to offer that goes beyond medicine or nursing, but combines both. However, given physicians' attitudes, the utilization of nurse practitioners, even those constrained by medical models, remains a critical issue; as long as nurses do not develop their own private practices, male-controlled employment may force their dependence. In 1976 Eric L. Herzog, a research specialist in management, investigated the underutilization of nurses in ambulatory care, noting that almost a decade had passed since the early positive reports on increasing skills for nurses in physical assessment, interviewing, and the care of acute and chronic diseases, and on the effects of placing nurses in settings of demonstrated need. Herzog reviewed several empirical studies, finding that the delegation of functions, although endorsed in theory, was not practiced by physicians; the work of graduates of nurse practitioner programs had also not substantially changed. Herzog deplored this waste of valuable resources, claiming that research findings demonstrated that "pediatric nurse practitioners alone can provide care for about three-fourths of the children seen in an office" (p. 26). Citing research conducted by Silver and Hecker (1970), Herzog noted that nurse practitioners managed 82 percent of 2,735 patient visits, consulting physicians by phone for only 11 percent of them. Such increases in productivity were achieved without loss of quality and with substantial patient approval.

Given these data, Herzog asked why nurse practitioners were so underutilized and concluded that a physician may not know how to delegate or blend skills since he has no training to do so. In earlier research, Herzog found the physician "almost always felt less efficacious in his work and less satisfied with his organization when the nurse assumed more responsibility" (Herzog, 1976, p. 27). To put it bluntly, when a woman takes responsibility for more than menial tasks, the man feels a "lessening of control" (p. 27). Herzog also suggested that nurse practitioners may have different desires and expectations. Another cause for underutilization may be the "lack of adequate support and acceptance" (p. 27) from other nurses, who may not see the nurse practitioner as a nurse, and from physicians, who certainly do not want her as a competitor. Hospitals did not provide even basic sources of support, such as examining rooms, for nurse practitioners; this simply reflected the overall lack of a suitable organizational structure for collaborative primary health care. Finally, Herzog found that the nurses were overtrained for prevailing legal or professional structures; organizations refused to pay them the salaries they deserved, and many insurance companies refused third-party payments.

To Herzog, the challenge in closing the gap between the potential and actual utilization of women health workers requires improving nurses' low self-image by training them to "deal with a social system, negotiate roles . . . build a team and manage change" (p. 27). A second solution was to build educators' roles into the system, using preceptors or clinical supervisors to facilitate students' transition to work. A third solution, improving the curriculum, required focusing on functions that increase student responsibility. Critically important was the need to increase the awareness of medical and administrative men and, where present, women. Ironically, Herzog suggested "teamwork," an organizational approach that certainly has not provided substantial *systemic* change in previous decades.

The Latter 1970s: Lagging Physician Use of Nurse Practitioners

Herzog called for more research, and in the following year, Robert Lawrence and his associates published the results of their study on physician receptivity to nurse practitioners (Lawrence, DeFriese, Putnam, Pickard, Cyr, and Whiteside, 1977). North Carolina physicians rated thirty-five clinical tasks, which were varied by level of difficulty and responsibility, according to their willingness to delegate them to nurse practitioners. These responses were correlated with questions on recruitment, training, reimbursement, and willingness to hire nurse practitioners. Over half the physicians would *not* hire a nurse practitioner. About 68 percent were willing to share their load in their offices, but only 3.3 percent preferred that the nurses work independently in satellite clinics. The researchers reported sexist assumptions; for example, the physicians wanted their "own" nurse practitioners trained on the job in medical centers. Clearly, educational control by nursing schools and credentialing through usual academic programs for nurses were not preferred. The researchers concluded that nurses must be trained only for tasks that physicians are willing to delegate; this, of course, negates the nurses' perceptions of their profession as distinctive and separate from medicine, with its own values.

The issue of gender, though inherent, was simply excluded from the analysis. Although it was noted that female physicians responded at a disproportionally high rate, Lawrence and his colleagues claimed that "this factor is of little practical significance since females constitute a small proportion of the total physician population" (p. 300). It is impossible to see how gender might affect, even qualitatively, physicians' acceptance of nurse practitioners when it is so summarily excluded from even a descriptive analysis.

Those physicians who approved of but would not hire nurse practitioners asserted that other personnel were already doing what nurse practitioners could do. Those who did not approve of nurse practitioners claimed that "standards of care" (p. 301) would be reduced—despite the absence of research evidence to support such judgments. Curiously, few physicians attributed their rejection to nurse-physician relations. It is also interesting to note that the functions most highly approved were those already done by nurses, such as recording the results of laboratory studies, while little approval was expressed for new functions, such as delivering babies or following uncomplicated pregnancies, already done by a few nurses, but outside hospital and medical control. The gender differentiation, although not analyzed, was also apparent in the 18.5 percent of physicians who would delegate functions to physician's assistants, who were more likely to be male and under direct male-medical control, but not to nurse practitioners, who were almost totally female in a female-dominated profession.

The one hopeful finding was that physicians who had experience in working with nurse practitioners indicated a higher likelihood of task delegation and of hiring. Still, most physicians saw the nurse practitioner as "a co-worker sharing responsibility for the total patient load, rather than as a person operating independently in a satellite setting" (p. 305). Further, one-third of the physicians, those preferring to send their "own" office nurses for short, on-the-job training, stated they would not reimburse their nurses at as high a rate as those physicians hiring fully trained NPs. About three-fourths of the physicians wanted to pay NPs a straight salary, with no incentive reimbursement and no percentage of practice income. Clearly, many of the physicians had no intention of paying appropriate market value for the nurse practitioners' enhanced skills and capabilities. Despite the emphasis on job training, many physicians thought it should be paid for, in whole or in part, by the nurses themselves. Of the specialties represented, the family or general medicine groups were *least* likely to employ nurse practitioners. Perhaps physicians in these practices were most threatened by nurse practitioners, who can do much of what physicians do in these areas.

Pediatric Nurse Practitioners: Competitors, Not Partners?

In a report on Arizona physicians' attitudes toward pediatric nurse practitioners, Paul S. Bergeson and Dori Winchell (1977) subtitled their article "Rejection of the Concept." They noted that an earlier national survey of the Fellows of the American Academy of Pediatrics (Yankauer, Connelly, and Feldman, 1970) found almost 60 percent of 4,203 respondents considered "the lack of trained allied health workers with whom they could share patient care tasks as very serious" (Bergeson and Winchell, 1977, p. 679). Of these mostly male pediatricians, 41 percent claimed they would hire such adequately trained persons, but 22 percent would hire only on a part-time basis. To help alleviate this perceived shortage, a pediatric nurse practitioner program was initiated at a local Phoenix hospital and existed from 1971 to 1975. Unfortunately, only seven of sixty-six graduates could find employment in the private sector, even though there was excellent utilization in public and nonprofit institutions, such as county and Indian health services, universities, and the military.

Why was there such poor utilization by physicians in the private sector? Bergeson and Winchell distributed a questionnaire to all 150 pediatricians in Arizona, and 89 responded. Of these, most felt that hiring a nurse practitioner rather than a "regular" registered nurse would not reduce their workload or allow them to accept more patients. Practitioners were valued in rural or low-income areas, obviously places where the physicians did not want to practice. Their written comments were very revealing: "Most were outspokenly negative though a few were equally positive" (p. 680). Some noted that the number of well babies referred to them had declined over the past five years; one physician noted a 300 percent reduction. Others wanted to associate only with other physicians in order to cover night work, since this relieved them of the obligation to be on call for backup.

Those who actually worked with a nurse practitioner "were most pleased with her performance" (p. 680). However, other physicians were afraid that nurse practitioners who diagnosed and treated common childhood disorders might fail to detect more serious problems. Bergeson and Winchell concluded that their survey did not support the idea of "an overextended and distraught pediatrician, deluged by bothersome and unimportant tasks he feels over-trained to do" (p. 680). To the contrary, many of the tasks the nurses were trained to do were "precisely the tasks the physician enjoys doing most" (p. 680). The researchers concluded that the nurse practitioner role is "perceived as competitive rather than collaborative" (p. 680). Bergeson and Winchell ad-mitted that "The literature is replete with articles describing ready acceptance of PNAs by patients, economic feasibility in practice, the advantages of a col-laborative working relationship with pediatricians, and other positive aspects" (p. 680), but research had not dealt with physician acceptance. Indeed, they asserted that the research is somehow not impartial because it is conducted by "workers committed to the concept" (p. 680). Presumably, their survey consti-tuted, in contrast, an "objective appraisal" (p. 680). Since no statistical data were presented and the response rate was relatively low, it is, ironically, some-what difficult to assess the impartiality and objectivity of this research. Cer-tainly, negative reactions of physicians to nurses' independence are not new. Bergeson and Winchell concluded that pediatric nurse practitioners were suit-able only for particular hospital and government institutions. This conclusion is evidently based on what physicians want, not on what nurses can actually do competently and safely.

Nurse Practitioners: A Matter of Medical Functions or Nursing Values?

Sporadically, the media had reported information on changing nurses' roles. For example, Donna Buys (1977), a health and medical journalist, pub-lished an article on nurse practitioners in *Modern Medicine* that was more in keeping with the medical model. She described the clinical nurse specialist in terms of caseload and institutional location. The nurse practitioner was de-scribed in terms of functions within the medical model: for example, two nurse practitioners are in complete charge of diagnosis and treatment in a hospital hypertension screening clinic; however, their protocols are approved by the hospital and a physician, who visits the clinic every week, presumably providing the usual medical control (supervision) of women's work. As a lay observer, Buys noted that some women practice the functions of nursing inde-pendently and that these have increased in scope: taking histories, doing physi-cal examinations, prescribing over-the-counter drugs, removing stitches, and so forth.

Since nurses have traditionally "obeyed orders without question" (p. 51), never making a statement without qualifying words, and physicians have historically thought nurses incapable of "independent (or even cooperative) decision-making" (p. 51), how did these changes come about? Buys credits the changes to the women's movement, education, need, and technological advances. The proof for successful women's independent practice can be traced to the rural Frontier Nursing Service in Kentucky, which since 1925 has handled maternal and child health-care needs, delivering 18,000 babies (94 percent of all births in the area) with a much lower mortality rate, despite poverty, than for the nation as a whole. In 1970 the nurses extended their services to family care, again using medical protocols to work with patients in rural areas that physicians avoid. Similarly, the Colorado pediatric nurse practitioner program, started in 1965, is noted, but credit is most often given to the physician (Silver) and not to the nurse (Ford) who co-developed the program. Buys claimed that the AMA-approved PA programs pushed nurses into reactively developing their own programs, rejecting PAs. As noted previously, the ANA, for example, advocated in 1971 a moratorium on the licensing of PAs. Like Bonnie Bullough in her 1975 article, Buys recognized the changes in state laws and acknowledged that these "legitimized what many nurses were already doing" (p. 52). She believed that physicians have had "the greatest influence in encouraging nurses to start private practices" (p. 52). She cites M. Lucille Kinlein (1977) as evidence of this, but how could the actions of this courageous independent woman, who even refused to check with physicians before setting up her practice and described nurses as too dependent on the medical model, be ascribed to physicians' influence?

Buys acknowledged that nurses have difficulty receiving insurance reimbursement. Organized medicine, for example, the California Medical Association, opposed the state assignment of separate provider numbers that would allow a fee for nurses' services. Ongoing attempts to sustain a medical monopoly and control nurses' independence cannot be justified when research indicates that 80 percent to 90 percent of patients want their subsequent exams done by nurses and that 95 percent believe the nurses' exams are more thorough. Returning to the question of gendered and professional threat, Buys claimed, "The question that bothers most physicians is, where does the nurse's domain end?" (p. 53). Still, Buys believed that collaborative practice has won over some physicians and predicted that Congress in the late 1970s would provide education funds for nurse practitioner training, an optimism that was not sustained by subsequent denial of resources in the 1980s. Buys concluded that "nurses emphasize that they are not in competition with doctors, because they cannot practice in isolation" (p. 54). Thus, competent nurses do not scare physicians, but how long will they continue to accept medical restrictions on their independence? Buys did not address this question, but many nurses did.

Who Owns a Body? Reordering Knowledge and Changing the Division of Labor

In Shirley Smoyak's view (1977), interprofessional relations are directly connected to women's status, which historically is colored by very early association with the helpless and less than fit, often doing what the male view considers "demeaning" work. In this century men doing women's traditional work are now accorded some status. While one can decidedly take issue with Smoyak's assumption that a century ago nurses and physicians did not experience the discord, disharmony, and distrust common today, it is possible to agree with her on the broadening gulf associated with education and technology: "Men went to universities and women nursed babies. Medicine developed with leaps and bounds; nursing barely crept along" (p. 53). By the 1940s, when nursing challenged the established order, physicians were "comfortably fixed in their views of nurses as subservient, nice-but-not-too-bright individuals," useful to have around if they "knew their place ... were available to do what anyone ... forgot or did not want to do" (p. 53). By the 1960s the two professions agreed that the hostilities and miscommunications were "straining the already limping system" (p. 53). Team effort was touted by the AMA and the ANA, which jointly sponsored three conferences, as noted earlier, in 1964, 1965, and 1967, and, in 1971, formed the National Joint Practice Commission.

What precisely constitutes joint practice or, more fundamentally, a team? Smoyak contrasted Type 1, highly task-oriented, specific work groups in which very differentiated functions lessen territorial disputes, with Type 2, work groups from different disciplines whose functions overlap and create many conflicts. Within Type 2 groups, conditions of allocating work undergo a dramatic shift: from assignment by skill, typical in Type 1 groups, to negotiations on time available, productivity for task, costs, available numbers of types of professionals, supply and demand, seniority and status, locus of care, nature of required care, and consumer's views of patient roles.

In these latter Type 2 groups, boundary battles over women's roles are basic: "May she or should she use her eyes only? How shall she report what she sees? Must her observations always be attenuated ... by words such as 'appears,' 'seems,' and 'perhaps'? Or should she say, 'The patient is bleeding'?" (p. 54). May the nurse use her hands? To soothe a fevered brow or palpate an enlarged liver? May she use an instrument? Or use only her eyes to visualize a retina, an eardrum? If she uses an instrument, can she interpret results, and act on the interpretation? Can a nurse name? "Naming requires conceptual activity," but, asked Smoyak with bitter satire, "Is the nurse an automaton? A person with a functioning brain? Do only physicians think? Is cerebral activity masculine?" (p. 55).

For that matter, who owns a body? Who has the right to what information? What does the right to know really mean? Smoyak relied on the proceedings of the National Joint Practice Commission to define major impediments to collaboration between nursing and medicine: (a) bureaucratic entrapment of nurses who are victimized by institutions but instead blame physicians, who, in turn, respond with anger and blame the nurses; (b) poor communication;

(c) excessive demands on both professions; (d) unjustified inequalities in payment and compensation; and (e) continuation of male domination and chauvinism. Joint practice is recommended, but Smoyak believed this involves a reordering of knowledge and division of labor. Fundamental change requires mutual agreement on goals, trust in competence, a shared basis of knowledge, equality in status and personal interactions, and shared equalization of fees for service. Institutional, not simply individual, consciousness-raising would be necessary. Such consciousness-raising would be required of nurses, as well as of physicians and hospital administrators.

The High Cost of Freedom: Nurses' Rejection of Nurse Practitioners

Even in the late 1970s, nurses' acceptance of other independent, self-employed women was still an issue, caused by the mixed reactions to AMA-supported PAs and the confusion about the ANA-supported alternative, nurse practitioners. Karon White Gibson (1977), an independent nurse practitioner, noted, "Those who choose such a career suffer from a shocking degree of discrimination and prejudice—and the 'shots' come mostly from fellow nurses" (p. 38). Gibson and another nurse opened their own office to bridge a gap in health care and release nurses from "their traditionally subservient role vis-a-vis doctors" (p. 38). She was sure they accomplished the first goal, "but we made very little headway on the second, except where our own identity was concerned" (p. 38).

Gibson claimed that the flak did not come from physicians, but from nurses; for example, an office nurse "spurned my request to speak with the doctor," saying, "Dr. A. doesn't practice mail-order medicine" (p. 39). The hospital director of nursing criticized them for having outside interests and fired them, causing "great embarrassment in the community" (p. 39). The nurses went to the newspaper editor, who accused them of vindictiveness, a "typically 'feminine' trait" (p. 39). They then went to the Equal Employment Opportunity Commission, which ruled that sex discrimination had occurred. At the time that Gibson's article was written, they were still fighting for third-party payment from insurance carriers. Gibson stated that local government agencies refused "even to consider my partner and me for ambulance duty and emergency care" (p. 40), hiring nonprofessionals instead and paying them more than nurses. Although their practice was successful: "We're saddened because we haven't made much of a dent in the mind-set of nurses who feel threatened by the profession's expanding role in health care.... It's time for nurses—especially if they're women—to stop discriminating against nurses" (p. 40). Obviously, the confusion over unilaterally imposed PAs and nurse practitioners was impacting nurses, who were still uncertain about the functions they could or should perform.

A Full-Scale Study: Satisfied Patients, Mixed Reviews from Physicians

Part of nurses' confusion was directly related to physicians' attitudes and actions. To clarify functions actually performed, a research study on nurse practitioners was reported by Jules I. Levine, Suezanne Orr, David Sheatsley, Jacob Lohr, and Barbara M. Brodie (1978). Though nurse Brodie had studied nurse practitioners trained in programs at the University of Virginia, a full-scale study of the entire nurse practitioner population in Virginia and a sample from Philadelphia ensured a wide variety of practitioners in different settings. Also included was a small but significant number of practitioners who were unemployed or not working as practitioners. Physicians with whom the nurse practitioners worked most closely were also contacted. The nurse practitioners completed a questionnaire and produced an activities log specifying patients seen and administrative and other activities. They were also interviewed, responding to a list of 50 tasks covering a variety of duties and roles. Physicians were interviewed with the same list of tasks, and patients also received comparable questionnaires.

Survey responses revealed that nurses were involved in obtaining patient histories, and ordering laboratory procedures and X-rays, although they were seldom allowed to read the results. The more independent the nurse, the less likely she was to prescribe medicine. The practitioners were more likely to evaluate outpatients; few were allowed to evaluate inpatients. Physicians obviously controlled the latter. The nurse practitioners were very likely to counsel patients, but infrequently advised them on health insurance or the availability of community resources or physicians.

Physicians rated the quality of the nurses' counseling, physical examinations, and history taking as excellent, while evaluating them as unsatisfactory on X-ray and EKG readings, hardly a fair assessment if they were not allowed to read them. The physicians and nurse practitioners were incongruent in their perceptions of actual work done: for example, 60 percent of the nurse practitioners reported they did no counseling on health insurance and community resources, while only 4 percent of the physicians reported no work by nurses in these areas.

The majority of patients (80 percent) seen by nurse practitioners were *not* referred by physicians; few consultations with physicians were requested by the nurses, who cared for patients with communicable diseases; neoplasms; diseases of blood, skin, and bones, and of early infancy; mental and psychoneurotic disorders; allergic or related metabolic, endocrine, or nutritional problems; accidents; poisoning and violence; and other problems. Although the nurses dealt with a wide array of problems, the most frequently occurring activity involved routine physical and well-baby examinations.

Non-patient care primarily involved administrative tasks, including conferences and charting. Nurses were also involved in telephone calls, laboratory work, housekeeping, travel, and home visits. The average amount of time spent on the additional 421 non-patient-care tasks was about 47 minutes a day.

Women physicians accounted for 25 percent of the respondents, again a disproportionately larger number than found in the total population of physicians at the time. Unfortunately, a complete comparative analysis by gender was not reported by Levine and his colleagues. Pediatricians were overrepresented, but most other specialties also responded. Few physicians were in solo practice, and over half classified their practice as in public settings. Clearly, the physicians were not representative of the general medical population. Usually they had no previous experience with nurse practitioners, but the majority who had experience said they would work with another nurse practitioner. This, despite the finding that some physicians felt some nurses lacked training in physical diagnosis (34.8 percent), needed more clinical expertise (8.7 percent), or lacked general experience (6.5 percent) and pharmacological knowledge (4.3 percent).

A majority of patients knew they were treated by a nurse; most had not previously been seen by a nurse, and had not seen a physician during the same visit. Only 9 percent expressed disapproval at being examined by a nurse; 13 percent thought she asked questions only a physician should. The majority of patients were happy with the nurses, feeling that they were in good hands. In short, the nurses were able to do competent work in their expanded roles. Physicians reported such benefits as expanded practice; more time for reading, professional meetings, and education; and increased clinic efficiency. Whether the nurses received equal benefits is questionable!

Bestowing Approval Only under Certain Conditions

From the responses of 88 family practice physicians out of 140 surveyed in California, Marilyn Little (1978) found that those more receptive to nurses in expanded roles were more likely to have practiced for shorter periods of time, to have had previous experience with nurse practitioners, to have a large number of female patients, and to be located in rural areas. Little did not back off from exposing the issue of greatest threat to physicians: "nurses are asking for more of a share of all resources. . . . They are going directly to the source of these resources, the patient" (p. 28). Recognizing that the patient-physician relationship has been somewhat of a "sacred cow," jealously guarded by physicians, "partly out of a genuine concern" (p. 28) for the patient, Little nevertheless stated that protection of this relationship has "controlled the flow of resources in health care" (p. 28). By providing direct patient care, nurses have "interrupted the flow of resources from patient to physician" (p. 28). Despite the fact that physicians may benefit through greater income, any increase in nurses' financial rewards, or even in provision of information, may be seen as threats: "A gap in knowledge provides opportunity for social control and induces dependency" (p. 28), but nurses' health teaching reduced the gap, giving the patient more opportunity for responsibility. According to Little, "The nurse practitioner who attempts to share information reduces the social distance between provider and client and jeopardizes the lofty position of the medical practitioner" (p. 28).

In her study, Little found that 48.9 percent of the family practice physicians had decided *never* to employ a nurse practitioner. Of the 18 independent variables studied, 12 accounted for 47 percent of the variation in the MDs' willingness to employ nurse practitioners. Gender analysis was omitted by excluding the three women physicians from even qualitative analysis. Little's findings support previous studies on other clinical specialties: physicians who were more receptive to nurse practitioners had practiced a shorter time; had prior experience with nurse practitioners; were located in group, not solo, practices; and lived in rural, not urban, communities. Physicians with greater numbers of female, infant, medical, and elderly patients were more willing to employ nurse practitioners. The interesting question is why nurses as late as 1978 were still viewing their independence as contingent on physicians' approval, rather than as separate practice.

Nurse Autonomy: Female Physicians More Willing to Delegate Functions

In their series of four articles analyzing fifty graduates of the Washington University Pediatric Nursing Practitioner Program, Lawrence Kahn and Patricia Wirth (1978) focused one article on the perceptions and expectations of physician supervisors. Whether nurses should be trained by physicians, rather than by other nurses—certainly a controversial issue—was not addressed in the study. Of the thirty-one physician supervisors, twenty-two were male and nine female, a disproportionately high number of women. The majority were located in agencies and institutions, not in private practice.

Tasks were delegated to nurse practitioners, for example, obtaining patient histories, but physicians wanted joint control of even minor illnesses and of sick-child examinations. Other functions, even visits involving parental counseling or determining whether X-ray or lab tests were needed, were also not shared with nurses. Kahn and Wirth's research, one of the few studies to compare, even minimally, male and female physicians, found several gender differences: male physician supervisors were unwilling to delegate *any* activity exclusively to nurse practitioners; thus, they maintained control of *all* nursing tasks. In contrast, the women physicians delegated to the nurse practitioners independent management of minor tasks.

That physicians would not allow nursing autonomy is clear: "most were not willing to grant independent status to the PNP as indicated by only 40 percent agreeing that PNP's should manage clinical problems alone and only

13 percent indicating that they view independent private practice as a viable professional option for PNP's" (p. 28). Further, the physicians believed there should be a clear separation between the level of earnings, with nurses' incomes substantially below those of the physicians; some physicians even believed that pediatric nurse practitioners should not earn more than the usual salaries of nurses with no advanced education.

There were also wide differences on whether nurse practitioners should substitute for nurses and whether nurse practitioners were equal to PAs, but there was little disagreement that medicine should control medicine *and* nursing. Despite these attitudes, most physicians felt the volume and range of patient services had increased and the quality of care had improved. Patient and physician satisfaction were also increased. Indeed, in well-baby care, 55 percent of the physicians felt the nurses' services were superior to their own!

Kahn and Wirth admitted that most differences center on the degree of autonomy: nurses, for example, want "exclusive right to well child care and the management of minor illness while the physicians insisted these responsibilities be shared" (p. 30). Gender did to some degree differentiate the physicians on a few issues, as noted. In contrast to the physicians, "Over 90 percent of the PNP's felt they were capable of managing patient problems without the direct personal supervision of a physician while only 41 percent of the supervisors agreed with this level of independence" (p. 30). The nurses saw themselves as distinct from "regular" nurses, but the physicians did not. Perhaps the clearest and most important difference was the disagreement on who should provide primary care, an area the women claimed as their own. Although Kahn and Wirth were optimistic, the depth and breadth of disagreement between nurses and physicians is substantial and central to role definitions and functions.

Sharp Distinction between What Physicians Think and What They Actually Delegate

The contrast between what a physician *thinks* he or she has delegated and what is *actually* delegated is central to research by Shirley V. Connelly and Patricia A. Connelly (1979), who published a study of forty residents and interns working with nurse practitioners in a Veterans Administration hospital primary-care medical clinic. Questionnaires were administered at the beginning of the physicians' rotation and responses were compared with actual behaviors. Despite expressing some positive attitudes, the physicians actually referred patients to nurse practitioners at a rather low rate, even for chronic but stable patients for whom the nurses were particularly well qualified to care: "only two physicians referred more than 50 percent and 34 physicians referred less than 30 percent" (p. 74). Critically important is the Connellys' finding that there was no significant attitudinal differences between the physicians with highest referral rates and those with the lowest. After more than twenty years of change in nurses' practice, the verbal acceptance by physicians of expanded and more independent roles for nurses simply was not reflected in their behavior. Not even verbal acceptance could be assumed, however, as organized medicine became increasingly overt in attacking nurses' independence across the nation.

Physicians Attack Nursing Autonomy: Nurses Fight Back

Typical of the national coverage on medicine's attack on nursing was a 1978 article in the *American Journal of Nursing* (*AJN*) entitled "Nurse Practitioners Fight Move to Restrict Their Practice." Accompanying the article was a drawing of a very large man in plaid pants and white jacket with large bare arms folded over the stethoscope on his chest. He had a broad grin on his face and his nose, which looked like a pig's snout, was pointed up toward the light reflector on his head. Potbellied and smug, he stood in front of a high iron fence, behind which were picketing female and male patients, one holding a sign: "Quality Nursing Now." The woman nurse, at least two feet smaller than the physician, appeared haggard and dejected as she looked beyond the physician to the patients behind the iron fence. Once again, the gendered nature of the struggle was more than obvious in the nonverbal message in the drawing.

The *AJN* article reported the national alarm of nurses to recent actions by the New Jersey Board of Medical Examiners to limit or curtail the nurse practitioners in the state: "In the most severe action taken, the medical board has charged two nurse practitioners who work in a health maintenance organization with practicing medicine" (*American Journal of Nursing*, 1978, p. 1285). On investigation, the New Jersey Board of Nursing disagreed and ruled the nurses were practicing nursing. The four physicians with whom the two nurses worked were supported by the nurses, but were accused by the state medical board of aiding and abetting the nurses in the supposed illegal practice of medicine. The ANA also investigated and supported the New Jersey nurses; they charged the medical board of overstepping its legal jurisdiction in calling the nurses before the board, since the nurses were accountable only to the state Board of Nursing. In addition, the nurses claimed that New Jersey law governing health maintenance organizations excluded the HMOs from regulation by the state Board of Medical Examiners and placed them directly under the control of the state health commissioner. In turn, the HMO in question had filed a suit against the Board of Medical Examiners before the New Jersey Supreme Court.

Regardless of the rulings and support in favor of the nurses from the state Board of Nursing and the ANA, the medical board ruled against the nurses, Joyce Adler and Ann Hirschman. Adler was accused of giving the drug erythromycin to a child with a cold. The record showed the child to be allergic to penicillin, but she had previously had other antibiotics. The two pediatricians who saw the child afterward said that "'she was having the usual side effects, not an adverse reaction'" (p. 1308). A family physician accused Hirschman of examining his patient and finding a lump in her breast. The physician later claimed there was no lump. The nurse countered that the patient herself had also palpated the mass and both agreed on the need for a mammogram. The radiologist could not feel a lump; the test did show mild changes of mammary dysplasia, but no indication of current malignancy. Clearly, there was evidence for the nurse's diagnostic skill and against the physician's judgment.

Both women were vehement in their denial that they had been practicing medicine. Adler said she in no way wanted to be identified with the medical establishment and further stated that if she had wanted to be a physician, she would have become one! A strong advocate of preventive self-care, she also indicated that the majority of people, presumably with prior education, should be able to take care of their health needs most of the time, without medical or nursing intervention.

This was not the only attack on nurses. For example, in the 1977–1978 academic year, four school nurse practitioners were ordered by the school principals to discontinue the physical assessments they had been conducting since receiving certification the previous year. The school district medical director, William Chase, MD, had ordered this change after he "had been called before the medical board and told his license was in jeopardy unless the nurses stopped practicing medicine" (p. 1308). When contacted by the *AJN*, Chase had no comment.

The four school nurses—Nora Dixon, Frances Edelstein, Dorothy Fredericks, and Alice Hobbs—all stopped conducting examinations, hoping that the case of Adler and Hirschman would resolve their problems. Although the four had done their practitioner training at Rutgers University and had received no salary increases for it, an anonymous letter to the medical board led to the actions that prevented the nurses from using their additional training on behalf of the schoolchildren, the ultimate losers in this gendered battle, which was being repeated in other states in the nation. Edwin Albano, president of the New Jersey Board of Medical Examiners, was quoted in the New Jersey *Sentinel* as saying that he personally had "'no need for any nurse . . .' and that in New Jersey no such entity as a nurse practitioner existed" (p. 1308). With such blatant opposition expressed by physicians, nurses could hardly maintain positive levels of satisfaction with their jobs and working environments.

Nurses' Job Satisfaction: Ambivalent to Say the Least!

Numerous studies of job satisfaction or dissatisfaction of nurses have been conducted. One informal study was reported by Marjorie Godfrey (1978). From a survey of 17,000 readers who answered a magazine questionnaire,

Godfrey found these nurses to be "*ambivalent,* to say the least" (p. 90). In addition to the questionnaires, the editors received 800 unsolicited letters from the nurses. These could be represented by one writer, who loved "taking care of sick people" (p. 90), but cursed administration that habitually forced nurses into double shifts, working on their days off, and was "so bent on cutting costs it can only see dollar signs lying in the beds" (p. 90). Godfrey concluded that nurses are "not willing to make all the compromises anymore" (p. 90).

The nurses no longer would tolerate unsafe practices, dangerous under-staffing patterns, retention of incompetent nurses, alcoholic physicians "prac-ticing medicine," and patients "stacked in hospital halls like so many sausages" (p. 90). The nurses rejected the poor leadership of head nurses who scheduled improperly; of inflexible supervisors "determined to preserve the status quo" (p. 90); of nursing directors too removed from patient care; and of "authori-tarian administrators concerned only with cutting costs—at any price" (p. 90). The nurses noted communication problems in learning about hospital changes thirdhand, being transferred to another unit without notice, going through channels and getting no response at all, and hearing supervisory promises that were forgotten.

The majority of nurses were dissatisfied, although they rated nursing as better than most or one of the best professions. Unfortunately, the *higher* the nurses' education, the *lower* the rating given to the profession: 94 percent of the licensed practical nurses versus 50 percent of the PhDs rated nursing favor-ably. Some nurses complained that their peers denigrate the profession: "I will see 30-year veteran nurses running to clean up the mess left by a medical stu-dent when we're really here to take care of patients, not medical staff" (p. 91). Others felt that professionalism was used against them by administrators on issues of money or working conditions, yet "we receive none of the benefits of professionals" (p. 91).

According to Godfrey, many nurses felt that sex discrimination was the real reason nursing was not valued or respected, even though nurses perform an essential societal role: "We're there when people are born, when over-whelming crises strikes them, and when they die. Yet I make less money than my uncle who's a garbage collector" (p. 91). Would male nurses improve a "woman's profession?" Already, said Godfrey, the numbers of male nursing administrators are disproportionate to their numbers in the profession, and male nurses receive higher salaries directly out of school. Therefore, many nurses believed this was a woman's battle. The male nurses felt that their pres-ence is beneficial to the profession; however, they believed they faced hostility from other professionals and even from patients. One man "developed a sense of being better than they [women] are, and not feeling sorry or guilty for it" (p. 92). The nurses were devastatingly critical of incompetent or uncaring nurses (whatever their sex), and only 32 percent expressed a great deal of trust in their supervisors; some were dissatisfied with the lack of leadership or the abuse of authority or bureaucratic rigidity.

On physicians, nurses stated that some did not belong in medicine at all: "Why can we be fired for one mistake, but a doctor can continue injuring and maiming patients forever!" (p. 95). This woman and her peers reported an alcoholic physician who was subsequently discussed at a medical meeting, but nothing was done about him. Another nurse resigned after an inebriated physician performed cutdowns (vein incisions for intravenous therapy) for over four hours, had three misses, and contaminated two cutdown trays. She reported him to the county medical association with no results. The physician finally overdosed on pills and alcohol and died. How many of his patients died before his death?

About 76 percent of the nurses responded positively to relations with individual physicians; the majority rated them as good, not excellent or poor. Again, the university-educated nurses were most critical. One nurse commented on an emergency room team of highly skilled nurses and physicians: "I realize our situation is not the usual" (p. 96). Only about half of the nurses reported that physicians respected them—38 percent said they received some, little, or no respect. This, coupled with the lack of clarity with their supervisors about job descriptions and, more importantly, inadequate constructive feedback, left a lot of room for job dissatisfaction.

Nursing administration was evaluated even more poorly, particularly for the absence of positive feedback, especially in large hospitals. The administrators, however, were evidently unaware of the nurses' feelings; they rated communication as good to excellent. But if the nurses' communication among themselves was not ideal, it was nonexistent with hospital administrators: "They weren't even credited with *one-way* communication" (p. 98). Nurses were not involved in decision making or informed of decisions, even those that immediately affected them. Nurses who brought problems or reports to leaders received no responses from the hospital hierarchy; by the time the issue went through various levels, it had "snowballed or it's dissolved. And the one who had the problem never knows what happened—if anything" (p. 98). Godfrey claimed the situation was totally demoralizing; "66% of the respondents told us that nursing administration is usually unresponsive . . . and 70% believe they're usually frozen out of the decision-making process" (p. 99). One nurse stated it clearly: "There's no such thing as an individual here. We're just a rack of white uniforms with no thought for the person underneath" (p. 99). Committees of staff nurses were also ineffective because hospital administrators did not act on their recommendations: "We weren't asking for much—a few extra eggs on the breakfast cart for patients who'd been admitted too late [for a menu selection] . . . that sort of thing. We never got any of it, and we never heard why" (p. 99).

Even worse were the reports that female administrators took the side of patients or physicians against the nurses. The trust level was so low that nurses said they wanted everything in writing. But, said Godfrey, "the process is not so much won't support as can't support" (p. 100). One nurse pinpointed the problem: "Most of our problems result from lack of professional courtesy from doctors. They put us in a double bind by giving orders not acceptable morally or ethically. . . . We have no cooperation . . . from the administrator. Our director of nursing backs us but she's being frozen out by the doctors and the administration" (p. 100).

Nursing leaders often had no voting rights on committees that had direct control over nursing; furthermore, they may have had no idea of how to take power into their own hands. In the words of one nurse, "We need a DN [director of nursing] with a commitment to *nursing*, not medicine-dominated administration. We need help" (p. 102). Unfortunately, this help was not immediately forthcoming, despite the accumulating evidence that many nurse practitioners were capable of providing such leadership.

Quality of Care of Nurse Practitioners: A Decade of Research

Between the end of the 1970s and the mid-1980s, a number of writers published reviews of the research to date on nurse practitioners. For example, Harold C. Sox, Jr. (1979), a physician, reviewed from a ten-year perspective literature on the quality of patient care provided by nurse practitioners and PAs. The remarkable development in primary care of "new" practitioners who diagnose and treat a wide variety of health problems had been researched in more than forty studies from 1967 to 1978 that specifically evaluated nurse practitioners' clinical competence. Of these, twenty-one studies directly compared care given by nurse practitioners or PAs with that given by physicians. Sox asserted: "These studies show that nurse practitioners and physicians' assistants provide office-based care that is *indistinguishable* from physician care" (p. 459; italics added). Sox qualified this assertion by saying that the studies were limited in scope; therefore, he provided no extension of this conclusion to care outside an office, to unsupervised cases, or to care of seriously ill patients. In addition, his assertion does not draw on data from public health nurses conducted over many years. As noted previously, the Frontier Nursing Service, in operation since the 1920s, has been consistently evaluated, and the evaluations have shown that the nurses working in the Appalachian area with little direct supervision have produced lower maternal and child-death rates at birth, despite primitive conditions, than those of physicians in urban areas. This and similar research is not included in Sox's review.

Indeed, Sox focused only on the twenty-one studies that specifically compared physicians' and "new" practitioners' care on process, outcome, patient satisfaction, and agreement with physician. Sox admitted that perfect agreement with a physician may be an unfair expectation since it assumes that other practitioners could equal but never exceed the physicians. This is obviously a problematic assumption. Certainly, no other profession could assume such a standard; even though it appears to be "a widely accepted standard of comparison" (p. 459), it assumes the omniscience of the medical model and excludes alterative models.

Another problem, of course, in reviewing clinical competence over time is the widely varied length and breadth of nurse practitioner education programs, which were only recently becoming standardized at the master's degree level. In addition, changes in state practice laws, as previously discussed, would affect the scope of NP functions by expanding or restricting them. Certainly, the breadth of care activities and their acceptance by physician supervisors may also have changed. In this regard the importance of differences in independence and autonomy, stressed by Lewis and Cheyovich (1976), may be critical to the kinds of care provided.

Sox established eleven methodological standards and found none of the studies he reviewed met all of them; five of eight of the studies with randomized trials and three of the nine nonrandomized studies met at least seven criteria. Unfortunately, Sox did not specify gender of participants as a criterion; evidently, he could not even conceive that the gender of patients, nurses, assistants, or physicians would be an important variable that should at least be described if not analyzed. This omission of groups that can be clearly differentiated by sex and have been subject to gender stereotyping is unfortunate indeed. Letters to researchers would have helped to clarify this dimension by obtaining appropriate demographic data, even when inadequately presented in the original studies and even if it were not ultimately reported. Similarly, race and socioeconomic variations in the research subjects and their patients should also have been considered. In any research, the inclusion of basic sociological categories of membership, reflecting at least some demographic characteristics of the subjects studied, is a standard data collection procedure.

We can only assume that most nurse practitioners were female and white; that PAs were somewhat more likely to be evenly distributed between males and females; and that most of the physicians were male. Thus, when Sox asserts that there were essentially no differences in care provided by different types of providers, one can only infer that nurses were equally competent as physicians in the care they gave. No refined comparisons can be made between male and female physicians and nurses; nor can one specify what nurses *added* to the usual care given by physicians. In short, if the medical model is considered the standard, then the measurements are conducted against a male-defined model of health care, which itself has been under severe attack by health reformers and consumers. This issue was also not addressed by Sox.

Sox did suggest caution when viewing measurements of outcome because these could be caused by other factors, such as access to housing, food, medication, and education. It should be noted that these socioeconomic factors are also heavily influenced by race and gender. Demographic variables would have allowed for some indications of such factors and their influence on caregiver-patient interactions and outcome. Sox also analyzed studies that had focused on *processes* of patient care; these dealt primarily with technical aspects, not decision-making dynamics. Sox recognized that the style of care could affect communications with and compliance by patients. He noted that the process of care was evaluated in eight of the twenty-one studies and that no measurable differences were found between physicians and nurse practitioners or PAs. One study (Duttera and Harlan, 1978) attempted to relate the severity of the patient's problem to the appropriateness of care. Even with severity of illness stratified, there were, remarkably, *no* differences between physicians' care and that of PAs. Even with methodological problems, Sox concluded that "This study provides the strongest evidence that nurse practitioners and physicians' assistants can provide office care the process of which is comparable in quality to that used by physicians" (p. 461).

Outcomes of Care and Patient Satisfaction: Nurses Equal to or Better Than Physicians

In his review of outcomes of care, despite insufficient numbers of seriously ill people among office patients, Sox found that in randomized trials of 1,529 patients of nurse practitioners and 2,796 patients of physicians, the two groups had "similar outcomes as judged by physical, social, and emotional status at the end of 1 year of study" (p. 461). Again, with studies of well-child care, acute minor illness, and stable chronic diseases, the alternative practitioners had "illness outcomes identical to those of patients of physicians" (pp. 461–462), although ideal conditions in definition of outcome were not achieved.

Reviewing patient satisfaction with their care, Sox again found that all alternative caregivers "uniformly gave satisfaction that was equal to or greater than satisfaction resulting from care given by physicians" (p. 462). Nevertheless, he called for more precise measures, such as patients' knowledge of disease and medication, compliance with a therapeutic plan, and concordance between what patients were told and what patients remembered. Unfortunately, Sox did not provide any results showing higher compliance by patients cared for by nurse practitioners. He did agree that patient satisfaction was a good measure of acceptance and that there was a high level of acceptance of alternative practitioners. He also did not analyze results that showed a *higher* acceptance of these practitioners than of physicians.

Ideally, valid designs would require that both practitioners studied would see the same patients, but this, Sox claimed, might disrupt the physicians' practice. This approach might be more useful for assessing a single episode of acute illness, rather than a series of visits for chronic illness since previous information given might affect subsequent providers. Furthermore, it would be difficult to distinguish the separate influences that two providers had on patient outcome. Obviously, random allocation of patients is a reasonable alternative, provided that the frequency of types of patients are equally distributed. In six of the randomized studies, these conditions prevailed, and in four of these, patient dropouts were also controlled. Again, the finding from such studies was that "nurse practitioners were indistinguishable from physicians in general ambulatory family practice, care of acute low back pain, and infant well-child care" (p. 464).

Sox considered ten of the controlled studies that compared nurse practitioners to physicians. PAs were not considered because the allocation of patients was not altered; however, he admitted that some studies assessed the pretreatment state of patients and several measures of quality of care. Again, Sox was most impressed by the studies that controlled for the severity of patients' health problems; even when these were controlled, the results were, again, essentially similar.

Of the studies that Sox claimed were sound, could the findings be applied to primary-care practice? Sox excluded consideration of all other types of practice in all other institutions. From only the smaller set of studies selected, he concluded that there was inconclusive evidence on differences between PAs and nurse practitioners, but admitted that the differences in care given by them are probably small or nonexistent because of the equivalent care proved in comparison to physicians. Sox also wanted more studies of "new" practitioners in emergency rooms and hospitals in order to assess their behavior with more seriously ill patients. He recognized that legal definitions vary, but most require "new" practitioners to work under physicians' supervision; nevertheless, "a large proportion of the care that they give does not involve a physician directly. . . . [They] are often the sole source of coverage of emergency rooms, especially in rural areas" (p. 465). Sox cautioned that solo practice was not studied; obviously, reports on this do exist in some form in the nursing literature. These reports do not constitute experimental data, but they are, nevertheless, important, if only to show the extent of physicians' cooperation or control.

According to Sox, highly motivated physicians were more likely to be studied because of self-selection; thus, above-average practices were also more likely to be studied. Sox concluded that the indistinguishable quality of care may be "very good indeed" (p. 465). However, he speculated that this quality would be achieved only when working with physicians of above-average ability. The assumption here is that the physicians, not the intelligence, education, and experience of the "new" practitioners, were the critical factor. This is certainly debatable! Sox concluded that there was enough information to assure physicians that the "new" practitioners would give favorable and comparable care. However, he recommended more supervision for those in settings not yet reported, for example, in hospitals and emergency rooms. This again assumes that independent practice of "new" practitioners was not occurring and that dependence on physician supervision would continue.

Questioning the Underlying Assumption: Is Physicians' Care Adequate as a Comparison Standard?

How did nurses themselves deal with conceptual and methodological issues in nurse practitioner research? M. W. Edmunds (1978) reviewed 471 publications on nurse practitioners, focusing particularly on 47 formal research reports and concluding that the nurses had been fully accepted by patients and that they were competent in delivering quality care. A year later, Donna Diers and Susan Molde (1979) reviewed the studies and considered certain research problems, particularly those pertaining to ambulatory or primary care. Diers and Molde claimed some conceptual issues could be traced to the history of the development of the practitioner role. Conceived as a solution to physician shortage, "the definition of the problem was *only* the problem of access to care. Underlying the definition was an unstated assumption that primary care services as defined and provided by physicians were adequate in every respect except quantity. . . . [T]he direction of the early politics set the framework for nurse practitioner research" (p. 73). According to Diers and Molde, this led to problems in the definitions of independent and dependent variables and in the theory of nurse practitioner practice.

Early research, couched in terms of access, measured the number of patient visits before and after the introduction of the nurse practitioner. As noted in the Sox analysis, the comparisons between physicians and nurses *assumed* medical care to be the standard and seldom studied the nursing care provided. In short, the nurse practitioner, *not the practice*, became the variable. The medical orientation was exaggerated in studies in which standard protocols were required; thus "the conceptualization of care seems even more narrow, restricted essentially to following the medical protocol" (p. 74). Furthermore, "When medical diagnostic categories were used to define nurse practitioner practice . . . very large proportions of patient care needs seen by nurse practitioner students were unclassifiable by medical definitions" (p. 74).

Indeed, technical aspects of care have often been analyzed only in terms of cure, palliation, or rehabilitation, but process evaluations require that the art of care be related to patient outcomes. A high level of care, noted Brook, Williams, and Avery (1976), promotes "willingness to discuss sensitive problems; use of medical services benefiting the patient's health; increased compliance with regimens directed at controlling or alleviating chronic diseases; and adoption of health habits conducive to longevity and decreased morbidity" (cited in Diers and Molde, 1979, p. 74). Diers and Molde asserted that even studies that measure process have not related art-of-care to patient outcomes.

Diers and Molde called for independent variables that are based not simply on the discipline of providers, but on better definitions of primary care as first contact, coordinated, continuing, comprehensive, and family-centered. From a gender point of view, what they recommended was an androgynous approach to independent variables that did not rest on male-medical conceptualizations, but incorporated female nurses' foci—for example, on patient teaching, counseling, or advocacy—as essential components of primary care rather than simply as traditional nursing activities. These could then be combined with routine medical procedures for "*any* group of practitioners." Diers and Molde urged that the system of care be the independent variable to be studied in the context of practice; this, in turn, requires a theoretical definition that "transcends, but does not ignore, the discipline of the practitioner" (p. 75). To get to new definitions, the authors recommended the study of actual collaborative processes to develop more systematic descriptions of "those aspects of primary care outside the boundaries of traditional medical practice" (p. 75).

Demanding Research That Incorporates Nurses' Worldview

Diers and Molde also analyzed definitions of the dependent variables. While nurse practitioner practice, the independent variable, has been conceived largely as a subset of medical practice, the dependent variable, patient outcomes, has also been defined in traditional medical terms. From a gender perspective, male-dominated medical conceptions of health and illness create the worldview for everyone, simply excluding female views or subsuming them as peripheral aspects of care. Diers and Molde asserted that the foci of nurses on, for example, health teaching must be incorporated into research, which should include not only what patients know about diseases and treatments, but what they learn to do for themselves without having to rely on clinicians— thus reducing reliance on office or emergency room visits or hospitalizations. Clearly, the combination of both women's and men's conceptualization of the world of health and illness fosters a better understanding. This new worldview would not simply be additive; the criteria for the *process* of health care would also have to change.

Diers and Molde analyzed the literature on nurse midwifery for help in sorting out the conceptual problem of defining patient outcomes that reflect actual processes of care. The authors noted that infant birth weight is not just another measure of medical care, but the function of nutrition counseling and finding nutritional supplements when needed. Infant mortality may also be a sensitive indicator of the detection of early difficulties in pregnancy and the provision of appropriate resources. Indeed, the authors noted that "significant decreases in prematurity and neonatal mortality, as well as improved quality of prenatal care" (p. 76), were attributed to nurse midwives in one California study (Levy, Wilkinson, and Marine, 1971). The usual obstetrical risk factors are insufficient, since nurses' work is often focused on social and environmental risks as well.

Clearly, the explanations for why nurse practitioners tend to produce equal or better results are inadequate. Diers and Molde asserted that the "results of studies are most often interpreted as justifying the nurse practitioner's employment or advocating more responsibility for the nurse practitioner" (p. 76). Obviously, women are being forced to prove they can perform as well or better than men. For this reason, most research has been couched in male-defined outcomes; what women do is often not measured. This leads to the "alarming but not surprising consistency . . . of atheoretical results" (p. 76).

Diers and Molde did not note the importance of gender in the research on differences and similarities of practice. Logically, the values and practices of nurses reflect those of women in general. Maybe the system of care given by nurse practitioners can tell us much about female perceptions of and actions in healing. Perhaps nurse practitioners are producing androgynous systems of care that go beyond, but also incorporate, male medical and traditional female nurses' approaches to health and illness. Sex-segregated disciplines require a theory, a system of explanation, that reflects not only professional but gender differentials. By focusing on the processes of care, Diers and Molde help us understand not only nursing and medicine, but women and men as they interact with clients of both sexes.

Disease Entities or Environmentally Embedded Measures of Outcomes?

Research conducted through the 1970s and into the 1980s was constrained by the issue of physician delegation; thus, the nurses who were studied often dealt with well patients or with those who were chronically ill. It is difficult to measure outcomes for these patients. Diabetes and hypertension are often best treated through effective management, and this depends on patient compliance; thus, Diers and Molde noted that the nurse deals "not only with an intractable chronic condition but also with a condition that is assumed to be well fixed in a life style not easily amenable to change" (p. 77). In addition, her patients are more likely to be poor, "subject not only to physical illness but to living circumstances that may make them vulnerable to environmental variables (poor housing) or to a lack of control over their circumstances that could have an impact on their disease and/or its treatment" (p. 77). Thus, nurses take on people whom the physicians see as economically valueless. Again, the results of sex-segregated disciplines are obvious, but often not taken into account. As Diers and Molde recognized, nurse practitioners are more likely to work with people over fifty, members of minority groups, and people on public assistance. They are also more likely to work with women, who are statistically more likely to live longer and more likely to be poor, particularly if divorced or from minority groups.

Diers and Molde recommended different measures than simple medical care indices, such as "multifactor measures of level of function that would appropriately tap several facets of patient condition, including, but not restricted to, the patient's medical problem(s)" (p. 78). Clearly, they are attempting to set standards of function that are not based on arbitrary medical indices, but those "empirically different for different people yet conceptually the same so that comparisons may be made" (p. 78). For example, the highest level of function might be capability to engage in work. Diers and Molde attempted to conceptualize measures of outcome that respect the individual, particularly in her or his context. Disease entity would not be the single factor considered. The authors' emphasis on embeddedness is congruent with many studies on women's interpersonal and even moral processes.

Because nurse practitioners traditionally have been given patients, problems, and functions that physicians have found economically unprofitable, Diers and Molde were particularly concerned with comparison groups. They emphasized the importance of a full description of the kind of practice the actual care provided. They also urged more clarity on types of practitioners: Are practitioners employees or fee-paid? Are they in training or full-time clinicians? Are they specialists or engaged in primary care? To compare nurse practitioners working in low-income housing projects with physicians in private offices with upper-middle-class patients is unfair unless private practice is held as the ideal. Even studies that make these unfair comparisons have proven that nurses are as competent as physicians, but "[t]he more appropriate interpretation is that the nurse practitioner practice was considerably better than that, given the high probability that the nurse practitioner patients were more ill and had fewer personal or social resources" (p. 78).

Unfortunately, the effects of nonmedical aspects of nurse practitioner practice are unclear. For these, there are few clear criteria. As noted previously in this volume, the overlap between professionals is substantial: "Even physicians and nurses who define their practices within the traditional boundaries of their respective professions act outside these traditional boundaries" (p. 78). Nurses, as previously noted, often make implicit and at times explicit decisions on diagnosis and treatment in their advice to patients. Diers and Molde suggested that the focus shift to descriptions of *systems of care,* to criteria from *actual practice.* This obviously involves going well beyond the doctor-nurse game.

Most studies of nurse practitioners have been conducted primarily on those who are new to practice. Nor are they controlled for the extreme variations in length and depth of the nurse practitioners' educational programs. However, the authors noted that nurse midwifery is more developed and standardized; therefore, there is more research on the effects of midwifery on both medical outcome (morbidity, mortality) and nursing outcome (compliance with postpartum recommendations, prenatal visits, or dietary advice). If the influence of nurses' healing can be defined, described, and empirically assessed, there may be greater clarity on the intersection of gender and professional roles.

Medical Records as Primary Sources of Data: Incomplete and Unstandardized

In their review, Diers and Molde attacked the primary, mostly male-defined sources of data in nurse practitioner research and decried the use of medical records, which are "notoriously incomplete and unstandardized" (p. 79). In addition, most outpatient records do not contain data on nursing care and are often "only indirect measures of the art-of-care" (p. 79). When nurse practitioners do chart, for example, their patient teaching activities, these data cannot be easily compared to those of physicians, who normally do not chart such activity. According to Diers and Molde, if nurse practitioners continue to be evaluated with medical records as the sole source of data, results will "inherently be biased toward a traditional view of medical practice" (p. 80). Unfortunately, by the late 1970s, they had found no studies that provided a wider view of clinical practice. Certainly from a gender point of view, this means that nurse practitioners may not be able to bring the female perspective to their practice or to their patients. Indeed, physician control of charting requires research on the nature of charting itself.

Diers and Molde noted that in most research studies, nurse practitioners were assigned patients in already established medical settings and practices; thus, random allocation of patients could not be totally achieved. In addition, there is the "undocumented feeling that their patients are older, more often dependent on public assistance, more often members of the Black or another minority, and more often female than are the patients assigned to physicians" (pp. 80–81). Furthermore, the standards of care established for properly randomized patients may not be adequate even within the medical model.

In the Canadian Burlington studies, reported by Sackett, Spitzer, Gent, and Roberts (1974) and by Spitzer, Sackett, Sibley, Roberts, Gent, Kergin, Hackett, and Olynich (1974), standards for the management of simple hypertension did not require control of blood pressure. To assess the adequacy of care for anemia in women over forty-five with a hemoglobin between 10 and 11 grams and vaginal blood loss, the research standard required "no diagnostic evaluation. Instead, it mandated a dilation and curettage *or* a gynecological consultation" (p. 81). How adequate, asked Diers and Molde, is this medical standard of care? They questioned the adequacy of the findings from the Burlington studies: did nurse practitioners and physicians achieve the same low standards of care? Did neither provide exemplary care and use the same inadequate standards? Clearly, research on nurses' adequacy leads to questions about physicians' standards as well.

Similarly, Diers and Molde questioned the superficiality of measures to assess costs of care: "The number of patients seen is at best a false unit of analysis unless patient condition and provider process are also taken into account" (p. 82). In a 1978 study, even "the time the nurse practitioner waited to consult with a physician was charged against the nurse practitioner" (p. 82). Obviously, the physician or institution should have been charged because that is who monopolizes and restricts the right to prescribe. It is clearly inappropriate to rate this as a component of the nurse's efficiency. In contrast, studies often charge equally for ancillary personnel or space, but Diers and Molde claimed such presumed equality does not exist. For example, "evaluation of nurse-midwifery costs must account for the fact that nursing service is provided more often for physician patients, in part because of the necessity for a female chaperon, than for nurse-midwifery patients" (p. 82). Finally, nurse practitioners remain nurses and can perform some activities for themselves that nurses regularly do for physicians. This fact is also not included in cost estimates. Quite clearly, the two gendered groups do have more than superficial differences in practice and in costs. And these differences required basic changes in group and institutional practices and structures.

Shifting Gender Templates: Increasing Nurses' Authority, Using Physicians as Consultants

By the end of the 1970s sociologist David Mechanic (1978) had created an *organizational* solution based on *systemic* change. Admitting that physicians dominated the division of labor, he nevertheless asserted that "the quality of nursing care may be the single most important factor affecting successful patient care in the hospital context and in patient outcome" (p. 360). Given the changes in health tasks, nursing was in a state of turmoil, particularly as a result of broader social changes, "including the women's movement, modifications in sex roles and a new professional militancy in the nursing profession itself" (p. 360).

In contrast to Friedson (1970), Mechanic recognized the shifting gender templates and tried to systematically interrelate personal and professional roles. He noted the movement of baccalaureate-educated nurses to administration and the pursuit of more autonomous and responsible roles, but saw these latter changes as primarily related to specialized functions—for example, in intensive care or dialysis nursing or in the shift to nurse practitioners, particularly in the care of chronic and ambulatory patients.

Again in contrast to Friedson, Mechanic recognized that good nursing care involves judgment, sensitivity, and decision making about patients' needs, communications, concerns, and responses, particularly in emergencies. Despite this, "The authority system of care in the hospital, however, is designed to make it appear that the nurses' responses are reactive to physician judgments and orders" (p. 361). Thus, said Mechanic, although "nurses frequently exercise important power of decision, they must do so subtly, avoiding the appearance of being in command" (p. 361). To Mechanic, nurses, in much closer contact with patients, have access to information that might "argue against certain physician assessments and decisions . . . [but] if the nurse is to "get on" in the system she must learn to express her opinion unobtrusively, to suggest alternatives, rather than contest physicians' views, and to show deference to doctors' expertness and authority" (p. 361).

Some nurses can function this way successfully, but others may be "immobilized and lose confidence in their ability to act independently" (p. 361). To Mechanic, some nurses resolved the dilemma by seeing nursing as an occupation secondary to the primary role as wife and mother, even leaving nursing after marriage or during child rearing, maintaining little identification with the profession. Thus, gender roles define sex-stratified behaviors and power, and these, in turn, may determine the degree and extent of commitment to professional identities.

Low hospital salaries also influence commitment. Even as wages increase and attitudes toward working women change, the larger number of nurses returning to work have not been supported by hospital authorities, who have often been quite inflexible in providing opportunities for part-time employment or in creating scheduling or conditions that would make work and family responsibilities compatible. Given the difficult hospital hours, nurses with children and families find scheduling difficult. These factors are exacerbated by the move by many nurses to college education. The increased social class and educational status of college-educated women in nursing gives a "better sense of the difficulties that are likely to arise as these new nurses come face to face with physician authority and control" (p. 363). To Mechanic, relationships were in ferment, arousing "considerable emotions among practitioners in both groups" (p. 363).

As long as women were considered interchangeable units to be rotated according to hospital demands, Mechanic perceived that both administrative and medical persons would deal with them according to organizational convenience rather than sound patient care. In agreement with Hans Mauksch's 1957 assertion, considered in chapter 6, Mechanic saw the history of nursing and the history of women as clearly interwoven; thus, physicians and administrators, primarily male, "tend to view the nurse as having the attributes of wife and mother, doing whatever home and family require, responding largely to others' definitions of her tasks" (p. 363). To him, the conflicts between physicians and nurses "reflect the growing attack by women in the society at large on these assumptions implicit in the cultural history of the sexes" (p. 363).

Mechanic speculated on what nurses' optimal patient-care domain would be if it were stripped of the gendered context. He believed that greater specialization was needed to obtain command over work. But the most important, and key, issue was responsibility for overall care. Physicians, who in theory held control, were "poorly located from a situational standpoint to exercise it effectively" (p. 364). The private physician, located outside the hospital, "does not have the continuity of contact necessary to monitor the patients success-fully, to perceive and respond to their emotional upheavals or to coordinate among all the personnel involved in the care of the patient" (p. 364). Under heavy work pressures, most residents and interns attend to medical tasks, rather than communication and coordination. Thus, the logical person to take over these functions was the nurse; the "situational location of the nurse is ideal for overall coordination of patient care and responsibility" (p. 364).

With a more specialized definition of their role, Mechanic believed that nurses could have a more specific role and responsibility. They would have to assume twenty-four-hour care and would have to be available when needed. Mechanic perceived the physician as a *consultant* to the health-care team; "he would give up some of the autonomy and control," but these "he cannot suc-cessfully exercise in any case" (p. 364). Mechanic recognized that he was chal-lenging traditional cultural assumptions and vested interests; nevertheless, he still asserted that it was time to rethink nurses' functions in a manner better fitted to technological advances.

As Mechanic recognized at the end of the 1970s, the need for change in nurse-physician relations and for shifting gender templates was a significant trend in thinking which would garner more attention in the 1980s. Increas-ingly, nurses would vocalize their distress with traditional nurse-physician roles and assert their right to autonomous practice and action. As usual, how-ever, their increased demands for equity and professional recognition would not go unchallenged; conflict between the professions of medicine and nursing would continue through the 1980s and into the 1990s, often with little observ-able improvement in their professional relations. In addition, the political con-servatism of the 1980s, the resurgent backlash directed toward feminists, and medicine's determined efforts to maintain its monopoly over health care, in-cluding initiatives to replace nurses with less-qualified personnel, would all contribute to nursing's increased dissatisfaction with their status in the health-care system.

PART III

An Outdated, Burdensome Model of Monopolistic Control: Entering the Twenty-First Century with a Fractured Health-Care System and Continuing Medical Opposition to Nurses' Autonomy

8 | Who Needs the Autonomous Professional Nurse?
Gender Stereotypes Remain Central to Nurse-Physician Relations

By the 1980s the backlash against the reemergent feminist movement was very apparent in the return to a more conservative political agenda. We begin this chapter with the resurrection of the traditional stereotype of the nurse as mother surrogate, brought back to life to reduce the widespread dissatisfaction with the impersonal health-care industry. Nurses recognized the impersonal and fragmented care, but strenuously objected to a return to powerlessness, pointing out that they could not be advocates for patients or affect their care if they were again relegated to a peripheral role. Central to the debate was the question of female versus male value systems, still expressed as caring versus curing.

The circular reasoning of some sociologists about nursing as a semiprofession continued; however, others advocated a cooperative agenda between nursing and medicine. Still the main reason for physicians' cooperation continued to be their need for nurses to meet MD obligations. This need was particularly obvious given the decline in the number of hours physicians worked, down substantially from the 1940s to fewer than 50 hours a week in 1980. There continued to be a considerable overlap among different types of nurses in the performance of their functions regardless of educational preparation; therefore, many tasks were beneath the level of the capabilities of more highly educated nurses. Rigid ritualization, standardization of procedures, and explicit orders for every action, although often unnecessary and sometimes deleterious, were still common. The evidence presented in this chapter shows a continuing devaluation of nurses and their work.

Organized medicine continued to control or even eliminate some nurses by underutilizing nurse practitioners, relying on physician's assistants (PAs), and threatening to replace registered nurses with yet another category of women, the registered care technologist, to be considered more fully in chapter 9. Sociologists stressed the limited threat posed by the small number (20,000) of nurse practitioners in comparison with the 450,000 physicians in the United States. Although a substantial number of nurses had achieved greater clinical competence and taken on more specialized roles, physicians were openly asserting that they had few economic incentives to accept more autonomous nurses, and would hire other workers to do the nursing care. Physicians repeatedly stressed the need for their own approval of any changes made by nurses in their practice. Yet physicians claimed to be "dismayed" when they learned from the National Commission on Nursing that they themselves were a major cause of nurses' dissatisfaction. Despite this dismay, the National Joint Practice Commission collapsed in 1983 because of the withdrawal of support from the American Medical Association (AMA).

Interprofessional problems caused by the medical monopoly were apparent, not only in the United States but in other countries. For example, in Great Britain some physicians continued to question whether nursing was or should be a profession, and one even asserted that medical dominance had lasted so long because women had *chosen* to be subservient. Traditional attitudes were also still apparent in the division between the "intellectual" physician and the "intuitive" nurse. In published work, it is clear that the key fear of physicians was the potential loss of their role as sole diagnostician and of their control over patient admissions to hospitals and other institutions. Indeed, one physician even deplored the exclusion of physicians from control over internal nursing affairs—for example, the appointment of nursing administrators—and stressed the need to reintroduce physicians as nursing instructors.

British nurses, like their American counterparts, were not pleased with renewed medical efforts to control the nursing profession. Some feared they were giving into traditional stereotypes because they were too tired to fight; some studied the views of nurses and physicians; some continued the struggle to keep a women's hospital alive. Others, deploring the lack of respect or even common courtesy, simply left clinics or moved to education, and still others stressed improving clinical skills and changing the valuation of female-associated work.

The views of American nurses and physicians continued to diverge. For example, at one convention, a nurse panelist concluded that medicine would not give up power voluntarily, nor would nursing limit its growth voluntarily. Given the gains created by feminist actions, nursing could no longer entice women into a segregated female profession that was totally subordinated to a predominantly male profession. At the same convention and at the same presentation, a male physician claimed that the conflict over professional turf was not with physicians, but between nurse practitioners and PAs. Ironically, physicians could now sit back and watch a struggle they themselves had helped to create.

How did the views of *women* physicians and *men* nurses compare? One female physician acknowledged that medical territoriality and monopoly continued, despite the research from 1965 onward that proved no differences in patient outcomes in the primary care provided by nurse clinicians or practitioners, PAs, or physicians. Gendered subservience of nurses was wrong and potentially dangerous to patients. In contrast, a male nurse viewed the discussion of gender as counterproductive, preferring to emphasize research on actual nursing functions and stressing mutual interdisciplinary goals in patient care. Indeed, at least one sociological study provided evidence that interdisciplinary rivalry was due to varying levels of organizational complexity. However, given the extreme gendered segregation of nurses and physicians, greater overt *intra*professional conflicts among nurses or among physicians could be a product of the amount of time that each spent together with members of their own occupational group.

As this chapter makes clear, legal experts in the field of health-care ethics who worked with interprofessional groups did not consider the complexity of health-care institutions to be the key factor in nurse-physician conflicts. Instead, the role perceptions of nurses and physicians were at the core of ethical issues, particularly in conflicts of interests about patient care. Despite the desire of some to ignore gender as an aspect of the problem, it would not go away. Research presented in this chapter proved that there was still an entrenched sex-defined hierarchy in the health-care workforce. Furthermore, traditional cultural images of nurses and physicians continued in both the public and professional imagination. This is particularly evident in the research that includes investigations on a range of topics—for example, physicians' and nurses' attitudes toward each other in their own fictional accounts; their portrayal in advertisements and in television programming; their depictions in key nursing and medical journals; the presentations of female nurses and patients in cartoons appearing in a major medical publication; and the degree of acceptance of nurses compared to physicians as authoritative sources in the media. From these variegated and usually longitudinal studies, it is more than amply apparent that gender stereotyping and discrimination continued to be central to nurse-physician relations.

Mother Surrogate or Autonomous Professional: Subordination Necessary for Tenderness, Warmth, and Sympathy?

The efforts to change nurses' roles were not without controversy, both in and outside of the profession. In 1981, for example, Lisa H. Newton asked: "If hospitals value employees who abide by the rules, and physicians want subordinates who follow orders with no back-talk, and patients need emotionally expressive caretakers—who needs the autonomous professional nurse?" (p. 348).

Newton, a philosophy professor, asserted that the skilled and gentle caregiver's role in health care "requires submission to authority as an essential component" (p. 348). Newton took great care to justify her use of female pronouns: "The whole question of autonomy . . . arises because nurses have been and are, by and large, women, and the place of the profession in the health care system is strongly influenced by the place of women in society" (p. 349). However, to Newton, the controversy over autonomy has its roots in the discrepancy between the public's view, which is still mired in the traditional image of the nurse, and the actuality of nursing. To nurses, the public ideal is used to justify their inferior status, low wages, and work at less than full capabilities.

Furthermore, nurses claim that the traditional role permanently bars them from being professionals; thus, a reform of the power base is needed, because subservience simply serves physicians' power needs and hospitals' economic needs. Everyone agrees, said Newton, on the removal of the "Lady with the Bedpan: an image of submissive service, comforting to have around and skillful enough at her little tasks, but too scatterbrained and emotional for responsibility" (p. 350). However, according to Newton, no one asks whether the public has *good* reasons to retain the traditional nurse.

The hospital is a bureaucracy, which by its nature has to have workers who do their tasks, report to supervisors, avoid initiative, and adhere to set procedures—particularly in conditions of urgency and emergency. According to Newton, only physicians know how to deal with serious medical situations and they are not always able to explain their actions. Therefore, said Newton, all others must be completely subordinated to medical judgments; they have "no right to insert their own needs, judgments, or personalities into the situation" (p. 351). Newton concluded that the general characteristics of hospitals and medicine create a negative situation for upgrading nursing. This, of course, assumes these institutional characteristics are unchanging or at least unlikely to change.

Patients' needs must take priority; these include specialized care that the physician has no time to give. Thus, he needs an assistant to perform simple tasks and to help with serious emotional needs. To Newton, the person "who would be capable of taking care of all these [patient's] problems is obviously his mother, and the first job of the nurse is to be a mother surrogate" (p. 351). Given the dictionary definition of "nurse," which is to nourish or suckle, Newton concluded that "the function of the nurse is identical with that of the mother, to be exercised when the mother is unavailable" (p. 351). This transposition excludes the father or any other male as caregiver; indeed, Newton specifically justified *women* as nurses, because they were really surrogate mothers for sick, injured, very old, or helpless adults. This, of course, assumes that all children and adults have positive feelings toward mothers and motherhood, despite the obvious fact that not all women are "good" mothers. It further assumes that all females, whether or not they want or are competent to be mothers, are available, able, and willing to be mothers.

Newton admitted that the mother role needs modification when transferred to hospitals, since maternal authority—total, diffuse, and unlimited—would be incompatible with "the retention of moral freedom" (p. 352). Having justified the elimination of *real* maternal authority, Newton, without analyzing the parallel paternal medical authority (fathers evidently do not count), concluded that the nurse must be free from any attribution of authority. Thus, the subservient role is necessary in order for nurturing to be expressed and received.

Nurses must be available to talk to the patient, because the physician is too busy. Presumably, physician as "father" requires *no* analysis to justify his business. Because the woman "can do absolutely nothing to change [the] course of treatment" (as if she gave no care of her own), she is therefore perfectly safe to talk to! (p. 352). According to Newton, "Neither bureaucracy nor medical professional can handle the human needs of the human beings involved in the process" (p. 352). Ironically, there is nothing inherent in, or "natural" about, a health system or a medical profession that cannot meet human needs. Indeed, if health is the reason for the system and for physicians, then humane care for human beings would seem to be a logical expectation. Nevertheless, to Newton the woman nurse was humane, but her medical colleague was coldly professional. The nurse's so-called maternal role allows feminine tenderness, warmth, and sympathy; these break through "the cold barriers of efficiency" (p. 352). How nurses were supposed to accomplish this without power to change bureaucratic rules and inappropriate medical orders remained unclear.

The need for institutions and physicians to function as they do leads to an admittedly unattractive conclusion that argues against nurses' autonomy, because "the tasks of making objective judgments and of expressing emotion are inherently incompatible; and since the nurse shows grief and sympathy on behalf of the system, she is excluded from decision-making and defined as subordinate" (p. 353). If this analysis is correct, only women can mother and exhibit maternal behavior, which includes sympathy and grief; thus, all mothers should be subordinate because they cannot make "objective" decisions and, therefore, cannot be allowed to act within family or public systems in authority positions.

Indeed, Newton argued that feminists of this generation, whom she does not name, have stated that the traditional housewife and mother role, though useful to others, traps the woman because the "profit of others is not a sufficient reason to retain a role that demeans its occupant" (p. 353). This assertion is, of course, only one aspect of a multifaceted feminist explanation, much of which is far more complex than admitted or perhaps even known by Newton, who seemed to assume that women, mothers, and nurses have occupied unchanging "traditional" roles over the centuries. Instead of historical accuracy, there is stereotyped assertion. Nevertheless, Newton claimed that the traditional nurse role is analogous to the roles of slave and housewife. Having drawn this analogy, Newton then claimed it could not be sustained, because people may be in subordinate roles without losing integrity. Indeed, some slaves and housewives, said Newton, have shown signs of personal integrity and autonomy. Without any acknowledgment of decades of complex research on gender roles, Newton's assertion on the nature of human freedom seems a glib generalization.

Some (unspecified) advocates wanted to abolish the "traditional" nurse "because it preserves the sex stereotypes we are trying to overcome" (p. 353).

Some (unnamed) feminists say that a nurse is a purely "feminine" role, histori-cally derived from "mother," embodying "feminine" attitudes of emotionality, tenderness, and nurturance. Ironically, the value-laden concept "feminine" is a term often avoided by feminist scholars, whose historical evidence, as dis-cussed in chapter 1, supports the interpretation that nurse and physician roles were previously *combined* for many women within families and communities. Intellect was then and is now part of good health care, whether given by mother, nurse, or woman healer. Indeed, to dichotomize feeling and thinking is not part of recent feminist thought. This polarization is Newton's own cari-cature of scholarship on women.

To Newton, sexism does not derive from the fact "that some roles are au-tonomous, calling for objectivity in judgment, suppression of emotion, and independent initiative" (p. 354), while other roles reflect an absence of these and the presence of obedience to superiors. Sexism derives from the fact that men are eligible for the first group and women for the second. Newton's defi-nition relies on civil libertarian feminism, which is concerned with role expan-sion, the opening of *all* roles to *all* people. Cultural feminist theory, however, questions the nature of hierarchy itself, among other things. The assumption that current organizational structures are appropriate to provide good health care is highly questionable. There is nothing "natural" about a sex-stratified health-care system that cannot deal humanely with human beings unless a class of subordinated women is present. Indeed, there is something distinctly unnatural and even illogical in such an assertion.

Newton did question the idea that warmth, gentleness, and loving care, expected of the nurse, are not possible for males. But how males, incapable of giving birth, would partake of the "maternal" was not discussed. Nor was the fact that male nurses are hired for higher salaries immediately out of nursing school; and that male nurses assume positions of greater power to a much higher degree than female nurses. Evidently, subordinate status, even within nursing, is neither appreciated nor needed by many men in nursing.

What was Newton's solution for nurses who do not accept subordination? They "will clearly have to do something else" (p. 354). Presumably these women will get jobs that do not have the nurse label and, thus, they will not need to combat "the traditional nurse" image. They will not have to fight ste-reotypes which "they find degrading and unworthy of their abilities [and] should seek out occupational niches that do not bear the label, and the stigma, of 'nurse'" (p. 354). So all strong women who value freedom, according to Newton, are to leave the profession; only those stereotyped as "maternal" would remain, and these females, and the males who agree with them, would accept their subordination. Newton's plea was for a "traditional nurse" to re-tain humanity "in a system that will turn into a mechanical monster without her" (p. 354). How, from a position of powerlessness, women nurses are to keep this monster from becoming even more monstrous is a central and unanswered question.

Outraged Reactions to "Traditional Nurse"

Nurses' responses to Newton and her assertions were immediate. The September 1981 issue of *Nursing Outlook* published numerous reactions to her article. Ken Zwolski, RN, from New York, said, "I strenuously object to what I surmise is the essence of her text—that is, the opinion that subservience is a required, indeed a crucial, condition for the fulfillment of our professional nursing ideals" (p. 500). The promulgation of the idea that autonomy is incompatible with nursing, which is to be valued because of subordination, was for this nurse harmful both to nursing and to the public. Zwolski asserted that a profession must have the right "to alter the traditional if the traditional is no longer adequate or has never been" (p. 500). Indeed, he said that it is very doubtful that subservience has ever been of any real value to best serve patients' needs: "The nurse may at times be perceived as a mother surrogate of the patient, but this is not her major intent or function. Her first job is to be a professional caregiver, one who protects as well as stimulates, one who fosters well-being through whatever professional therapies, activities, or educational endeavors her assessment deems necessary" (p. 500). Of course, the patient needs kindness and sympathy, but "What the patient does not need . . . is a subservient attendant who threatens his self-esteem by treating him as a baby" (p. 500).

A second nurse, Ellen D. Baer, also took issue with Newton's conception of the traditional nurse, who historically submitted to medicine only in pharmaceutical and therapeutic interventions. She referred to Florence Nightingale's paper, read at the 1893 nurses' meeting at the Chicago World's Fair, that specifically argued against servility and advocated the independent sense of responsibility to secure genuine trustworthiness. Baer claimed that Newton had not questioned the authenticity of the so-called traditional nurse. For example, the nurse did *not* evolve in the hospital context, which "did not become a primary locus of nursing practice until the post-Depression and World War II years" (p. 500).

Diana Mason accused Newton of erroneously assuming that autonomy requires suppression of emotions, which are supposed to be antithetical to rationality: "Does Dr. Newton not expect a physician to be warm, gentle, and compassionate? And if she came upon such a physician, would she view him as incapable of 'objectivity in judgment . . . and independent initiative in action?'" (p. 501). Mason asserted that *all* health caregivers should be compassionate, humanistic, and rational thinkers.

Why, asked Mason, did Newton not see distinct, even though overlapping, disciplines? Why did she not advocate collaboration? To this nurse, physicians were not trained to nurse; therefore, they could not tell nurses how to practice. Furthermore, physicians were primarily involved in the diagnosis of disease or the prescription of medicine, a narrow range of practice with limited patient contact. Mason disagreed with Newton's conceptualization of disciplines and institutions: "Medicine and the hospital, in particular, are not 'devoted to the saving of life and health'; rather they are largely devoted to profit making, which will become blatantly obvious to anyone in the position of needing health care without the means to pay for it" (p. 501). Mason stated unequivocally that perpetuation of the current hospital power structure would continue the "cold, mechanical aspects of health care which Dr. Newton decries" (p. 501).

Arizona nurse Phyllis Fitzgerald asked why the affective function would be lost if the nurse acted as a patient advocate. In medical crises, physicians do sometimes direct actions; "patients are not consistently in medical crises, however, [so] why should physicians expect continual subordination?" (p. 501). If the nurse finds problems brought on by a patient's hospitalization, "Is she to listen and not attempt to do something about such a situation?" (p. 501). Using the maternal analogy, Fitzgerald said that mothers of children with problems can speak for the children or tell the children to solve their problems themselves. A mother needs to know when to speak in behalf of the child and when the child can handle the problem alone. In a telling statement, this nurse suggested that Newton spend some time in hospitals, where she would find both traditional and autonomous roles coexisting. Patients need the "expertise of everyone involved in their care" (p. 501).

Nancy Creason, Illinois nurse, accused Newton of erring in her assumption that physicians make all the important decisions about patients and that "the nurse's only function is to do what she is told" (p. 501). As Creason noted, in acute care settings, "the need for highly capable decision making is ever present. The problem, of course, is that physicians are not" (p. 501). Who, she asked, cares about and for the patient all the hours when doctors are not present? To advocate the mother surrogate role, "implies that mothering behavior is something women do naturally without need for thought or knowledgeable judgment . . . [but] mothering children is not an inborn female ability" (p. 501)—nor is nursing, which Creason hoped had gone beyond mothering and the treatment of patients as children.

Newton said people in pain deserve sympathy; Creason claimed they deserve to have their pain treated by both nurses and physicians. To her, sympathy is the least potentially successful measure of any that can "be performed by a competent, intelligent nurse independent of anyone" (p. 501). Nurses seek autonomy so they can better perform their functions as nurses, not as mother surrogates, slaves, or housewives.

Jeffrey M. Rossman, a Connecticut nurse, acknowledged the importance of helping patients deal with "a faceless and threatening alien environment . . .

[even] [o]ffering a degree of 'mothering,'" but he asserted that "nurses . . . have a legitimate right to seek autonomy" according to their hard work, responsibilities, and education (p. 502). Rossman attempted to combine both "tradition" and autonomy by emphasizing patient education and patient advocacy. Two other nurses, Bobbi Jean Perdue and Margaret Lunney, both from New Jersey, did not agree with Rossman and certainly not with Newton, whose article "introduced a new breed of nurse, not heretofore recognized in the nursing literature—surrogate mother and caretaker of patients, physicians, and hospitals too" (p. 502). Not only a provider of feeling, but an obedient servant as well! "Which nursing schools," they asked, "can recruit a supply of students who want to function in this romantic version of 'traditional' nurse?" (p. 502). These nurses argued that "the origin of a word does not establish its present function" (p. 502).

To Harriet Rosenman, Newton set up a situation of suffering and death when she advised no one should question the physician even when serious situations arose without warning. Unfortunately, said Rosenman, physicians are human and, as such, prone to error. Furthermore, nurses have considerable knowledge, which Newton seemed to nullify. As a nurse for twenty years and an administrator for ten, Rosenman said, "I have frequently seen patient safety ensured by an astute nurse interfering with an erring physician" (p. 503). She concluded, "What an awful world the world of health care would be, if Dr. Newton had her way" (p. 503).

Nurse Marguerite B. White also concurred with the need for humane nursing care, but she totally rejected "the assumption that submissiveness is the key to the fulfillment" of humanistic care and charged that it "has been and still is a barrier to providing the care Dr. Newton describes" (p. 503). Indeed, White noted that Newton, not being a nurse, seemed unaware that "the majority of hospital rules are for the efficient functioning of the bureaucracy and not necessarily in the best interest of the patient" (p. 503). Most nurses in the past and present were not permitted, nor did they have sufficient time, to sit and listen to patients or families; rather, they have been and continue to be kept busy with tasks. White claimed that only when the autonomous nurse insists on humane care will it be provided. She also took Newton to task for assuming that humanistic care and autonomy are incompatible. Relying on twenty-five years as an educator, White said that neither she nor her colleagues have advocated relinquishing skilled and gentle care; however, they have urged students to be patient advocates against hospital rules if these compete with patient welfare. Indeed, White asserted, "hospital policies have become more humane through the efforts of caring nurses who refused to be submissive to bureaucratic authority and blindly follow regulations" (p. 503). White flatly rejected the premise that hospital effectiveness depended on unquestioning adherence to procedures.

Betty G. Harris, RN, of North Carolina agreed and stated it is not the fact of the nurse's powerlessness that made patients share their fears and concerns: "I suggest that the patient confides in a traditional nurse not because she is powerless, but because he perceives her as *having* power" (p. 503). When nurses cannot act to create change, sharing becomes an exercise in "futile commiseration without progress or relief" (p. 503).

Delores A. Gaut, in a sharp rejoinder to Newton, said, "The task of philosophical analysis is clarification, not obfuscation" (p. 502). Gaut acknowledged that her so-called objective view was shrouded with anger about an article that was filled with truisms but overlooked the real history of nursing. Indeed, Nightingale created a profession as an "outcry against the forced idleness of Victorian women in subservient roles" (p. 502). To accept Newton's truisms was to return to the Victorian view of woman as man's inferior. If humanism in health-care systems is so desperately needed, "it is the nurse, with power and authority to protect the patient's rights and control the patient's environment, that is desperately needed" (p. 502).

Unmasking the True Intent: Expansion for Physicians or Nurses?

Did the expanded roles for nurses really provide for more power and authority to allow them to protect patients, or were these "new" roles simply a product of medical manipulation? The latter interpretation is clear from Dorothy Fiorino's (1980) research (cited in Lovell, 1982) on the development from 1973 to 1978 of the National Association of Pediatric Nurse Associates/Practitioners (NAPNAP). The parent organization, the American Academy of Pediatrics (AAP), had ostensibly worked with the nurses' association, which presumably functioned independently, supposedly receiving only guidance and advice from the older, "wiser" medical group. In reality, Fiorino found that the AAP, under the guise of generous paternalism, had exerted power by imposing controls that medical men thought to be essential. The United States Labor Department, after conducting a national survey which found a shortage and maldistribution of physicians, mandated medicine to solve this problem. The shortage was more acute in pediatrics, so the AAP moved quickly to create pediatric nurse associates or practitioners because this, according to Fiorino, was a quick, cheap, and accessible way to delegate physicians' tasks. Despite these advantages, some pediatric physicians still did not approve; one wrote in a letter to his colleagues that he feared losing control over *his* nurses, and criticized the medical profession for allowing nurses' education to come under the control of nurses, who had only limited practical experience and thus could not be really aware of what was needed.

Despite such objections, the pediatric nurse association, according to Fiorino, was created primarily by physicians, who developed, approved, and accredited the nurses and thus avoided nursing input because knowledgeable nurse leaders would not have allowed such exploitation of other nurses. From

Fiorino's research, Lovell (1982) stated that most nurses had "no way to distinguish between benevolent or malevolent motives for physicians' interference" (p. 219) in nursing and did not sufficiently question the chain of events. The nurse was so "eager for their [physicians'] guidance and control that she unquestioningly (but wrongly) assumed is always for her own good" (p. 219). Clearly, expanding nurses' roles would not lead to more power and authority for nurses if such expansion was introduced *by* physicians *for* physicians. However, if nurses *thought* they were achieving more autonomy and if this was *not* forthcoming, conflict was sure to result.

The Continued Devaluation of Nurses and Nursing

Clearly, nurses did believe that new roles would bring more authority. Unfortunately, in the 1980s nurses were still subject to gendered subordination. To Ada Jacox (1982) problems in role restructuring in hospital nursing were still traceable to the discrepancies in the definitions of nursing, which

> clearly are the result of social and political factors in which an occupation made up almost totally of women has tried to define its role in relation to medicine, an occupation traditionally composed primarily of men and commonly viewed as near the top of the occupational hierarchy in social prestige. In more recent decades, nurses have been confronted by hospital administrators, a professionalizing group also largely made up of men, who have assumed it their prerogative to manage and control the practice of hospital nursing. (pp. 75–76)

The gendered system has resulted in low economic status for nurses; erroneous expectations that their primary responsibility is to follow physicians' orders; acceptance of any tasks and hours allotted; and lack of authority in policies and decision making. Jacox warned that without role restructuring, nursing would remain a "low level, poorly reimbursed occupation capable of attracting primarily those persons who have limited options for pursuing more interesting and satisfying work" (p. 76).

Nurses were still likely to perform a variety of roles "ranging from housekeeper to housestaff" (p. 77). This role variability existed at the same time that hospitals were more likely to be populated by very seriously ill patients. Indeed, in the 1980s, 30 percent of nurses provided intensive care, which requires substantial technical and clinical knowledge. For example, coronary unit nurses must be able to diagnose six to eight different common conditions, take appropriate immediate action with medication, resuscitation, or other measures— all of these must often be accomplished *before* calling a physician for assistance. As Jacox stressed, these actions are *normal* expectations for nurses in all intensive care units. According to a study of five Boston hospitals (Goldstein and Horowitz, 1978; cited in Jacox, 1982, p. 78), a continuum of simple to complex care activities existed; there was, however, a "great deal of overlap in the performance of various functions regardless of educational preparation. . . . Considerable overlap was apparent among levels of nursing personnel in tasks performed, and there was similar overlap with physicians" (p. 78). For example, 77 percent of nurses spent 28 percent of their time on simple, level 1 activities (locating and setting up simple equipment or moving patients to another floor), while nearly one-half of physicians spent 23 percent and 81 percent of nurse's aides spent 57 percent of their time on these activities.

During the 1970s a direct substitution of nurses for nurse's aides occurred, made possible by low salary differentials; thus, nurses are clearly likely to do tasks beneath their level of educational training. In contrast, from 5:00 P.M. onward, nurses are likely to take on the work of many other professionals, including the tasks of physicians. Further, the women were also usually responsible for accident and incident reports, ensuring patient safety. All of these tasks were completed in an atmosphere of "rigid ritualism and standardization of procedures accompanied by an absence of decision-making freedom" (p. 80). Jacox concluded that *explicit orders are required for practically every action.*

At the same time, the devaluation of women's work continued, as in previous decades. Other professionals continued to receive reimbursement for what nurses do; for example, under third-party indirect payment, physicians could earn up to 54 percent profit from employees who are nurse practitioners and, at the same time, ensure their dependence. Another way to make money from women's efforts is to require nurses to do admission histories, order routine medications, and carry out diagnostic and treatment procedures in hospitals; however, these acts must be "validated" by the physician, who countersigns and then collects a fee for "authorizing" the work of the nurse, who is paid by the hospital. In addition, the hospital classifies diagnostic treatments and procedures as revenue-generating, but skilled nursing care is classified as a cost or liability. Ironically, as Jacox stressed, hospitals provide *both* diagnosis and nursing care as the reasons for their existence.

Registered nurses were still devalued economically; nurse's aides' salaries had *increased* from 65 percent to 71 percent of registered nurses' salaries, but simultaneously *decreased* from 33 percent to 20 percent of physicians' income. The mistreatment of administrative nurses, said Jacox, was widespread and obvious in a Colorado lawsuit involving a director of nursing who had a master's degree, twelve years of administrative experience, and responsibility for a budget of $3.5 million. She was classified not with equivalent administrators, but in the graduate nurse 1 category; thus, she was paid $457 less than similarly prepared administrators. The judge ruled that "we are confronted with a history which I have no hesitancy at all in finding discriminated unfairly and improperly against women" (p. 84). But men—for example, those in the clergy—were also underpaid; therefore, the judge ruled against the nurses, claiming that the disruption of the entire American economy was at stake!

As noted previously, devaluation was also apparent in sociological research, which establishes male professions as the norm. To Jacox, the circular reasoning asserts that autonomy is not granted women; therefore, a woman's profession can never be autonomous; thus, nursing is a semiprofession. The further implication is that the work is inferior; yet, as Jacox properly noted, a review of studies comparing nurse practitioner and physician performance found that the nurses scored higher on twenty variables, from completeness of histories to control of blood pressure.

Different definitions of professional expertise are often used "as a mask for privilege and power" (p. 86) rather than a means for promoting the public interest. This is obvious in the historical efforts to deny education to nurses and, at the same time, to refuse to delegate authority because of "inadequate" educational preparation. There was even then, according to Jacox, a call for reduction in education of nurses while all other health professionals were extending their training.

What were nurses doing to offset their devaluation? Jacox pointed to role restructuring in primary-care nursing, which started about 1970 and involved twenty-four-hour responsibility for patients. In addition, temporary service agencies allowed nurses to be hired for specific nursing homes, as clinical specialists and nurse practitioners. Altering institutional practice arrangements and placing nurses through independent organizations are important, but it is unclear how these changes are to be enacted without modifying the medical monopoly.

Nurse Dissatisfaction and Physician Resentment: Is a Cooperative Agenda Possible?

Perhaps appealing directly to physicians would help redress the power imbalance and nurses' dissatisfaction with their lack of autonomy (see Godfrey, 1978, and Mechanic, 1978). This strategy was used in 1982 by David Mechanic, sociologist, and Linda H. Aiken, nurse researcher, who urged a cooperative agenda for medicine and nursing. They claimed that the competitive strain between the two professions had been "unnecessarily exaggerated," taking attention away from mutual interests and patient care. Given that medical sociologists had historically paid little attention to nursing, and even in the 1980s continued to sustain their identification with medicine by the title of their disciplinary specialization, it was refreshing to finally see an article that incorporated nursing concerns published in the *New England Journal of Medicine*. The initial assertion of an "exaggerated" stress on competition was followed by the delineation of very serious problems, particularly those related to changing women's roles.

Mechanic and Aiken recognized the stresses on physicians from biomedical advances, their medicalization of everyday problems, and their need to deal with technical, psychosocial, and behavioral problems: "Many physicians deeply resent the growth of regulation and increasing criticism from patients and the mass media. Some fear an erosion of their economic status and clinical autonomy" (Mechanic and Aiken, 1982, p. 747). The degree to which physicians can face multiple, conflicting expectations and stresses, and remain technically expert while expressing a humane attitude toward patients depends, said the authors, on physicians' arrangements with other health professionals, particularly nurses.

Nursing must be perceived in terms of "broad social changes in sex roles and in women's conceptions of themselves" (p. 747). These include the dramatic increase of women in the workforce; increased female expectations for comparable opportunities, incentives, and rewards; and the expectation of lifelong paid employment with opportunities for growth and development. Indeed, women are "increasingly dissatisfied with episodic work, with an absence of rewards and career ladders, and with expectations that they will be deferential and perform tasks not relevant to work that are not expected of men" (p. 747). Thus, women may increasingly bypass nursing for law, medicine, or business.

To Mechanic and Aiken, nursing exemplifies the limitations of "women's occupations." It involves a growing knowledge base with technical demands, but also "plain hard work in terms of physical labor, night and weekend work hours, social stress, and continuing responsibility . . . [which is] poorly remunerated in comparison to other occupations demanding similar levels of education, skill, and responsibility" (p. 747). In addition, the dramatic increase in the gap between nurses' and physicians' salaries is accompanied by few rewards for increased education and experience. Consequently, competent nurses exit the profession, leaving inexperienced nurses overwhelmed.

Finally, Mechanic and Aiken got to the main issue: "Nurses have lacked the authority to make many simple decisions necessary for the safety and comfort of patients, and they have been expected to defer to medical authority, even in situations in which they possess greater experience" (p. 748). Undervaluation of knowledge and experience leads to dissatisfaction, which is paralleled by patients' dissatisfaction with the absence of physicians, who cannot easily coordinate office and hospital time to deal with patients and their families. Thus, collaboration with nurses is obviously needed to meet physicians' obligations.

Aiken and Mechanic stated: "The number of hours worked by the average physician has declined from over 65 hours a week in 1943 to less than 50 hours a week in 1980. Moreover, most physicians spend less than two hours a day in making rounds in the hospital" (p. 748). Given the reduction of 20 percent in average length of hospital stays and the increase of 74 percent in the number of intensive care patients, it is clear that nurses must deal with sicker patients, more complex technology, more difficulties in coordination of more specialized caregivers, and with physicians "not present in the hospital or easily accessible for direct consultation. . . . Nurses are left with the continuing responsibility for acutely ill patients, but their authority to act in the absence of the physician has not been formally modified" (p. 748).

These factors contribute to the reality of hospital practice in which medical tasks are shared by nurses, causing confusion over nurses' functions. Although overly optimistic about relations being well-defined and nonconflictual in intensive care, the authors are correct that survival rates have been positively affected by better interprofessional relations. In noncritical care, nurses experience the greatest ambiguity and the most need for "authority to act in matters within their spheres of competence" (p. 748). It is important to list a few of the functions for which nurses need authority: "Changing inappropriate special diets; modifying medications when indicated, including dosage and mode of administration; rescheduling strenuous diagnostic procedures as warranted by patient's conditions; changing surgical dressings if needed; deciding on the frequency of vital sign monitoring; inserting catheters for patients unable to void; and contributing to decisions . . . on hospital discharge" (p. 748). These are only a few of many that cause nurse dissatisfaction and patient inconvenience, suffering, and even anger.

Another major national concern, according to Mechanic and Aiken, is the state of nursing homes, which care for an increasing number of patients for whom neither nursing nor medicine has taken undisputed leadership. The absence of physicians is clear: "Only 17 percent of physicians participate in nursing home care at all. . . . Primary-care physicians . . . spend on the average less than 1½ hours a month caring for their patients in nursing homes . . . [Thus] a promising strategy . . . is to strengthen the role of nurses as primary providers, with physicians in consultative roles" (p. 749).

Mechanic and Aiken stressed that perceptions of economic threat from 20,000 nurse practitioners—out of more than one million nurses—compared to 450,000 physicians is "more symbolic than real" (p. 749). This is because nurses obtain their remuneration primarily from hospitals or nursing homes, not from fees from services. This assertion excluded those nurses who were entering private practice. It also excluded nurses' demands for independent access to patients to break the medical monopoly. Writing for physicians, the authors instead emphasized the benefits to physicians from nurses' expanded clinical responsibilities, freeing physicians for uniquely and more remunerative medical functions. The authority of advanced nurse specialists in making clinical decisions must be within a differential structure that defines nurses by expertise, allowing physicians to have greater confidence in nurses' clinical decision making. In addition, primary nursing is needed to establish continuity of care, limit turnover, and reduce the wasteful expenditures caused by the average annual turnover rate of 30 percent among hospital nurses. Indeed, research shows that fewer experienced nurses can manage more efficiently than "transitory personnel or those with fewer skills who require continued supervision" (p. 750).

The most important factor creating interprofessional conflict was, said Aiken and Mechanic, the increasing isolation between nursing and medical schools. They called for closer academic connections involving collaboration between medical and nursing faculty and models of interaction that included, for example, young medical students learning from experienced nurses. Such partnership models would require that the traditional sex-stratified, monopolistic system be substantially modified; thus, a cooperative agenda demanded an overt explication of the gendered systemic factors involved.

Neither Side Should Be Surprised by the Opposition of the Other

To set a cooperative agenda, the participants would have to have perspectives that were at least somewhat congruent. Such congruency was not immediately apparent, however, in two perspectives on nurse-physician relations presented at a 1982 meeting, Conflicts and Collaboration: Nursing and Medicine, sponsored by the Subcommittee on Nurse/Physician Relations of the Committee on Medicine, Society of the New York Academy of Medicine. Barbara J. Stevens (1984) presented the nursing perspective and Conrad Rosenberg (1984) the medical view.

Stevens could find only four articles on interrelations written by physicians in the last few years, but many by nurses, attesting to the salience of the problem for them. Indeed, research studies confirmed that nursing was perceived as unsatisfactory because of low economic compensation, poor work environments, and undesirable relations with physicians. These facts were recognized by the National Commission on Nursing in 1981, which recommended collaborative partnership, involvement in clinical decision making, and sufficient authority for professional practice. Stevens clearly understood that relations are "not problematic merely on a one-to-one, psychological-sociological basis" (Stevens, 1984, p. 800). As a group, physicians were still more likely to be males, who were older than nurses, exceeded their education levels, and came from higher social classes. In Stevens's view, physicians had the edge; nevertheless, competition between them and advanced practice nurses had increased. By the 1980s, organized medicine had allowed the overproduction of physicians; thus, they had given little support for nurses' advanced preparation. This had shocked nurses, who should have, however, recognized that "no group gives up status, power, or control voluntarily" (p. 801). Similarly, physicians should realize that "No aspiring professional group voluntarily limits its growth potential" (p. 801). Stevens claimed that "In this power conflict, neither side should be surprised by the opposition of the other" (p. 801).

Complicating the conflict is the shortage of nurses, to which the Department of Health and Human Services attested in 1982 in the *Third Report to the*

Congress, which specified aspects of the work environment that led to dissatisfaction, turnover, and shortage, such as inadequate salaries, inability to define and control practice, exclusion from decision making, and lack of opportunity for professional growth. If nurse shortages are to be eliminated, collegiality from physicians is necessary; yet many may yearn, said Stevens, for the nurse who "smiled and stood at attention until dismissed" (p. 803). Pointedly Stevens noted, "It is always simpler to relate by giving orders than by negotiating" (p. 803). However, the "Stepford nurse" is wishful thinking because today's women "just do not accept a subservient role," nor a "pseudoreligious substitution" (p. 803), nor a stopgap job until marriage.

Stevens bluntly asserted that nursing has to appeal to *today's* women: "One simply cannot 'sell' a role in which one profession is subjugated to the service of another profession" (p. 803). Nor can one sell positions in which a nurse with a BS degree has an average salary equal to that of a secretary with no college degree. Nor jobs for which a nurse retiring at sixty-five receives $2,500 more than a beginning nurse. Nor work for which a nurse in 1945 earned one-third the physician's income but earned only one-fifth in the early 1980s. Nor can working conditions be used to sell nursing because of rotating shifts, weekend work, unsafe locations, increasingly acute illness of patients, more technological demands, and staffing crises. Added to these factors is the undervaluing of nurses' contributions by physicians and administrators.

Stevens called for radical changes in this "dreary picture." According to her, two options were available: one, respect and cooperation for real accountability in nursing judgment, requiring physician acceptance of nurses' autonomy; or, two, exclusion of professional nurses and their replacement by licensed practical nurses. If the latter option is selected, "it is likely that physicians will, by default, find themselves doing some nursing for their own patients" (p. 805). Although some physicians were hinting at the second, subservient solution, they may still "expect further pressures to change their patterns of interface with nurses" (p. 805).

From the medical perspective, Conrad Rosenberg saw salaries, sexism, and self-image as possible explanations for conflict, but contended that solutions to the "nursing problem" are as varied as those who propose them. Unlike Stevens, Rosenberg provided no research evidence, but relied on his personal experience and concluded: "There is too often a mismatch between training and responsibility" (Rosenberg, 1984, p. 809), with some women overeducated for menial tasks and others undereducated for complex ones. Failing to see that many physicians have historically denied the need for fully educated nurses or manipulated their "training," he stated that the nurse-physician relationship is not the problem, nor is it an important symptom of the problem. Physicians tend to have strong egos, but the ego turf fight, he believes, is between nurses and physician's assistants. Again, he failed to see that physicians created the new category of PAs, which, in turn, forced nurses to fight for their turf and profession. Rosenberg predicted increasing future conflict with midwives over fewer health dollars, but did not say that this group of women had already been *purposefully* excluded by men. Fortunately, the midwives were still unwilling to die a professional death at the hands of physicians.

We Are Advocates for Patients, Not Physicians

A comparison between Stevens's and Rosenberg's views would hardly suggest a high degree of congruence. In the daily work of the nurse and physician, however, there were in genuine emergencies sometimes true cooperation, cohesiveness, and mutual interdependency. Some day, said nurse Margaret McGuire (1980), such interaction would be an everyday reality, but until then, "You and I, as professional nurses, must learn to speak out. Not next year! Not tomorrow! Today!" (p. 39). To speak up, to keep a sense of humor, to take responsibility for further education, to document events in writing—all these are necessary. McGuire stated flatly: "We are patient advocates. . . . Speak for patients. . . . Intervene for them, if necessary. . . . Never hold a grudge" (p. 39). While being diplomatic, insist that physicians treat nurses with respect, for they are human beings who also feel anger and frustration. McGuire envisioned individuals responding to individuals, but how nursing *groups* were to respond to medical *group* pressures remained unexplored. What is clear is that some nurses were no longer willing to protect physicians and now saw themselves as patient advocates.

Physician Response: We'll Get Someone Else to Do Nursing

How did physicians respond to nurses as more autonomous professionals and patient advocates? One trend is clear in a presentation by James Levy, MD (1981), at a conference of the Maryland, Virginia, and Washington, D.C., Hospital Associations. Levy claimed that physicians have *no* economic incentive to prevent doctor-nurse conflicts. He did admit that maximizing hospital efficiency to keep patient volume high might involve physicians, who may want to cut down on "poor communication" that results from "excessive telephone calls and messages between physicians and nurses" (p. 47). Levy also acknowledged that physicians from countries "where women are subservient may be especially tough for nurses to talk with" (p. 47), but he simply advised nurses to be "pragmatic."

Reminiscent of Stein's 1967 analysis of the doctor-nurse game, Levy believed nurses should consider having physicians formally approve any practices that the nurses decide to pursue. This would allow the physicians to feel they were making all of the decisions that nurses, in reality, were making: "Remember that physicians have no experience in personnel management" (p. 47). Although nurses' self-esteem was important, Levy wondered whether the nurse could accept her role as it is. Clearly, Levy wanted "good communication," but only if it is based on the status quo.

It is obvious that physicians such as Levy were still advising nurses what to do and how to behave. Physicians also continued to form their own committees on nursing. In 1982 William Y. Rial, president-elect of the AMA, writing on the shortage of nurses, referred to Donna Deirs, dean of Yale University School of Nursing, who said, "I hope to live long enough to see nurses hire physicians to perform that small piece of health care that is the medical surgical treatment of disease when patients need to be admitted to nurse controlled institutions" (p. 22). Rial then contrasted Deirs with A. D. Roberts, MD, who acknowledged that nurses may have mastered technology, but warned that "they should not be overtrained and overly licensed for what hospitals need . . . basic traditional nursing" (p. 22). This assertion sounds almost identical to those of physicians from the nineteenth and early twentieth centuries, a very familiar refrain, as noted in chapters 3 and 4.

The National Commission on Nursing, chaired by a physician (a fact that did not seem peculiar to Rial), was "dismayed to hear that nurses who testified perceive that the treatment afforded nurses by physicians is a significant part of the problems relating to job dissatisfaction" (p. 22). It is astonishing how, after a long history of trying to subordinate women in order to create a medical monopoly, the men could *still* be so oblivious to nurse dissatisfaction with this strategy. In a blunt statement of arrogant power, by now very familiar, Roberts stated: "In patient care, somebody must give the orders—that's the physician. And somebody must translate orders into patient care. That's the nurse. If the nursing profession has problems with that, we've got to get somebody else to do it" (pp. 22, 24).

Rial engaged in the usual rhetoric: better communication and collaborative partnership. He hoped that nurses would leave the profession only when pregnant or when their husbands were geographically transferred. Obviously, Rial seemed unaware that male nurses exist; or that patrilocality may be unacceptable to female nurses, who valued their own careers; or that they may not marry or, if married, may decide to remain childless. Clearly, traditional gender stereotypes were still basic to physicians' beliefs about nurses.

The Collapse of the National Joint Practice Commission

In contrast to Rial, Ann P. Morgan and Janice M. McCann (1983) pointed clearly and unambiguously to male dominance and female compliance as the central issue in physician-nurse relations. As women nurses refused to be subservient, there were increased efforts by organized medicine to sustain its monopoly and impede changes in laws that would give nurses more autonomy. The medical monopoly was under attack, and an unsolicited report on nursing education by the New York Academy of Medicine provided "considerable evidence . . . that doctors feel threatened by educated nurses" (Skoblar and Amster, 1977; cited in Morgan and McCann, 1983, p. 2).

To Morgan and McCann, the lack of integrated education of nursing and physicians kept artificial distinctions in knowledge alive. Furthermore, gross economic disparities in income enforce a social class distinction, even when both physicians and nurses enter from comparable family backgrounds. Therefore, despite the threat to physicians, nursing must capitalize on the women's movement, accentuate independent roles, demand equality, and force physicians to give more than lip service to female liberation. The authors reviewed the work of the National Joint Practice Commission on Nurses and Physicians Practice, and concluded that many issues were not resolved by the nurse and physician commissioners. Still hoping for mutual collaboration at the local level, Morgan and McCann focused on reducing economic disparities and increasing research on work roles.

Evidently, nurses were insufficiently docile for organized medicine because in 1983 the AMA broke away from the National Joint Practice Commission. One member, nurse Shirley Smoyak (1987), focused on the factors that led to nurses' dissatisfaction, such as the dramatic gap between physicians' and nurses' income: "Just after the Second World War nurses' incomes were one-third of doctors'. By 1980, the figure was one-fifth" (p. 36). However, said Smoyak, the most significant achievement of the commission was the dialogue among the members themselves, which was honest but uncomfortable and involved discussion about the nature and reimbursement of work: "What was fair and not fair?, What was good for patients?, and What was not?, and How work could be defined, re-defined, and managed" (p. 36). For example, if the nurse observes, can she make interpretations? "Interpretation, of course, is simply a process of naming. What is it that the nurse may or should name?" (p. 37). Since interpreting requires conceptual activity, "How fully may a nurse use her brain?" (p. 37). This question is tied to the role of woman, since a "fairly common belief was that thinking was masculine, and women might damage themselves if they did too much of it. Decision-making was even more masculine, and clearly not for women" (p. 37).

Indeed, Smoyak advised: "Nursing is best viewed within the context of broad and far-reaching social changes in sex roles and women's perceptions of themselves" (p. 37). As women enter the workforce in increasing numbers, expect the same opportunities and rewards for comparable work, and demand better career ladders, they are going to move to other kinds of work than nursing. Bureaucratic entanglements make gendered work relations even more difficult or cause unjustified and angry attacks between nurses and physicians, characterized by poor communication, misinterpretations, false assumptions, and lack of follow-through. These are exaggerated in systems now under cost containment that place excessive demands for performance on both groups.

In addition, the gross disparity in pay "continues to grow and furthers the disenchantment of nurses" (p. 37).

Lastly, noted Smoyak, "there is chauvinism. The women's movement has exerted a tremendous positive influence on work settings, yet a substantial core of both sexes remain unconvinced. Anger, game-playing and superficial interaction are very costly, but hard to measure" (p. 37). Certainly by the 1970s these problems were identified, joint practice defined, and the division of labor rethought and replanned, leading nurses to perform functions previously under the physician's jurisdiction. Indeed, the commission had agreed on collegiality, equality in status, shared scientific and professional base of knowledge, mutual trust and respect; however, Smoyak was forced to conclude that all their work and thought

> proved too threatening to the American Medical Association. The AMA had become increasingly displeased with what it saw as its appointees "giving ground" to the nurses. Several times, it pulled its commissioners off the commission and replaced them with men (no women doctors were ever appointed) who were thought more able to adhere to the "party line" of "captain of the ship" philosophy. The final straw came when three officers of the AMA were appointed to the commission and they, too, spoke publicly and articulately about the values of joint practice, collaboration and collegiality. The AMA not only withdrew its funding, it did not allow the medical commissioners to participate in seeking outside, corporate or philanthropic support. (p. 37)

The commission was subsequently disbanded and Smoyak concluded: "A structure may be demolished, but not an idea" (p. 37).

A Woman Physician on "Us" versus "Them" Interaction

Was the idea alive in the minds of those who were not male physicians, female nurses, or even members of the two professions? For a different perspective, we turn to a female physician, Victoria A. Cargill (1986/87), who briefly traced the history of nurse-physician relationships because significant forward steps require that "we need to look at where we once were" (p. 33). In her view, nurses previously wore caps, whispered in the presence of physicians, and finished every sentence with "yes, doctor." Although these behaviors had changed, "there has been tacit acceptance and perpetuation of the subservience principle" (p. 33). Indeed, even by the mid-1960s, research showed the deleterious effects of the exaggerated subservience of women nurses (Hofling, Brotzman, Dalrymple, Graves, & Pierce, 1966). As noted in chapter 7, the research of Hofling et al. involved a verbal order from an unknown physician for an unknown drug at twice the maximum dosage; twenty-one of the twenty-two nurses set out to give the drug. To Cargill, this was clear evidence of the negative effects of nurses' subordination.

According to Cargill, "Feelings of inexperience, fear, inequality, and responsibility contribute to this volatile relationship which often triggers an unfortunate incident" (p. 33). When two physicians cannot agree, another consultant is brought in, but, said Cargill, a difference of opinion between a nurse and a physician has an "us" versus "them" quality, in part, because the physician sees the nurse as a helper to carry out orders and not a colleague or partner with different skills. There was, said Cargill, ample historical evidence on the territoriality of physicians; for example, the thermometer, initially used as early as 1625, was denied to nurses even in the late nineteenth century, because "physicians distrusted thermometer readings taken by nurses or others to whom the task was delegated, yet were unwilling to spend time making the observations themselves" (Reiser, 1978; cited in Cargill, 1986/87, pp. 33–34).

Cargill charged that nurses today are seen as task-oriented helpers, if not simply women "whose real desire in life is to file her nails and marry a doctor (not necessarily in that order)" (Cargill, 1986/87, p. 33). Indeed, in one university hospital's employee health clinic, the nurse takes vital signs, checks vision, makes appointments, and records chief complaints, but "A physician's assistant sees patients and treats minor/stable illnesses!" (p. 34).

This occurs despite the evidence for nurse practitioners' competence, which had been clearly demonstrated in research from 1965 onward. In these studies, there were *no* significant differences found in outcomes for nurse practitioners, PAs, or physicians, and there was proof of lower cost for nurses' care under certain circumstances. In some studies where continuity of care was important, the nurses have improved patient compliance. Cargill concluded that physicians need "to temper the authoritarianism taught in medical school . . . medicine and nursing need to join hands instead of fists" (p. 34). How this was to occur in the context of the gender-defined hierarchy is unclear.

A Male Nurse on Nursing Diagnoses and Treatments

Where did a man in nursing stand? Dr. Edward Halloran, RN (1986/87), traced the aims and efforts of the National Joint Practice Commission, but noted that it "was eminently unsuccessful and was disbanded" (p. 35). Perhaps it would be more accurate to say, as Smoyak did, that the AMA withdrew its support from the commission. Instead, Halloran blamed its demise on dialogues that were "reduced to dealing primarily with issues of gender and economics" (p. 35). He viewed these as preventing dialogue, rather than as genuine, fundamental, and still unresolved issues. Clearly, he did not identify with the nurses on the commission. As far as he was concerned, dialogue should have focused on patient care. Although such dialogue is necessary and important, it is difficult to see how focusing on it alone would change sex-stratified systems or insufficient nursing authority or inequitable economic levels. Nevertheless, Halloran stressed his own research, which provided evidence on nurses' actual functions, and asserted these could be used as the basis for dialogue, thus narrowing the scope of nurse-physician relations to mutual concerns about patients.

Halloran's study, of 2,500 patients in an Illinois hospital, specifically focused on nurses' motivations in their decisions to spend more or less time with patients. Was there a nursing ethic? Or simply a correlation between physicians' prescriptions and nurses' time? The patients in his study usually had four or five conditions, such as anxiety, discomfort, immobility, pain, or negative feelings, in each day and often a total of twelve such conditions over their hospital stay. Nurses did not deal with these in relation to a patient's age, gender, or race: "We found that less than 4% of the variability in the amount of nursing care could be explained by these factors" (p. 35). Although age was somewhat more correlated than gender or race, it was statistically insignificant. Unfortunately, the measures of patients' social class, such as occupation, income, or education, were not provided. It is, however, clear that a predominantly female professional group was not giving care based on racist or sexist decisions—at least in the quantity of care.

Over 50 percent of the variability in the amount of nursing care given was traceable to nursing diagnoses. Thus, nursing care was somewhat different from medical care: Halloran hoped to reduce the confusion about medicine and nursing, separate the professions more distinctly, and make clearer the benefits from dialogue on patient issues. Thus, his finding that over half the variability in the time that patients spend in a hospital was related to factors associated with nursing care, not simply to medical orders, led him to make the case for greater nursing autonomy; for example he recommended that nurses, not physicians, should discharge patients. Although this recommendation is sensible and logical in terms of better patient care, how physicians could be forced to give up their power over patient discharge was not clear. Presumably, rationality, based on the research data, would prevail. Clearly, Halloran, as a male nurse, deemphasized gender and stressed instead the functions involved in care. Indeed, his view of the collapse of the National Joint Practice Commission is distinctly different from those of the women nurses involved.

Organizational Complexity and Professional Conflict

Halloran's deemphasis of a gender-defined system seemed to be indirectly supported by research conducted by political scientist Mary Ellen Guy (1986), who found organizational complexity to be a more salient factor than gender. Comparing two psychiatric hospitals, she found more conflict within rather than between professions. Guy asked respondents to list the factors they used to rate quality of patient care and then determined the conflict in terms of incompatible preference ratings. Comparing the responses, she found that physicians and nurses had about the same level of conflict, but each had more *intra*professional conflict than with any other professionals. As organizational complexity increased, conflict increased not only across professions, but also within professions. Guy concluded that members of a profession do not necessarily agree with their peers more than with someone from a different profession.

Although the range and type of nurse independence in action is central to the current *inter*professional debate; Guy's research did not clearly focus on who is going to do what in terms of quality of patient care. Nor did she focus on the amount and type of sex segregation. If this were high, then *intra*professional conflicts on patient care would be expected because the group members had more interaction with others in their own profession, thus heightening the possibility of differences in perceptions of patient care.

A Professor of Ethics: Role Perception at the Core of Ethical Issues

Unlike political scientist Guy, attorney Robert P. Lawry (1986/87), director of a center for professional ethics, drew from his experience in bringing together diverse professional groups to improve communication on ethical issues that cut across disciplines. From his experience, Lawry found *inter*professional differences in approach to seemingly identical issues, for example, confidentiality or conflict of interest. Unlike the communication patterns of engineers and lawyers, the unique difficulty in discussions between nurses and physicians is that "the role perception in each group is constantly at the core of the ethical issue itself" (p. 36). If this is true, centering on patient care, as Halloran suggested, would not alone resolve problems between nurses and physicians, since the basic unsolved issue was the roles themselves. Even if, as Guy found, organizational complexity increased conflict over patient care, the gender-segregated roles would still not necessarily change, and the role perceptions, according to Lawry, would be at the core of conflicts.

As an outsider to nursing and medicine, Lawry said the most striking aspect of nurse-physician roles is their changing imagery over time. The physician as general and nurse as foot soldier in wars on diseases demanded immediate and unquestioning obedience; in his view this image was still frighteningly alive, as detailed by Cargill. In more recent familial imagery, "Mom [nurse] took care of the child during the large part of the day that dad [physician] was away, but he was still clearly in charge whenever he returned" (p. 36). Both Halloran and Lawry noted how atypical, even in 1987, male nurses and, to a lesser degree, female physicians were, given the lopsided gender ratios in both professions.

To Lawry, the current ethical implications of the doctor-nurse game are legion: "Neither blind obedience to orders nor subtle psychological manipulations to win the war between the sexes can possibly be the way we want good medicine practiced, nor good people to behave" (p. 36). Strangely, Lawry stated only "good medicine," not "good nursing"; thus, even with the best of intentions, he could not overcome the tendency to subsume nurses within medicine.

Although uncertain about how to eradicate past imagery, Lawry called for joint education: "To allow the stereotypical images, prejudices, and jokes, to be perpetuated as the two groups grow from fumbling rookies to mature professionals is to miss the opportunity to develop a team or collegial approach" (p. 37). To Lawry, the latest image of nurse as patient advocate, protector against threatening forces, was unsatisfactory: "Is it not clear that one obvious threat comes from the doctor?" (p. 37). This new image, said Lawry, did not capture the joining of hearts and minds of independent professionals. He cautioned against being enslaved by imagery, but then ironically used sports imagery—the corporation, previously pictured as a football team, was now being depicted as a basketball team! Since female physicians and nurses have in the past rarely engaged in either sport as professionals, it is difficult to follow Lawry's suggestion that, like basketball players, health professionals have to be more flexible and adapt to quickly changing circumstances.

Lawry sensed something was wrong: "it may be that this imagery is just as bad as any other?" (p. 37). However, he did not catch the gender problem and simply noted that health care is really unique and unlike athletics. He was at a loss to come up with any other imagery, stressing instead that both nurses and physicians are only professionals part-time, but are human beings full-time. He urged respect in decision making and the recognition that "we are prone to error, and inevitably, we do make some mistakes" (p. 37). Again, how the system-wide gendered structure might change in order to achieve such respect was not discussed.

The Views of British Physicians and Nurses

If the views within a single culture varied according to gender and occupational position, would perspectives also vary across cultural lines? We turn next to British physicians and nurses to answer this question and find considerable similarity in their perspectives to those of the Americans. In 1983 general practitioner Ian Stanley asked, "Where do we (or rather you) stand with doctors?" (p. 46). He answered that at best medical men were lukewarm to nurses and, at worst, they were hostile. Since 1977 the General Nursing Council alterations in the "training" syllabus indicate "you have taken a decision to become something different; no longer (to use the cliché) the handmaidens of the medical profession, but aspiring professionals in your own right" (p. 46).

To Stanley, medical dominance had lasted so long because physicians jealously guarded their monopoly and nurses had "chosen to be subservient"

(p. 46) and to defer to doctors. Nurses who see the relation with dominant physicians as a power struggle are really distorting or denigrating the traditional roles of nurses. In fact, the "new" academic (university-educated) nurses are describing activities that were "yesterday's intuitive behavior" (p. 46). Nevertheless, he admitted that to some nurses the "relationship between medicine and nursing has reflected a social imbalance in decision-making and in turn limited the development of the role of nurse" (p. 47). However, the real question was not how far nurses had moved toward a profession, but why nursing would want to be a profession, since it is now a devalued status, attacked by Ivan Illich (1976), for example, in *Medical Nemesis*.

Did nursing militancy arise from a genuine concern for patients' long-term welfare? Admitting that the question is "probably unfair," Stanley nevertheless says that "we are entitled to ask whether the new expertise [of nurses] . . . is appropriate and sufficient" (Stanley, 1983, p. 47). Medical judgments were particularly appropriate when nurses' actions and criticism involved more than just "getting above their station" (p. 47). After justifying the medical right to pass judgment on nursing, he proceeded to do so: "much of your theory is half-baked . . . [a] plethora of jargon . . . borrowed from sociology and educational psychology" (p. 47), heady stuff with which nursing journals seem intoxicated. Indeed, physicians feared that nurses risked the patients' welfare because of the nurses' emphasis on holism or interrelatedness, which, as a theoretical idea, is "pretentious" and "the practice [of the theory] is likely to harm you and your patients" (p. 48).

"The second fear of the medical profession is in many ways more fundamental"; it, said Stanley, is "the fear of having our magic stolen" (p. 48). Why do nurses need to be autonomous and skillful? To take over the traditional medical activity of diagnosis: "Here then is potential for real conflict: two parallel diagnostic processes, not necessarily reaching identical conclusions" (p. 48). Thus, patients may suffer from a lack of professional congruence. To Stanley, diagnosis is presumably instrumental and not expressive. Therefore, the third fear of physicians is that nurses' emphasis on the intellectual and diagnostic will lead to a loss in their intuitive, expressive skills.

Of the four characteristics of an established profession—expertise, autonomy, commitment, and responsibility—the first two, says physician Stanley, are confused by nurses. Autonomy, yes, but expertise that denies nursing history and seeks to usurp the role of the doctor would simply produce the duplication of the medical role of diagnostician. Stanley's views are reinforced by those of British physician J.R.A. Mitchell (1984), who asked, "Is nursing any business of doctors?" During the 130 years since Florence Nightingale, physicians had seldom been forced to examine nurse-physician relationships, simply taking them and the nature of nursing for granted. This, said Mitchell, was no longer possible because of the American import called the nursing process, which involved identifying patient's problems, developing and implementing plans, and evaluating their effectiveness. The differentiation between nurse as authority on daily living activities and physician as specialist in diagnosis and treatment of disease is rejected by Mitchell, who claimed these could not be separated. He further objected to the nurses' assertion that a nursing evaluation is different from a medical diagnosis except in an emergency, when both nurses and physicians share the same actions and goals. He also rejected the idea that physicians are primarily concerned with disease, and not with the whole individual. Next, he objected to the nurses' plan because it included referrals to *other* health professionals: "no nurse is allowed to assume such an extended technical role without adequate training plus a certificate of competence from medical staff who are prepared to delegate such tasks to her" (p. 217). After rejecting any independence in referrals, Mitchell did the same for any nursing "evaluations," which, although presumably devoted to the improvement of patient care, merely covered the deeper purpose of achieving independent decision making. How, he asked, can nurses evaluate an expected outcome without the medical diagnosis and the known history of a disease?

Mitchell doubted the motivation of the advocates of the nursing process. Indeed, "some nurses see it as a bid for independence from what they regard as medical domination" (p. 217). To him, the nursing process "formalises what many of us have felt anxious about for some time—namely, the progressive exclusion of doctors from nursing affairs" (p. 217). In many hospitals (not, he is delighted to say, his own), "doctors have been removed from the appointment committees which choose ward sisters and nurse managers . . . and have been virtually excluded from nurse teaching" (p. 217). Mitchell contended that the nursing teachers did not have the necessary background to teach diagnosis and outcome and therefore could not act as substitutes for physicians. This assertion totally excludes the historical evidence on the neglect of nursing students' education and the misuse of free student labor by both medical and hospital authorities. Nevertheless, physicians, said Mitchell, care about nursing and want to be more involved in educating and evaluating nurses' education and practice. (This, of course, would also bring nursing under even more medical control.) Mitchell continued by rejecting nurses' rights to admit patients to hospitals, saying that the nurses are "confusing rights with responsibilities" (p. 217). Employing authorities are alarmed at the suggestion that patients on a ward may be admitted by nurses, without being under the care of a doctor, or that there may be nursing documents, containing a nursing diagnosis and a nursing plan which are independent from or even in opposition to the medical diagnosis and the medical plan. He did not believe that two people could be equally in charge of one patient. At no point could Mitchell accept more highly educated nurses taking over hospital care with physicians acting as consultants, a change recommended by medical sociologist David Mechanic (1978), as noted in chapter 7. Indeed, Mitchell rejected any increase in nurses' authority and reasserted the need for *more* medical control over nursing, thus reinforcing the medical monopoly.

Too Tired to Fight

Under such pressures, British nurse Libby Thornton (1983) asked whether nurses were giving in to the traditional stereotype because they were tired of fighting physicians and degrading prejudices. Referring to American philosopher Lisa Newton (1981), who, as noted earlier, advised nurses who were unhappy with their stereotyped roles to leave nursing, Thornton wondered if this was not already happening. As evidence, she contrasted the dropout rate of 40 percent for nursing students with the 13 percent rate for other university students in Great Britain. To test whether nurses were leaving precisely because of traditional stereotypes, Thornton distributed an informal questionnaire listing fourteen characteristics, half favorable and half unfavorable to nurses. These were completed by forty-five nursing students, fifteen staff nurses, fifteen physicians and medical students, and fifteen patients. She also asked who affected nurses most and the reasons for wastage in nursing. Thornton found a high correlation within the nursing groups about the ideal nurse's image—intelligent, interesting, patient, understanding, and observant. The nurses rejected authoritarian, obedient, and submissive characteristics. Even though the nurses expressed a congruence between the ideal image and their perceptions of themselves, 39 percent were planning to leave nursing because of role pressures and working conditions.

There were clear discrepancies between the perceptions of nurses and patients, with the latter expecting nurses to be submissive, unquestioning, obedient, and unemotional. There were also low correlations between the views of nursing students and those of physicians. Thornton then analyzed those nurses who wanted to leave nursing and found that they believed physicians, not senior nursing staff, were "preventing them from reaching their full potential . . . [and] expected nurses to be submissive, obedient and unquestioning, in short to conform to the old stereotype of the handmaiden" (p. 12). Physicians themselves did not necessarily want this stereotyped nurse. Why, then, did the nurses perceive the physicians as having this view? Perhaps from nursing education? asked Thornton. Unfortunately, there were no behavioral measures, so it is difficult to know if physicians actually acted in a less stereotyped manner. Regardless of the interpretation, one thing is certain: some women who felt they were expected to be traditional handmaidens were indeed leaving nursing. Given ongoing shortages despite the increased actual number of nurses, the perceptions of subordination did indeed affect nurses' dropout rates.

What happens to those who stayed in nursing? Judith Canham (1982), another British nurse, accused nurses of being "dull and reluctant to speak their minds in defense of themselves and their patients" (p. 50). Admitting that nurses are underpaid and work in a "badly developed, poorly structured organization" (p. 50), Canham nevertheless accused them of being apathetic, even when they should protect the National Health Service from "commercial medicine."

Unfortunately, British nurses found communication with physicians "next to impossible. This is our main problem ... making it impossible for us to offer complete care to the patients" (p. 51). Indeed, a research study conducted by the Royal College of Nursing found that 80 percent of physicians accepted nursing as a profession, but with many reservations and with expectations very different from those of the nurses. One physician, for example, felt that common sense, not intelligence, was necessary, saying: "They should be willing to help the doctor and have a pleasant personality" (p. 51). Canham retorted that women in nursing have a great deal of intelligence: "so why do they possess that unique ability to be belittled by doctors ... nurses themselves feel unable to change even with the backup of feminism, equal pay rights and an upsurge in unionism. We still have an almost pre-suffragette standing" (p. 51). The physician still had ultimate control of the patient, allowing the nurse some importance but only in relation to physicians.

Nurses experience inward grief and grumble when patients are improperly treated, but, Canham asked, do the nurses have the courage to wade in and confront the physician or do they "comply unquestioningly"? If they comply, "Our own standards of care are in doubt" (p. 51). Unfortunately, many nurses are frightened to voice their opinions, but Canham insisted that nurses should "feel free to remark casually, suggest knowingly or demand insistently" (p. 51). With practice, the nurse can "direct her own conversation, without cowering, or apologizing for stepping out of line and without expecting rebuke" (p. 51).

Become an Anarchist or Get Out!

British nursing educator Lorraine Smith took on the issue of power directly in her 1987 article, which was accompanied by a large picture showing a man's hand holding crossed sticks with attached strings connected to a marionette nurse, a woman all askew. On the last page of Smith's article, the picture is reversed: a female hand controls the strings from which a physician dangles. Smith noted that the two professions are divided by terms such as "dominant and submissive, male and female, active and passive, independent and dependent, upper class and lower middle class, academic and vocational" (p. 49). In Smith's view, physicians are supported by the patriarchal system that gives them their power base to make decisions, but nurses are crushed by this system.

Smith questioned physicians' belief that they have the right to head the interdisciplinary team. Nurses were beginning to focus on power, and physicians, though powerful, felt threatened and moved to protectionism and insularity. Still, nurses allow a physician to sit at their desks while the women work around him trying to get at drawers or speak to a relative on the phone: "Does the doctor get up and offer her his seat? No, he continues to sit and write up his notes" (p. 50). If the situation were reversed, the nurse, said Smith, would probably get up. The man's action shows lack of respect, implying that the woman is not important enough to be offered the usual courtesies even in her own office. Smith gave another example in which a nursing Kardex (a card-filing system) was adopted by the entire health team in a move to foster multi-disciplinary teamwork; over time, however, "the name of the nursing Kardex is now the *doctors'* Kardex!" (p. 50).

In Smith's view, power is men's condition and lack of it is women's condition. Even with men entering nursing, and women entering medicine, the overall characteristics of the professions had not changed. Indeed, it was not unusual for physicians to insist on being included in interviews for sister/nurse posts: "Who concedes them that privilege? And why do nurses not command the same right to sit in on interviews for psychiatrists? If they seriously tried to follow through that suggestion they would be laughed out of court" (p. 50).

To Smith, it was very annoying to hear physicians speak of *their* nurses and *their* wards; this "smacks of possessions, to be controlled and manipulated and used to serve one's needs" (p. 50). She admitted that power through a higher standard of education encourages forceful, analytical, assertive, and articulate expression. Physicians, she believed, have role models that are strong, masculine, and intelligent. Historically, women nurses have not had a high level of academic achievement; some are now entering with grades that would be acceptable for admission to medicine. But these women do not often have strong clinical role models, since powerful nurses often leave nursing because they cannot function in such a hostile environment. Research suggests that there seem "to be three alternatives: join the system and sacrifice the values and standards which you know to be good; become an anarchist within the system and suffer the consequences; or get out" (pp. 50–51).

It Is Remarkable Not That There Is Conflict but That There Is Any Cooperation at All

If physicians have gained a monopoly over defining what is "true," then nurses who challenge this monopoly are also contesting physicians' authority to define reality. British nursing historian Philip Darbyshire (1987) wrote that medical authority is derived from charismatic authority, connected to healing and fate; to sapient authority from highly valued knowledge; to moral authority from the idea that their actions must be for the sake of patients; and to Aesculapian authority associated with the "quasi-mystical powers of healing and association with God, life and death" (p. 32). Given these sources of authority, even if originally taken from earlier women healers (see chapter 1), it is hardly surprising that many physicians believe they must always be right or, at least, never admit to being wrong. This belief mitigates against democratic work relations. Add to this differences in length and depth of training, plus the sex-segregated arrangements in which there is little if any contact between medical and nursing students, and it is, said Darbyshire, little wonder that there are problems.

Although medical omnipotence, omniscience, and interpersonal relations are increasingly criticized, most physicians know only that nurses are physicians' helpers, assuming that they practice a lower level of medicine instigated by medical orders. As noted previously, research tends to indicate that nurses and physicians, even at the patient's bedside, do not acknowledge the presence of each other: "This is a sobering thought: that the extent of our ability to work together has risen to the level of parallel play exhibited by toddlers" (p. 33). If nurses engage in passive complaining, hold no constructive conception of their roles, and if, as other British nurses allege, have not changed their conceptions in thirty years, then nurses can hardly expect physicians to change their views.

To Darbyshire, what is remarkable is not that there is conflict, but that there is cooperation. But at what price? Students today still instantly recognize the nurse-doctor game described by Stein (1967) almost three decades ago; young nurses still word their recommendations so that they appear to originate with the physician. Nevertheless, changes have been forced by the women's movement, consumer demands, organizational change, and, not least, the development of nurse practitioners' clinical roles that presumably increase autonomy and specialization.

Darbyshire claimed that the negative effects of interprofessional relations continue despite sporadic attempts at dialogue, even though research indicates collaboration produces better results for patients. To expect that "paternalistic domination will end after a few meetings" (p. 33) is unrealistic. However, he sees one clear change: "The 'Stepford Nurse/Wife' of yesteryear is gone and has taken with her unquestioning obedience, her hero-worship, her dowry and the camp bed from the duty room" (pp. 33–34). Somewhat skeptical of joint education, Darbyshire looks instead to increased clinical competence through better nursing education, which would also include the history of nurse-physician relations and the meaning and manifestations of sexism as researched in the women's movement. In the final analysis, the problems go beyond dyadic interrelations: major changes are needed in how kinds of work are valued in society and how shifts can occur from male-stereotyped high technology and illness-orientation to female-associated work involving long-term care, health maintenance, and the quality of life. Unlike American male nurse Halloran, Darbyshire asserted that to change the public's valuation of female-associated work demands a change in fundamental gender images.

Sex and Status: Hierarchies in the Health Workforce

Not only images but the structure of the health-care system itself would have to be changed. Turning to American research in the mid-1980s, Irene Butter and her colleagues stated: "Female health workers outnumber men by three to one yet they continue to be clustered in occupations which are lower paying, less prestigious and less autonomous than those which are predominantly male" (Butter, Carpenter, Kay, and Simmons, 1985, foreword). Gender-based segregation reflects the traditional roles of women in the general society, even though the full extent of female secondary status in health care has not been fully documented and is available only in "diverse, fragmented, multiple sources which invariably provide inconsistent data" (p. 1).

The increased number of women in medicine has "not significantly altered the overall gender imbalance and has produced an incomplete integration of women into elite professions" (p. 2). Indeed, as the health delivery system has grown, the gender-based inequities are more glaringly apparent and so are their negative effects on health care. Women and men are not only separated by occupation, job function, work setting, level of autonomy, educational attainment, and economic reward, they are also structurally segregated *within* occupations, for example, in "departmental affiliation, specialties, type of professional practice and roles" (p. 5).

With nursing 95 percent female and medicine 85 percent male in 1990, gender segregation is obvious in those occupations. However, within nursing, males, for example, are more frequently administrators and females more often involved in supervisory personnel work. Specialization is more pronounced in health care than in most other areas of the labor force, even involving segregation by specialties. In 1985 female physicians were more likely to specialize in psychiatry, pediatrics, and public health, areas related to traditional female concerns. Some later researchers claimed this pattern was weakening slightly (Kletke, Marder, and Silberger, 1990), although in 1998, the top five specialties in which female MDs practiced—psychiatry, pediatrics, internal medicine, OB-GYN, and family practice—indicated little significant change. In contrast, males are more likely to enter surgery or pathology, and technical specialties. Very pronounced sex segregation is associated with varied levels of autonomy in relation to occupations classified as psychosocial, somatic-diagnostic, or technical. In psychosocial healing, Butter and her colleagues found that nurse practitioners, 87.9 percent female, had mixed autonomy; however, in the somatic-diagnostic category, women made up only 3.8 percent of dentists, 5.7 percent of optometrists, 6 percent of osteopaths, 11 percent of chiropractors, 5 percent of podiatrists, 12.3 percent of veterinarians, and 12 percent of physicians. Only PAs, originally mostly male but increasingly female, countered the general trend between gender, autonomy, and professional roles.

The health labor force is known for a high degree of differentiation; indeed, the degree of inequality is greater than in other industries, exhibiting wider disparities in power and wealth. As Butter and her colleagues noted, blockages in interoccupational mobility cause a vertical gap in the hierarchy, which is rigidly enforced by special interest groups. From one perspective, the gender hierarchy is *superimposed* on the occupational structure. From another perspective, the gender segregation has, in part, *created* the occupational hierarchy.

Certainly, the historical closure of formal education to women, the refusal of organized medicine to support full professional education for nurses, and the medical quota systems, historically designed to keep the number of women and minorities very small—all these contribute to the present differentiation by education and income. In 1985 women workers were more likely to be found in occupations associated with the five lowest educational levels—87 percent, compared to 31 percent of all males. At the four top levels, one finds 69 percent of all male workers, compared to 13 percent of all females. Unfortunately, these figures do not tell the whole story. Nurses, for example, have increased their educational levels, but their income as a proportion of physicians' income has not risen to the same degree. Nor do years of experience necessarily correlate with increased income for nurses.

Feminist researchers as early as the 1970s had established the extreme income inequality in the health occupations hierarchy, and by the mid-1980s women were still severely underrepresented (only 11 percent) in the six most lucrative occupations that equaled only about 12 percent of the entire health workforce, and they were overrepresented (87 percent) in occupations earning under $20,000. In 1983, $40,000 to $94,500 was the median income range for the most lucrative occupations. In contrast, 53 percent of health workers had median incomes below $20,000, and only 35 percent earned between $20,000 and $26,500: "Notable is the absence of health occupations between $26,500 and $40,000, a reflection of the vertical gap" (Butter, Carpenter, Kay, and Simmons, 1985, p. 13). Although there were three times as many female health workers, "men outnumber women more than 8 to 1 in the six most lucrative health occupations, and only 2% of all female health workers earn the higher levels of income realized by 46% of all male health workers" (p. 13). The gendered hierarchy is obvious: 4 to 13 percent of females in the most lucrative occupations, compared to 56 to 98 percent of females in the least lucrative.

This pattern was sustained in the 1980s even for women in male-dominated professions, who earned 42 to 64 percent of the men's incomes. In female-dominated occupations, men also earned more: "health therapists and registered nurses earned about 85 percent of the weekly earnings of men in these occupations, and the same earning ratio applied to licensed practical nurses, nurses aides and non-professional health service workers" (p. 14).

The move toward equal pay for jobs of comparable worth had, by the

1990s, forced many states to engage in job evaluation studies and, even with underestimations of wage discrimination, female-typed jobs have consistently paid less than equivalent male-dominated jobs. Whether the legal route will provide redress is, according to Butter and her colleagues, highly questionable given increasingly conservative courts.

What has been the effect of feminist activities on this sex-segregated system? First, there has been a rising trend of female entrants in male-dominated fields, such as pharmacy, health administration, and veterinary medicine. In medicine, women constituted 9.6 percent of first-year students in 1970, but about 33 percent in 1982. The number of women physicians increased from 7.1 percent to 15.3 percent between 1970 and 1986 (Kletke, Marder, and Silberger, 1990); in pharmacy from 12 percent to 21 percent, and in veterinary medicine from 5.7 percent to 12.3 percent. However, there were few comparable increases of men in the female-dominated fields; thus, by the end of the 1980s the gendered hierarchy remained largely intact. Even for those entering elite occupations, the differential in rewards continued. As noted previously, female physicians tend to be located in lower-status specialties. Although some have entered internal medicine and surgery, they are more likely to be in salaried employment and bureaucracies. According to Butter and her coauthors, the differences in reimbursement cannot easily be traced to differences in hours worked or numbers of patients seen. Indeed, gender segregation is also obvious in the minor roles assumed by women in the leadership of national professional associations and in academic institutions. Clearly, "gender integration into influential positions and decision-making roles has scarcely begun" (Butter, Carpenter, Kay, and Simmons, 1985, p. 31).

In health administration, the effects of feminism were also apparent: from 1970 to 1980, female first-year students increased from 14 percent to 52 percent, a shift both remarkable and sustained, according to Butter and her colleagues, who, however, argued that extreme heterogeneity of the category suggests overrepresentation in middle levels. They concluded that relevant information is "severely limited in quality, quantity, and coverage" (p. 31). However, there are sufficient studies to show internal sex segregation, with more women in technical and more men in management areas; thus, women are likely to be in staff rather than line positions, limiting their upward progress toward higher administrative levels. Indeed, two Canadian studies in the late 1970s found "women comprised 18.6% of chief executive officers, 11% of the senior executive officers (below chief executive officers), 17% of all assistant administrators, and 36% of administrative assistants" (p. 32). In addition, of the three top administrative posts, 80.5 percent were held by males in Ontario hospitals, 97.3 percent in the Ministry of Health, and 94.1 percent in consulting. Only in nursing homes were there any substantial numbers of top female executives.

Salary differentials and functional differentiation both exist: more females were involved in research, planning, and program analysis and more males in management. Gender typing was also evident in the higher numbers of women administrators in female-defined jobs: housekeeping, personnel, dietetics, and nursing. The problems of females in power are clearly reflected in their continued exclusion from the highest levels of executive power. Indeed, even with a larger minority of women physicians and a trend toward gender equity in health administration, "Numerical representation alone may not suffice without integration across all status levels and activities ... gender-linked differences in career paths of men and women ... suggest that widening the entry opportunities for women into male-dominated occupations does not necessarily imply equal access to functions, roles and positions within an occupation. ... Upward mobility of a relatively small group of female health workers affirms the hierarchy and leaves the skewed power structure intact" (pp. 33–35).

In the view of some researchers and commentators, licensing and credentialing, required to a much higher degree of health workers, has rigidified the sex-segregated structure of health care. By the mid-1980s around 51 percent of health workers were legally required to be licensed; 62 percent were legally required to be licensed and/or certified. As many as forty-five health occupations were licensed or registered in one or more states. Of these, eight, the elite male-dominated groups, were licensed for autonomy. In contrast, women made up most of the licensed practitioners who could function only under supervision. Similarly, state boards have often been composed of male supervisors, not females from each of their respective occupations. Particularly difficult for nurses is the comprehensive definition of medical practice acts that mean "almost any health care function can be defined as within physicians' purview" (p. 40). Unfortunately, the gendered and segregated occupational hierarchy is reinforced, for example, by the Joint Commission on the Accreditation of Hospitals, composed of physicians, hospitals, and other health professionals. The commission, because of the nature of its institutional memberships, "is a primarily male-controlled organization" (p. 43).

Certainly, nurses are largely unable to provide the full range of services that they currently or potentially are able to give. Because medicine is so broadly defined, nurses are constantly subject to the charge of practicing medicine without a license. Butter and her colleagues suggested a restructuring toward equivalency and proficiency assessments of competence; however, they warned that if medicine and dentistry retain legal monopolies through licensure, while women-dominated occupations are decredentialed, then nurses and other women health workers would be in double jeopardy in such a dual system.

In 1989 Dr. Butter published an update of her earlier work, again noting the rapid increase of women workers in the health-care system, who remained, however, in lower-level positions and income levels and continued to have relatively little control over standards of practice, institutional resources, or values and conceptual frameworks governing work. Nevertheless, the shrinkage of the population group of 20- to 30-year-olds became apparent in the mid-1980s, and their number was projected to decline from 47 to 39 million between 1986 and 1997. In health disciplines, between 1980 and 1987 there was a drop of 22 percent in applicants in medicine, 44 percent in dentistry, and 30 percent in veterinary medicine. Nevertheless, between 1980 and 1986, female entrants increased from 31 percent to 35 percent in medicine, 20 percent to 30 percent in dentistry, and 40 percent to 59 percent in veterinary medicine. Entering university male students are showing greater preferences for business, engineering, and computer sciences, while young women are choosing highly remunerative health professions.

In nursing, the reduction in the size of 18-year-old cohorts has also impacted the field; it is partly responsible for the 20 percent decline in nursing school enrollments since 1983. But the drop was also caused by changing attitudes: between 1974 and 1986, said Butter, there was a 50 percent decline in the proportion of full-time freshman women who planned nursing careers. The drop was particularly sharp from 1983 to 1986: from 8.3 percent to 5.1 percent. Indeed, in 1986, a survey of the American Council on Education found that the number of female freshmen planning to enter medicine was larger than the number wanting to enter nursing by a ratio of 10 to 8. In contrast, in 1968, three times as many female freshmen were interested in nursing than in medicine.

Young women are now evaluating financial rewards, recognition, respect, and autonomy commensurate with responsibility. Although, as Butter noted, nursing salaries had increased, there was still no salary structure to compensate nurses adequately for their education, experience, and skills. Thus, despite increases in the early 1980s, the average hospital nurses' salary was in 1985 19 percent lower than that of teachers and 10 percent lower than that of female professional and technical workers in general. Lack of autonomy, respect, and recognition continued to be major complaints of nurses that were reinforced by the systematic media portrayal of nurses as handmaidens to male physicians, as severe or cruel task mistresses, or as sex objects. Nevertheless, Butter was guardedly optimistic that gender balances could improve in the future if salaries and autonomy for nurses increased.

Nurse-Physician Relations Portrayed in Fiction and the Media

The gender-defined hierarchy was also reflected in multiple professional and lay publications studied by researchers from the beginning of the 1980s and into the 1990s. For example, Beatrice J. Kalisch and Philip A. Kalisch (1983) analyzed the impact of the occupational identities of authors on the image of nurses presented in novels. In a very thorough research study, these historians engaged in content analysis of 201 novels, published from 1843 to 1980, that had important nurse characters. The Kalisches compared the images of nurses and nursing produced by authors who were nurses, physicians, and non-health-care providers. They concluded: "Of all authors, physicians presented the most negative nurse images; they were least likely to endow nurse characters with positive personality and behavior traits. On the other hand, physicians were the most likely to show nurses valuing and being engaged in sexual activities" (p. 17).

Nurse authors, such as Mary Roberts Rinehart, were "most active during the first 60 years of this century . . . [but] the physician authors dominated the past 20 years" (p. 18). Between 1843 and 1980, 268 nurses' and 87 physicians' characters were presented by nurses who authored 35 novels; physicians, 29 novels; and non-health-care providers, 136 novels. In demographic characteristics all authors depicted nurse characters similarly: "They were almost always female (99%), single (71%), childless (92%), under 35 years of age (69%), and Caucasian (97%)" (p. 19). However, from the multivariate analysis of variance, differences emerged. Nurse authors were more likely to emphasize nursing activities; physician authors were *least* likely to emphasize nurses' skills in physical comforting, technical procedures, or emotional support. Non-health-care providers, as authors, were less likely to portray nurses as resources to others or as engaged in educational activities.

On the variable of professional competence, nurse authors were more likely to depict nurses as contributing to patients' welfare and providing help to non-patients. In contrast, physician writers were *least* likely to portray nurses as contributing to patients' welfare and were *most* likely to portray nurses as harming patients. There was even a statistical difference in the likelihood of praise—nurse authors showed nurses being commended for their professional performance, but physician writers were least likely to show nurses as recipients of praise. Autonomous judgments by nurses were statistically more likely in nurses' fictions and least likely in physicians' novels. Indeed, the nurse writers were more likely to show male physicians as consulting nurses and treating them with respect.

In career orientation, the statistical results showed that the nurse authors were *most* and physician authors *least* likely to portray nurse characters as expressing altruistic motives for being nurses or satisfaction with their careers. In the portrayal of personality attributes and values, nurse writers, according to the Kalisches, were statistically more likely to depict nurse characters as having more drive, empathy, nurturance, power, and intelligence. In comparison, "Physician writers were the least likely to attribute these qualities to nurse characters in novels" (p. 20). While nurse authors depicted their characters as valuing service to others, physician writers focused on nurses as valuing sex: "The propensity for physician authors to present nurses in sexually demeaning terms was reinforced by other findings. Physician writers, for example, were more likely to present nurses as having wider sexual experience than other women . . . and as engaging in more sexual activity" (p. 21). The overall image of nurses was most positive in nurses' novels and most negative in physicians' novels. The nurse authors presented nurse characters as more central to the plot, but physicians portrayed them in more peripheral positions.

How were physicians portrayed in novels? Compared to other writers, the physician authors were more likely to depict MDs as central to the plot, and these characters were more likely to value integrity, a better world, home and family, order and scholarliness, and helping others. Women in nursing were more generous in their depiction of physicians, not differing significantly from medical novelists in portraying, for example, physician characters as valuing intelligence. Physicians deemphasized the nursing profession, depicted more negative nurse characters, and "displayed a predilection for presenting nurse characters as sex objects . . . [however] nurse writers depicted physician characters just as positively as did physician authors" (p. 22). A number of the novels were used as the basis for performances in the mass media, for example, in such television programs as *M*A*S*H;* thus, some fictional work was highly influential in the general culture.

The Kalisches next researched nursing images and sex-role stereotyping of nurses and physicians on prime-time television. In another research report (Kalisch and Kalisch, 1984b), the dichotomy in occupational portrayals was glaringly apparent. Again, using content analysis, the researchers statistically contrasted the portrayal of nurses and physicians from 1950 to 1980. Using a 20 percent sample of 28 relevant sources, they studied 320 individual episodes, 240 nurse characters, and 284 physician characters. The Kalisches concluded: "Results show extreme levels of both sexual and occupational stereotyping" (p. 533). The nurses, 99 percent female, were depicted in "an image of the female professional nurse as totally dependent on and subservient to male physicians" (p. 533). In contrast, male television physicians "not only have outstanding medical competencies but also embrace all the attractive competencies of professional nurses" (p. 533). Indeed, "Television nurses largely serve as window dressing on the set and have little opportunity to contribute to patient welfare" (p. 533).

The Kalisches recognized the stunning amount of research on sex roles produced in the 1970s, during the rise of the women's movement. Nevertheless, sexual stereotyping, even though degrading to women, has been considered "less blatantly offensive than racial or ethnic stereotyping and has therefore persisted on television while the other stereotypes have disappeared into the netherworld of 'bad taste'" (p. 535). In general, previous research proves that women characters are less likely to issue directions, orders, or even advice; and less likely to dominate men, either at home or in criminal situations, where they are often pawns controlled by others. More likely to be portrayed at lower stages of value development, women are concerned with personal happiness and interpersonal harmony, rather than the general social good and people's rights, the provinces of men. The Kalisches also noted that women in the media are less likely to be pictured as exceptional, particularly in specific professions, such as medicine, largely populated by men.

The most pernicious effects of gendered stereotypes are on children, who, after seeing a videotape or film presenting a male nurse and a woman doctor, reported they had seen the opposite (Mankiewicz and Swerdlow, 1977–1978, pp. 7, 14; cited in Kalisch and Kalisch, 1984b, p. 536). Indeed, children tended to rank the attractiveness of an occupation according to power over others. From this research, M. DeFleur (1964; cited in Kalisch and Kalisch, 1984b, p. 537) ranked occupations in terms of relative power, finding that nurses were "virtually at the bottom of the scale, with a −100 rating and a rank of 32 out of 34 occupations . . . physicians ranked relatively high—in ninth place, with a power rating of 96" (Kalisch and Kalisch, 1984b, p. 537).

The Kalisches pointed out that the majority of females are shown having no jobs (40.1 percent), but when they are shown in an occupation, nurses occupied, after secretaries, the second most frequent women's occupation (7.2 percent) (U.S. Commission on Civil Rights, 1979; cited in Kalisch and Kalisch, 1984b, p. 537). Therefore, the portrayal of nurses is critical to *all* women. The Kalisches concluded that television glorifies the medical profession and that the physician "perhaps more than any other professional—has benefited from this process" (p. 537). In contrast, the Kalisches found in their own research that the typical female nurse—single, childless, white, and under thirty-five— had not significantly changed in thirty years. When exceptions were present, they were often presented unfavorably; thus a male nurse is the subject of sexual innuendo and an older nurse is depicted as sadistic toward patients. Over the same time span, physicians were older, more often parents, and over-whelmingly male (95 percent). However, there was a *small* change in gender over time: no female physician in the 1950s, two (2.8 percent) in the 1960s, and thirteen (6.9 percent) in the 1970s. However, only 3.9 percent of physi-cians were from racially different groups.

As in the historical study of novels, physicians were in central roles while nurse characters were "typically relegated to supporting roles, which conveys a message to the viewer that nurses are simply not essential in health care" (p. 541). A factor analysis of twenty-three personal attributes produced four interrelated factors: nurturance, individualism, benevolence, and assertive-ness. In the 1950s nurses and physicians were shown as equally nurturant, but in the 1960s nurses were significantly more and in the 1970s less nurturant than physicians. Physicians were portrayed as more individualistic and more assertive in both the 1960s and 1970s. Nurses were consistently depicted as more benevolent. Physicians were portrayed as placing higher valuation on service to others in the 1950s and 1970s, and as valuing scholarship and work, more than nurses across *all* decades. Similarly, physicians were pictured as more dedicated to career, more likely to be commended for professional behavior, and more likely to receive positive attitudes from other characters, including nurses, throughout all decades.

In professional competencies, "Nurse characters were shown helping patients significantly less than their physician counterparts" (p. 548). In addition, in all decades, nurse characters on television used their own judgment in patient care much less than television physicians. Indeed, nurses were more often portrayed in the traditional role (giving physical comfort or making beds) than in progressive roles (taking histories or resuscitating patients), or in both traditional and progressive roles (such as giving medicines or taking vital signs).

The Kalisches concluded that nurses' roles had been underplayed and physicians' roles were "exaggerated, idealistic, and heroic" (p. 550). The nurses' roles seemed stuck in the 1950s, hardly reflecting the change and diversity in actual nursing activities. Physicians maintained not only the male traits of individualism and assertiveness, but also the traditional female values of service to others: "No concomitant gain in the portrayal of nurses is evident: nurses on TV have not assumed a more androgynous personality and value system" (p. 551). Indeed, TV physicians in the 1960s shifted more toward "omniscient, omnipotent, ubiquitous, and self-righteous" portrayals (p. 551). *The Nurses,* on CBS from 1962 to 1965, was "the only series to actually focus on the profession of nursing in the three decades studied, and it offered television audiences a view of nurses at work minus the domineering presence of physicians" (p. 551). By the 1970s, although nurses' actual technical competence, knowledge, and education had increased, "the television image was largely one of the nurse as subservient to the physician and the nurse as a sex object" (p. 551). The Kalisches concluded that television had cemented nurses into the role of handmaiden to physicians.

Gendered Isolation and Ritualized Displays in Nursing and Medical Journals

Clearly, nurses' roles, not only in television but in fictional portrayals by physician-authors, were hardly positive and were largely gender-stereotyped. Would these images produced for the general populace be sustained in the professional journals of medicine and nursing? To answer the question, we turn to the research of Nora J. Krantzler (1986), who analyzed media images in the advertisements of the *Journal of the American Medical Association* (*JAMA*) and the *American Journal of Nursing* (*AJN*). Using an anthropological approach to advertisements as ritualized displays, Krantzler found these reflected and reaffirmed widely held societal stereotypes and beliefs. Historically, trends in medical ads shifted from traditional symbols, such as white coats and stethoscopes, to symbols of science-in-action and high technology. The trend for nurses was toward using symbols previously used by the medical men.

The sex segregation was very clear: "Both physicians and nurses are depicted in their respective journals as existing largely independent of one another" (p. 933). Thus, the segregation of professional men and women is noticeable, even in advertising, which is propped up with considerable sums of money: pharmaceutical companies, said Krantzler, spend over $2 billion a year. Indeed, the *JAMA* had at one time revenues for advertising that exceeded $8 million. These substantial sums support advertising images that influence the perceptions of illness; of medical and nursing practice; of patients, nurses, and physicians; and of their interrelationships.

From her research on the predominant symbols and their change over time, Krantzler found that even the cover of each issue of the professional journals was different: the medical journal had photographs of classical art with a one-page commentary inside; the nursing journal had photographs of people, often nurses, or cartoon-like drawings. The physicians present their journal as high culture; the nurses present a "more mundane, everyday appearance" (p. 934). This parallels other research findings that male tasks are often considered upper-class, even exploitative, while female work is often symbolically thought to be lower-class, or even drudgery.

As Krantzler noted, editorial policies of the *JAMA* and the actions of the AMA's advertising committee had since the early 1950s allowed physicians to have "almost complete control over drug products and drug selection" (p. 934). It is thus not surprising that drug ads most often show physicians and their work. Indeed, Krantzler found that the rendering of a prescription was a predominant symbol of the exchange between physician and patient; sometimes it was used to placate the patient, or to buy time for the physician, or to ensure return contact, or to check on progress and represcribe an old drug or start a new one. The prescription legitimizes the exchange and increases both dependence and the likelihood the patient will return. Drug ads were frequently one full page, but often much longer, even including a completed sample prescription form, symbolizing MD authority.

The white coat and stethoscope predominated from 1965 onward, but by 1982, physicians were often shown in street clothes, particularly when business matters were at issue. Currently, when physicians are depicted as prescribing drugs, they are still somewhat more likely to be represented in the older symbols, in white coats, not in street clothes. This separation, said Krantzler, suggests a symbolic division between healing and making money.

In the medical journal, Krantzler found, in both the 1960s and 1980s, few ads that depicted nurses: "those which did showed a male physician with a female nurse" (p. 935). Indeed, "a major symbol of physicianhood has been maleness" (p. 935). In the 1960s "all of the physicians shown were male"

(p. 935). With increasing numbers of female physicians, particularly as students, Krantzler found that "like male nurses, female physicians are rarely portrayed as the sole physicians in an advertisement. This suggests that the medical and nursing roles have taken the form of gender-based social identities. In this sense, all physicians are male and all nurses, female, regardless of their anatomy" (p. 935).

The white coat, now often worn by non-physicians, was *never* worn by anyone except physicians in their ads, and this stereotyped them as scientists in laboratory coats, possessing the authority of science. Similarly, the stethoscope, said Krantzler, symbolized the physicians' ability to make definitive diagnoses. Even medical students were depicted with stethoscopes draped over their necks and shoulders, and attending physicians had theirs in their pockets. In the nursing journal nurses were depicted with their stethoscopes prominently displayed.

In ads in the most current issues of the medical journal, working physicians are evidently no longer required to deal with patients. Indeed, they are "manipulators of technology behind the scenes. They are rarely shown talking to patients, more rarely yet talking to nurses or to each other" (p. 937). The exception was military ads, where there is a clearly defined social hierarchy. In nonmilitary ads, brightly colored, high-tech imagery, stressing computers and scientific evidence, was present. When physicians were shown with patients, they were often "depicted looming large in the background of a patient's life. For example, the physician's hand may be shown superimposed over the patient, symbolically protecting or encompassing the patient" (p. 937). Drugs were depicted, said Krantzler, as extensions or even substitutes for physicians, who became powerful agents who could solve problematic life events, often those presented by stereotyped patients, who were "older, overwhelmed and depressed. . . . The notion is fostered that life problems can be treated using drugs" (pp. 937, 939).

When physicians are depicted with patients, Krantzler found they were usually positioned higher than others, thus reaffirming their authority. In contrast, "Nurses are almost never shown; the few who are are still depicted in subordinate roles—for instance, looking on as the physician acts, or working in a clerical capacity" (p. 939). Touch, whether by male or female physicians or even male nurses, was utilitarian, but touch by female nurses was ritual, feminine. To Krantzler, the significant trend for physicians was the move toward dominance through technology and away from social interaction; thus, the physician has become a technocrat, a businessman, and even an extension of the machine.

Nursing advertisements showed a critical difference: there was a clear tendency to emphasize the nurse as woman. Recruitment and personal products—shoes and lotions, for example—reflected "the association of nursing with the female gender—indeed, 'nursing,' by definition, is something only women can do" (p. 939). Nursing ads reflect the fact that women are socialized to be consumers. Nevertheless, Krantzler did note a "recent trend toward rejection of some of the trappings of traditional, gender-based nursing roles—the outward symbols—yet pose the problem of maintaining nursing's core identifying features" (p. 939). Indeed, the nursing ads have, said Krantzler, become more affirmatively professional, taking on the power symbols of the medical men.

In contrast to the prevalence of drug advertising for physicians, the nurse uniform business has been a key advertiser in the nurses' journal. Thus, in 1952 for example, the white uniform and cap predominated, and "All the nurses depicted were women" (p. 939). In that year, *no* white coats or stethoscopes were depicted. By the 1980s, Krantzler observed that uniforms still predominated, but were presented in a variety of so-called wardrobes of professional fashions. She found a definite emphasis on the professional and the feminine in both the 1950s and 1980s, but in the latter, the focus was also on "fashion." By 1982 a few male nurses were shown, but usually with female nurses; however, one male nurse with a male child as patient appeared in 1984. By 1982, new symbols, previously associated with physicians, had appeared—the white coat and stethoscope. In only one issue and only one ad was a nurse shown with a physician, and this was in an army recruitment ad, which presented both as professionals, probably because their relative power was clearly defined.

Krantzler found an almost fourfold increase in recruitment ads from the 1950s to 1980s. Earlier ads stressed salary, benefits, and hours; the later ads focused on benefits, career opportunities, and recreation. In addition, the emphasis on creative nursing philosophy in the 1980s was never conceptualized in the 1950s. Krantzler also found an emphasis on the idea of nurses leading a double life. Unlike physicians, nurses "are portrayed as being both 'women' (in the social sense) and 'professionals'" (p. 946). Krantzler noted that in "a recent survey by *R.N. Magazine*, 3 out of 4 physicians were found to regard nurses as nothing more than their assistants" (p. 947). She continued: "[M]any writers assume that because 30 percent of new medical students are female and 2 percent of nurses are now male, this situation will change. This perspective assumes a 'natural' inclination by gender—i.e., a female physician will be less likely to regard nurses in a sexist or subordinate way, and male nurses will be less likely to experience gender-based prejudice" (p. 947). But Krantzler claimed that when the professional roles are perceived as gendered *social,* not *biological,* identities, "the physician is still 'he' and the nurse 'she,' in articles in the mass media" (p. 947). It is important to grasp this distinction. Simple *biological* identity is insufficient to force systemic change in health-care institutions. It is the social construction of the biological identity that is the critical issue.

Although Krantzler found increasing symbols of professionalization, she also found in the 1980s a continuation of feminine gender displays, such as ritual touching and smiling. There was also a high likelihood that the nurses' patients were depicted as children, not adults. Physicians were peripheral, "if indeed, they exist at all. . . . The nursing world is just that: nurses are shown alone, with other nurses or with patients. They are subordinate only to other nurses" (pp. 947–948). In one ad, the nurse did consult with a physician, but no gender pronoun is given for the physician and his/her role is "dismissed as virtually irrelevant" (p. 948). Similarly, nurses were portrayed with patients in a direct relationship, without any third-party intervening. Krantzler concluded from her research that the ads in both professional journals "paint a picture of physicians and nurses working almost totally independent of one another" (p. 950). To her, the research shows "increasing isolation of medical and nursing traditions from one another" (p. 951).

"Doctoring the Media"?

Problems with public imagery of women nurses and patients were not restricted to the United States. In both the United States and Great Britain, even daily news reports underrepresented women in general and overrepresented medical men to the exclusion of women and even men nurses. Indeed, slanted news coverage was the norm in both countries. Ann Karpf, author of *Doctoring the Media: The Reporting of Health and Medicine* (1988a), traced recent news events in a separate article (1988b), noting the slow strangulation of the National Health Service by the conservative British government. Evidently, this trend was not initially considered to be particularly newsworthy. As late as 1987 "a hospital consultant blamed a staff shortage for the death of a 62-year old woman in a busy hospital ward, because she bled to death after a tube became disconnected from her ankle" (Karpf, 1988b, p. 16). However, this event was reported in only *two* newspapers. A year later the media were replete with stories about patient deaths due to a lack of staff in intensive care, of deferred surgery on babies with heart conditions, and other stories about the negative effects of inadequate funding.

What had created this change? Karpf traced it to concerted intervention by the medical establishment in December 1987, when 1,200 physicians and medical professors signed a petition which was presented to the prime minister by five physicians. From Karpf's research, it is clear that only physicians had the power to capture the media's interest; "ironically nurses, though at the sharp end of the cuts and the subject of much of the coverage, couldn't have initiated it" (p. 16). Why? Because "nurses are not considered authoritative commentators on health matters" (p. 16). When the British press reports on nurses, they are still stuck with the angelic label and treated as "unqualified geysers of nurture rather than staff working at full tilt under pressure" (p. 16).

Indeed, English television focuses on physicians to an excessive degree. Although nurses constitute 92 percent of hospital staff, they represent only 7.5 percent of health workers on the small screen.

Physicians, said Karpf, have legitimate power, defined as the authority to certify something as true, because of the widespread belief that scientific and medical knowledge are objective and neutral, untainted by human fallibility and self-interest. In contrast, nurses are not perceived as part of men's science, but exist instead in the "very feminine realm of caring" (p. 17). Reporters are unlikely to turn to nurses, even on topics for which they have *more* experience or on the range of *nonmedical* topics upon which physicians are called to pronounce. Karpf claimed nurses are falsely "protected" by the media. To her, even nurses on strike in 1982 were differentiated into "good ones" with valid problems and others who were "bad and invalid."

As a medical sociologist and journalist, Karpf found that the media draws on cultural beliefs and continually reproduces stereotypes. In British television, the nurses' roles are limited; they function, said Karpf, as if time is no object; sitting behind desks, becoming infatuated with doctors, they seem to require few qualifications beyond average intelligence and cosmetic makeup. The influence of the American media is also apparent in Karpf's contrast between the excessively good American nurses working with *Marcus Welby, MD* and the excessively bad one in *One Flew over the Cuckoo's Nest*. Evidently, the media cannot accept women nurses exerting control over dependent male patients, so the nurses are turned into battle-axes or sex objects, which then reverses female power and male dependence. Ironically, Karpf warned against nurses who may want to resemble real-life doctors. However, it is, according to the Kalisches, media-portrayed physicians who often resemble real-life nurses.

Nurses are challenging media presentations by organizing and speaking out against their images; thus, the incorporation and assumptions of women's characteristics and roles was the more likely portrayal in fiction, on television, and in the print media. The Nurses' Media Watch, modeled after earlier feminist groups, was specifically formed by nurses in the United States to monitor the coverage of nurses in all media forms.

A Profession in Caricature

Ironically, nurses and women in general may even have to monitor medical humor, as evidenced in an article by nurse researcher Judith A. Chaney and historian Patrick Folk (1993). They investigated physicians' attitudes toward nurses, choosing to study cartoons, since public expression of hostility toward women that could not be publicly voiced might be acceptable if presented as "humor." The only major medical publication aimed at all physicians which has included cartoons since its inception in 1958 is the *American Medical News*.

The official publication of the AMA, it was read by about 89.6 percent of American physicians in 1960. By the 1980s, the weekly readership of 300,000 was more than the combined number of subscribers of the AMA specialty journals, which totaled only 215,000. Consciously seeking to advance physicians' interests, the *American Medical News,* given the numbers and loyalty of its readers over time, could be assumed to reflect the attitudes of the clientele.

The researchers analyzed every cartoon from May 1960 to August 1989, studying 3,045 cartoons, of which 416 (14 percent) contained nurses or female patients. Of these 416 cartoons, 109 contained members of both groups. From content analysis by both researchers, 7 categories emerged—3 negative, 1 neutral, and 3 positive. Only 11 (2.6 percent) portrayed the nurse as sex object, but 9 of these were published after 1979. A second category of 22 (5.3 percent) cartoons portrayed nurses as performing menial or unimportant tasks. The third and largest negative group (42, or 10 percent of the cartoons) depicted nurses as incapable of professionalism, which was ascribed to traditional female "characteristics," such as emotionalism and inability to think rationally. In the neutral category nurses were used as set decorations or simply as indicators of a medical setting. Of the three positive categories, 35 cartoons (8.4 percent) show nurses engaged in medical activities, although under physicians' supervision; of the second and largest category, 112 cartoons (27 percent) portrayed nurses in joint collegial efforts with good-natured jousting and nurses delivering the punch lines; and the third and smallest group (9, or 2.2 percent of the total) depicted nurses as superior to physicians, who were portrayed as absent-minded or ineffectual. Obviously, these were unpopular since only 2 of the 9 had been published since 1969.

The cartoon nurse was female and the physician male. In thirty years of cartoons, the researchers found only one male nurse and two female physicians. The male nurse and one of the female physicians were in the same cartoon, which depicted a male patient's confusion with the sex-role reversal. The other female physician, a pediatrician, faced a small male patient, who refused to undress for her.

Comparing cartoons about women patients and women nurses to see if these jointly reflected changing gendered attitudes toward women in general, the researchers were "shocked to discover that the cartoon view of female patients *never* changed. In thirty years the *News* published 267 cartoons showing female patients. *Not one of those cartoons was positive.* Female patients were depicted as overweight, illogical, ignorant, hypochondriacal, pampered, self-indulgent, and generally mindless" (Chaney and Folk, 1993, p. 188). To determine if this hostility was due to gender or the role of patient, the researchers compared a random sample of cartoons portraying male patients, who appeared far less frequently but were also depicted negatively; however, "serious differences became obvious" (p. 188). Sometimes portrayed neutrally as helpless patients, but not as the butt of the joke, the male patients were also usually their own advocates and were occasionally also viewed with more compassion. In addition, "It was also male patients, not doctors, who primarily saw nurses as sex objects" (p. 188). The researchers concluded from these comparisons that the "unswerving hostility toward female patients was clearly sex-linked" (p. 188).

Did the frequency of hostile cartoons featuring women patients increase over time? Yes, skyrocketing from 5.5 percent in the early 1960s to 14.5 percent in the later part of the decade and in the early 1970s to 17.5 percent; it dropped in the early 1980s, only to increase again from 1985 to 1989. The cartoons depicting nurses peaked from 1965 to 1974. Indeed, almost half of cartoons involving women were concentrated in this decade, when the women's health care movement was making negative critiques and strong demands for more power in women's medical treatment. However, Chaney and Folk found feminism was "largely ignored by the *News* editorial columns until 7 October 1974, when they devoted five pages to explaining 'what these women want' to a readership described as suffering from 'simple confusion'" (p. 195). The researchers did find one cartoon in 1970 in which the women's movement was recognized, but women's issues were solved by violence. In this cartoon, the female nurse asked the male physician where was the woman patient, who had a sign advocating women's liberation. The physician said that she had left by the side door. The nurse responded, "We don't have a side door." And the physician replied, "We do now" (p. 196).

Even with societal changes, Chaney and Folk noted that this did not "change the unremittent nature of that hostility" (p. 195). Interestingly, the three combined negative categories involving nurses rose from 3 percent in 1964 to 8 percent in 1969; almost half of the negative cartoons were printed between 1965 and 1969. By the early 1970s to the late 1980s these had dropped to 2 percent; in fact, after 1985 only three negative cartoons appeared. The positive cartoons peaked in 1970, in contradiction to the consistently and highly negative cartoons of women patients at that time. As the nursing profession created change in practice and education, cartoons doubled, but these mirrored the ambivalence of physicians. Following the enactment of civil rights legislation, the incidence of collegial cartoons increased and provided the bulk of those after 1975. However, only two cartoons since 1969 "dared to suggest that nurses might be good enough to replace physicians. Perhaps some jokes strike too close to find humor in them" (p. 199).

Chaney and Folk found that in the 109 cartoons depicting both female patients and nurses, the empathic nurse appeared in only 1 percent of the samples. After 1974 only one cartoon depicted a nurse who showed compassion for a female patient. Indeed, one way to achieve a collegial relationship with physicians was by showing disdain for female patients: Cartoons showing nurse hostility toward women patients "peaked in 1970 to 1974, when positive views of nurses also reached their apogee" (p. 199). Unfortunately, the category that is larger than all others combined includes cartoons depicting nurses' neutrality to the hostility shown toward women patients. The researchers suggested that this may indicate that physicians are uncertain about how nurses feel toward their sisters who are patients, or it may indicate that physicians assume that nurses share, but do not usually express, similar hostile feelings. From this perspective, the nurse is a silent accomplice. Ironically, nurses appeared in only 17 of 60 cartoons hostile toward women patients, which peaked between 1965 to 1969, but, with the portrayal of greater collegiality, 36 of 73 hostile cartoons from 1970 to 1974 included nurses.

In contrast to the Kalisches' earlier finding of the predominance of nurse as sex object in the mass media, in the medical cartoons the nurse was asexual or antisexual: overweight, postmenopausal, and disinterested in sexual activity: "She was almost as unappetizing and uninterested as her frumpy sister, the female patient" (p. 200). With fat, loutish, male patients making passes, the sex-ogled nurses were very attractive. Rarely did male physicians appear as attractive or attracted.

The researchers concluded that nursing was perceived as a dependent, gender-determined occupation throughout the thirty-year period. At this same time, there was unrelenting disgust and hostility toward female patients without one positive cartoon in three decades. Hostile cartoons did peak as feminism reemerged and as changes in the nursing profession were initiated. Increasingly, said Chaney and Folk, more collegial and fewer negative cartoons in recent years suggest that despite continued stereotyping of nursing as feminine, the profession is not closely identified with the hostility toward women in general or women patients in particular. This finding is problematic, however, since the price of such "collegiality" may be collusion in this medical hostility.

Is Gender Still Central to Nurse-Physician Roles?

Some observers have argued that gender, given the increased number of women in medicine and the larger number of women PAs, is no longer a critical determinant in nurse-physician relationships. Clearly, the data from studies of media images do not support these views. Indeed, the research reported in the 1990s continued to produce gender-typed results. Cynthia S. Aber and Joellen W. Hawkins reported in 1988 and again in 1992 that the content of advertisements in medical and nursing journals continued to distort the image of women and, to a lesser degree, men nurses. Studying 1990 issues of thirty-five nursing and forty-eight medical journals, the researchers investigated the images of nurses and the extent to which these reflected their actual roles and the differences between the images of nurses and physicians in the same advertisements.

Aber and Hawkins (1992) found that 79.4 percent of the nurses were pictured as women under thirty years of age. Only 6.31 percent of the nurses were male. All of the nurses portrayed as sex objects were female, but only 4.2 percent were depicted as spouses and 4.2 percent as parents. When any women were portrayed as health-care workers, they were almost always nurses, rarely physicians. Of the physicians depicted, however, only one (1.75 percent) was female, and the remaining 98.25 percent were male. When any individual was pictured as simply ornamental or decorative, the person was more likely to be a woman or a female nurse. Statistically, they were more often shown as just "being there"; the reverse was found for men and physicians.

Female nurses were still shown assisting physicians. Not one physician was depicted helping a nurse. Indeed, "In one picture, the male physician was looking very angry and the female nurse was wringing her hands. Five other ads pictured a male physician looking angrily at a female nurse. The male nurse in four ads was engaged in a nursing activity and the female nurse was observing" (Aber and Hawkins, 1992, p. 291).

The researchers found that the nurses' images did not reflect the actual roles of nurses: 95.6 percent were giving hands-on care, but few ads showed administration, teaching, or research. Indeed, only one ad depicted research at all, and this involved a female nurse and a male physician. Most advertisements for job openings (52.7 percent) focused on recreation in off-duty hours and by implication "getting a man." When on duty, portrayal of nurses' uniforms partially continued the stereotypes: 43.7 percent wore white uniforms and 12.4 percent white nurse's caps, although some were shown in white lab coats with stethoscopes. From the research, the investigators found several major stereotyped themes: Nurses are always clean and white; do not make important decisions or do important things; are sex objects, not spouses, or significant others, or parents, or caretakers of parents.

To the researchers, nurses still exemplified sex-role stereotypes; were often decorative or were merely "being there" in some form of decorative idleness; and were still portrayed as handmaidens to physicians. Indeed, they were also depicted as needing the protection of others: "All the ads for malpractice insurance depict female nurses. In one ad, a nurse in a white cap and white uniform was in the defendant's box in a courtroom wringing her hands and looking helplessly at her male lawyers. Considering that a very small percentage of nurses as compared to physicians are ever sued . . . these characterizations are particularly over-dramatic and unwarranted" (p. 292). There was by the 1990s a freezing of the image of nurses in the print media of both the medical and nursing professions. Clearly, gender remained a central issue, despite changes in the proportions of sexes in different caregiver roles.

Throughout this chapter, we have presented information and research from a wide variety of perspectives that clearly establishes the salience of gender in nurse-physician perceptions, attitudes, expectations, and behaviors. Extending from 1980 into the 1990s, it is readily apparent that gender and professional relations intersect in a health-care "system" that requires system-wide change. How this can occur without a substantial weakening of the medical monopoly remains the central issue, and in the next chapter we see nurses engaging in a more overt, frontal attack on this monopoly.

9 | Challenges to the Medical Monopoly
Nurses' Gains in Direct Payment, Hospital Privileges, Prescriptive Authority, and Expanded Practice Laws

By the 1980s it was possible for nurses to attack the medical monopoly directly. Following the U.S. Federal Trade Commission's ruling in 1975 that antitrust laws also applied to professional workers in the health-care system, unfair laws and practices affecting nurses could now be legally challenged. In this chapter we consider the monopolistic medical practices that limit nurses' access to facilities, exclude them from direct or third-party reimbursements, force them to use backup physicians, deny them hospital affiliations, and limit their prescriptive authority. Clearly, physicians had been engaging in group boycott, tying, and bottleneck agreements, all of which were now subject to attack under the new antitrust ruling. Efforts by nurses and others to weaken these monopolistic practices were countered by physicians with a quality-of-care defense; thus, proof of the equal or superior patient care provided by nurses compared to physicians was imperative. Fortunately, the strategy of shifting nursing education to colleges and universities had paid off as more nurse researchers were capable of and involved in investigating the comparative outcomes of patient care and providing proof of nurses' competence, particularly in primary care.

Increasingly, economic competition between nurses and physicians was openly discussed, but the future of advanced practice nurses (APNs)* and, of course, physician's assistants (PAs) was still tied to the profits they provided physicians, who, given the projected physician surplus, had few incentives to give nurses greater autonomy. Studies of the cost-effectiveness of APNs proved that their contributions were substantial, although varying according to different work situations. In aggregate, the nurses' positive economic impact on the nation's health-care system was or could be considerable. Although physicians continued to stress any weaknesses in the research studies, there were numerous reports by the early 1980s on the comparative costs and productivity of APNs that provided evidence that they could successfully substitute for physicians in primary care.

Despite these findings, federal education funds for APNs began to dry up

---

*In the early 1990s, the term "advanced nurse practitioner" (ANP) was replaced by the term "advanced practice nurse" (APN or APRN) to describe those nurses with advanced and/or master's level preparation in a variety of clinical specializations. The more generic term "nurse practitioner" (NP) continues to be used widely by many authors and is used in most legislative titles, e.g., state nurse practice acts.

under the Reagan administration in the 1980s, and evidence began to accumulate proving that institutions, not consumers, had profited from the services of the APNs. Indeed, as we see in this chapter, some researchers were asking whether the nurses were floundering without a constituency. Given the backlash against feminism in the 1980s, it is hardly surprising that a predominantly female group of professional workers would be under attack, particularly given research evidence that APNs infrequently needed to consult with physicians. In contrast, the physicians were more satisfied as their control over nurse practitioners increased, and thus they were still more inclined to accept PAs, over whom they had complete control.

Physicians asserted that a stalemate on APNs had been reached; they accused nurses of being more concerned with power than patient care and claimed that "gender politics" obscured rather than clarified problems. All these accusations are very similar to those expressed by physicians in the early twentieth century, but by the end of the century, such assertions were substantially weakened by the research on nurses' cost-effectiveness and on their quality of care, evidence too often missing in physicians' pronouncements. Despite the dismissal of "gender politics," some physicians admitted that they would accept only those APNs who were sexually and politically "nonthreatening." Thus, in the 1980s and into the 1990s gender remained a central problem despite shifts in the gender mix within professional groups.

Research on the practice characteristics of male and female PAs revealed significant gender differences: More male PAs were in surgical and family specialties and more females in internal, pediatric, obstetric, and gynecologic specialties. Furthermore, the women were more likely to be in clinics than in physicians' offices and to work in urban areas. Additional research on male-female differences in descriptions of the self and of the ideal of PAs produced results that were very similar to those found in earlier research on male and female physicians. The latter described themselves as more "feminine" than the ideal physician. Similarly, female PAs described themselves in a way that was more divergent from the "ideal" and as more "feminine," a finding that did not change with increased educational levels. There was, however, proof that the male PAs were more likely to include stereotypic "feminine" characteristics in their description of themselves, suggesting a shift to more androgynous perceptions.

Certainly the stereotyped "feminine passivity" of female nurses was missing in their assertive efforts to create nurse-managed health-care centers. As noted in chapter 7, nursing had worked to change the legal definition of nursing to include the diagnosis and treatment of human responses to actual or potential health problems, thus allowing them to try to work more independently of physicians. By 1982 the first national conference on nurse-managed centers was convened, and the issue of nurses as substitutes or additive health-care providers was central, along with issues of quality control and financing of the centers. Docility was specifically rejected as incongruent with the estab-lishment of nurse-controlled centers.

Physicians again raised the issue of "quality of care" to reject autonomy in nurse-run centers, but this defense suffered a severe loss of potency with the publication of a study by the U.S. Office of Technology Assessment (1986). Experts in medicine, nursing, and related disciplines surveyed and analyzed 268 studies and found that APNs' care was *equivalent to or better than* physi-cians' care. As in the past, the key problem, according to the report, was physi-cians' opposition, although their acceptance of APNs increased as medical control increased. Again, cost-effectiveness was considered, and repeatedly nurses were less costly in their training and education; in their patient care, depending on work situations; and in their specialties, for example, the care of normal pregnancies and deliveries provided by nurse midwives. These con-clusions were obtained on nurses as physician *substitutes,* but excluded the full range of care that nurses could provide if nurses' own indices were used.

What was the response of organized medicine to the increasing evidence of nurses' competence? Resolutions passed by the American Medical Association (AMA) in the 1980s called for eliminating federal funding for "mid-level" practitioners, restricting hospital staffs to physicians, limiting patient admis-sion histories and physical examinations to physicians, and opposing legisla-tion that would allow non-physicians to provide "medical" care to patients. In short, organized medicine moved to maintain a monopoly regardless of the cost to patients and to restrict the predominantly female professionals, regard-less of their competencies in helping patients at less cost. Nevertheless, the research in the 1990s on the quality of care provided by APNs continued to support the findings from the 1960s onward.

In 1990 the AMA continued the attack on nurses' autonomy by approving a resolution that opposed "unsupervised" primary-care providers and rejected direct reimbursement to these nurses for their services. Nevertheless, nurses continued to chip away at monopolistic medical practices, particularly those involving prescriptive authority, the right to diagnose or treat under state nurse practice laws, the right to be directly reimbursed for services, and the right to admit patients. As nurses obtained legislative changes on prescriptive authority, organized medicine worked to oppose or water these down; thus, in the fifty states a hodgepodge of laws resulted, characterized by a variety of unnecessary restrictions—despite the research results that proved nurses' pre-scribing behavior was similar to physicians'. Regardless of whether the nurses' authority is legally mandated, the key issue is judgment about the patients' conditions, not medical supervision. Furthermore, only a small percentage of nurses who prescribe found it necessary to consult with physicians or to refer patients to them. Indeed, as we shall see in this chapter, 98 percent to 99 per-cent of nurses' prescriptions are safe and effective when the nurses use a for-mulary that lists 90 percent of the most commonly used drugs. Nevertheless, a majority of physicians disapproved of the nurses' prescriptive authority, even when severe restrictions were placed upon it; in contrast, almost all APNs approved. Physicians' opposition once again resulted in a mass of contradictory laws, which nurses often circumvented, writing prescriptions with or without enabling legislation. Research in the 1990s substantiated the positive findings from the 1980s, and in one study only 2 percent of the nurses' prescriptions for new medications were changed by physicians and these changes were minor—for example, a shift from one antibiotic to another. In contrast, other research by Philip Sloane and Deborah Lekan-Rutledge (1988) indicates that the current system of obtaining prescriptions from physicians by telephone is a key factor in polypharmacy, or the improper introduction of multiple drugs without adequate consideration of drug interactions.

Indeed, it is no longer a question of whether nurses will prescribe but one of whether physicians will stop monopolizing prescriptive authority through lobbying for restrictive state and federal laws. The obstacle course that nurses are forced to run is obvious in their efforts at the federal level to obtain prescriptive authority and in their struggles in all states, despite positive research findings which prove that APNs provide appropriate prescriptions regardless of the presence or absence of medical supervision or of legal requirements for additional pharmaceutical education.

The mass of inconsistent and restrictive state legislation was also apparent in the scope of nurse practice laws, particularly in regard to their right to diagnose and order treatments. Again, because of the opposition of organized medicine and through their political lobbies, many nurse practice laws were controlled by joint boards of nurses and physicians. These mixed regulatory boards have ensured medical control over nurses' practice. To get around severe limitations on nurses' practice, approved protocols have been used in some states; in others, disclaimers on APNs' diagnoses and treatment have been added to existing laws; and in still other states delegation of authority by physicians has been specified or medical "supervision" mandated. Regardless of the efforts to change practice laws, hospitals have continued to blur practice lines through "standing orders," a practice that sustains physicians' authority and income, but forces nurses to conduct medical functions even without a state nurse practice act that would give them the legal and independent authority to do what they are already doing.

Medical monopolistic meddling with nursing has resulted in multiple roles, titles, procedures, and laws, which are likened by one legal expert to the rubble from the Tower of Babel (Safriet, 1992). From the legal viewpoint, what was needed was a simple designation, "advanced practice nurse," and control of such nurses by all-nurse boards of nursing. Mixed regulation schemes lead to biased and confusing policies that favor medical monopolies and that produce, because of medical political lobbying, restrictive formal practice arrangements and unnecessary medical supervision. Indeed, the AMA passed resolutions in the 1990s that illogically equated collaboration with supervision and demanded restrictions that were potentially harmful and more costly to consumers.

Legal problems arise when states give over their power to individual physicians, who decide whether a nurse practitioner can practice. State laws that allow independent nurse practice, but only in undesirable geographical areas, predicate their range of practice on where, not what or how, the nurse practices. Clearly, these restrictions protect physicians from competition but do little for consumers. Indeed, malpractice suits against APNs are quite rare, suggesting greater consumer satisfaction with nurses than with physicians. Nevertheless, by the late 1990s, the state nurse practice acts were, although somewhat improved, still in a state of flux.

Another way to maintain a medical monopoly is to refuse direct payment to nurses for their services and to tie their income to physicians. As we shall see in this chapter, only a minority of states had legislated direct reimbursement to nurses through insurance companies by the end of the 1980s. Previously, Medicare and Medicaid direct payments to nurses were possible in rural areas, but only if there was a physician shortage there. By the mid- to late 1980s there was some possibility of direct payments; however, at the end of the 1990s, there were still restrictions, although all states and companies were *supposed* to accept direct payment to nurses through federal programs. Nevertheless, for most patients the general practice continued: physicians received money and then paid nurses at very reduced rates, pocketing the difference as their profit. By the 1990s nurses had achieved some success, but as is evident in this chapter, there were still wide variations among states in direct payments, despite federally mandated directives.

Even at the federal level, unequal treatment of nurses was evident, for example, by the federal Physicians Payment Review Committee (PPRC), established in the late 1980s to rein in physicians' costs. A resource-based relative value scale was created that established the same rate of payment for the same service, regardless of educational level for physicians, dentists, optometrists, and chiropractors; however, when APNs were considered, educational level was included and used as the justification for reduced payments. In these and other federal actions, collaboration was again illogically equated with medical direction and supervision. The American Nurses' Association (ANA), however, contested these provisions and lobbied for legislation to provide direct and equitable payments regardless of medical supervision and geographic location. Clearly, the efforts of the two professional groups continued to be in direct opposition to each other. Indeed, some medical societies were refusing membership to any physicians who used the new practice laws for APNs, and the AMA also increased lobbying efforts against the application of antitrust rules by the Federal Trade Commission, which was, in contrast, supported by the ANA.

Organized medicine not only engaged in efforts to control APNs at the top end of the nursing hierarchy by utilizing PAs, but also through proposals designed to provide bedside care by minimally trained non-nurses. The AMA moved to establish yet another new category of health-care provider, the registered care technologist (RCT), a high school graduate who was to be trained in hospitals and who would be responsible not to nurses but to physicians. Clearly, between the RCT at the bottom end and the PA at the top end, nurses would be squeezed into an increasingly ambiguous position somewhere in the middle and possibly be largely eliminated as potentially independent professionals and as economic competitors.

Nurses were understandably enraged by this unilateral decision that would, like the establishment of PAs in the 1960s, give physicians direct control and power over bedside nursing, which could signal a return to the situation in the early twentieth century. Once again, hospital training would be the norm, and physicians would simply get rid of or rename nurses at the bottom and at the top of the health-care hierarchy. Some twenty-nine national nursing associations strongly objected to the RCT proposal, and their presidents were sharp in condemnation. The physicians began pilot programs for RCTs anyway. Indeed, as discussed in this chapter, an extensive interview with a high-level AMA official provides ample evidence of the arrogant assertion of medical monopolistic power on this and other issues. Although the nurses were able to block implementation of the RCT proposal, they soon faced a variant: minimally trained "unlicensed assistive personnel" (UAPs), who would threaten both the employment of many nurses and the safety of patients (see chapter 10). Given the surplus of physicians, the various new modes of health-care delivery systems, most notably health maintenance organizations (HMOs), were not likely to increase nurses' centrality. The impact on nurses of "new" organizational structures and the rise of the corporate ethos in health care is considered more fully in chapter 10.

By the end of the 1980s nurses were publicly criticizing the health-care "system" and recommending, as in the past, a national system of maternal, child, and school-age preventive and primary care, and of community-based and long-term care of the disabled and elderly. The ANA produced *Nursing's Agenda for Health Care Reform* (1991), which again insisted on greater nursing autonomy for advanced practitioners and a national system of primary and preventive health care. As usual, the major obstacle to nurses' goals was organized medicine. We turn now to a more detailed consideration of the issues outlined in this brief introduction.

Cracking the Medical Monopoly

To gain any semblance of autonomy, nurses and other health practitioners would have to challenge the medical monopoly directly by using federal antitrust laws to lessen physician dominance. According to Andrew K. Dolan (1980), at least three specific practices were susceptible to antitrust legal remedies: "the denial of admitting privileges, third-party reimbursement, and physician backup to nonphysician practitioners" (p. 675). Dolan stated that after decades of medicine's almost unquestioned authority, omniscient behavior, and godlike image, media reports of medical abuses, reformers' studies of limited access to care, and research on the self-protective machinations of the medical profession now cast doubt on the value of medical dominance. Government-sustained monopolies had produced economic inefficiencies and outrageously high medical costs: "A disgruntled public, tired of long waits in doctors' offices, high copayments and indifferent professionals, are turning to other practitioners, although that would have been unthinkable even ten years ago" (p. 675).

Some of the "newer" reformers included feminists, who were even challenging the strategies of previous reformers, maintaining that "the dominant therapeutic ideology in the United States unduly favors inpatient care, hospital-based outpatient care, extravagant use of pharmaceuticals, high-technology therapeutic interventions such as surgery, and continued and frequent contacts with the delivery system" (p. 676). This medical ideology escalates health costs, limits availability of care, and produces iatrogenesis (medically created problems), which then leads to malpractice suits from a previously passive population dependent on physicians, who had furthered that dependence by medicalizing normal conditions, such as pregnancy. This ideology was linked "to the training, socialization and self-interest of physicians" (p. 676).

The new reformers were initially dismissed as kooks and fanatics, but, wrote Dolan, "Much of what they claim has been substantiated. Much surgery is unnecessary and ineffective. Drugs do cause adverse side effects which often are inadequately explored before the drugs are widely used. Childbirth can usually occur without anesthesiology, use of devices, and exclusion of the family" (p. 676). Patients have shown increased willingness to consult alternative practitioners, for example, in community clinics and women's heath centers. Unfortunately, "the organizational constructs by which they [physicians] obtained and have maintained a central position over the decades remains largely intact" (p. 676).

Until the 1970s the medical system was considered beyond the reach of federal antitrust laws; however, as noted in chapter 7, the United States Supreme Court in 1975 ruled there were no exceptions for professionals, and in 1976 it held that hospitals were within the jurisdiction of the Sherman Act. Thus, there is "no longer any doubt that the federal antitrust laws apply to the health care delivery system in much the same way as they do to other industries" (p. 677). These rulings would prevail only as long as or until organized medicine was able to force new legislation reinstating a medical exclusion. Indeed, attempts to do just that were initiated and sustained by the AMA (see chapter 10).

The major impediments to a more eclectic system, specifically to the use of APNs, included unfair professional licensing laws, limited access to facilities, control of third-party reimbursement, and requirements for backup physicians to control other practitioners. Indeed, "Physicians constitute the only class of health practitioners whose licenses are virtually unlimited; others can only legally perform specified functions under certain circumstances" (p. 677). The participation of physicians with nurse practitioners is often mandated, forcing the patients "to subsidize the undesired practitioner in order to obtain access to the preferred one" (p. 677). Obviously, this also destroys competitive price advantages that nurse practitioners could offer and excludes "one-stop" care.

Access to facilities, hospitals, long-term-care institutions, and clinical laboratories, has also been controlled by physicians to eliminate competition. For example, "Midwives may have patients who wish to have their births in hospitals even though the midwife's scope of practice does not permit her to utilize hospital equipment or perform inpatient procedures incidental to some childbirths" (p. 678). Admitting privileges have traditionally been limited to physicians or occasionally to affiliates of physicians, but most others, including APNs and nurse midwives, "are simply ineligible for independent privileges across the country" (p. 678).

Federal antitrust laws notwithstanding, hospital and commercial laboratories, fearing physician reprisals, have refused to process requests from other professionals. Indeed, hospitals have given to medical staffs the right to reject changes in admissions policies, and when overridden, physicians have even gone on strike in the past to exclude, for example, osteopaths. Clearly, "it is the patients of these practitioners who are also being restrained in their choice of otherwise lawful alternatives" (p. 679). These alternative practitioners are usually not denied privileges because they are practicing outside their lawful scope of practice, but because one group of competitors believes it knows what is best for patients.

Another way to eliminate competition is to restrict third-party payment to coverage only for medical expenses. Throughout the 1980s and into the 1990s, PAs could often be reimbursed for covered costs, but nurse practitioners and midwives were frequently ineligible, even if the service itself was covered. For example, a New York City outpatient birthing center had great difficulty in obtaining eligibility from insurance carriers, even though "there was no record of untoward episodes in excess of those of hospitals" (p. 680). Feminist groups were especially hard hit: "A Seattle birthing clinic was recently denied eligibility under Medicaid because birth centers are 'somewhat new'" (p. 680). Health maintenance organizations that limit covered services to staff providers may be very restrictive, particularly to nurse practitioners and midwives. The legal issue is whether third-party carriers can refuse to hire or reimburse classes of lawful practitioners operating in their legal areas of practice. Insurance businesses have been insulated from antitrust attack because of state regulations, but they are now more vulnerable because of recent litigation.

A fourth obstacle for limited license practitioners is created by eliminating access to physicians: "to maintain its hegemony, the medical profession has discouraged its members from cooperating with these competing groups" (p. 681). However, it is the patients of alternative practitioners who are the actual targets: "the medical establishment seeks to crush the competing providers in order to force their patients back into mainstream medicine" (p. 681). Medical associations pressure physicians to conform by depriving those who work with other professionals of medical society membership, malpractice insurance, and hospital admitting privileges. Although medical organizations are now legally constrained, Dolan noted that they use more subtle intimidation, often related to control of the network of referrals and backups. Physicians who have departed from the economic code, particularly those working with feminist groups or low-income patients or counterculture groups, have, said Dolan, been the targets of vigorous repression by their medical societies.

The medical establishment will go to great lengths, Dolan said, to squash even modest competitive threats. For example, a Florida women's health group started a clinic offering low-cost first-trimester abortions, using local physicians for such services. When the lower cost of their services became known, the obstetrical staff of the community's only hospital filed charges with the state medical disciplinary board and threatened the physicians with exclusion from referrals. The cooperating physicians backed out, but physicians from another community were brought in by the women. Again, the local obstetricians filed charges with the state board, claiming "outsiders" were working without local support. Since they had already quelled the local physicians, the attack on the "outsiders" was successful. One physician stated the real issue was income and practice, but "he masked his concern to others with ethical and quality-of-care language" (p. 682). Indeed, little formal action by organized medicine is usually required because physicians, said Dolan, know how relentlessly dissenting physicians can be pursued, how easily informal networks can be manipulated, how difficult it is to restore cooperation, and how costly legal battles can be. Certainly, nurse practitioners and midwives could expect that cooperative physicians would be subject to strong pressures from their medical colleagues.

Medical Monopolistic Practices

According to Dolan, physicians use at least three monopolistic practices to eliminate competition: group boycott, tying mechanisms, and bottleneck arrangements. A monopolistic boycott is a practice in which one group refuses to do business with another in order to crush competitive potential or to obtain customers' patronage on terms favorable to the boycotters. Translated, this means that physicians seek to eliminate non-physician practitioners, particularly nurses, as threatening competitors and to obtain patient patronage on terms favorable to the medical cartel.

Tying agreements are those in which people who control a highly desirable product condition its receipt on the purchase of a less desirable product. For example, hospitals who refuse patients of nurse practitioners tie highly desirable inpatient services to less desirable—from the patient's view—physicians' services. Insurance carriers who limit reimbursement of covered services only to physicians are "tying the highly desired product of risk sharing intrinsic to insurance to less desirable physician services" (p. 684). A tying agreement in medical care occurs when physicians and their allies control highly desired ancillary services and use this control to coerce patients to purchase medical services.

A bottleneck arrangement is a strategy in which "a highly desired facility is either denied to a group of consumers or made available on discriminatory terms unrelated to the cost of the service" (p. 685). In health care, the hybrid of boycott and tying arrangements involves a bottleneck caused by the control of hospitals, clinical laboratories, third-party reimbursement, and ancillary physician services; thus, nurse practitioners experience a form of boycott when they are "denied admitting privileges, specimen analysis, third-party reimbursement, or necessary physician backup" (p. 685). For clients who are forced to patronize physicians to gain access to backup services, the situation is similar to a tying agreement.

Although "it has been relatively easy to prove that the medical care industry has committed an antitrust offense" (p. 685), there is a wide array of defenses, including the right of governments to make laws favorable to the public even if they limit competition, unless these are a sham to provide cover for anticompetition. The most troubling issue has been "the slow movement toward a quality-of-care defense" (p. 685). Since virtually all anticompetitive measures have been defended as measures to ensure quality of care, this defense, if successful, "would virtually have repealed antitrust laws' applicability to the health care industry" (p. 686).

Courts, said Dolan, must resist the argument that quality of care can *only* be found in medical practice that is congruent with the dominant medical ideology. Instead, courts must demand proof for a clear difference in *outcome* from competing schools of thought and therapies. Even if legally successful, nurses face the discretion of organizations in applying favorable rulings in health-care systems; therefore, courts should retain continuing jurisdiction of cases as "they have been forced to do in racial discrimination situations" (p. 687). Clearly, this shift to a frontal attack on the medical monopoly represented a distinct change from previous approaches, bringing into the open the issue of competition between nurses and physicians.

A Momentum of Its Own: Emerging Economic Competition of Nurse Practitioners

What happened to nurses when they were perceived to be in direct competition with physicians? A nurse practitioner with twenty-five years' experience as a pediatric nurse, well-known in the local community, joined the office of a leading pediatrician. The practice size almost doubled, and the nurse carried a large caseload. Without warning, the physician informed the nurse that there was no longer room for her, even though the office had eleven examining rooms. According to Marilyn Edmunds (1981), the receptionists reported that there had been a 25 percent increase in the number of patients, formerly seen by the physician, who were now asking for appointments with the nurse practitioner. Clearly, this was unacceptable to the physician.

Edmunds attributed competition to deliberate or unconscious acts to overcompensate for feelings of inadequacy, unclear role definitions of the nurse practitioner, and ambiguities and overlap in roles. These combine with territorial possessiveness, communication breakdowns, and deliberate attempts by nurses to obtain power, the latter "not always unjustified" (p. 47). As nurses gained skill and confidence, they (perhaps not as unconsciously as Edmunds believed) rebelled against the authority of the "Captain of the Ship." However, even small actions or words were often interpreted as assertive or threatening and led to defensive actions from physicians. Given the nurse-physician game, described in previous chapters, almost any nurse's direct assertion of even simple facts might lead to physician rejection or even retaliation.

The fundamental issue, said Edmunds, is access to patients and economic profits. The greatest area of competition is the one in which nurse practitioners and physicians are perceived to be doing the same things with patients. But this is exactly what nurse practitioners must do to demonstrate their competency and skills. For these reasons, Edmunds predicted increased competition in the 1990s, exacerbated by the physician surplus. Research was already showing that pediatricians perceive nurse practitioners as competitive, not collaborative. In a 1981 report, the Graduate Medical Education National Advisory Committee (GMENAC) recommended that the training of "physician extenders" not be allowed to increase substantially; that physicians should be the only ones to see patients in 80 percent to 90 percent of patient visits; and that 80 percent of all checkups for pregnant women, 84 percent of office care for children, and 88 percent of office adult care should be handled by physicians.

As reported by the advisory committee, the future of PAs was more positive, because of greater acceptance by physicians, who perceived the PA as a role enhancer, not a competitor. As noted in the report, sexual bias and stereotypes also led physicians to believe that male PAs were more committed to careers. Critically important was the fact that PAs acted under *medical,* not nursing practice acts.

Edmunds also noted that some physicians believed there was *no* need for any type of physician "extenders," unless they could "improve the profit margin" (Edmunds, 1981, p. 49) for physicians. Many nurses reacted to the committee's report with incredulity and outrage: "Who is the Graduate Medical Education Committee [*sic*] that they should be deciding how many nurse practitioners should be educated? Physicians haven't done such an overwhelmingly sparkling job in the health care system themselves. The consumers are the people who should decide who is to meet their health care needs" (cited in Edmunds, 1981, p. 49).

According to Edmunds, the nurse practitioner role was out of physicians' control and had a momentum of its own; however, APNs must act immediately before the physician surplus overwhelmed forward movement. She recommended several strategies: First, make the nurse practitioner indispensable by working in areas where *nursing* roles are emphasized; by making the role strong, visible, and desirable to patients; by documenting and recording the nursing component of care; by selecting physicians and agencies that emphasize the role as physician complement, not substitute; and by focusing on younger physicians. Second, standardize APN functions and differentiate these from physician functions. Third, bypass physician support if it is not positive, and go directly to consumers, administrators, and legislators. This last recommendation represented a distinctly different approach from those of previous decades.

Organized nursing's emphasis on university education and advanced degrees had by the 1980s also produced positive results. Thus, Edmunds could recommend that nurses continue to conduct research and present results on nurse practitioner performance and the economics of their care. The advantages of cost-effective, competent, and sometimes superior care should encourage employers to hire APNs instead of more physicians. Nurses should directly enlist consumers' support, present statistics about advanced practice nurses' care in legislative hearings, bargain on third-party payments, and use the media to achieve visibility and obtain support.

Edmunds also recommended that nurses strengthen professional credentials through national unity, develop leaders in nurse practitioner programs who would ensure comparability in training at the master's degree level, and create a respected certification examination. The constant historical intrusion of physicians and hospital administrators into nursing had created a wide variety of educational backgrounds over which nurses continued to fight. Whether the short-term training by physicians or the full master's degree credentialing by nurses would prevail was really a question of whether nurses could stop organized medicine from intruding into nursing affairs. Finally, Edmunds recommended a power shift by urging nurses to capture the practice sites which serve the socially deprived, the poor, the elderly—the groups that physicians avoid and do not want. If physicians do not want to practice in areas of urban or rural poverty, then nurses should manage these along with more generic substantive areas, such as patient teaching, disease prevention, care of nursing home patients, obesity, and substance abuse. To be successful, nurses would have to prove to the public and to politicians that they were a cost-effective alternative to physicians.

Economic Advantages of Utilizing Independent Nurse Practitioners

The economic benefit of utilizing nurse practitioners should have been, given political efforts to control health-care costs, a critical factor. In 1979 the Congressional Budget Office had evaluated this issue and published the results in *Physician Extenders: Their Current and Future Role in Medical Care Delivery.* Cynthia M. Freund and George A. Overstreet (1981) were well aware that in the federal debates the nurses had powerful adversaries and had to prove their economic usefulness. After reviewing the research, the authors found the overall trend on utilizing nurse practitioners was positive, but warned that opponents would stress specific negative studies without considering the aggregate research findings; thus, nurses must be aware of the total research done in order to defend their own interests.

Most of the economic studies primarily assessed female nurse practitioners (NPs), although PAs, originally predominantly male but increasingly both male and female, had also been studied. Unfortunately, the gender of practitioners and assistants was not consistently controlled, reported, or analyzed; thus, the effects of gender are difficult to assess. However, by the 1980s, the majority of all the "new" health practitioners (NHPs) were female. (Freund and Overstreet use "NHP" to include *both* NPs and PAs.) The economic impact of these practitioners was assessed using various measures: productivity, profitability, cost of care, and hospitalization patterns. The last of these was assumed to measure lower or increased costs.

Field studies in actual settings were conducted primarily by nurses, physicians, and health-services researchers, and "these findings suggest a positive overall economic impact attributable to the NHP" (Freund and Overstreet, 1981, p. 28). However, these studies varied in sampling and in pre- and post-observations, and they often lacked experimental control groups. A second set of studies involved computer simulation analyses by economists and operations researchers, often using mathematical models that reflected actual practice settings. Although these involved better manipulation of variables, they often did not include or control for factors identified in field studies. Most of these studies were conducted early in the development of NHPs, when they were more restricted and experimental.

The effects on productivity, as an increase or decrease in services provided or patients seen, focused primarily on number of patient visits relative to physician output; *no* consideration was given to "the qualitative aspects of output nor to the fact that NPs contribute more than just 'physician services'" (p. 29). In a review of some seventeen studies, the productivity ranged from a 12 percent to 74 percent increase, as very narrowly measured. The variations were related to practice type (solo or group), practice history (length of time in practice, roles and utilization patterns), the scale of practice (number of patients weekly), and the degree of practitioner autonomy. Most research focused on practitioners during training or after less than one year in practice—only two even studied up to two years—thus, the effects of experience are absent or greatly underestimated. Critically important is the fact that only one study specifically focused on autonomy, although other studies indirectly contributed to the finding that greater increases in productivity were found in conditions of maximal autonomy and full utilization.

Profitability was defined as the extent to which practitioners generated income that covered their own costs and exceeded expenses incurred in their employment. A correlated question dealt with incremental profit to physicians, who presumably kept the profit rather than passing on savings to nurse practitioners or consumers. Different formulae were used, but despite these differences, "all but one study reported a positive income generation potential, providing a positive incentive for NHP utilization" (p. 29). A wide variation was found, probably associated with practice settings, utilization, and types of practitioners.

The cost of care was primarily measured by comparing the cost of care provided by NHPs to that of physicians. These measurements were also variable: costs for both inpatient and outpatient services; costs per person per year; cost per visit or cost per hour or fees charged. In addition, practice settings and levels of NHPs' education varied from no additional training, to on-the-job training, to extensive formal education. Freund and Overstreet found that cost for care per year "ranged from 4 percent to 23 percent less than the cost for care provided by physicians. . . . A per-visit cost for NHPs ranged from 20 percent to 41 percent lower than the per-visit cost of physicians and the per-house cost of NHPs was 44 percent less than the per-hour cost of physicians" (p. 29). These costs decreased as the scale of practice increased. Even for those of comparable size, cost of care was lower when NHPs were employed. Various studies have demonstrated decreased hospital utilization in numbers of admissions and length of stay for patients of NHPs compared to those cared for by physicians. However, the authors noted, other factors were not controlled nor were patients followed over more extensive time periods.

The differential economic impact of NPs and PAs was, by the early 1980s, an unresolved issue, since only one study had directly addressed this issue. Comparing studies in which NPs or PAs were the sole subjects should allow for cross-study comparisons, but Freund and Overstreet noted that research designs and a multitude of variables were inconsistent. In research involving *both* NPs and PAs, either there was a lack of differentiation or the sample sizes were too small for comparison. From the single study that could be analyzed, PAs had more weekly patient encounters, generated more income, but spent less time with patients and charged higher fees per encounter. However, setting, patient mix, practice history, utilization patterns, and autonomy were not considered. Nor could cost-effectiveness be ascertained since most comparisons on this issue were with physicians, not NPs. Furthermore, goals other than productivity and income generation were absent; thus, the cost definitions considered were inadequate.

Freund and Overstreet concluded that results taken in aggregate supported a *positive* economic impact of NPs; however, they warned again that opponents would emphasize the methodological weaknesses of selective studies. The authors concluded: "It is crucial to point out that NP autonomy, a factor affecting productivity identified in many previous studies, was neither controlled nor manipulated" (p. 32). It is equally important for a predominantly female group, historically underpaid in relation to physicians, to determine where the positive profit incentive should go: to themselves, to consumers, or, as in the past, to physicians. If women achieve greater autonomy and take on greater responsibility, but find no increased reimbursement for these, how has the sex-stratified system been affected? If all measures are quantitative and the value system basic to nursing is not studied or even considered, how will women's concerns impact on health delivery?

The Uncertain Future of Advanced Practice Nurses

By the early 1980s the growth in the numbers of nurse practitioners had slowed. Organized medicine had created a physician surplus; tried, with very limited success, to increase the number of physicians in primary care; and resisted giving more independent authority to nurses. Given the shift to a more conservative political agenda, federal support for training of APNs was in jeopardy. In 1982 Alfred Yankauer and Judith Sullivan considered the future of these nurses and concluded that, although it was uncertain, nurse practitioners, clinicians, and PAs were not likely to disappear, but were probably going to work in positions that physicians did not want, or in institutions that needed high quality services at the least cost, or as midwives because of consumer preference.

This pattern was certainly not new. Even without formal and separate licensure, public health nurses, particularly in rural areas, have performed midwifery functions for decades. However, public health nursing in the United

States, in contrast to district nursing in England, was "inhibited by a free enterprise tradition and the opposition of the medical profession" (p. 251), restricting services even for well-child care to only a small proportion of the poor. These restraints on nurses continued, despite research on physicians, specifically pediatricians, that continued to prove that a high proportion were "performing tasks which clearly did not require a medical degree; a quarter of them carried out vision screening and urinalyses personally, half gave their own immunizations and parenteral drug injections, and 13% weighed infants and children themselves" (p. 252). As the authors noted, in hospitals all these tasks were delegated to nurses. Similar studies produced comparable results for family physicians and internists. Clearly, physicians were familiar with task delegation, but sharing the role of diagnostician and therapist, even under physician control, was difficult for them. Given the gendered professions, this also meant sharing authority with women. To keep control, a variety of different health workers were created, but all the various names had been dropped except the two major categories of APN and PA, although there was still debate over the status of nurse clinicians.

As noted in chapter 7, by 1971, sixty-one physician's assistant programs existed; forty-seven did *not* require nursing degrees, but of these only twenty-eight were fully devoted to preparing PAs. As previously discussed, nurses largely ignored the new PAs until they were legitimized by licensure, AMA accreditation, enabling state legislation, and federal funding. By 1981, fifty-six accredited programs for PAs existed, and many of these had survived ten or more years; however, the composition of students had changed dramatically. The original military corpsmen, who formed two-thirds of the earlier student group, had decreased to 30 percent by 1977, replaced by medical technicians/technologists or registered nurses, many with college degrees, who represented 62 percent of PAs in 1979–1980. The gender ratio had changed considerably, with women about half the graduates by the beginning of the 1980s.

As discussed in chapter 7, nurse practitioner programs developed quickly in the 1970s, partially in reaction to moves by the AMA, which, "acting on its own initiative and without consulting the nursing profession, issued a statement to the effect that, as a stop gap measure, the physician shortage could be alleviated by training thousands of nurses to practice as 'physician's assistants'" (p. 257). As noted in chapter 7, the AMA's well-publicized statement (*American Medical News*, 1970), by its wording and later interpretation, "clearly placed the nurse in a position of a girl Friday who functioned only at the doctor's beck and call. Nurses, having endured identification with such an image for many years, were understandably enraged" (pp. 257–258). By the 1980s the fracture between the AMA and the ANA was still not healed.

In countering the AMA's initiative, nursing fostered the rapid growth of nurse practitioner programs. By 1976, 5,800 graduates had been produced, and by 1980, an estimated 16,000, with a wider, better balanced distribution in practice areas of family, pediatrics, adult and geriatric, maternity, and family planning: "A few nurse clinicians had opened independent private practices, but without third party reimbursement, the financial viability of these practices was limited" (p. 259). The proportion of master's degree programs increased from 34 percent in 1974 and 1977, to 60 percent in 1980, with the highest number in family practice. That the nurses themselves were producing competent practitioners was obvious from several research studies and reviews of these; however, the role overlap between nurses and physicians continued, although the practitioners focused more on prevention, common health problems, and long-term care. It is, of course, difficult to know what the nurses were actually doing since the measures in research were predominantly defined by using medical indices. Considerable overlap with PAs continued, although in their own programs the nurses focused more heavily on counseling patients and preventive care.

Theoretically, nurse practitioners were able to function independently of physicians, but the PAs could only execute medical orders. Actually, the balance between independence and dependence appeared to rely heavily on practice settings and relations with individual physicians. Although nurses reacted favorably to their advanced roles, they, too optimistically, believed that physicians had more favorable attitudes toward nurse practitioners than toward physician's assistants: "In the Victorian past one might have been tempted to align PAs with a male-like role and NPs a female-like role, but in the androgynous present this is no longer tenable" (p. 263). However, it is clear, as noted in chapter 8, that gendered issues were still unresolved. Although Yankauer and Sullivan hoped androgynous care might be the direction of the future, it certainly had not been achieved by the 1980s, even in the measures of care, since they relied on medical, not nursing, indices.

Indeed, by the 1980s, the quality of nurse practitioners' practice had received "far more attention than the quality of services delivered by physicians had ever received" (p. 263). Although methodological problems existed in research on nurse practitioners, "A reliable and valid baseline for physician error is nonexistent and probably nonattainable" (p. 264). In general, nurse practitioners and PAs had been positively evaluated and had not been involved significantly in legal claims, except as accessory appendages to physicians—not as central figures.

Nurses' Cost-Effectiveness and Competence Proven; Their Potential Still Not Fully Recognized

Though costs and quality of care and services provided by physicians have been virtually ignored, the evidence on the comparative productivity and lower costs of APNs has been substantial (Record, McCally, Schweitzer, Blomquist, and Berger, 1980), involving over 1,000 published and unpublished studies and reports. From these, "About 90% of routine pediatric visits appear to be safely delegatable, with 80% a reasonable figure for adults" (Yankauer and Sullivan, 1982, p. 264). Furthermore, Record and her colleagues found a substitution ratio for both types of advanced health professionals that fell in the range of .50 to .75, leading Yankauer and Sullivan to conclude that "the bulk of evidence indicates that substantial societal cost savings are attainable from the substitution of new health professionals for physicians in the delivery of routine primary care" (p. 265).

Although nurse midwives were included in studies of "new" health professionals, the Frontier Nursing Service had, as previously discussed, prepared nurse midwives from 1925 onward, and the Maternity Center Association from 1931. These were the first of only seven programs still operating by the end of the 1960s. The women's movement and nurses' move toward autonomy in the 1970s focused greater attention on nurse and lay midwives. Thus, by the beginning of the 1980s, twenty-four accredited midwifery programs existed, and "Full practice for nurse midwives (including labor and delivery) was legal in every state except Kansas" (p. 266). Nevertheless, the medical monopoly of childbirth continued: before the 1970s "only about ⅓ of the employed nurse midwives were practicing their profession" (p. 266), and many of them were doing it in foreign countries. By 1977, 49 percent were unemployed; of those working, about two-thirds were working as midwives, but about a sixth of these were in foreign countries. This was the situation despite the fact that midwives could care for difficult problems. In rural areas where midwives usually substituted for physicians, the women manually removed placentas, repaired fourth-degree lacerations, managed multiple births and breech deliveries, used vacuum extractors, and performed circumcisions. Clearly, nurse midwives were capable of doing far more than giving prenatal and sexual counseling and performing uncomplicated deliveries.

Even the 1981 *Report of the Graduate Medical Education National Advisory Committee (GMENAC)* admitted that 64 percent of the annual well-care exams and 60 percent of family planning exams could be delegated to non-physician providers. Furthermore, the report predicted that nurse midwives would handle 5 percent of all deliveries by 1990. Recommendations were made to remove restrictive state laws, eliminate exclusionary reimbursement policies, and forestall physicians' unwillingness to delegate.

Given these facts, what did the future offer? Congressional funding for "new" health providers began in the 1970s, but "the production of PAs peaked quite early in the decade; a few years later nurse practitioner production peaked" (Yankauer and Sullivan, 1982, p. 268). Certainly, the nurses' objections to PAs affected the latter's growth, but both types of practitioner were influenced by the scarcity of government education funds in the conservative 1980s. In addition, the government did nothing to stop the influx of foreign medical students, and by 1976 they "filled almost one out of every three training and staff positions in hospitals and comprised one-fifth of all physicians delivering patient care in the United States" (p. 269). At the same time, the supply of American physicians was not stemmed, leading to the current over-supply of physicians, which had been predicted years before.

Although the "new" health professionals were "to reduce the costs of health care, counteract the geographic and specialty maldistribution of physicians, and repair what was seen as physician shortage" (p. 269), these predictions were not supported: the cost of health care to consumers was not reduced, although institutions profited. Reduced education costs had been offset by the increased costs of educating more physicians, and the geographic maldistribution had been only partially affected. Even in primary and ambulatory care, the outlook for the future remained uncertain. Indeed, the potential of the "new" professionals had not been fully recognized and the health-care system remained inflexible even though "the delivery of health care might have been revolutionized in the United States, the costs of care reduced, and the quality of care improved" (p. 270).

The vast majority of primary care could be handled as well or better by the "new" professionals, but they had been "tolerated as a second best solution rather than seen as a means of improving efficiency and effectiveness in the delivery of primary care" (p. 270). Yankauer and Sullivan concluded that "one cannot expect revolutions to occur in a nonrevolutionary climate" (p. 270). Even so, nursing education has become more realistic, medical and nursing practice acts have changed, and primary care is the subject of increased attention and study. Even with the physician oversupply, "the new health professionals are here to stay" (p. 271). Unrealistically perhaps, the GMENAC projections assumed that "distribution and roles will remain fixed in their present state" (p. 271), but the "new" health professionals were continuing to take roles that physicians were "unable or unwilling to assume in nursing homes, residential care institutions, and prisons" (p. 271). They would also fill the gaps left by foreign medical graduates in hospital-sponsored ambulatory-care centers and emergency services and eventually replace interns and residents in some hospitals when residency training or physician coverage was discontinued because of cost.

The "new" health professionals were still operating under a number of constraints, and if physician resistance became more acute, this could pose a serious threat. In addition, government funding of education has "wavered between full funding and a completely hands off policy . . . [but] PA and NP training programs can never stand entirely on their own feet financially any more than medical or other nursing education" (pp. 272–273). Given the conservatism of the 1980s—which reappeared in the mid-1990s—severe budget cuts and restraints on federal funding initiatives were likely to create difficult problems in the future. These would have national as well as international ramifications.

Floundering without a Constituency? Worldwide Variations in "Allied" Health Professionals

What happens to advanced practitioners in the United States has serious global repercussions, given the widespread dissemination of the gender-stratified medical model to developing countries. In 1982 David D. Celentano tried to estimate the future for advanced nurse practitioners and create a global model for "allied" health professionals. He initially used Eliot Friedson's (1970) definition of a profession as incorporating legitimate, organized autonomy with the right to control its own work (see chapter 7). Given the gendered subordination of women in many Western and non-Western cultures, this definition automatically excluded many "allied" health workers. Thus, he was forced to use a definition that included traditional healers, paramedical health workers, physician substitutes, and primary health practitioners. But even this definition is difficult to use in many non-Western cultures where formal education, especially of girls and women, is limited, making Western sociological ideas about health professions inappropriate, particularly given the fact that many of the "allied" health workers provide the *only* "medical" resources for large populations. Indeed, are these health-care providers, very often women, "allied" (meaning joined or connected) and, if so, to whom? One need not go to developing countries; one can find such relatively independent women workers in the Frontier Nursing Service in the Appalachian Mountains. As noted previously, these nurses have provided services for more than seventy years, producing lower infant and maternal mortality rates than those achieved by physicians nationwide. Are these women "auxiliary" or "paramedical" personnel? Are they providing medical care or *health* care?

Indeed, Western cultural definitions of professionals do not make sense, in part because the terms are expressed in bureaucratic hierarchical models. Physician's assistant, for example, is a term based on a model of lines of authority and division of labor: "The name itself, 'assistant,' directly implies a subservient role; legal statute bars independent practice and mandates direct control by physicians" (Celentano, 1982, p. 689). Cross-culturally, many health workers are not located in bureaucracies; they work with little or no supervision, guidance, or collaboration. Even within Western cultures, the degree of supervision varies from day to night and from weekdays to weekends, times when nurses especially are unofficially expected to work with little physician direction. In different historical periods, community or public health nurses have functioned with considerable independence, particularly in rural or poor urban areas. Clearly, terms such as "allied" are *ideological*, actually representing control and power relationships.

"Responsibilities" is also a difficult term; even if they are defined in part by education and training, these vary so much worldwide that the criteria for appropriate functions are also variable. Indeed, actual practice settings can lead to "under utilization of skills and over dependence" (p. 689). In short, the context is "the central determinant of what is deemed to be appropriate clinical behavior" (p. 689). If the context is gender-defined and if the sexes are channeled into superordinate and subordinate roles, then the model can hardly be helpful to the women who still do much, if not most, of the healing throughout the world. The traditional, obedient, submissive model of female nurse has certainly done more harm than good. Yet as Celentano observed, the American medical model has had a pervasive influence on other countries. Although "the model of the semi-autonomous health practitioner existed for decades in the form of the nurse-midwife and the public health nurse" (p. 690), this is not the model transmitted to other countries.

Celentano said there was "rapid acceptance" of "allied" health professionals; however, this assertion is certainly debatable. It is also doubtful if many nurses, even now, would accept the term "allied," precisely because of the hierarchal implications. The movement toward acceptance had slowed, but Celentano attributed this to a lack of foresight in restructuring the system, rather than to the refusal of organized medicine to accept nurse practitioners' autonomy. Indeed, Celentano further asserted that the major determinant of the success or failure of programs is the degree to which the hierarchy is kept viable. According to him, optimum utilization "can best be approached through an analysis of where they have been seen to be most useful to physicians" (pp. 690–691). His focus is not on the patient, but on the "benefits to physician employers or supervisors . . . [which] is most often conceived of as including increased income, decreased hours of work, and decreased amount of routinized activities" (p. 691). He did not discuss why nurses would want to take on additional responsibilities simply to make life easier and more lucrative for physicians and hospital administrators, who often provide minimal economic incentives for nurses. Nor did he discuss benefits for patients—a peculiar omission.

The Issue of Control over Resources and Opportunities

Most analysts agreed by the 1980s that research on nurse practitioners or physician's assistants showed decreased waiting time for clients, more available physician time, and increased net revenues, although some physicians claimed the economic benefits were overstated. How advanced practitioners themselves or their patients had economically benefitted was not analyzed by Celentano. Their productivity in office practices does increase the availability of medical (health) care services, although this varies widely, from 25 percent to 76 percent. From the research, job satisfaction of PAs was quite high, even without career ladder opportunities. Celentano did not present any data on nurse practitioners' satisfaction or careers.

Given the benefits for physicians that had been proven by research, "it is difficult to reconcile recent evidence that employment opportunities are narrowing, tasks are being withdrawn, rights suspended, legislation being changed to become more restrictive and job satisfaction dropping" (p. 691). Celentano specifically blamed the physician "who maintains control over resources and opportunities" (p. 691). With a potential oversupply of physicians, training monies for "allied" workers had been curtailed. Without a gender analysis, the irrationality of rejecting nurse practitioners and PAs, who were increasingly drawn from the ranks of female nurses puzzled Celentano, who considered the future of allied professionals to be uncertain, even though this could not be explained by utilization factors. From a gender perspective, however, it is clear that the societal trend toward conservatism in the 1980s and into the 1990s involved a backlash against women's increasing liberation in general and nurses' autonomy in particular.

Clearly, what constituted "appropriate responsibilities," or specific tasks, could not be separated from power and decision-making relationships with physicians. Indeed, "allied" professionals "can perform a wide variety and scope of tasks, and the limitations in practice appear to be a function of legal restriction or length of training. . . . The practice of an experienced pediatric nurse practitioner can be quite difficult to differentiate from that of a pediatrician in the normal working environment" (p. 692).

Autonomy and Role Performance of Nurse Practitioners and Physician's Assistants

To what extent do the "new" professionals function autonomously? Celentano surveyed a variety of health professionals—pediatric and adult nurse practitioners (PNPs and ANPs), physician's assistants (PAs), and health associates (HAs). About 200 respondents were asked to indicate their specific care activities and to estimate the number of occasions that involved physician consultation. Presumably, the higher the number of care activities and the lower the number of consultations, the more autonomy. Ironically, this is labeled the "index of Medical Autonomy," illustrating once again the centrality of physicians' language and perspective. Pediatric nurse practitioners were generally *more* autonomous than physician's assistants, but less than the health associates who had received post-baccalaureate education in general health care: "On average, PAs consult with their physician supervisors more than 65% of the time, while PNPs and HAs consult less than half of the time related to pediatric encounters" (Celentano, 1982, p. 693). Autonomy also varied according to the patient's need and type of visit, but "practitioners who can provide continuity of care are more autonomous" (p. 694). Acuteness of problems was related to a drop in autonomy; conversely, if problems were chronic, the degree of autonomy rose. Autonomy also decreased as the proportion of adults seen increased, compared to children. Finally, "the more unstructured the consultation pattern, the higher the level of medical autonomy" (p. 694). Structural variables affected independence, which in turn affected job satisfaction. "For NPs and HAs both autonomy and job satisfaction were quite high; a large variance was found for PAs on each measure, although their mean scores were not statistically different from the other ANPs" (p. 694).

Variation in role obligations and tasks was large, despite the fact that each index was based on the educational curricula of the respective training programs of the respondents. Therefore, the actual role performance of practitioners is "strongly affected by the positions they hold in various work settings and by the realities of the supervision characteristics of their physician employers" (p. 694). In other words, physicians control what others do and can restrain them from fully using their training, intellect, and skills. The result is "an increased tendency for practitioners to leave their professions and return to universities for alternative types of training; the principal reasons given for career changes are that they can no longer practice in the ways they have been trained" (p. 695). This happens despite the fact that "allied" health workers "can perform many medical care functions quite adequately and for most primary care situations they can handle presenting acute and chronic conditions" (p. 695).

These practitioners, most of whom are female, should have a promising future, but the situation is the exact reverse: "the competition between physicians and allied health professionals for resources has left the latter group floundering without a constituency and the support they had previously enjoyed" (p. 695). Thus, a gender-based struggle for control restricted the quality of care nurses could provide and patients could receive.

To emphasize a point made previously, the most distressing aspect of this situation is the global implications. If the patriarchal medical model continues to be transmitted to developing countries, the result can only be disastrous. Given low levels of wealth, the full use of "allied" health workers is required and the physician-centered American medical model is hardly appropriate. With no worldwide agreement on health-care models, the failure in Western cultures to use "allied" professionals effectively and the move to create a "doctor glut" forced Celentano to look elsewhere for solutions. Unfortunately, he did not challenge physicians' power, or condemn their refusal to cede power to nurses in order to provide quality care at lower costs.

Celentano focused instead on the feldsher in the Soviet Union and the barefoot "doctor" in China. These roles arose out of community need and involve local selection and participation; thus, they could provide a model that incorporates what already exists locally. Since the majority of community health providers are still women, Celentano's recommendation to enhance and retrain "manpower" would actually involve thousands of women. If the empowerment of nurses in the United States has met with rejection, what is the probability that the female power of traditional healers could be enhanced elsewhere? How would existing international nursing organizations be able to provide the needed health-care model when Western nurse practitioners have been blocked from independent, autonomous practice? If these nursing groups cannot influence the global model, then the only conclusion is that the distribution of health services will probably remain under medical control. This model will hardly solve the problems of delivering health care to the masses of people in developing countries. To give up the Western "allied" health model because organized medicine in America has limited alternative healers would mean premature closure for an ongoing process that continues to be hotly debated.

The Medical View: A Stalemate on Nurse Practitioners?

Premature closure is more than evident in the view of some American physicians. In 1983, S. K. Lapius, MD, noted that he had watched the ebb and flow of the debate about physician's assistants and nurse practitioners and its seldom-acknowledged financial and political overtones. "S. K. Lapius," is, of course, a pseudonym based on the name of Asklepios, the god of medicine who was discussed in chapter 1; however, the journal editors described this contributor only as "an academic physician who wishes to remain anonymous" (p. 95). To this coy physician, the original concept for creating PAs was simple: a physician shortage and high health-care costs led physicians to shed repetitive routine tasks that "didn't require prodigious amounts of knowledge or skill" (p. 94). Among their concerns were those that arose from the nurses' push for expanded roles. Peculiarly, this anonymous reincarnation of Asklepios seemed to overlook the nurses' objections to being again dictated to by organized medicine; to losing their nursing orientation if they functioned as PAs; and to taking orders from male medical corpsmen with fewer years of training and experience, but greater diagnostic and treatment prerogatives. This part of history eludes S. K. Lapius, who charged: "It was hard at times to distinguish between the legitimate aspirations of a profession striving for self-respect and the machinations of people who were less devoted to patients than to power. Issues of gender politics tended to obscure rational, patient-oriented considerations" (pp. 94–95). We would of course, argue the reverse: Unless gender politics *are* explicated, women, including nurses, will be unable to analyze accurately and adequately their subordination and will continue to use less than their full capabilities. Given his academic background, a better intellectual analysis could have been expected from S. K. Lapius; however, given the anonymous nature of his credentials, perhaps very little of a substantive nature could be anticipated.

Having dismissed the fundamental issue of gender, "Dr. Lapius" called for patients' interests to override territorial and financial interests. Since physicians' incomes were, by the 1980s, five to six times those of nurses, despite substantial increases in nurses' educational levels, this recommendation does seem a bit superficial, if not downright disingenuous. Evidently, patients' interests did not override the writer's primary concern: "Do midlevel practitioners save money?" (p. 95). The answer is probably too complex for private practice, but in the public sector, the physicians' choices may be between employing a nurse practitioner or physician's assistant and offering no treatment at all: thus, there is no "quarrel with the judgment of those few physicians who employ midlevel practitioners and find them cost effective" (p. 95). From this androcentric and medicine-centered perspective, there is no grasp of the continuing devaluation of women's labor; no perception that nurses may have a value system different from physicians'; no appreciation that nurses were demanding more autonomous practice, not merely employment by a few physicians; and no understanding of the fact that physicians are often overtrained, certainly overpaid, and, therefore, hardly cost-effective.

Could "midlevel" practitioners actually provide quality care? This issue is considered at great length in research studies and lengthy research reviews; however, none of these were covered by this physician, who simply said it depends on the definition of "care." If it is basic diagnosis and treatment of sore throats or urinary infections, then yes. If it is evaluating complex histories, then no. Without bothering with previous research findings, this "academic" medical man simply assumed that all physicians give quality care. The real problem is mutual monitoring of care from both nursing and medical perspectives. This already occurs informally without overt recognition or acceptance by physicians, including this anonymous man.

Indeed, the next question posed by "Lapius" is whether physicians can provide the "necessary supervision and policy direction" (p. 95). He considers this a tough problem, because physicians have not been trained to supervise nor have they had experience with the "new" practitioners, although they may get this if they work with nurse practitioners in residency programs. Note again the totally medical emphasis, not on collaboration with peers but on "cordial" supervision. He also wondered if patients would accept the "new" practitioners. In answering this question, he again provided no references to the substantial and positive research results about patient acceptance. He did admit that "in most cases it is the physician, not the patient, who is hung up on the issue. Most patients would rather be treated by a midlevel practitioner who takes time to care than by a physician who is 'too busy'" (p. 95). Although a refreshing shift of perspective, this conclusion is one that was adequately proven in a number of research studies; thus, hardly any other conclusion is possible.

Finally, having said that gender politics obscures rationality, "Dr. Lapius" asked if territorial, gender, and economic issues could be resolved. More accurately, his question should be rephrased as "gendered economic and territorial issues." In any case, he asserted, "It seems unlikely. Each feeds on the others.

A male physician might be willing to share his turf with a female nurse practitioner if she is non-threatening politically or sexually, but given the predicted physician glut, will he allow her to challenge him economically?" (p. 95). In contrast, hospital administrators will hire a PA (note that in this case the APN is *not* specified) who will work for half the money. How long this state of gendered imbalance will continue is not addressed by Dr. Lapius, but his prognosis is simple: "Stalemate." Whether nurses and consumers would accept this stalemate was not considered.

The Changing Gender Mix: Toward Androgyny or Continued Stereotyped Ideals and Practice?

To what extent was gender still an important part of nurses' analysis of nurse-physician relations and still related to the issue of autonomy? As noted previously, the original cadre of PAs were mostly male. Over time, some female nurses also became PAs; the numbers of women increased from zero in 1967 to approximately 44 percent in 1979. During this same period, women graduating from medical school increased from 6.8 percent, or 503, to over 21 percent, or 3,086, in 1978. Although medicine is still male-defined and -dominated, there have been changes in the gender mix, and how this will eventually affect medicine or health care in general is yet to be determined. Changes in the gender mix led some researchers to focus on gender and the personal and professional attributes of health caregivers. For example, the practice characteristics of male and female PAs were studied by Denis R. Oliver, Reginald D. Carter, and Joseph E. Conboy (1984), who published the results of a national survey of 3,294 PAs. From their survey, the researchers found that family medicine was the most common specialty in which PAs practiced. Males were more likely than females to be in this area and in surgery. Females were more likely to be in internal medicine, pediatrics, obstetrics, and gynecology. They were also less likely to be located in office-based practices and more likely to be in clinics and in urban communities. Males reported almost the same number of working hours per week (48.6) as females (47.9).

There were differences in the reasons given by both sexes for specialty selection. Since PAs must accept both training and employment simultaneously, their careers were dependent on the decisions of physicians and health-care administrators; thus, gendered difference in practice "may reflect, in part, preferences of the employer" (p. 1400). Oliver and his colleagues called for more research on the issue of employer preference, but concluded that "differences between male and female PAs are small and may not be of practical significance" (p. 1400). It is, however, significant that more men than women were working with physicians in surgery and in offices, not clinics. This suggests initial male bonding of potential partnerships.

Would gender biases in self and ideal descriptions of physicians and PAs persist as well? Early studies of medical students compared male-female differences in attitudes toward women and women medical students, finding more biases toward males (Gross and Crovitz, 1975; Giles and Williams, 1979; Williams and Best, 1982). More recent studies suggest an increased androgynous view of needed characteristics, combining dominance, independence, and problem solving with nurturance and interpersonal competence. However, women medical students' self-descriptions were more feminine than those of the ideal physician, but men students' descriptions were very similar to the ideal.

In 1984 Stephen Davis, D. L. Best, G. Marion, and G. H. Wall asked if similar patterns would be found among physician's assistants, since they presumably combined medical diagnostic and nursing psychosocial skills. Whether this assumption is correct for medical corpsmen has not been confirmed. The research was conducted on thirty-nine first- and second-year and twenty-eight graduating students, all of whom completed checklists for their own characteristics and those of the ideal PA. These were scored for degree of sex stereotyping, strength and favorability of affective meaning, and psychological need. Descriptions were similar across gender and class, containing both typically feminine and masculine stereotypes; however, the female students described themselves as more feminine and *less* similar to their ideal. This discrepancy did not lessen for graduating students. Thus, the female PAs were similar to women in other professional groups, including medicine, who also see themselves as further from the ideal practitioner in their fields. However, both male and female students in this study "described themselves as more nurturant and more dependent than their ideal" (p. 679). Males in particular considered themselves to have "more stereotypical feminine needs than physicians or men in general. These differences were amplified for PAs entering high interpersonal specialty fields" (p. 679). Clearly, more androgynous personal characteristics were being espoused by individuals, and although women saw themselves as more divergent from the ideal, androgyny seemed to be valued—although it was hardly the reality in organizational structures and professional interrelations.

Founding Nurse-Managed Centers, Controlling Practice, and Connecting with Other Women Practitioners

Though some nurses may have perceived themselves as far from the "ideal" practitioner in their field, many, even without independent authority, continued to set up nurse-managed centers. These were often started by faculty at schools of nursing to serve as model teaching centers for nursing students. Norma M. Lang (1983) noted that sixty-three nursing centers were in operation in the early 1980s and that most were adjuncts to universities, serving the campus or adjacent inner-city communities. In addition, forty-four more were in the process of planning to open. The first national conference on nurse-managed centers was held in 1982. In addition, ANA-sponsored legislation, the "Community Nursing Centers" bill, would provide for direct reimbursement for care delivered at the centers, which were sometimes associated with visiting nurse associations. The centers were completely managed by nurses and incorporated education and research. The key was controlling practice not simply through collective bargaining, but by internal control of definitions of care, peer review, political processes, and practice standards. It is remarkable that a traditionally subordinated group of women could contemplate not simply centers, but an organized national network of practice, research, and education.

Many questions still needed to be answered. Should centers provide only nurses' services or should they involve others, such as physicians or occupational therapists? Obviously, the inclusion of other female professionals could politically integrate women and broaden the power base for all. Should centers only be devoted to primary health care, involving prevention, screening, and routine health problems? Most consumers would opt for comprehensive services. How would the nurses "bring nurse-controlled services to public health departments, home health care, ambulatory care, hospice, primary care and elderly care . . . [and] institutional services, like nursing homes and rehabilitation units?" (Lang, 1983, p. 1292).

The key to these questions depended on the definition of nursing, and for this Lang used the ANA document *Nursing: A Social Policy Statement* (1980), in which society, not the medical or legal system, is claimed as the source of nursing authority. Nursing is defined as the diagnosis and treatment of human responses to actual or potential health problems. To Lang, this means that nurses must make decisions and take actions to test their autonomy. "How," she asked, "can we possibly ask for reimbursement for something we cannot describe?" (Lang, 1983, p. 1292).

Lang narrowed the issue to the decision on whether nursing is a substitute or an additive service. In agreement with Claire Fagin (1983), Lang said that studies on the lower costs and higher benefits of nurse midwives and rehabilitation nurses, for example, prove they are qualified providers. Barriers to nurses' services, particularly the exclusion of non-physician caregivers and the refusal of third-party payers to reimburse nurses, must be destroyed. Consumers can then have access to nurses, who will substitute for physicians by delivering equally safe, cost-effective, quality care.

To Lang, the key issue was quality control. There were 1.4 million nurses who might want third-party payments, and these would depend on assurance of quality care. Therefore, modes of peer review should be examined to determine responsibility for the provision of high-level nursing care. Another major issue was financing of the centers. To achieve funding assistance, what organized political action should be taken? Senator Daniel Inouye, a sponsor of the

Community Nursing Centers bill, said that nurses could have whatever they wanted—they could control the health-care system and have more power than any other group, including oil lobbyists. However, he feared the nurses might "go to your graves with 'docile' written on your tombstones" (p. 1293). Lang concluded, "It is time we proved him wrong" (p. 1293).

Evidently, organized physicians wanted to prove Senator Inouye right. In 1981, the AMA House of Delegates had adopted several resolutions that directed the AMA to work to eliminate federal funding for training any more "midlevel" practitioners and recommended that hospital staffs allow only physicians to do admissions histories and physical examinations (Health Planning Report, 1981). Then, in 1985, another AMA resolution was adopted that opposed any new legislation that would authorize "medical acts" by unlicensed persons or extend medical practice to "non-physician" providers (AMA, 1985). In 1990 yet another AMA resolution was passed that opposed "any attempt at empowering nonphysicians to become unsupervised primary medical care providers and be directly reimbursed for case management activities" (AMA, 1990a). If physicians were genuinely concerned about patients, instead of territorial and monopolistic power, they should, given the equivalent or superior care of nurses compared to physicians, have passed resolutions in support of advanced nurse practitioners. Their true priorities are obvious in the resolutions they did pass through the 1980s and into the 1990s.

Nurses' Quality of Care Equivalent to or Better Than Physicians'

Ironically, the medical attacks on nurses' autonomy occurred at the same time that the U.S. Office of Technology Assessment (OTA) issued a prestigious report that affirmed advanced practice nurses' competence. In 1986 the OTA, in response to the Senate Committee on Appropriations, published *Nurse Practitioners, Physicians' Assistants, and Certified Nurse-Midwives: A Policy Analysis*. Quality, access, and cost were evaluated from an extensive review of the literature and involved a panel of experts in health policy, medical economics, health insurance, medicine, nursing, and consumer advocacy, who defined the goals and conducted the research. Of some 268 sources, mostly published research studies, some were flawed by particular methodological problems; nevertheless, when combined with randomized, controlled studies, valid generalizations could be drawn. The first conclusion was that the APNs provided, within their areas of competence, *"care whose quality is equivalent to that of care provided by physicians"* (Office of Technology Assessment, 1986, p. 5).

Ten of the studies analyzing processes and outcomes proved nurses' equivalence, but fourteen studies showed a difference in quality, and of these twelve demonstrated that the care given by advanced practice nurses was *better* than that given by physicians, both in process, such as the thoroughness of diagnoses, and in outcome, such as the control of blood pressure levels. Of the other two studies, the only one favoring physicians involved technical solutions; the second was misinterpreted since the results were actually in favor of the nurses. In addition, the majority of studies provided evidence of patients' satisfaction with the nurses, and some proved that patients were *more* satisfied with the nurses than with the physicians. Successful malpractice cases against nurses were also extremely rare.

Given these findings, if physicians were genuinely concerned with patients, the level of medical acceptance of nurse practitioners should have been very high. Physician acceptance, although tangential to nurses' actual quality of care, was considered in the OTA report, which found that acceptance could be influenced by fiscal interests and financial competition. Although physicians who had worked with APNs expressed more satisfaction, the "level of physicians' satisfaction increases with the degree of their control over the activities of NPs" (p. 22).

The OTA report also found similarly positive results for certified nurse midwives (CNMs), concluding from the review of research that nurse-midwives could manage normal pregnancies as well if not better than physicians, and that they recognized deviations from the normal and quickly sought appropriate medical consultations. Low-risk pregnancies and deliveries managed by nurse midwives resulted in fewer low-birth-weight babies, fewer forceps deliveries, less fetal monitoring, less medication, and shorter inpatient stays for labor and delivery. At eighty-four free-standing birth clinics in which nurse midwives gave care in about 75 percent of the labors and births (Rooks, Weatherby, Ernst, Stapleton, Rosen, and Rosenfeld, 1989), there were lower rates of cesarean births and rates of infant mortality that were comparable to those in studies of low-risk hospital births. The midwives were equally capable of giving good care to high-risk patients in collaboration with physicians (Bell and Mills, 1989).

The OTA report also found high patient acceptance rates and in some studies greater satisfaction with nurse midwives than with obstetricians. Women particularly appreciated the quality and quantity of information and the sharing of control. Despite the formal support of the American College of Obstetricians and Gynecologists, there was resistance from general and family physicians, who saw the nurse midwives as threatening the physicians' sole control of this specialty. Again, physicians' approval increased as their control over nurse midwives increased.

The positive results from CNMs' care and their competence are sustained in evidence from more recent research studies. In 1991, for example, the National Center for Health Statistics studied all single, vaginal births in the United States, delivered at between thirty-five and forty-three weeks of gestation by either certified nurse midwives or physicians. Controlling for many social and medical risk factors, the results were impressive: "the risk of experiencing an infant death was 19 percent lower for births attended by certified nurse midwives than for births attended by physicians. . . . The risk of neonatal mortality . . . was 33 percent lower, and the risk of delivering a low birth weight infant was 31 percent lower" (American Public Health Association, 1998b, p. 12). Analysts attributed the CNMs' excellent performance to spending more time with their prenatal patients, emphasizing preventive and supportive care, counseling, and providing care throughout the entire labor and delivery process, while physicians' care is more episodic. It was also noted that the proportion of births attended by CNMs in the United States increased from 3 percent in 1989 to 6 percent in 1995. Though the growth in using CNMs is frustratingly slow, their cost-effectiveness and competence is now fully documented.

Cost-Effectiveness of Nurses Confirmed

Many of the problems in assessing cost-effectiveness previously discussed by Freund and Overstreet (1981) were still apparent in the OTA report; nevertheless, the evidence presented confirmed the nurses' cost-effectiveness as physician substitutes with equivalent or better outcomes, particularly given their patients' greater adherence to care plans, and the nurses' considerably lower costs of training. The analysis by Jane Record and her colleagues (1980), followed by that of Lauren LeRoy (1982), had also established the same general conclusions. As Diers and Molde (1979) had previously observed (see chapter 7), the OTA report also pointed to the continuing problem of patient/time measures that overvalued medically oriented services at the expense of the treatment and prevention of health problems. To overcome this, costs per episode, not simply per visit, proved that NPs were at least 20 percent less costly than MDs. And in 1989 a national survey of maternity-care costs found that the average cost of a normal pregnancy and delivery by a nurse midwife was $994 but for a physician, $1,492—about a third more (Minor, 1989).

A second continuing problem is that the research was based on substitution practices, not on the full use of nurses' capabilities since these are constrained by restrictive legal requirements. Critically important was the central constraint: physicians' willingness or unwillingness to delegate tasks. As the OTA report asserted, some physicians admitted that they could safely delegate *more* tasks; thus, estimates of the nurses' potential productivity were underestimated, and cost-effectiveness would be higher if legal and physicians' restraints were withdrawn.

The direct costs of education were much easier to ascertain; nurse practitioners' education cost about 20 percent as much as physicians' education: in 1979, $10,300 compared to $60,700; and in 1986, an estimated $14,600 versus $86,100. Clearly, several nurse practitioners could be educated for the cost of educating one physician. Following education, the direct cost of provider compensation differs substantially, and on average primary-care physicians earn four times as much as nurse practitioners. According to a 1989 analysis for the Institute of Medicine, nurse midwives earned an average of $30,000 compared to $296,000 for obstetricians (S. Cohn, 1989). Obviously, the overvaluation of physicians can be directly traced to their state-sanctioned monopoly and to the unregulated fee-for-service type of compensation. Clearly, nurse practitioners were cost-effective.

Continuing evidence from 1987 and into the 1990s sustained with qualifications the earlier data on cost-effectiveness of nurse practitioners. This is apparent in Dr. Claire Fagin's 1990 review of the research from 1981 to 1990. It was also obvious in other analyses (McGrath, 1990; Kearnes, 1992; Nichols, 1992; Safriet, 1992). Similarly, evidence continued to support the positive findings in the OTC report. For example, Bezjak (1987) studied physician-perceived incentives for association with nurse practitioners, and Feldman, Ventura, and Crosby (1987) reviewed studies of nurse practitioners' effectiveness and analyzed issues in practice and theory in research. Kane, Garrard, Skay, Radosevich, Buchanan, McDermott, Arnold, and Kepferle (1989) studied the positive impact of geriatric nurse practitioners on the process and outcome of care in nursing homes. Most significantly, using meta-analysis, registered nurses Dr. Sharon A. Brown, RN, and Dr. Deanna E. Grimes, RN, (1992) focused on the process of care, clinical outcomes, and cost-effectiveness of nurses in primary care. Meta-analysis is a statistical method for synthesizing research data from a number of studies; in Brown and Grimes's research, it involved some thirty-eight investigations of nurse practitioners and fifteen studies of nurse midwives, using physician care as the standard for comparison. Adjustments for sample size and heterogeneity were included. The obvious advantage to meta-analysis is that it allows an exact estimation of statistical results, a decided improvement over previous descriptive comparisons. It is now possible to assert *statistically* that the fifty-three studies *proved* that NPs provided more health-promotion activities, such as patient education and exercise recommendations, than physicians. The nurses ordered laboratory tests for 36 percent of their patients, compared to 30 percent of physicians' patients, but the costs of the nurses' tests were 8 percent *lower*. Both the NPs and physicians were equivalent in their rates of prescribing drugs. On clinical outcomes, the nurses achieved statistically equivalent outcomes or scored more favorably than physicians on most variables. Compared to physicians' patients, the nurses' patients demonstrated equivalent or greater satisfaction, more compliance with recommendations, and greater knowledge of these and of their health status. Finally, the nurses scored higher on the measure of quality of care, which involved diagnostic accuracy and/or completeness of the care process, for example, in taking comprehensive medical/health histories.

Although the nurses had two years of experience, compared to seventeen years for the physicians, they still achieved equal or better results. And although they spent more time with patients (an average of 24.9 minutes compared to the physicians' 16.5 minutes per patient), the average cost per visit was significantly lower, by 39 percent, a difference confounded by providers' differentials in salaries. The numbers of visits per patient were equivalent, but the nurses' patients experienced somewhat fewer hospitalizations than those of physicians. All of these studies and analyses added more evidence to support nurse practitioners' effectiveness and competence (as if any more were needed!) and some began to pinpoint more precisely the *processes* of nursing care that accounted for their superiority.

The Rise of the Corporate Ethos

Despite evidence of competent care and cost-effectiveness, changes in the delivery of health care were making the nurses' quest for greater autonomy more problematic. Nurses such as Diane Feeney Mahoney (1988) warned about the effects of rapid changes in the health-care system on nurses, who faced increasing competition and pressures for cost-effectiveness. For example, the retrospective system of payment had been changed in Medicare reimbursement to a prospective payment system in which costs are preestablished for different health problems (diagnostic related groups, or DRGs). Significantly, Mahoney warned that nurse practitioners who "focus only on obtaining traditional third-party reimbursement can become eligible only to find acceptance in an outdated payment methodology" (p. 45). Thus, efforts must shift to obtaining positions on HMO and PPO boards to ensure utilization of nurse practitioners.

Mahoney asserted that the rise of the corporate ethos in medicine would make nurses' problems more difficult and complex, particularly since a surplus of 145,000 physicians was projected by the year 2000. Economic theory usually predicts that increased supply will lower consumer demand and providers' prices; however, physicians' services, seen as a necessity, lead consumers to demand the same quantity of services regardless of price. This phenomenon, noted Mahoney, is termed inelasticity of demand, but it can be threatened by the availability of substitutes, such as nurse practitioners, who can decrease the inelastic demand for medical services: "Predictably, the group in control does not desire to see their power diminished by a substitute group" (p. 45). Thus, an increase in the supply of providers will "cause those in control to react defensively against encroachment" (p. 45). Physicians will try to mandate themselves as primary providers and, given a surplus, will move from specialties to general practice and to practice outside of traditional practice settings. To struggle against these trends is difficult because APNs and PAs are constrained by physician and institutional independence, legal restrictions, and problems with direct reimbursement.

Indeed, in 1986, a representative of the AMA claimed that the market forces that promoted physician extenders no longer existed. By allowing a surplus of physicians, organized medicine could exclude PAs. Nurse practitioners,

however, are independently licensed, certified, and authorized to practice under state nurse practice acts: they are based in nursing and not subject to direct
medical control. Given the confused and contradictory status of state laws, the
multiple restrictions, and the involvement of state medical boards, the possibility of medical control was, nevertheless, still very likely. Mahoney urged
APNs to align not with medical, but with nursing administration, who should
use the nurse shortage to decrease physicians' influence and nurses' dependence.

Institutional dependence, particularly in hospitals, may be increasingly inappropriate as some of the surplus physicians locate in hospital-based clinics
and ambulatory-care facilities. Thus, Mahoney recommended that nurse practitioners move to community settings, such as industrial health services, hospitals, home care, and elderly housing units. Given the trend toward releasing
hospital patients "quicker and sicker," community programs were increasingly necessary.

Again the Old Canard: "Practicing Medicine without a License"

How can nurses, if legally restricted, practice independently in these settings if medical challenges in the legal system are likely to continue and even
escalate. For example, a suit—*Sermchief v. Gonzales,* 600 SW 2nd 683, 1983—
was brought by the physicians and osteopaths of the Missouri Board of Registration for the Healing Arts against two nurses for practicing in expanded
roles. Neither woman had caused any injury or patient complaint; nevertheless, "the initial trial court ruling found the nurses' actions, such as history-
taking, performing physical examinations and giving birth control counseling,
constituted the unlawful practice of medicine" (Mahoney, 1988, p. 48). Fortunately, "the Superior Court recognized that the intent of the state's Nurse Practice Act revision was to substantively change the law" (p. 48). The nurses' actions were authorized under the Missouri Nurse Practice Act. Because of the
national efforts by nurses to change such laws, the two nurse practitioners
were exonerated.

Mahoney urged nurses to support changes in nurse practice acts to expand
roles and to give authorizing power exclusively to the Board of Registration in
Nursing. Nurses had previously compromised to obtain legislative reform by
accepting reviews by interdisciplinary boards, which included medical personnel, presumably to ensure safe care. By the beginning of the 1990s there was
enough research that "clearly substantiates the quality of practitioner services.
Complex multiboard review is no longer necessary" (p. 48). Thus, nurses were
again urged to take full control of their profession.

Like many others, Mahoney noted that the final barrier, independent payment, requires that nurses' services, previously billed under physician charges
or agency fees, must be clearly and separately designated. This would "allow

the system to separate out the contribution made by each provider and allow more accurate monitoring of their respective cost impacts" (p. 49). Thus, said Mahoney, a consumer faced with a charge of $20 for a nurse practitioner and $35 for a physician could choose the least costly provider, benefitting both consumer and insurer.

The categorical fee structure now prices service according to the most efficient service, regardless of the kind of provider. Using this system, routine services, such as the monitoring of common episodic problems, would be priced at a lower rate than those established for complex, acute diagnostic evaluations. Obviously, nurse practitioners would have a good chance of being the least costly alternative. Furthermore, freed from dependence on physician referrals, nurse practitioners could charge lower fees. But would they? Mahoney noted that nurse midwives, as recipients of third-party payments, have continued to charge lower fees than obstetricians. To gain entry or maintain a market share, nurse practitioners will have to charge lower fees. Mahoney urged nurses to lobby for reimbursement based on *both* cost reduction and consumer choice.

Critical to Mahoney's recommendation is a central issue: Do nurses function as complements to or substitutes for physicians' services? Traditionally, the coordinating, facilitating, and clarifying roles embrace, but do not substitute for or replace, physicians' services. From this perspective, claimed Mahoney, nurses (predominantly women) are seen as dependent on physicians (predominantly men). The alternative—substitution—allows women to be independent from men in order to foster their own values. Thus, they could emphasize healthy lifestyles, early detection of problems, treatments to minimize hospitalizations, and coping with the effects of chronic illnesses. Mahoney was urging nurse practitioners not only to be physician substitutes, but to use their nursing orientation to create something more than what is usually offered by physicians. Obviously, nurses, predominantly women, come from a different subculture and bring with them different approaches to health issues.

Research on APNs was needed that went beyond simple measures of consumer satisfaction, quantity, or even quality of care. Rather, research that differentiated nurse and physician practitioners and established productivity measures appropriate to nurses' approaches to health needs was critical. Advanced practice nurses must insist on measures of *nursing* and medical interventions: "Otherwise, NPs appear to use more time than physicians in treating similar diagnoses and may wrongfully be considered inefficient" (p. 50).

Studies that focus on seeing a large volume of clients during brief, multiple visits do not, said Mahoney, provide appropriate measures of nursing care. Additionally, complex clients, particularly those in lower socioeconomic groups who are medically underserved and often served by nurses, cannot be equated with the usual caseload of most physicians. Mahoney urged nurses to insist on comparability of patients in any research conducted. Indeed, she recommended productivity measures that go beyond the per-visit emphasis, considering instead the entire course of treatments. From this perspective, nurses' concerns about continuity of care can be demonstrated in fewer visits, less hospitalization, and more effective outcomes. As one example, a nation-wide survey conducted by Everitt, Avorn, and Baker (1987) presented similar case situations and provided the opportunity to ask for more information on clients. Mahoney noted: "While the MDs were quick to prescribe medications without obtaining detailed histories, NPs took more complete histories and more often favored non-drug therapies" (p. 50). Mahoney believed that nurses' backgrounds favor active listening to clients' concerns. Translated, women are traditionally supposed to listen to others and to be concerned with interpersonal relations. Certainly, the differences found in research are related not only to professional but to gender-role socialization as well.

New Organizational Structures: The Latest Threat to Nurses' Autonomy

In agreement with Mahoney, Linda V. Walsh (1988) said that emerging alternative health-care systems "pose a potential threat to the growth of autonomous nursing practice" (p. 56). Unfortunately, these newer systems continue to retain the physician as the primary provider and to restrict direct access to nurses. Walsh reviewed two separate developments in the provision of alternative health care: direct-service providers, such as home health agencies, ambulatory surgical centers, dialysis centers and birth centers; and mechanisms for financing health care, including health maintenance organizations (HMOs), individual practice associations (IPAs), preferred provider organizations (PPOs), and exclusive provider organizations. Walsh claimed that it is "difficult for the nurse practitioner to keep abreast of the administrative aspects of each organization and the impact that the organizational structure will have on professional nursing practice" (p. 56).

As those in power respond quickly to cost-containment mandates, nurses may be forced into a reactive position, thwarting their initiative and momentum to change sex-stratified systems. HMOs providing comprehensive care for fixed prepaid premiums were stimulated by the 1973 congressional actions and subsidies for startup costs. Preferred provider organizations vary widely, but consumers retain freedom of choice, usually of physician providers. There are often financial incentives, such as discounted fees, to use these providers; geographic or population limitations also encourage use of PPOs, which range from a single provider to a corporation formed to provide a discount rate. These PPOs differ from HMOs in that they do not restrict consumers to participating providers. Consumers or groups purchase the care so there is no financial risk to providers.

Traditionally, physicians assume an entrepreneurial and nurses a salaried, institution-based approach; however, nurses who seek independent practice threaten physicians as the nurses move from service and charity to compete in one of the largest business empires. The physician surplus projected for the 1990s and beyond, claimed Walsh, creates an economic incentive to restrict nursing practice and to retain gatekeeper status through control of third-party payment, hospital privileges, referrals, and diagnostic services: "Even in HMOs and PPOs where economic incentives should support the use of nurse practitioners, the future participation of nurses is questionable because of the difference in focus of care" (p. 61). Walsh noted that HMOs have "increasingly moved to the medical model of provision of episodic or acute care, rather than retaining their original provision of services supporting 'health maintenance'" (p. 61). Since nurses have been particularly effective in long-term care and continuity of services, the medical control of alternative systems will keep "nurses in a dependent role to physicians" (p. 61).

Walsh urged nurses to monitor federal and state regulations and stop proposed revisions that include any restriction of nurses to dependent roles. She also recommended membership on nurses' legislative committees, subscription to publications on legislative activities, regular contact with legislators on health-care committees, use of professional consultations on financing of new structures, and coalitions with other professional and community groups, such as those dealing with women, children, and the elderly. For example, PPOs can be challenged by antitrust laws if they create a monopoly in health care. As advocates for clients, nurses need to be certain their rights are protected. Clearly, rapid changes in organizational structures and in profit-making institutions would create major problems for nurses if these alternatives sustained or even enhanced the medical monopoly. Indeed, as discussed in chapter 10, the increase in HMOs' influence over the structure and provision of health care in the United States grew at an astonishing rate in the 1990s, affecting both physicians' and nurses' practices as well as threatening patients' safety.

"Nursing Will *Not* Let This Happen": The RCT Proposal

As new health-care organizational structures emerged, there is no doubt that organized medicine again moved to exclude or subordinate nurses. The active opposition to nurses' autonomy by medical associations was very clear. Not only did the AMA break away from the National Joint Practice Commission, which had been devoted to improving nurse-physician relations, but it created physician's assistants, giving them greater power than nurses when the nurses refused to conform and take on medical "leftovers" under increased medical control. The physician's assistant classification was established *unilaterally*, without the involvement of organized nursing. Organized nursing countered with nurse practitioners, whose expanded roles were fought by state medical groups in the clinics and courts. Medical schools began to admit larger numbers of students, creating a surplus that countered the increased clinical sophistication of the nurse practitioners. As if these measures were not enough, by the late 1980s, the AMA and their state associations had rejected additional federal educational funds for nursing, fought nurses' prescription rights, and forced restrictive alterations in the new nurse practice acts. The attack on nurses from the top down is clear. But the attack by physicians from the bottom was also obvious. Organized medicine recommended still another category of health worker, the registered care technologist (RCT), who would be, like the PA, directly under medical control. With this latest move, physicians' strategy of eliminating or totally subordinating women nurses could not be mistaken.

In 1988 *The American Nurse* published a report entitled "Nursing Opposes RCTs," including the full press release from the ANA which "expressed outrage at a recent move by organized medicine to solve the nursing shortage by introducing a new category of health-care providers called 'Registered Care Technologist (RCT)'" (p. 2). Despite the objections of *sixteen* national nurses organizations, the AMA House of Delegates moved to establish pilot training programs for RCTs. American Nurses' Association president Dr. Lucille Joel stated that nurses were appalled at medicine's lack of concern for consumer safety. Given increasing hospital admissions of the acutely ill, the very old, high-risk infants, and persons undergoing massive medical and surgical procedures, "What we need is for physicians to spend more time with us at the bedside rather than to send us technicians to carry out doctors orders" (p. 2).

Once again, physicians were involved in directly controlling the practice of nursing; this time, by creating a position for high school graduates, trained in the hospital, to carry out physicians' orders: "They would be accountable to physicians and be extended the right to practice by state medical boards" (p. 2). For all practical purposes, physicians would directly resume control over bedside nursing.

Nurses viewed this plan as both shortsighted and ill-conceived, and saw no reason why nurses should supervise and train such persons since a new category of health workers would not solve the nursing shortage, "which medicine has chosen to ignore" (p. 2). Instead, nursing organizations called for maximizing the efficiency of existing registered professional and licensed practical nurses through support staff, nurse's aides, clerical help, dietary aides, and transport personnel. Furthermore, they called for better compensation and working conditions for nurses themselves. Pointedly asserting that physicians had achieved control and substantial financial gains for themselves, Joel insisted that they support similar economic gains and control of practice by nurses: "In 1986 physician income increased by 10 percent with average MD earnings at $112,700. The average maximum salary for hospital-employed RNs was $27,744 in 1986 and $29,088 in 1987, a 4.8 percent increase" (p. 2).

Holding nothing back, Joel asserted that physicians ought to look to their own practice: "'The increasing number of lawsuits filed against the medical profession is evidence of a major problem in the delivery of care'" (p. 2). She concluded: "Medicine needs to clean up its own house before it looks to intervene in the practice of other professionals" (p. 2). To introduce minimally trained people would jeopardize patient care, and "Nurses will have no part in jeopardizing the quality of patient care or in escalating the cost of care in this manner" (p. 2). Again, in a hard-hitting assertion, Joel concluded that the AMA action was still another effort to control the health-care delivery system. "We refuse to stand and watch medicine add confusion and costs to an already fragmented and costly health care system" (p. 2). To her, "one of the primary effects of the proposal will be to enhance the monopoly power of physicians in the health care marketplace. Nursing will not let this happen" (p. 2). If nurses had to take on the AMA, she affirmed that the nursing organizations would do so.

These assertions are a far cry from nursing's mild and respectful statements of the past. No holds were barred, and the power game was defined and explained in a public press release. Organized nursing claimed that the AMA was attacking from both ends; the least educated caregivers would be directly controlled by physicians and the higher educated nurse practitioners would be eliminated through active opposition to legal changes in their practice and by creating excessive numbers of new physicians.

The AMA began the move toward the RCT proposal in 1986 when a board of trustees report on nursing education and personnel again recommended support for *all* levels of nursing, not for the efforts by the ANA and other nursing organizations to establish specific educational entry level requirements and limited categories of caregivers. The trustees called for the RCT, who would care for the chronically ill, the frail elderly, and the less critically ill. In short, they would be under *direct* control of physicians. At joint meetings of the AMA and ANA executive committees in 1988, the nurses stated their opposition to the proposal. Later, AMA officials decided that the RCT report would go through without further input from the ANA.

By May 1988 representatives of twenty-nine national nursing organizations reached consensus on strategies to deal with the nursing shortage and subsequently sent a joint letter to William Hotchkiss, AMA president. By June the nurses had voted unanimously at the ANA House of Delegates to oppose the RCT. Nevertheless, by the end of June, the AMA moved to proceed with the pilot projects. By mid-year the press was notified, and nurses met to deal with the nursing shortages by themselves.

"The Nurse Is the Doctor's Right Arm": A View from the AMA

In an interview conducted by Richard Froh (1988), a member of the editorial board of *Nursing Economics,* AMA vice president James Sammons asserted that the RCT would not duplicate nursing efforts. Froh noted that nursing leaders had developed their own strategies for easing the nursing shortage: reallocating resources, designing new staffing systems, and drawing on established nursing education. Why, he asked Sammons, couldn't the AMA concentrate on supporting funding for nursing education rather than the RCT? In a response that challenges the credulity of any informed reader, Sammons stated, "The AMA has always been and will always be a vocal supporter of increased funding for nursing education as well as higher salaries for nurses to attract and retain quality individuals" (p. 221). The AMA's historical record on this issue certainly does not support this assertion! Sammons then validated the AMA's support of the RCT, no doubt aware that women, who were most likely to assume the new role, would do the work under the control not of nurses but of predominantly male physicians.

Froh, who was also vice president of the Kaiser Foundation Health Plan in Washington, D.C., pointedly asked why the AMA believed it could resolve a shortage in another profession external to medicine. Sammons skirted the issue of professional independence and focused on patient care, claiming that RCTs would not take away jobs from nurses because of the void caused by shortage. One can only wonder what Sammons's response would have been if nurses had suggested that an RCT be trained to do the jobs of physicians, despite their objections and ignoring the issue of medical professional control and authority.

Sammons viewed the reason for the shortage as simply the absence of trained but inactive nurses, and again asserted the AMA's support for "the most underpaid professionals . . . of any group in this country ever" (p. 221). Failing to acknowledge the historical facts which led to the increasing disparity between physicians' and nurses' salaries, particularly in the last few decades, he simply suggested that corporations and school systems could outbid hospitals for nurses' services. This ignores the fact, of course, that the majority of nurses are employed by hospitals, not by schools or industries. Indeed, Sammons believed that today's "women have open to them any and every opportunity they choose to take advantage of, I think that the salary level of nurses is badly in need of updating" (p. 221). Certainly, he was overly optimistic about opportunities for women and chose not to recognize the roughly one-third less that female workers make compared to men; yet he is correct that women can choose other work. However, he did not address how nurses' salaries could be increased or how physicians' salaries could be decreased to achieve greater parity in income levels.

Sammons finally got to the heart of the issue: "the nurses themselves have done something that truly troubles me. They have finally convinced themselves that people do not appreciate the fact that they are professionals . . . nurses are concerned about their image and that they do not think the public appreciates them. They think that doctors do not really appreciate what they do. They do not have the standing in the community that they used to have" (p. 221). Sammons disagreed with the nurses' perceptions, evidently unaware of the medical sociological studies and pronouncements on nursing as a "semiprofession." Admitting "isolated instances" of negative MD perceptions, he nevertheless stated that any sick person in a hospital or any physician who has practiced more than twenty-four hours knows that "the nurse is a very vital, integral part of the care of that patient. I do not think they are looked down on. I do not think they should talk themselves into that, but they certainly seem to have done so" (p. 221). In short, Sammons blamed the victim: the nurses themselves are at fault, deluded, evidently, in their views of themselves.

Sammons acknowledged the need for career ladders in nursing, but said nothing about nurse practitioners; indeed, he concluded that with hospitals losing money, it would be difficult to appropriate funds for nursing career ladders. Thus, the AMA's support for better reimbursement for nurses was superficial at best if Sammons's prognosis on current economic conditions held.

Froh moved logically to the AMA's consistent opposition to nurses' expanded practice. Given tight economic constraints, he asked, why shouldn't consumers have the opportunity to have qualified nurse practitioners' care for them rather than be forced to visit more costly physicians? Obviously, if physicians could give substantial medical functions to medical corpsmen, why should they think nurses unqualified to do the same functions? This was not Sammons's position. Instead of drawing on the research which proved nurses' competence as practitioners, Sammons questioned their qualifications and voiced the old canard: "If nurses want to be practitioners of medicine, they should go to medical school. If doctors want to do bedside nursing, they should go to nursing school. Clearly, there is an in-between stage that nurses have always fulfilled" (p. 222).

What constitutes the "in-between" stage? Sammons is unclear about this, or sees it as medically defined, since he stated, "Nurses have always been the doctor's right arm," and concluded, "I do not believe the nursing profession can take over the practice of medicine" (p. 222). At no point did Sammons admit that medicine has encroached on another healer's territory, or that physicians had taken over women's traditional healing activities, or that they have sharply restricted nurses from doing what they are able to do, or that medical corpsmen were given diagnostic and prescriptive rights denied to better qualified nurses.

Instead, Sammons concluded: "What you have is a group of very vocal nurses who want to do more in terms of medical practice than nursing practice" (p. 222). He again advised them to go to medical school. He admitted that nurses' expanded roles were an area in which "the AMA and organized nursing have had disagreements and will probably continue to do so" (p. 222). In an echo of historical rhetoric, Sammons essentially said that physicians would not allow nurses to expand their roles because they were "unqualified," but at the same time, allowed no possibility for them to become qualified unless they became physicians. At no point did Sammons recognize this as a sexist restriction, which was leading many women to reject nursing as too subservient, or to leave nursing because the field is too restrictive.

Froh asked Sammons about the role of the AMA in representing physicians' interests, but Sammons denied that the AMA places medical self-interest over the public's health and welfare. Again, the historical record does not fully support this assertion since the AMA has traditionally rejected many efforts for social reform and legislation, in contrast to the ANA, which has usually supported them. Sammons ignored this history and concluded that the AMA was doing well in representing the public. He claimed that the "biggest problem today . . . [is] the right of the physician to continue to exercise that professional judgment" (p. 223). He connected this to problems with Medicare and Medicaid policies. Still, to him, "the real major, screaming, crying concern today is the ability to make professional judgments . . . and not get second-guessed by a whole series of alphabet soups that are out there" (p. 223).

Sammons complained that physicians were receiving more insulting letters in which their professional judgments on medical matters were second-guessed. He rejected the new fee system based on diagnostic related groups (DRGs), and rejected Medicare and other government restrictions on physicians' incomes, even asserting that "there is a significant part of the Medicare population that can afford to pay more" (p. 224). However, when asked about a government proposal to compel physicians to refund to Medicare patients all monies related to denied Medicare claims, Sammons stated the AMA was contesting the legality of such a proposal on the basis of who had the right to define what is necessary care. What is clear is that the AMA was fighting to retain physicians' privileged economic position and rejecting any efforts, particularly governmental, to control physicians' power.

Froh asked Sammons why the AMA refused to support Senator Edward Kennedy's 1987 Nursing Shortage Redirection Act. Sammons claimed that it was far too expensive and would not solve the problem. The AMA's lack of support for money for nursing was not explained further. Froh pursued this issue, however, and asked why the AMA had also refused to support legislation introduced by Senator George Mitchell to provide support for graduate education costs for nurse clinical training in teaching hospitals. Sammons said physicians were "opposed to the tinkering being done with graduate medical education funding" (p. 225). He stressed integration of such sources for what he termed "aspects of medicine" and rejected individual concerns without appropriate input. "Appropriate" obviously meant from medical schools or other bodies, all controlled, one may assume, by physicians or by hospital or university administrators.

Nevertheless, Sammons insisted: "We are not anti-nursing. Let me hasten to say that. Unfortunately, there seem to be a lot of people in this country who think we are. Nothing could be further from the truth; that is absurd" (p. 225). Indeed, he claimed the AMA's position was not anti anything; it was "pro"— a plea for integration. It is truly extraordinary that this physician would assert this and think nurses were so naïve as to believe it! If physicians could stop funding for educational programs for professions in which they had *no* membership, and if they could "integrate" funds which they could then divert for their own interests—surely the power play is obvious even to the most apolitical person.

Nurses were not the only women to be excluded or subordinated by Sammons. When asked about the 1986 Massachusetts law requiring hospitals to make public data on the frequency of cesarean sections done on women, Sammons replied: "I think that is almost as dumb as Hitler releasing the mortality statistics" (p. 226). He completely ignored the position of the women's health movement and the appalling findings presented in well-researched books, such as *The Silent Knife* (Cohen and Estner, 1983), which showed a shocking increase in unnecessary C-sections, many having substantially negative effects. Sammons simply noted that patients themselves influence physicians' choices for surgery, and that some studies support the incidence of cesarean sections. To blame women for a rise in the rates of unnecessary surgery is simply not acceptable. Since he had previously argued for no governmental intervention in physicians' judgments, it was illogical for Sammons to turn around and blame women for unnecessary cesarean surgeries. The weight of research is now overwhelmingly negative on unnecessary cesarean sections. Surely, AMA leaders should be responsible for knowing the trends of the latest research and taking a moral and professional position on improper surgical intervention into women's bodies.

No Need to Reinvent the Wheel! Nurse Leaders Reject the AMA-Sponsored Technologists

Several nursing leaders were interviewed and asked to respond to Sammons's assertions. Dr. Lucille A. Joel, ANA president, stated that nurse practitioners were not medical practitioners but nurses with advanced preparation, often holding master's degrees. These nurses performed physical examinations and health assessments, recognized acute recurring disease symptoms, managed chronic diseases, coordinated patient services provided referrals to other health caregivers, conducted patient counseling and education, and offered services to improve and maintain peoples' health status. Significantly, Joel did not list the specific functions already given over to physician's assistants in the 1970s. She pointedly asserted that nurses "collaborated" with, but presumably no longer obeyed, physicians and others.

To Joel, advanced practice nurses were needed as medicine became more specialized, particularly given the geographical maldistribution of physicians and increased cost-containment efforts. How well did the nurse practitioners function? What, in Sammons's terms, was their "quality"? Joel referred to the review by the Office of Technology Assessment (1986) discussed earlier, which concluded that "the quality of care provided by nurse practitioners functioning within their areas of training and expertise tends to be as good or better than care provided by physicians" (as cited in Froh, 1988, p. 228). From the review of comparison studies, the report further claimed that patients were more satisfied with the nurse practitioners in "personal interest exhibited, reduction in the professional mystique of health-care delivery, amount of information conveyed, and cost of care" (as cited in Froh, 1988, p. 228).

The layperson may well ask why Sammons, the executive vice president of the AMA, did not know these research findings. Or, if he was aware of them, why did he choose to ignore them? If he was genuinely concerned about the qualifications of nurses, why did he not seem to know or acknowledge the studies that provided an answer to his concern? Furthermore, why did he seem so uninformed on the realities of the nursing shortage?

In contrast, Dr. Joel asserted that more nurses were working then ever before: Almost 1.6 million of the 2 million registered nurses were employed, representing a labor force participation rate of 80 percent, a higher rate than other predominately female occupations. Thus, Sammons's assertion that not enough nurses were working could not be the central issue. Rather, said Joel, the demand for nurses had escalated. As evidence, she said: "Hospitals have increased the use of RNs from 50 to 100 patients in 1972 to 95 per 100 patients in 1986—a 92% increase" (p. 228). More nurses are used because more education and expertise are required as technological demands increase, patient activity levels worsened, and shorter lengths of stay put more demands on nurses, whose "salaries and working conditions have not improved to keep pace with increased demands" (p. 228). Added to this is the increased need for nurses in skilled nursing facilities, home-care agencies, and health maintenance organizations, and for public health needs. Joel challenged physicians to cooperate in creating collaborative relations, to become true partners, to help nurses achieve salaries commensurate with their actual responsibilities, and to support efforts to enhance nurses' image.

In contrast to Joel's pointed but restrained response to Sammons, Patricia Jordan, president of the American Nephrology Nurses' Association, took direct issue with Sammons's misconception of the nursing shortage, which to her represented the AMA's fundamental lack of understanding or acceptance of professional nurses. Referring to nursing's very low (0.9 percent) unemployment rate, Jordan claimed that the demand for professional nursing services has "simply outstripped the current supply" (p. 229). Furthermore, the supply of RNs will continue to be inadequate for two major reasons: first, a decrease in the number of college-age people; and second, a change in the value systems of America's youth. Thus Jordan warned: "[C]areers demonstrating poor working conditions, noncompetitive salaries, compressed salary structures, and poor professional image will not be attractive to individuals who value money, status, and power . . . [this applies] not only to nursing but also to individuals whom the AMA thinks will be attracted into RCT programs as opposed to existing nursing programs. The last insult our complex health-care system needs is another health-care worker" (p. 229). Calling for a *simplification* of the health-care system, Jordan urged the AMA to abandon the RCT concept, stating there is no need to "reinvent the wheel."

To Susan W. Salmond, president of the National Association of Orthopaedic Nurses, "The practice of nursing is NOT restricted to the 'bedside.' Nurses with advanced education and certification are *qualified* to specialize in expanded roles and work in a variety of health-care settings" (p. 230). The "in-between" stage does represent an overlap in services, but these are implemented differentially by members of the two professions. The size and responsibility of the overlap are "NOT dependent on what physicians decide to define it as (that is, what they don't want to do)" (p. 230). Indeed, Salmond pointed out that many functions in the "in-between" area are "gladly delegated by physicians to physician assistants—a group of health-care workers with less education, training, and experience. In this regard, 'qualified' takes on a new meaning—'that which is determined and controlled by medicine'" (p. 230). Salmond claimed that nurses *are* operating legally within their own autonomous scope of nursing practice. In her view, the determination of quality must be based on the type and outcome of service, data on complications, and consumer satisfaction: "These are objective criteria by which the public can judge 'qualified'" (p. 230).

Dr. Salmond then turned to the nursing shortage, agreeing with Dr. Joel that more nurses than ever are employed but new markets for home care, ambulatory services, and specialty care now exist: "These jobs often are innovative and flexible, allowing for a more autonomous expression of nursing" (p. 230). In addition, the women's movement has helped create more opportunities for women who are not choosing nursing: "This is an image problem—not one that nurses have talked themselves into!" (p. 230). Also, the shift among young people from human services values to financial rewards is also well-documented. The quick fix solution—increasing starting salaries substantially, but providing inadequate financial remuneration for experienced practitioners—is no solution: "People will not be drawn into nursing when they can expect only a 36% salary increase over their lifetime as compared to a computer programmer at 106% and an accountant at 193%" (p. 230).

Even more fundamental, said Salmond, is the view that nursing is not an autonomous profession: "This image of nursing is encouraged by medicine's continued portrayal of nursing as the 'right arm of medicine' as stated by Dr. Sammons" (p. 230). To which Salmond retorted: "The image of myself as the nurse dangling from the physician's glenohumeral joint is not only comical but describes the inaccurate dependent image of nursing practice that makes it unattractive as a career choice" (p. 230). Medicine should support nursing as an independent and interrelated profession that "requires scientific and technological expertise combined with extraordinary depths of feeling and compassion" (p. 230).

These national nursing organization presidents represented the positions of thousands of men and women nurses. They were not a handful of dissidents, but elected leaders of well-established, respected nursing organizations. By the end of the 1980s it is clear that they were no longer accepting a subordinate position in the health-care system, but demanding the right to function as a central force in patient-care delivery. Ironically, in 1990 AMA leader Sammons was forced to resign a year before his expected retirement, not because of any arrogance and intransigence toward nursing, but because of a scandal involving him within his own organization (Wolinsky and Brune, 1995). And although organized nursing was largely successful in blocking full implementation of the RCT proposal, nurses still were forced to fight for their right to practice independently—with prescriptive authority, third-party reimbursement, and hospital/staff privileges.

Medical Attacks on Nurses' Prescriptive Authority

If nurses were to shed their subordinate position in the health-care delivery system and function as a central force in patient-care delivery, it is clear that certain barriers to their independent practice and autonomy must be broken. One such barrier, prescriptive authority, had been jealously guarded by physicians for decades. Their monopolistic control over prescribing drugs and devices was staunchly defended by the medical community and increasingly opposed by the nursing profession. In the allocation of more medical functions and prerogatives to PAs, primarily male medical corpsmen, prescriptive authority was allowed, but not to the mostly female APNs. The first limited prescriptive authority for nurse practitioners was achieved in 1975 in North Carolina and by nurse midwives in 1977 in Maine.

By 1979, most state licensure bodies and third-party carriers required nurse practitioners to act under physician supervision, presumably to ensure quality of care, but this also resulted in duplication of health-care costs. By 1980 statutory amendments granted prescriptive authority to nurse practitioners in seventeen states. These were implemented in thirteen states through regulations that varied markedly, ranging from an extension of medical authority to recognition of autonomy based on education and RN licensure; some regulations required medical supervision or limited drug prescription to an approved formulary for nurses. Even these changes were hard-won. Indeed, in 1981, a medical attack in Oregon on nurses' prescribing privileges was reported that was typical of actions throughout the nation. The Oregon Medical Association moved to limit the nurses' authority, won only two years previously in 1979. The Oregon legislature had also granted nurses the right to receive direct reimbursement for their services. But the medical association sponsored a bill to cut sharply the scope of independent practice achieved under the new state law, which gave qualified practitioners "permission to prescribe, under their own license, a wide range of medications without any specific protocols or working relationships with physicians" (*American Journal of Nursing*, 1981, p. 653).

The physicians never accepted the legislation which gave nurses prescriptive authority and continued efforts to repeal or restrict or to limit the number of drugs prescribed by the nurses. This attack occurred despite the requirement that the nurses meet criteria set by the Nurse Practitioner Prescription Advisory Council, which was composed of three physicians, three pharmacists, and three nurses. In addition, further education in pharmacology was required of the nurses before certification, and subsequent continuing education was mandated every two years. By 1981, seventy-eight nurse practitioners had been approved to prescribe from a formulary that included about 280 medications, but excluded experimental and narcotic drugs.

Women, both as practitioners and as patients, would have been directly affected if the MDs' bill had passed. Typical of the new independent practice, the Nurse Practitioners Community Health Clinic in Portland was run by women's health-care and pediatric nurse practitioners in an underserved area of the city. Women could receive routine gynecological care, including physical exams, Pap smears, vaginitis treatments, tests prior to birth control, prescriptions of birth control pills, and diaphragm fittings. Pelvic inflammatory disease was treated with medication after a phone consultation with a backup physician. Children were treated from birth to twenty-one years, and many were seen in home visits. Many patients were new emigrants from Vietnam, Laos, and Cambodia; therefore, the nurse practitioners dealt with problems such as tuberculosis, ova and parasites, and bacterial conjunctivitis.

All these activities of the nurse practitioners would have changed if the medical association's bill had passed. It would have restricted the prescriptive council to advising the medical board, which would have had "the ultimate authority to define the nurse practitioners' relationship with physicians; to determine the protocol for practice; to establish the formulary from which practitioners prescribe; and to set all the educational requirements for prescription-writing privileges" (p. 653). The physicians would have screened and approved nurses and the board would have approved their credentials. It is very important to understand that this struggle was gender-based and to recognize that in 1990 95 percent of nurses were women and 85 percent of physicians were men. From this view, men simply want to control women. That the issues of female and nursing autonomy were both at stake is obvious.

Nurses' Prescriptive Actions Based on Judgment, Not Mandate

Research on nurses' prescriptive practices was urgently needed to block physicians' assault on the nurses' newly won legal authority. In 1983 and again in 1985, Marjorie V. Batey and Jeanne M. Holland published results from their study of the impact of structured autonomy, accorded through state regulatory policies, on nurses' prescribing practices. The researchers sought to determine the degree to which varied structural arrangements influenced prescribing behaviors and to compare these with medical practices reported in other studies. A total of 401 nurse practitioners in five states with varying regulations were asked to keep prescription logs for ten clinical-practice days. The study reported on the 188, or 46.7 percent, who completed and returned their logs. These were classified into four groups, from lowest to highest, according to the autonomy allowed by the various states.

The proportions of patients given prescriptions did not vary consistently across these conditions, but in total the nurses gave somewhat fewer drugs per visit than physicians (1.82 versus 1.87). The level of autonomy seemed to have little influence on whether new drug therapies were initiated or old ones continued. Of all the drugs given, 56.2 percent had a generic option, and the researchers found that the higher proportions of generic prescribing occurred in the two conditions that did *not* require physician supervision. For example, in the most autonomous groups, 66 percent used generic drugs, but this usage did not correlate consistently among groups. The largest drug repertoire was associated with the highest autonomy, but again the variation across groups was inconsistent. The kinds of drugs by type, as categorized by Batey and Holland, did vary somewhat from physicians—who prescribed more analgesics, antidepressants, sedatives, hypnotics, and tranquilizers—to nurses, who prescribed more antibiotics, hormones, and respiratory drugs. The variations among nurses seemed to be related more to their distribution by type of practice, rather than to their degree of autonomy.

A critically important variable was the nurse practitioners' use of physician consultation or referral. The researchers found an 8.9 percent rate of consultation prior to prescribing and a 5.9 percent rate of referral of clients, who received prescriptions and were then sent to a physicians. Again, little association was found with level of autonomy among the independent decisions (85.4 percent) or those involving consultation or referral (14.6 percent). Certainly, these data provide evidence that nurses, *regardless of restrictions,* prescribe drugs without great reliance on physicians. Indeed, the nurses with lowest and highest regulatory autonomy were both only somewhat more likely to consult and refer. Batey and Holland concluded that prudent judgment regarding patients' needs was the most likely explanation of these findings. Judgment, not mandate, determined prescribing practices, which were quite comparable to those of physicians.

Probably the most important finding was that 85.4 percent of all prescriptions were made independent of medical involvement, which means "a high proportion of people seeking primary care could be managed by NPs alone" (Batey and Holland, 1983, p. 89). Obviously, significant savings in costs for patients would result, since the additional fees for physicians would not be charged and the cost of work time lost to get confirmation of nurses' diagnoses and prescriptions would be unnecessary. The finding that over half the prescriptions could be generic is also a potential cost-saving factor. Certainly, the data showed that nurses did not rely on physicians or state regulations to determine actual prescriptive judgments. Prudent patient care seemed characteristic of the nurses across all conditions of autonomy, making excessive state regulation an unnecessary as well as potentially costly factor, primarily useful to physicians at the expense of patients' income.

These findings were further supported by other studies on prescriptive authority. Janet Rosenaur, Dennyse Stanford, Walter Morgan, and Barbara Curtin (1984) researched the prescribing practices of 18 primary-care nurses with 1,683 patients over a six-month period. In earlier research (Munroe, Pohl, Gardner, and Bell, 1982), nurses had prescribed about one-third the number written by physicians: 98 percent to 99 percent of these were appropriate and safe. As noted previously, the patterns of prescribing in Batey and Holland's 1983 research were comparable, but again nurses were somewhat less likely than physicians to prescribe drugs and tended to prescribe somewhat different drugs.

The critically important aspect of the study conducted by Rosenaur and her colleagues is the information provided on nurse-physician consultations in relation to *specialization*. The nurses were family, women's health, pediatric, and adult-care practitioners, who were limited to prescribing from a formulary of 257 drugs or devices, representing 90 percent of commonly used drugs but excluding controlled substances. Consultation with a physician regarding the drug selections occurred in *only 5 percent* of all patient encounters and consultations with a pharmacist in *less than 1 percent*. The pediatric nurses were most likely to consult, and the women's health group least likely. The researchers stated: "The relatively low percentage of consultation activity with the physician is an interesting finding" (Rosenaur et al., 1984, p. 12). This may have been an underestimation, but it is equally likely that these results were accurate because the nurses simply did not need the physicians' assistance.

A second 1984 study may help to explain the low number of nurses' requests for help from physicians. Jeri L. Bigbee, Sharon Lundin, John Corbett, and James Collins compared the attitudes of pharmacists, physicians, nurse practitioners, and other selected nurses toward prescriptive authority for nurse practitioners. Recognizing that there was "considerable controversy" (p. 162), the researchers sent opinion questionnaires to 1,219 professionals in a state that, unlike fourteen others, had not yet legally permitted prescriptive authority for APNs. Of the 510 respondents, most physicians disagreed with, most nurses supported, and most pharmacists straddled the fence on prescriptive authority for nurse practitioners. Of the physicians, 66 percent disagreed somewhat or strongly with nurses' prescriptive authority. Among the nurses in general, the proportions were almost exactly reversed, with 70 percent agreeing that nurse practitioners should have prescriptive authority. Thus, the lines of opposition between the two groups of professionals were clearly drawn. Yet a few nurses crossed these lines to deny prescriptive authority to their colleagues. Physicians' opposition occurred even given a set of restrictive regulations that limited nurses to physician-approved protocols, a drug formulary of approved drugs, and interdisciplinary control by state medical, pharmacy, and nursing boards. Few would argue with mandatory education and certification, but given these assurances of competence, it is questionable whether restrictions on nurse practitioners are creditable, except as a way to placate physicians and sustain their monopolistic power.

A Mass of Contradictory and Restrictive Legislation

What did these interprofessional conflicts mean for the health consumer in the 1980s? How did regulations placed on nurses affect their capacity to act independently in behalf of their patients? Claire LaBar (1986) reviewed the national changes in prescriptive authority for nurses and found a slight increase; nineteen states allowed nurses to prescribe, but the regulations created a mass of restrictive problems. LaBar gave an example of a Georgia nurse midwife in private practice who could telephone in prescriptions, other than narcotics, only on behalf of her collaborating physicians and only for drugs listed on protocols developed with the physicians. Is this private practice? Under these limitations? In Missouri, nurse practitioners were restricted from prescribing by the pharmacy practice act, which did not list nurses among those who could prescribe. In South Carolina, the board of nursing approved nurse practitioner prescriptions according to protocols, but even with this limitation the attorney general did not agree. To get around this nonsense, nurses had to call in prescriptions as though they were from physicians, thus inconveniencing everyone.

Even what appears as nurse practitioners' autonomy was in practice severely limited by their status in particular specialties as regulated by a variety of state boards. In some states nursing boards regulated, but in others medical boards were in control. In still others, supervising physicians were required. In some states, such as Mississippi and Utah, even written agreements and practice protocols had to be state-approved. Similarly, the types and forms of pharmacological education required varied widely by experience and by type of degree credentials. Sometimes the laws required the authority, supervision, direction, or delegation by a physician. LaBar asked, "How many nurses have run the obstacle course?" (p. 32). She concluded that the transition period should be over; legislation that requires too many regulations and restrictions must be repealed.

It is this confusing mass of contradictory and inconsistent legislation designed to control nurses that led Linda J. Pearson (1986) to publish an editorial on prescriptions written by nurse practitioners regardless of enabling legislation. A questionnaire was included with the June 1985 issue of the *Nurse Practitioner;* 1,929 nurses responded from all regions of the country, but more heavily from the Northeast. Dividing the respondents into two groups, those from states with some sort of prescribing law for nurses and those from states without such legislation, the researchers found that the practices of calling prescriptions in to pharmacies or writing prescriptions on presigned prescription pads did not vary according to absence or presence of state prescriptive laws.

More nurse practitioners who reported writing a prescription and then obtaining a physician's signature or signing the physician's or nurse practitioner's name came from states *without* enabling legislation. More practitioners who used their own prescriptive authority came from states *with* enabling laws. But even nurses without state-sanctioned authority used this method if they were located in institutions that gave nurses authority to prescribe. Thus, even without state legislation, many APNs were using institutional regulations to justify prescriptive authority.

From the states with prescribing laws, Pearson found that the numbers of nurse practitioners who prescribed on their own authority varied regionally: 10 percent in the West, 59 percent in the Mountain states, 14 percent in the Midwest, 27 percent in the South, and 57 percent in the East. According to Pearson: "Even though the percentage of respondents from states with prescribing laws in the East is almost as high as in the Mountain states region, the NPs in the Mountain states use their own prescriptive authority more often" (Pearson, 1986, p. 7). Midwestern nurses were least likely to use their own authority without physicians' signatures.

The initial analysis of the data collected led Pearson to conclude, "One thing is very clear from the responses we received. Nurse practitioners who need prescriptions for their clients find ways to obtain them regardless of the laws" (p. 7). Pearson urged nurses to make legislators aware of the tremendous burdens that restrictive laws were placing on nurse practitioners, who must continually circumvent restrictions in order to provide safe and cost-effective health care.

Indeed, Linda J. LaPlante and Freda V. O'Bannon (1987) reported on research which examined the influence that nurse practitioners, even without prescriptive authority, actually have on the selection of prescription and non-prescription drugs. The researchers asked nurse practitioners to provide information on diagnoses and recommended drug therapies over a three-day period in adult ambulatory-care settings. LaPlante and O'Bannon found that

"Nurse practitioners recommended 2,081 new over-the-counter and prescription drugs during this study. Of these over-the-counter and prescription drugs, only 50 (2 percent of all recommended drugs) were changed after consultation with supervising physicians. Of the 50 changes, only two drugs (0.1 percent of all recommended) were changed to different drug categories" (p. 52).

This finding is particularly important since only those prescriptions requiring *new* medications were included in the study. Over three days, the 59 nurse practitioners treated 1,632 patients with 1,711 health-care problems requiring *new* medications. Of these, 1,646 (79 percent) were prescription and 435 (21 percent) over-the-counter drugs; thus, the majority of recommendations made by the nurses were those requiring prescriptive authority. Of the 50 changes made by physicians, 21 were for alternative antibiotics.

It is also important to note the wide range of health problems the nurses diagnosed in order to recommend prescriptions. These included respiratory, genito-urinary, skin, musculoskeletal, gastrointestinal, ear, eye, cardiovascular, neurological, endocrine, and health-maintenance problems. It is obvious that nurse practitioners had to diagnose first in order to have a basis for prescribing; thus, the nurses were having an impact not only on writing prescriptions, but on diagnosing types of illnesses involving a broad range of health problems.

From the research, it is clear that the number of drug recommendations made by nurse practitioners without prescribing privileges were quite similar to those of nurse practitioners with privileges and to physicians' rates reported in other research. Furthermore, the studies showed no major differences in the types of drugs given by practitioners with and without prescriptive authority. This research concurs with Pearson's findings on a much larger national sample. LaPlante and O'Bannon concluded: "Nurse practitioners who need prescriptions for their clients find ways to obtain them regardless of the laws" (p. 58). They too called for an end to piecemeal restrictive legislation.

By the end of the 1980s, research continued to support nurses' prescriptive practice. Sloane and Lekan-Rutledge (1988) studied drug prescribing by telephone as a potential cause of "polypharmacy" in nursing homes, finding that physicians too often prescribed inappropriate drugs for their patients, some of whom were rarely seen or visited, and harmful drug interactions were not uncommon. Gene E. Harkless (1989) debunked common assumptions about prescriptive authority, noting nurses' appropriate prescribing behaviors were based on more than a decade of research.

By the 1990s there were statutory or regulatory provisions in forty jurisdictions. As Linda Pearson (1992) and Karen Fennell (1991) stated, these varied quite widely in degree of independence *and* types of drugs and devices *and* requirements for written protocols and drug formularies, or types of drugs allowed, *and* the legal need for physician supervision and direction. *All* of these varied by geographic or practice settings. In a cogent analysis of nursing, health-care dollars, and regulatory sense, Barbara J. Safriet, associate dean, Yale

Law School, noted: "Oddly enough, the first question is not whether these providers *can and do* prescribe, but rather, whether the state will *acknowledge and authorize* their prescribing practices" (Safriet, 1992, pp. 456–457). Without legal authority, many advanced practice and other nurses called in prescriptions using physicians' names, used presigned blank prescription pads, asked physicians to sign prescriptions, wrote prescriptions and signed physicians' names, prescribed according to protocols, and co-signed physicians' prescription pads (S. Cohn, 1984).

Which nurses can prescribe? What can be prescribed? What is the degree of independent authority? Should the scope of authority vary? What state agency should regulate? What qualifications beyond RN licensure are required? What form should the authorization take? Again, there are widely varied answers to these questions in different states, but, said Safriet, two predominant patterns, differing in the degree of autonomy and range of drugs, were apparent in the early 1990s. In some states, such as Alaska, Oregon, and Washington, advanced practice nurses could prescribe without any physicians' involvement from a formulary including controlled substances, but only with Board of Nursing approval. Independent or "substitutive" authority, first allowed in Oregon, was extended to Washington and Alaska; all three required advanced training, continuing education, and specific education in pharmacology and clinical management as a condition of authority.

In sharp contrast, several states had physician involvement and supervision as the central requirement. Both the Board of Medicine and the Board of Nursing in Virginia, for example, regulated licensure of nurse practitioners, and allowed prescriptive authority only if the nurses had written agreements with physicians, who supervised and directed the nurses, who could only use a formulary approved by both boards and subject to written protocols with the supervising physicians, who must make periodic site visits to locations where there was no physician present. The number of nurses a physician could supervise was limited, and the 1991 statute prohibited nurses except midwives from establishing separate offices.

It should be stressed that "organized medicine has played a central role in shaping the states' current provisions . . . and lobbied against any legislative efforts to acknowledge prescriptive authority" (Safriet, 1992, p. 461). Indeed, in April 1991 the AMA distributed "An Act to Grant Prescription-Writing Authority to Nurse Practitioners and to Regulate Such Prescription Practices" to state medical association executive directors and to national medical specialty organizations. The model for legislation was *not* encouraged, but was to be used only when legislatures were considering the issue to ensure that resulting statutes would reflect the conditions and limitations specified in the medical model.

Such restrictive and anticompetitive legislation had detrimental effects on the public's access to health care: "Even the most basic common illness, a sore throat or an ear-ache, for example, often requires medication of some type, such as a simple antibiotic" (pp. 462–463). A nurse practitioner is well qualified to diagnose and prescribe for these common illnesses, but even this would require in some states written protocols and physician supervision or referrals, raising direct and indirect costs that are then imposed on the patients. Given the rapidly expanding pharmacological requirements for nurses, said Safriet, and the quickly changing array of drug interventions possible, rigid statutory restrictions through multilevel, multiprofessional bureaucracies make little sense.

This is exemplified in the confusing mess with the Drug Enforcement Administration (DEA), which had provided DEA registration numbers that allowed prescriptive authority to APNs. In 1989 the agency refused to provide New York State nurses with *independent* numbers since a nurse practitioner's prescriptive authority depended on the protocol developed with a supervising or collaborating physician (New York State Nurses Association, 1992). The terms of these could not be easily assessed by the DEA. Therefore, only physicians would be assigned numbers, which they could then assign to their "affiliates." Clearly this was a monopolistic tying mechanism, which would deny patients direct access to nurses. Furthermore, the DEA equated RN-MD collaboration with medical control; thus, not only were nurses denied prescriptive authority but their reimbursement was also restricted because insurance companies used the DEA assigned numbers to provide payment to providers.

By January 1992 nurse Melinda Mercer reported that the ANA was monitoring the Drug Enforcement Administration on the development of a final rule defining an "affiliated practitioner." Two separate systems for DEA registration were proposed that depended on state laws. In the first, "plenary" authority would allow, as in the past, the APN to obtain a prescriptive registration number, but in states authorizing "collaboration" (such as New York), the nurse would be an affiliated practitioner, who could obtain a number only from a "collaborative" physician. The ANA was lobbying for direct reimbursement at least in states where it was already allowed. By October 1992 nurses had successfully lobbied the DEA and forced a July 1992 proposed rule that would allow "mid-level practitioners" to receive their registration numbers directly. The DEA asked each state to submit an interpretation of its law and noted in its April letter withdrawing the previous ruling that it would have impeded accessibility and negatively affected quality of care. However, this new rule would be operative only in states whose attorneys general had determined that eligible nurses actually had authority (*American Nurse,* 1993d).

Obviously, there was, as attorney Winifred Carson (1993c) observed, inconsistency even by the mid-1990s in nursing practice; some states (e.g., New York) recognized nurse practitioners, but not clinical-nurse specialists; others allowed prescriptive authority without physician supervision, but others limited nurses to such supervision; others limited authority to certain sites or special communities; still others limited nurses to formularies and some to specific drug schedules. As if this were not sufficiently confusing, some states limited nurses' prescribing to noncontrolled substances; others merely allowed nurses to write prescriptions under physician cosignature, but others required a variety of physician controls. Some allowed nurses to "order" drugs.

In Carson's view, there were three major trends: first, expansion of prescriptive authority in states that currently allowed nurses to prescribe in some form; second, use of prescriptive authority legislation to acknowledge advanced nurse practice; and third, the use of educational requirements to obtain prescriptive authority. Offsetting these positive trends, many states had moved toward joint nurse-physician regulation of advanced practice and prescriptive authority. Clearly, organized medicine was not giving up the monopoly and was actively pushing nurses back into their previous dependent roles. Although 78 percent of states had by the early 1990s some degree of prescriptive regulations for some nurses, the mess created by medical meddling was glaringly apparent. By the end of the decade, NPs had prescriptive authority in all fifty states, but in four states (Pennsylvania, Georgia, Michigan, and Ohio) physicians had to co-sign the prescription. Wide variations continued in supervisory requirements and in types of drugs NPs and PAs were allowed to prescribe. Of the 2.5 billion prescriptions written in 1998, NPs wrote 15 million, up 66 percent from 1977, and PAs wrote 12 million, up 33 percent (Galewitz, 1999). These represent a small but growing fraction of the total prescriptions written.

Nurses Rate Higher Than Physicians on Appropriateness of Care

Research in the early 1990s added accumulating evidence for nurses' superior care. Diane Feeney Mahoney reviewed past research trends (1992) and in 1994 published her own research on the appropriateness of prescribing decisions made by nurse practitioners and physicians. Using three standardized geriatric-case vignettes, the NPs scored *higher* on an index of appropriateness of care than physicians—"a difference that remained whether or not the nurse had regulatory support to prescribe" (Mahoney, 1994, p. 41). Mahoney's research was particularly important because it was based on a national random sample, and because of the hypothetical nature of the vignettes, NPs without legalized authority could participate, making possible comparisons between nurses with and without such authority. Of the 296 NPs, 40 percent (118) had legal authorizations, and of these, 60 were dependent on physicians and 58 independent; of the 501 physicians, 140 were general practitioners, 151 family practitioners, and 210 internists. Of these, 373 were used in the analysis.

A multidisciplinary panel of experts—two geriatricians, two gerontological NPs, and two geriatric pharmacists from different geographic areas—determined the appropriate treatments for the patients in each of the vignettes and evaluated respondents' answers independently. The judges were not aware of whether the responses were from a NP or a physician. An index of appropriateness was constructed on the basis of unanimity on treatment modalities. There was no statistical difference between the nurses with and without legal authorization, nor between those with independent or dependent authority and those with no legal authority. However, there was a statistically significant difference between physicians and NPs, regardless of the latter's legal authority or their dependence or independence from physicians. In *all* cases, the nurses, whose gender makeup (mostly female) was the converse of the physicians' (mostly male), scored *higher* on appropriateness of care than did the physicians.

A comparison of the number of drugs prescribed showed that the NPs prescribed significantly fewer drugs and also recommended more nondrug therapeutic interventions. Prescribing experience and geriatric experience were found to be statistically related to appropriateness; graduate education was also related but not statistically so. As causal factors, the degree of legal dependence or independence were insignificant, clearly not affecting appropriateness in primary-care settings.

As Mahoney stated, regulations that refused or limited nurses' prescriptive authority were clearly not supported by the research data. Although requirements for additional pharmacological training for nurses are useful, they did not appear necessary, based on this and previous research studies. In addition, no continuing pharmacological education was required for physicians, despite research that proved suboptimal prescribing and drug monitoring (Avorn and Soumerai, 1983), irrational drug prescribing (Segal, Thompson, and Floyd, 1979; Bapna, 1989), and lack of knowledge in prescribing for the elderly (Ray, Federspiel, and Schaffner 1980; Ferry, Lamy, and Becker, 1985; Beers, Avorn, Soumerai, Everitt, Sherman, and Salem, 1988). Mahoney concluded: "The findings from this research should warn policy makers about adopting regulations that disproportionately burden nurses" (Mahoney, 1994, p. 45).

Indeed, policy makers should take a serious look at *physicians'* prescriptive actions. Sidney M. Wolfe, MD (1997), director of Public Citizen's Health Research Group, revealed research findings, for example, that showed that 70 percent of physicians who took an exam testing their knowledge of prescribing for older adults failed, despite the fact that they were currently treating Medicare patients. In fact, the majority of physicians contacted refused to even take the exam because of their lack of interest in the subject. Ironically, 40 percent to 50 percent of drugs prescribed for older adults outside hospitals were overused. And 48 percent of patients taking three or more drugs were given drugs with one or more harmful interactions with other drugs. According to Wolfe, who had worked with Ralph Nader since the early 1970s, falls caused by adverse drug reactions among the elderly were common (659,000 a year), as was drug-induced memory loss (163,000 a year). Before the Public Citizen group took action, more than 1,000 children in the past died or suffered brain damage from aspirin-induced Reye's syndrome. Several hundred diabetics died each year from adverse drug reactions to phenformin, sold under different brand names. Thousands of people, mostly under the age of fifty, suffered acute kidney damage from the widely used painkiller Suprol. Such evidence indicates that physicians should examine their own prescriptive practices and behaviors.

The Medical Monopoly and State Nurse Practice Acts

Just as nurses' prescriptive authority involved a mass of inconsistent and unnecessary legal restrictions, legislation affecting nurse practice acts was also in a state of flux. As noted previously, physicians had increased the supply of physicians, and this abundance could be used to eliminate or restrict nurse midwives and practitioners. Certainly, the production of 70,000 more physicians than were actually needed by the 1990s could not have happened without some deliberation. The physician backlash, said Bonnie Bullough (1986) in her review of state nurse practice acts, now centered on the restriction of hospital privileges and prohibitions in state laws on nursing. In these efforts, "medical societies routinely employ well-financed governmental relations teams to assist them with lobbying efforts" (p. 355).

Nevertheless, changes in nurse practices acts continued to be initiated by nurses to expand the scope of functions of the registered nurse and those of advanced practice nurse specialists. Some states, even prior to 1971, recognized nurse anesthetists, although their legal status forced them to depend too frequently on physicians. Nurse midwives were sometimes exempted in clauses in medical practice acts; thus, there were historical legal precedents. As noted in chapter 7, Idaho revised its state nurse practice act in 1971; following the prohibition against diagnosis and treatment, a clause was added, allowing exceptions as authorized by the joint rules and regulations established by state nursing and medical boards and implemented by nurses. According to Bullough, these boards set policies and procedures for agencies so they in turn could set up their own protocols for APNs.

By 1986, thirty-seven states had adopted changes similar to the Idaho model, empowering boards to draw up regulations from which agency-generated protocols were established. Only in Wisconsin, Delaware, and Tennessee were boards of nursing alone responsible without new statutory law. Bullough noted that fourteen states had mandated policies or protocols at local levels. Another approach was to expand the basic definition of nursing by omitting or limiting the 1953 disclaimer against diagnosis and treatment or rewriting, using broader language, the definition of the nurse's roles. As noted in chapter 7, New York became the first state to use this approach in 1972, which was followed in part by thirty-five additional states.

Still another approach appeared in the Maine practice act, which allowed individual physicians the right to delegate diagnosis and treatment. This pattern already existed in five other states before the latest phase in licensure began in the 1970s. As Bullough noted, PAs had no authority through licensure, so most states provided exemptions in medical practice acts for other workers—but under medical supervision.

Bullough evaluated the legislative changes, observing that expanding the definition of all professional nurses, for example, in the 1972 New York law copied in thirteen other states, had not been completely effective. The differentiation between nursing and medical diagnoses was not operationalized, and in both New York and New Jersey, the language of the new law had led to a doubtful legal status for nurse practitioners. By 1980 Colorado removed the word "nursing" before diagnoses; however, independent action was qualified by the addition of executing delegated medical functions and making referrals to medical or community agencies. Even Colorado's more precise law needed revision to cover specifically the APNs.

The incorporation into state laws of physicians' power to delegate had not held up well over time, because nurse practitioners' independent functions were already legally possible under separate licensure. The incorporation of mandated protocols had not been particularly effective because they took too much time to produce and were too rigid in actual practice. Although useful as teaching devices, protocols were not a sound basis for legal practice.

The major mechanism for legal coverage is a system for state certification, which is created by states, not by national professional bodies; thus, nurses must continue to work with state legislatures. Certification, continuing education, and career ladders also relate to the fight for the two-year and four-year entry-level educational requirements; this is complicated by the licensed practical nurses' lower education levels. Bullough concluded that a three-tiered system had developed: practical nurses, with one to two years of education; associate degree nurses with a two-year degree, usually from a community college; and nurses with a baccalaureate degree from a four-year university program, who may also become specialists at the master's degree level. Bullough urged that state certification should be determined by national criteria set by national nursing organizations. Clearly, the status of nurse practice acts showed a strong effort by nurses to gain autonomy, and an equally strong effort by physicians to restrict nurses and enhance the medical monopoly.

The Medical Backlash in New York State

Still another attack on autonomy has taken the form of institutional licensure. As Helen Mellett (1986) noted, "Historically, professional autonomy has been achieved through legally mandated individual licensure" (p. 56). Indeed, the 1972 amendment to the New York State Nurse Practice Act was seen by many nurses as sufficient to cover nurse practitioners. The state education department, however, disagreed, claiming that nurse practitioners were going beyond the legal definition of nursing. In attempting to amend the nurse practice act to "definitively recognize nurse practitioners. . . . They have been stalemated by lack of consensus on regulatory and philosophical issues" (p. 56), arising from difficulties in separating practice lines among various occupational groups and stalled by medicine's need for dominance.

Because of court rulings, physicians were trying to hold institutions responsible for physicians' negligence. In addition, quality assessment measures and payment systems arising from Medicare and Medicaid had also resulted in more institutional scrutiny. Hospitals also increased control by "blurring practice lines between occupational groups . . . to get the work done. Standing orders, for example, are a truly ingenious way to rationalize blurring of practice lines" (p. 56). As Mellett stated, a standing order to defibrillate patients is only one example of nurses carrying out a medical act allowed by institutions when no physician is present. The hypocrisy of the system is clear: "Both job functions and lines of authority have been blurred when necessary. The nursing supervisor may act as the night pharmacist; the L.P.N. nurse may function as an R. N. Now the practice of nurse practitioners overlaps with that of primary care physicians" (p. 56).

Mellett acknowledged that medical practice was the first occupation legally defined by statute; thus, physicians have insisted that all other health professions are simply amendments to medical practice acts: "The medical ideology allows physicians infinite possibilities to legally 'expand' and at the same time, prohibits nurses from approaching the practice of 'medicine' in any form" (p. 56).

According to Mellett, the 2,000 nurse practitioners in New York State (in 1986) were not informed they were illegally practicing their profession; instead, hospitals were informed that they were in violation. In 1985 the state health code was revised to allow nurse practitioners to practice, but authority was given not to them but to the institutions through *both* nursing and medical groups. Once again nurses' independence was thwarted. Indeed, institutional licensure takes away the power of nursing associations and state boards to control the licensing of nurses.

Although the New York State Nurses Association fought for several years to maintain the 1972 Nurse Practice Act, claiming it adequately covered all professional nurses, the battle was finally lost when Governor Mario Cuomo on July 11, 1988, signed into law the Nurse Practitioner Bill, which became effective on April 1, 1989. The law requires that a nurse must be certified by the state education department in order to practice as a nurse practitioner. Furthermore, "Nurses who want to *practice* as nurse practitioners must establish a written collaborative practice agreement with a physician. After April 1, no nurse practitioner, regardless of educational preparation or experience, may practice as a nurse practitioner without this connection to a physician" (New York State Nurses Association, 1989, p. 1). Thus, despite organized nursing's efforts to gain control over the practice and certification of members of their own profession, at least in New York State, the battle had been temporarily, but only partially, lost. Political pressure and manipulation from physicians, hospital administrators, and some nurses had turned an admirable effort to gain professional autonomy into another partial loss for nursing. It should be noted also that with the passage of the New York State Nurse Practitioner bill the requirement that a nurse practitioner hold a master's degree was eliminated!

Mixed State Regulatory Boards: A Wrong Approach to Nurse Practitioners

According to Safriet (1992), by the 1990s the most critical barriers to the effective use of advanced practice nurses were still the conflicting and restrictive state laws limiting their practice and fragmented federal standards for their reimbursement. The statutory definitions of the practice of medicine or surgery are extremely broad, and this breadth, combined with the provision making it illegal to engage in any acts in the definition, has resulted "in a preemptive strike by the medical profession to totally occupy the health field" (p. 441).

The defects in the current "system" were still multiple. Some states, said Safriet, had deleted the absolute prohibition on diagnosis and treatment or added nursing diagnosis: some added a clause on "additional acts" for specially trained nurses to diagnose and prescribe according to rules of state nursing and/or medical boards or as agreed by the two professions; some had generic or specific categories with definitions of scope of practice or authorization by medical and/or nursing boards to establish rules; some revised medical practice acts to include delegation of tasks to nurses with additional training. The multiplicity of roles and titles led Safriet to state: "When viewed from a national perspective, the resulting nomenclature begins to resemble the rubble of the Tower of Babel. Even the most sophisticated health care consumer or policymaker can easily be confused" (p. 446). Insurance provisions were also very difficult to handle nationally when titles varied so widely from state to state. Said Safriet, "The easiest solution would be to have a single statutory designation—Advanced Practice Nurse, or APN—in each state, and to leave any subsequent regulatory or professional designation to the state Boards of Nursing and the national professional associations" (p. 447). This simple recommendation is, however, made more complex by a second problem: the composition of regulatory bodies, which in a number of states, require the joint action by both the board of nursing and the board of medicine, or by the latter alone, or by joint committees: "Such a multiprofessional approach is unique in the regulatory arena" (p. 447).

These mixed regulator schemes, said Safriet, erroneously assume that physicians, who are not trained in nursing, and typically have never experienced the sustained practice of nurses with patients, can regulate nurses. However, it could also be argued that physicians do know what APNs do because it used to be called medicine. Yet this, too, is a fallacious argument: since general medical practitioners now do what only medical specialists did only a few years ago, changes in medical practices or regulations should also be required, yet none were even contemplated. Why then should nurses who take on health-care tasks be subjected to medical scrutiny? In fact, it is, said Safriet, easy to argue that physicians are doing nursing, not medicine, at least in regard to preventive and wellness care. Indeed, since normal pregnancies and deliveries are not diseases, it could be argued that physicians are practicing nursing, not medicine, under some state medical practice acts.

The pattern of mixed regulations "attempts to perpetuate the dominant position of the physician as the all-knowing, authoritative definer of all aspects of health care delivery" (p. 448), and this leads to biased policy making, which is usually related to professional territoriality and to financial or competitive opposition. Nurses have long engaged in functions technically done by physicians, but the enactment of advanced nursing provisions now shifts these from informal to more formal arrangements. Since APNs are now legally recognized as substitutes for physicians, "the only legal way to dampen the competitive effects . . . is to use the regulatory power to constrain as much as possible the definition of their scope of practice" (p. 449). With mixed regulators, "there is a strong possibility that anti-competitive motives will dictate restrictions that are not justified on public safety grounds" (p. 449). Thus, despite the proven capability of nurse midwives to practice independently in most pregnancies and deliveries, an anticompetitive regulation would require direct physician supervision that is unnecessary for safety reasons. Given the reality of nurses' cost-effective competition, "the potential for anti-competitive regulation will grow more intense" (p. 449). Safriet concluded that "consistent with other professional licensing systems, the regulation of nursing in all its aspects should be carried out by each state's BON [board of nursing]" (p. 450).

Collaboration: Joint Action or Supervision?

The multitude of statutory and regulatory restrictions can be divided into two related kinds: first, requirements for formalized practice relationships with physicians in written agreements, protocols, and collaborative guidelines, or for MD direction or supervision; and second, restrictions to certain sites or facilities. Elaborate definitions, said Safriet, distinguish between general, direct, or immediate physician collaboration, direction, or supervision of nurses' activities. "Other definitions surpass the elaborate and border on the absurd. For example, 'collaboration' generally connotes joint effort, people working together as equals" (pp. 450–451). However, one proposed definition in Virginia of "collaboration" defines it as the process of a nurse working with a physician "with medical *direction* and appropriate *supervision,* as provided for in jointly developed *protocols* as defined by law and regulation" (p. 451). Equality of contribution is totally eliminated in this approach, and the degree of mandatory direction and supervision make a "mockery of . . . the NP's professional expertise" (p. 451).

Such provisions, said Safriet, are both "needless and detrimental" because nurses, like other professionals, are trained to use independent judgment, know the boundaries of their competence, know when to consult with and refer to others, and have a legal and ethical duty to do so when needed. "These provisions are more than benignly redundant"; they are "harmful and costly" (p. 451). The nurse is forced to question and seek affirmation, and this has a corrosive effect on her or his sense of professionalism. Physicians are also forced into either winking at legal requirements that are deemed unnecessary or supervising even when it is not appropriate. Such game playing weakens the patients' confidence in the nurse practitioner and raises questions about the actual role of the physician.

After the state has legally recognized APNs, "it is odd indeed to condition practice upon the agreement or permission of a private individual . . . it conditions an APN's employability or fitness to practice upon the consent of a willing physician . . . [and] in effect mandate[s] a life-long apprenticeship" (p. 452). No matter how skilled or experienced the nurse or how inexperienced the physician, a physician's oversight is a legal requirement to define the competence of the nurse's practice: "Any state that adopts such a mechanism has in effect yielded its governmental power to one private individual, the physician, who is given almost complete discretion to assess the competence of another licensed health care provider . . . governed by no identifiable objective standards and limited by no procedural guarantees" (p. 452). This constitutes a wholesale privatization of a governmental function: assessing competence for licensure.

These restrictions when combined with limitations on geographical locations or types of practice sites create a regulatory and policy-making quagmire. Many states exempt physician supervision in medically underserved areas. These statutory affirmatives of the unsupervised practice are "hypocritical and fundamentally indefensible" because competence is determined by *where,* not *what* or *how,* the nurses practice and because poor people and those in rural areas are provided "second-class" care—these propositions, although false, are, said Safriet, the only possible bases, other than anticompetition, upon which states can exempt specific geographic or practice settings. The states must admit that they are permitting unsupervised or less-than-competent APNs to deliver care to mostly poor people in rural and inner cities. Or they must admit that if an APN is competent to practice where physicians do not or will not, then they must be competent to practice where physicians are: "it follows that the MD supervision mandated by the state is unnecessary to competent APN practice everywhere" (p. 453).

We are left, said Safriet, with a disquieting but compelling conclusion that the "continuation of these restrictions has more to do with protecting the competitive position of physicians than with protecting the public health" (p. 454). Trying to encourage nurses to practice in particular areas is an improper use of licensure, which should mean the same thing across all geographic boundaries as it does with all other professionals: "A gerrymandered scope-of-practice definition . . . is reminiscent of involuntary servitude" (p. 454). Safriet asked how the current national crazy quilt came to be and answered that legislators were overcautious and overreliant on the medical profession.

Third-Party Reimbursement: AMA Lobbies against Nursing Legislation

Even if nurses gained independence through expanded nurse practice acts and achieved the right to diagnose, prescribe, and treat, the success of their efforts still depends on their ability to break physicians' monopoly over reimbursement for work. In 1988 Mary T. Caraher reviewed the status of third-party or direct reimbursement for nurse practitioners. Although partially successful in getting reimbursement, "under some health care plans, barriers still exist, such as opposition by medical societies, procedural problems and restrictive interpretations of state licensure laws" (p. 50). By the late 1980s more than 85 percent of Americans were covered by varied forms of private insurance; 23 million were in federal Medicare programs, and half of these also carried private health insurance. A major cause of rising health-care costs was the lack of competition; physicians and hospitals were still the major health-care providers recognized by third-party reimbursers, who are not keeping "pace with the evolution of state legislation regulating the practice of NPs" (p. 50). By 1987, only fifteen states had passed legislation requiring health insurers to reimburse nurse practitioners directly for their services.

Congressional legislation in 1977 authorized Medicare and Medicaid reimbursement to nurse practitioners and physicians' assistants in rural health clinics, but such clinics were approved *only if* there was a shortage of medical "manpower" and *if* treatment plans were reviewed and approved by physicians. Thus, only 215 of the potential 2,600 rural health clinics were certified in the first year. By 1980 another federal act mandated payment to needy recipients under Medicaid and "specifies that physician supervision cannot be a condition of reimbursement" (p. 50). By the 1980s Medicare legislation provided coverage for nurse practitioners within health maintenance organizations. By 1982, between seven million and nine million dependents of active-duty military personnel and retirees could seek care from nurse practitioners, who were directly reimbursed. Clearly, nurses had been active politically to achieve these changes. Unfortunately, the state laws still often required physicians' signatures to release reimbursement.

As expected, the AMA consistently fought nurses' efforts to achieve third-party reimbursement. According to Caraher, physicians had influenced a wave of restrictive decisions and negatively influenced nursing legislation, for example, lobbying against third-party payment to nurses who treated federal employees under federal health insurance plans. Indeed, "Medical societies with a non-delegation-of-work rule have denied membership to physicians using NPs" (p. 52). Following the application of antitrust actions to professional groups, efforts by medical groups to restrict practice unfairly have been investigated, beginning in 1979, by the Federal Trade Commission (FTC). The AMA has responded to these inquiries "by heavily supporting legislation to prohibit the FTC from investigating restraint-of-trade activities in professions" (p. 54). In contrast, "The American Nurses' Association has opposed the exemption of professions in order to maintain the FTC's ability to protect health care professionals, such as nurse midwives forced to bring restraint-of-trade actions against physicians" (p. 54). Obviously, men in the most prestigious profession are directly pitted against women nurses. The fight is a gendered struggle and the odds are against the nurses, unless other women's groups provide much greater support.

Changes in modes of delivery also affect the nurses' struggle for autonomy through direct payments. The rules and regulations concerning reimbursement of HMOs could be enhanced by nursing directors in such groups. However, "collaborative" practice with physicians is increasingly difficult because some states refuse to allow nurses to incorporate with physicians, requiring, instead, that they be employed by physicians. That the legal system is stacked against women practitioners is an obvious and blatant example of what a sex-stratified society does to women.

Caraher faced the discriminatory problems squarely. For competition to exist, two conditions must be met: "Consumers must be actively involved in choosing alternatives, and qualified providers must have free entry into the system" (p. 54). Caraher urged nurses to educate their clients on the issues; to become involved in nurses' professional organizations; to influence current proposed legislation; and to initiate networking with other professional groups and consumer rights organizations. Unfortunately, Caraher seemed to subsume women's groups somewhere in these categories; nevertheless, the responsibilities of other women to nurses are obvious. If nurses achieve autonomy, they do so not only for themselves, but for all women.

Direct Payment: The Bottom Line Revisited

Obviously, nursing autonomy could never be achieved without third-party or direct payment to nurses. The ANA had advocated this as early as 1948 and incorporated the idea into the 1958 ANA Social Security resolution that called for nursing services to be included in health-insurance plans. The call for direct payment was strongly advocated in the 1980s and into the 1990s by Pulliam (1991), Etheridge (1991), and Sullivan (1992). According to Sullivan, nurses had achieved limited success through regulatory and legislative channels. Although nurse midwives and nurse anesthetists had received direct reimbursement under Medicare, APNs were limited to such reimbursement only in designated areas. Pediatric, family, and sometimes adult and geriatric nurse practitioners might be reimbursed, but again this was subject to wide variations in state statutes. Linda J. Pearson (1992) reported that twenty-five states, up from fifteen in 1988, had passed legislation to authorize third-party reimbursement; thirty-eight states allowed Medicaid payments to nurses, and eleven other states were expected to pass legislation by the end of 1992. Nevertheless, state and federal laws continued to discriminate against APNs, who, according to Safriet (1992), are paid at a significantly reduced rate for a narrow range of services and often are not even eligible for direct reimbursement. Usually the physician is able to bill for services at the higher MD level, pay the nurse's salaries, and pocket the difference.

At both the state and federal levels, reimbursement laws discriminate unjustly against APNs, who must have direct access to third-party payers if they are to enter private practice. The states regulate the insurance industry, and the nurses have been unable to get private insurance companies to cover services unless the reimbursement is contingent upon collaboration with or employment by a physician. Thus, of critical importance were changes in Medicaid and Medicare regulations on reimbursement and the reform of physician payments in the 1989 Omnibus Budget Reconciliation Act. Although nurse midwives working separately from physicians were covered under Medicaid since 1980, their practice was limited to the maternity cycle, excluding family or gynecological care. It was not until 1989 that some services by family or pediatric nurse practitioners were covered under Medicaid whether or not the NPs were under physicians' supervision. Almost all states were in compliance by 1992.

Reimbursement levels for Medicaid are subject to the discretion of the states, which have in the past used fee schedules or reasonable charges for reimbursement. However, with rising expenses in 1984, Congress developed diagnostic related groups (DRGs), allowing the federal government to pay hospitals only the amount an average patient would need for each category of diagnosis (Lake, 1992; Diers, 1992). As noted previously, by 1989 the Physicians Payment Review Commission (PPRC) had adopted a resource-based relative value scale to replace the reasonable charge system. Although some nurse midwives' services have been covered under Medicaid since 1980, whether they were working independently or collaboratively, their practice was still restricted to the maternity cycle and, although they were directly reimbursed, as of 1992 they received only 65 percent of the physicians' fee amounts.

Nurse practitioners were required to collaborate with a physician and were reimbursed for services related to a physician's services under HMO contracts and in skilled nursing facilities and in rural areas. They were additionally restricted to a percentage of the amount paid to physicians—75 percent in hospitals and 85 percent in all other settings as of 1992—but not in rural areas, where they could be directly reimbursed. Presumably, these differences in payments reflected the difference in actual costs of educational preparation of nurses and physicians. Collaboration was defined as working with a physician with medical direction and appropriate supervision as provided in jointly developed guidelines or other mechanisms as defined by each state. Clearly, this definition did not foster nurses' independence, even with direct payment.

Using the new payment system developed by the PPRC, each separate medical function would be given a value relative to all other services, adjusted by a geographical factor to achieve a regional value, and then multiplied by a national conversion factor. As Safriet (1992) stressed, "at the core of Medicare fee reform is the concept of paying the same amount to all physicians who provide a service, regardless of specialty" (p. 474). Thus, physicians should be paid the same when they provide the same services. Indeed, differential reimbursement based on differing training costs by specialties was explicitly rejected. There are still insufficient data or inadequate methods to determine differences in quality or competence of physicians, so these were excluded as determinants of the relative values of payments (Physicians Payment Review Commission, 1991).

When "nonphysician" providers were considered, the PPRC chose to ignore or forgot this principle of equality of payment for the same services. To Safriet, "It makes no sense to differentiate based on opportunity costs [foregone income caused by years of training] for one group, but not another" (Safriet, 1992, p. 475). When contrasting physicians' services with those of dentists, podiatrists, optometrists, and chiropractors, the PPRC found no differences and thus recommended they should be paid the same. However, when assessing rates for APNs, the PPRC looked for evidence of the *sameness* of services, and asserted that although the Office of Technology Assessment report (1986) proved equivalent *quality* to physicians' care, it did not say the *services* were the same. Thus, the PPRC did not recommend elimination of the payment differentials for APNs. Even the Health Care Financing Administration (HCFA) rejected bonus payments for APNs working in undeserved areas. Indeed, the commissioners, according to Edmunds (1991), were openly critical of the quality of the research on nurse practitioner performance and used the hearings "to soundly scold NPs for failing to answer basic questions" (Edmunds, 1991; cited in Safriet, 1992, p. 477) on what NPs did and how their care differed. Evidently the commissioners wanted to know in minute detail what the NPs did, rather than proof that the quality of care was equivalent.

Legal Changes Needed to Remove Barriers to Nurses' Scope of Practice

Safriet concluded that state and federal legislators should remove barriers to scope of practice by, first, eliminating all references to mixed-regulator entities and by vesting sole authority in each state's board of nursing, to which advisory committees might be provided. Second, nurse practice acts should be amended to acknowledge advanced practice nursing, with few if any designations of specific types of specialties. Because the overlapping roles of nursing and medicine will continue to expand, it is "difficult to distinguish neatly between nursing and medical diagnosis" (Safriet, 1992, p. 479). Third, practice acts of APNs should be included under regulations adopted by the state board of nursing, which should be authorized to promulgate all other regulations. And finally, all statutory requirements for formalized collaboration or practice agreements or physician supervision or direction should be eliminated. "Unnecessary" and "insulting," these restrictions are "an inappropriate intrusion" in nurses' professional judgment and expertise and create "unrealistic strictures" that are widely ignored or "too rigidly adhered to" (p. 480). By conditioning the advanced nurse's practice on the dictates of one physician, the "unfettered delegation of governmental power to private actors . . . poses fundamental legal and significant policy questions" (p. 480).

Removing physician supervision will also eliminate the numerous problems in prescribing. Legislatures should acknowledge APNs' right to prescribe drugs in schedules II through V of the Controlled Substances Act or leave this specification to state boards of nursing. Safriet recommended reimbursement reform in all states be enacted to ensure nondiscrimination for health-insurance plans and contracts and to forms of payment which should be of the same type for all providers. At the federal level, all restrictions on nurses' direct reimbursement should be eliminated, thus removing the practice of payment through billing physicians. Safriet noted that the unrestricted, retrospective fee-for-service has not worked because this system is immune to cost containment. The value of primary and preventive care has also been discounted in the old system, which has encouraged episodic, invasive, and technologically oriented care. Equity in payment must be a principle applied to all providers, and the propensity to use physicians and their care as the benchmark for valuing and paying all other health-care providers must be changed since it "perpetuates the now-discredited assumption that medicine and medical doctors are intrinsically the norm for the kind and quality of care delivered" (p. 483). Using medical services as the basis for payment treats as "other" caregivers who are lumped together as non-physicians: "Setting out to change the status quo, without questioning its underlying norms, is futile" (p. 483). Equal-pay-for-equal-services for all practitioners is necessary, and APNs must be grouped with other "non-physicians"—dentists, podiatrists, etc. Since the primary care provided by nurses is less costly than high-tech care, it is likely that even with pay equity the costs of care will be lower. Furthermore, lower costs could be anticipated based on research that found, for example, higher patients compliance with APNs than with physicians. Freed from restrictions, nurses, said Safriet, could cause fundamental changes in the health-care system, bringing preventive and primary health care to large segments of the population through home-health-care programs and nurse-managed community clinics.

Running the Federal and State Mazes for Direct Reimbursement

To what extent would Safriet's recommendations become a reality? Pamela Mittelstadt (1992a) reported that the new Medicare fee schedule would affect many APNs, who could expect increases in their fees. Medical specialists could experience a 10 to 14 percent reduction, but primary-care providers could expect a 15 to 20 percent increase. Nurse practitioners in nursing facilities would receive 85 percent of the fee schedule of physicians, and, if employed by physicians, they would be paid as if the physicians had delivered the service. There was also a reduction in fees for service provided in hospital outpatient departments. The ANA believed the fee schedule should be "based on the service and not on the type of provider delivering the service" (p. 2). In a second article in the same issue of *The American Nurse*, Mittelstadt (1992b) noted that increased Medicare reimbursement for APNs under S2103, proposed by Senators Charles Grassley and Patrick Moynihan, would improve payment rates from the 65 percent to 85 percent to 97 percent of the fee schedule. This action was contrary to the recommendations of the Physicians Payment Review Commission. The legislation, said Mittelstadt, represented a significant component of *Nursing's Agenda for Health Care Reform* (American Nurses' Association, 1991).

Throughout the 1990s, there were numerous efforts by nurses to obtain direct reimbursement. For example, Marjorie Vanderbilt (1992) reported that the ANA was lobbying in support of a bill (S1842) to provide direct Medicaid reimbursement to APNs, regardless of whether they were associated with or supervised by a physician and regardless of location or practice setting. The Omnibus Budget Reconciliation Act of 1990 (Public Law 101–508) had provided direct Medicare reimbursement. With the introduction of Medicaid bill S466, Senator Tom Daschle said, "[W]e must reevaluate outdated taboos and break down barriers that prevent nurses from caring for patients. This means reimbursing them directly and according them the autonomy and authority they deserve" (Vanderbilt, 1993, p. 11). To him, quality primary care did not "always mean being directed by a physician" (p. 11). Nurses were also pushing at the state level for mandatory third-party reimbursement; for example, in New York, legislation (New York Senate Bill 2492) was underway to require insurance companies to reimburse nurses for services provided (New York State Nurses Association, 1993a).

In June 1992 the ANA had been successful in changing the Health Care Financing Administration's definition of clinical nurse specialist, who were often not included in state laws. The ANA encouraged a broad definition of APNs, which would make them eligible for third-party reimbursement (Mittelstadt, 1992c). By 1993, HCFA had clarified Medicare payment under the "incident to" provisions, in which a physician is able to bill for services delivered by non-physician employees, including nurses. Payment is made to the physician as if he or she had delivered the services, which must be delivered under a physician's supervision. According to nurse-lawyer David Keepnews (1993), this provision had been widely used by insurance carriers to prohibit or severely hamper payment for nurses' services; the carriers refused to pay for services that involved independent evaluation or treatment or required that a physician independently evaluate the patient and the treatment provided by nurses. This meant in practice that some nurses could not provide services at all to Medicare patients, which restricted the types of services; indeed, "many advanced practice nurses feared that their ability to practice at all was in serious jeopardy" (p. 18). The HCFA produced new instructions that specified that non-physicians were eligible for coverage, but sustained the requirement for physician supervision; however, it was not necessary for a physician to provide services to a patient each time a nurse provided services. As Keepnews said, this action did not eliminate the need to press for direct reimbursement or to ease restrictions on payment mechanisms. Indeed, Robin Cassetta (1993) asserted that nursing groups had to work together to get away from the medical model and to get nurses recognized in health-care reform.

By mid-1994 direct Medicare reimbursement for APNs as provided in the Grassley-Conrad amendment was approved for *all* outpatient areas. Approval by the Senate Finance Committee was due in large part, said Vanderbilt (1994), to N-STAT, the ANA's grassroots organization of nurses across the country. However, by 1995, the Republican congressional majority was threatening to make severe cutbacks that would negatively impact on nursing, workplace safety, research, and health education programs. Nevertheless, the 1993–1994 health-care reform debate had allowed nurses to educate legislators, and there was still strong bipartisan support for "direct Medicare and Medicaid reimbursement for advanced practice nurses, graduate nurse education, removal of barriers and discriminatory practices to nursing practice and workforce and quality of care protection" (Vanderbilt and Reed, 1996, p. 10).

Independent reimbursement was closely tied to scope of practice, and in the late 1990s, states continued to enact new laws on nursing practice. For example, from January 1996 to May 1996, legislators in twenty-six states enacted eighty-one laws affecting nursing. Nevertheless, Wendy Fox-Grage (1996), researcher at the Intergovernmental Health Policy Project, asserted, "Despite the general trend to expand scope of practice and reimbursement, great inconsistencies across states . . . remain. . . . States cannot even agree on what name to use for nurses in advanced practice" (p. 1). Thus, advanced practice registered nurses, unlike physicians, still could not move from state to state and "know what their professional title will be, what procedures they can legally perform, what medications they can prescribe and whether or not an insurer will pay for their services" (p. 1). Certified nurse midwives had made some progress, but several state laws required the "attending provider" to make decisions based on medical standards; however, "Many lawyers and nursing professionals question the legality of requiring CNMs to follow guidelines from another profession" (p. 4). Indeed, these inconsistencies and irregularities have led the American Association of Colleges of Nursing (AACN) to work with the National Council of State Boards of Nursing (NCSBN) and other nursing organizations to develop an interstate compact for advanced nurse practitioners. Such a multistate agreement would allow APNs to practice in states other than the state in which the nurse is licensed without being required to obtain additional nursing licenses (American Association of Colleges of Nursing, 1998). Though a commendable effort, the NCSBN cautioned that this process might take several years before a model for APN multistate licensure was approved. Nevertheless, Utah became the first state to enact an interstate compact (*American Nurse,* 1998b), and several other states have subsequently considered and enacted similar legislation.

Obviously, third-party payment was also directly tied to prescriptive authority. By 1996, forty-six states had granted prescriptive authority to advanced practitioners, but sixteen of these still required a physician protocol, collaboration, or supervision. The other thirty also granted authority to prescribe controlled substances, but these varied from state to state. Most states allow "independent" practice, but only under some variant of physician control; however, Nebraska in 1996 changed its nurse practice law, giving APNs greater independence, for example, allowing pharmacists to fill nurses' prescriptions and allowing a Board of Advanced Nurse Practitioners to approve integrated practice agreements between nurses and physicians, a process previously controlled by the medical board. In Kentucky, after a sixteen-year fight by the state nurses association, pharmacists must now fill nurses' prescriptions without the co-signature of a physician.

In all states, but not the District of Columbia, direct Medicaid reimbursement rates for nurses are now allowed, but the rates range from 50 percent to 100 percent of what physicians receive. In about twenty states, the APNs receive the same rate as physicians for rendering the same service. Slightly more than half of the states guarantee third-party payment for nurses' services through their health insurance codes. Whether these laws pertain to HMOs is still at issue in many locales. Although significant advances had been made, the nurses in many states "had to fight the traditional medical community, as well as businesses and insurers" (Fox-Grage, 1996, p. 5). Nevertheless, President Clinton's budget request for 1997 called for direct reimbursement for nurse practitioners and clinicians, the first time in history that a budget request contained such a provision. The budget bill (Public Law 105–33) was enacted in August 1997, and as of January 1998, Medicare coverage includes direct payment for APNs regardless of the geographic area in which services are provided. Payments are authorized at 85 percent of what a physician would be paid for the same service. However, as recently as summer 2000, the AMA filed a "Citizens' Petition" with HCFA (which regulates Medicare), claiming that HCFA may be improperly reimbursing APNs for their services to Medicare recipients (*American Journal of Nursing*, 2000b, p. 23). As another example of the AMA's continuing effort to control nurses' scope of practice, the "Citizens' Petition" pressures HCFA to develop and regulate prescriptive authority protocols for all Medicare caregivers, to verify and document APNs' compliance with physician collaboration requirements, and to verify that all APNs are practicing within their state law's scope of practice requirements. Needless to say, nursing groups across the United States have rallied to oppose the "Citizens' Petition," crafting a "strong message for HCFA that reaffirms the nursing community's support of APNs' ability to bill Medicare without facing costly, burdensome, and unnecessary restrictions on their practice, including supervision" (p. 23). Indeed, as the ANA House of Delegates noted, APNs have been billing Medicare for many of their services since the early 1990s with no evidence that they are "practicing beyond their legal authority or inappropriately billing the federal health programs" (cited in *American Journal of Nursing*, 2000b, p. 23).

Hospital Admitting and Staff Privileges for Nurse Practitioners

Though nurses have seen positive gains in third-party reimbursement, their protracted struggle to gain hospital privileges has continued, due largely to the opposition of organized medicine. Nevertheless, some positive results for nursing have been achieved. The Oregon State Nurses Association and the Oregon chapter of the American College of Nurse Midwives won a major victory, after four years of effort, when on May 4, 1993, Oregon Governor Barbara Roberts signed Senate Bill 479 into law, which granted hospital admitting privileges to nurse practitioners. Previously, nurses had to go through emergency departments, a costly route, or be referred by a physician. Clearly, obstacles to access were high and the patients suffered. In 1992 the Oregon State Health Division had denied the nurses' petition for a rule change after the attorney general stated the division did not have the authority to make the change. In 1993 an amendment was introduced and passed by the Oregon legislature (Gies, 1993).

Russell Wesley Moss (1993) of the ANA legal staff said that privileging was essential as health-care reform opened the door for nurses' independent practice. Clinical privileging involves admitting patients to hospitals, but staff privileging is the process of becoming a member of the medical staff, as established in bylaws that lack specificity or uniformity across hospitals and states. Moss recommended that state nursing associations or boards of nursing educate hospitals and medical staffs about the problems. Some facilities require that an advanced nurse practitioner must become a member of the medical staff in order to obtain privileging—an obvious way for the medical monopoly to be sustained. Nevertheless, Moss recommended that the hospital nurses or a group of APNs establish criteria to guide the medical staff and work to ensure nurses' membership on hospital boards of directors.

In Florida the Nursing Service Clinical Privileging Board is vested with the authority to grant clinical privileges, but this is subject to securing supervisory physicians. By 1993, twenty-two states had some form of privileging for some types of nurses. Of these, only twelve allowed both admitting and clinical privileges, four allowed clinical only and two admitting only, and three were, as reported, unclear or unknown. The actual scope of practices varied widely and may apply only to certain hospitals, to rural areas only, or only under physician supervision.

By the second half of the 1990s, most states still did not regulate hospital admitting privileges for APNs. Typically, hospitals extend privileges only to nurses whose collaborating physicians also have staff privileges. Only Florida and Oregon had laws pertaining to hospital privileges, although a New York bill would make it illegal to refuse staff privileges to non-physician professionals, if they can provide patient care within their scope of practice. All hospitals would be required to establish written criteria and procedures to deal with applicants for hospital privileges.

Hospital admitting privileges were obviously closely connected to the protection of nurses' identity. According to Pearson (1997), in an annual update on legislative issues affecting advanced nursing practice, twenty-six states had nurse practitioner title protection and the board of nursing acted as sole authority in scope of practice with no requirement for physician collaboration or supervision. An additional sixteen states protected APN titles and granted the board of nursing sole authority, but required MD supervision or collaboration. Six states had title protection, but scope of practice was authorized by both the board of nursing and the board of medicine. Three states were with out title protection at all. Clearly, nursing had made significant gains, although much remained to be done.

Without prescriptive authority, hospital admitting privileges would be highly unlikely. By the late 1990s, there were nineteen states where nurse practitioners could prescribe (including controlled substances), independent of any required physician involvement. However, eighteen states allowed prescribing (including controlled substances) only with some degree of physician involvement or delegation. Another thirteen states allowed APNs to prescribe but excluded controlled substances and mandated physician involvement. In fourteen states, there was dispensing authority, but in one state, Illinois, nurses had no prescribing authority at all.

According to Pearson, the major obstacles to independent practice included potentially disastrous national policy proposals, physician abuse of power, political hardball realities, and exclusion from managed-care organization provider panels. Perhaps most insidious is the fact that advanced practice nurses are marginalized in their worlds of work—discounted, degraded, and demeaned in various ways, as proved in research by Dr. Patricia Martin, RN, and Dr. Sally Hutchinson, RN (1997). The marginalization would prove to be more, not less, evident as health-care organizations changed to profit-making business throughout the 1990s.

Whether working for changes in hospital privileges, state practice acts, prescriptive authority, or direct reimbursement, over the last three decades nurses have not given up their struggle for greater autonomy and have clearly made some progress toward these goals. However, as we shall see in the next chapter, in an era of cost containment, profit-making hospitals, and health management organizations, nurses would be sorely tested, forced to continue their efforts to sustain progress made, struggle to maintain their employment in a corporate environment geared to downsizing, as well as to defend their patients' rights and safety.

The Results of the Medical Monopoly
"A Regulatory and Policy-Making Quagmire"

By the end of the twentieth century, the results of the centuries-old medical monopoly were singularly unimpressive. In this chapter, focused on the last decade of the twentieth century, we consider nurses' and consumers' critiques of the health-care "system," discuss the efforts at reform by nurses, and document the continued rejection of nurses' autonomy by organized medicine. The politics of government efforts to reform health care and their impact on nurses are analyzed, particularly the Clintons' national health-care proposal and its collapse. With the election of a conservative Congress came an attack on social-entitlement programs; women and children were disproportionately affected. Following the lead of the political conservatives, organized medicine formally rejected advanced practice nurses' autonomy and actively lobbied to overturn the antimonopolistic rulings by the Federal Trade Commission.

In the absence of a national health care system and a rise in hospital and agency mergers, health maintenance organizations (HMOs) and profit-making corporations gained ascendance. Hospitals and other health agencies sought to reduce institutional costs by introducing minimally trained unlicensed assistive personnel (UAPs) to replace RNs. Efforts were made to eliminate primary-care nursing and reintroduce a form of functional nursing, to shift from state nurse practice acts to institutional or other forms of licensure, and to create multi-discipline professional regulatory boards instead of boards of nursing. Modification of existing nurse practice acts to foster greater autonomy continued to be challenged by medical societies and physicians; in its resolutions, the American Medical Association (AMA) equated collaboration with supervision. The possibility of nurses organizing to gain more power to deal with the changes in the delivery of health care was substantially weakened by a Supreme Court ruling in 1994 that defined most nurses as supervisory or administrative personnel, thus limiting their rights to organize in unions to improve their work conditions and control at least some aspects of patient care. Though the National Labor Relations Board (NLRB) ruled in 1996 that staff and charge nurses were not supervisory personnel and were thus protected by federal labor laws, many institutions attempted to ignore this ruling.

Despite all these negative shifts, the research continued on nurses' quality of care compared to that of physicians, confirming the positive findings from the mid-1960s onward. With support from foundations, APNs moved to create, sometimes with physicians, community-based health care centers and to expand their own nurse-controlled health centers. Yet the medical monopoly, given the collapse of the Clintons' national health-care program, seemed stronger than ever; therefore, the twenty-first century would probably be marked by the continuing struggle of nurses to gain even moderate autonomy.

Gender, although still critical, received less emphasis as increasing numbers of women became physicians and more women nurses and medical technicians became physician's assistants. By 2000, 27 percent of physicians were women, but nurses did not perceive women physicians to be substantially different from men physicians in their behaviors. However, women physicians reported that they still experienced sexist and discriminatory behavior. For example, in one of many reported cases, Dr. Frances Conley, a neurosurgeon, quit her tenured professorship at Stanford University Medical School in 1991, saying "she was fed up with demeaning comments and unwelcome sexual advances from male colleagues" (Conley, 1991). In a letter to the *San Francisco Chronicle,* she wrote: "Even today, faculty are using slides of *Playboy* centerfolds to 'spice up' lectures; sexist comments are frequent and those who are offended are told to be 'less sensitive'; unsolicited touching and fondling occur between house staffs and students, with the latter having little recourse to object. To complain might affect evaluation." Though Conley returned to Stanford as professor of neurosurgery in 1993, she noted that sexual discrimination and harassment toward female physicians and medical students were still evident: "you're not going to have the brash-type discrimination that women in my generation saw, but the verbal taunts, verbal degradation is going to continue" (Manning, 1998, p. 1D). Conley's perceptions were supported by Lynn Nonnemaker's recent study of women physicians who, although 10 percent more likely to pursue a career in academic medicine, were 26 percent *less* likely to be promoted, with few advancing to full professorships (De Angelis, 2000). Clearly, simple increases in numbers of women physicians or PAs were not an adequate measure of more fundamental changes in gendered value systems and practices. Even with a blurring of occupational gendering, the pattern of male dominance in higher-authority positions was still largely intact.

Indeed, this pattern was still evident throughout the work world, and was clear in a 1995 Roper Starch national opinion poll of 3,000 women and 1,000 men on gender issues, which is conducted every five years (Dobrzynski, 1995). Of the women polled, 84 percent agreed that, regardless of changes that may have occurred, women still face more restrictions in life than men do. A majority (77 percent) said that sex discrimination remains a serious problem even if it is more subtle and less open. And 76 percent said there was considerable or some sexual harassment in the workplace. Only 56 percent saw the role of women continuing to change, compared to 73 percent in 1990. Men agreed: 57 percent, down from 76 percent in 1990, said that women's roles would continue to change.

The poll indicates that 73 percent of women work because they must, up from 55 percent in 1990 and 46 percent in 1980. Only 23 percent worked simply to bring in extra money. Unfortunately, only 31 percent received great personal satisfaction from their jobs. Almost equal numbers of women (32 percent) and men (31 percent) wanted company-run, on-site day care for their children. Ninety-four percent of the women said that some or major changes were needed in their salaries, and 87 percent in their opportunities for leadership positions. When listing specific reasons why women were held back, 44 percent said they were given mostly low or midlevel jobs, while men held the real power; 44 percent said women faced the old-boy network in major corporations; and 38 percent felt that the doors have not been open long enough for women to get to the top. Indeed, in another poll, this one conducted for *Working Woman* magazine by Louis Harris, 54 percent of 500 female top executives described their work world as a very alien territory or a hostile environment; the women still felt like outsiders, whose achievements were downplayed and who were dismissed as the "other" (Dobrzynski, 1995). In the Roper Starch poll, 44 percent of the respondents said women are held to a higher standard than men. Changes were obviously necessary, but the one of particular interest to nurses is the substantial proportion of women (58 percent) *and* men (59 percent), who cited better health benefits as a key to greater job satisfaction. They had good reason to be concerned about this issue.

By the last decade of the twentieth century, the results of the sustained medical monopoly were not impressive. The United States spends over two billion dollars a day on health care, more per capita than any other society; in fact, costs for health care in the United States have risen 48 percent since 1990 (AARP, 1998). Still, some 60 million Americans receive only minimal health care, another 60 million have insurance inadequate for serious illness, over 42 million are totally uninsured, and more than 25 percent of these are children. Obviously, some form of a national health system is needed, but the AMA has opposed this for decades, as it opposed national maternal and child-health programs in the 1920s, Social Security in the 1940s, and Medicaid and Medicare in the 1960s. In contrast, the American Nurses' Association (ANA) has consistently over several decades supported such social legislation. Medicare and Medicaid are not enough; the latter, even by the early 1990s, provided care for only half of those eligible. Though many physicians are now blaming HMOs for a perceived loss of control and autonomy and reduction in incomes, they are themselves being accused of greed, since many refuse to care for Medicaid patients because they receive more money from patients with private insurance. For example, in 1991, 23 percent of pediatricians refused Medicaid patients and 39 percent limited the number they would take. When the government capped hospital costs for Medicare, physicians created outpatient services; by 1991, the costs for these had risen three times more rapidly than costs in hospitals. Without substantial cuts in physician and hospital costs, it is predicted that these programs may be bankrupt by the early decades of the twenty-first century.

Nurses' Views of the Health-Care "System": A Call for a Different Direction

Nurses are well aware of the inadequacies in the "system" of health care in the United States and have clear views on how they would change it. In 1988 nurse Florence L. Huey said that Americans had the poorest access to the most expensive health-care system in the world, paying $1,800 per person and 11 percent of the gross national product. In comparison, Canada offered universal access for $1,300 per capita and 8 percent of its gross national product. Of the $500 million spent each year in the late 1980s, American hospitals and physicians took 60 percent or $3 out of every $5 spent. And physicians' payments under Medicare were rising by 17 percent per year. Reducing the number of days spent in hospitals had only shifted the costs to ambulatory care. From 1980 to 1986, the number of hospital days had fallen from 68 million to 57 million, but the number of outpatient visits rose from 55 million to 67 million. Administration of health-insurance costs about 22 cents on the dollar in the United States compared to 2.5 cents in Canada.

From interviews with nursing leaders, said Huey, it was clear that there was "gerrymandering" of competition. Despite thirty years of research on the cost-effectiveness of nurses as primary-care providers, they were still shut out of competition. Instead of prevention, stressed by nurses for decades, there was continued emphasis on high-tech care and on cures. For example, for every $1 invested in prenatal care, $3 to $10 are subsequently saved; nevertheless, about $2 billion was spent on low-birth-weight infants, while only $500 million would provide prenatal care for *all* women who currently go without such care and, therefore, are more likely to produce the low-birth-weight babies.

The Medicaid maze, a means-tested obstacle course presumably designed to help the uninsured, has simply prolonged the "unbroken history of begging for health care in the United States" (Huey, 1988, p. 1484). Under President Reagan, the 1981 Omnibus Reconciliation Act caused a half-million people to lose Medicaid eligibility. This budget reform consolidated twenty-one health-care programs into four block grants to be administered by states; subsequently, federal funding dropped by 18 percent for a number of programs. "What we save by limiting access to health care, we spend to treat the complications" (p. 1486). The medical monopoly directly contributed to the problems: "In a 3-year demonstration project in California, for example, prenatal care doubled and prematurity rates fell by 40 percent when nurse-midwives provided access to prenatal care.... When the program ended (because of physician opposition to nurse-midwives), prenatal care again fell and the prematurity rate turned to the previous level" (p. 1486).

Nurses wanted to stop plugging the holes in the system caused by piecemeal coverage of specific populations. They recommended that universal maternity care for every pregnant woman be channeled to the appropriate level of care through neighborhood birthing centers run by nurse midwives, who could also handle about 75 percent of births. If only 25 percent of the 3.6 million pregnant women used birthing centers, between $717 million to $33 billion could be saved. For school-age children, an expanded system of care by school health practitioners could, according to research, "handle 87% of problems with 96% resolution, no duplication of services, and for one-quarter of the cost of conventional end-stage care" (p. 1491). Similar savings could be produced with community-based, long-term care, not only for the elderly but also for the people under 65 who represent 40 percent of those who need such care. Huey asserted that "nurses are painfully certain that our nation's health priorities are wrong: We need to shift emphasis away from the most expensive settings—institutions—and the most expensive providers—physicians" (p. 1493). Clearly, the nursing leaders interviewed by Huey had solutions to health-care problems, but whether they or others could act on their analyses remained the key issue.

Nursing was successful in stopping the development and widespread implementation of the registered care technician (RCT) that was proposed by organized medicine; however, as we shall see, it was replaced by another variation, unlicensed assistive personnel (UAPs), forcing nurses into still another struggle. Indeed, in the 1990s changes in the direction of health care happened so rapidly that nursing was hard pressed from many directions.

In 1991 the ANA published *Nursing's Agenda for Health Care Reform*, espousing a primary and preventive health-care system in which consumers could access the most cost-effective providers in community-based settings. Nurses again called for a shift from illness and cure to an orientation toward wellness and prevention, assurance of direct access to a full range of qualified providers, and the elimination of unnecessary bureaucratic controls and administrative procedures. Supported by the ANA, the National League for Nursing (NLN), and the American Association of Colleges of Nursing (AACN), the proposal positioned nurses as primary caregivers, provided new incentives to cut costs, decreased the emphasis on inpatient acute care, and increased preventive, primary, and long-term care. Subsequently approved by eighteen national nursing organizations, the plan included a federally defined standard package of essential health-care benefits available to all citizens financed through a mix of public and private sources but with federal enforcement. The nurses further advocated improving consumer access by delivering primary-care services in convenient settings, such as schools, homes, and the workplace. They recommended the control of health-care costs through managed care in which there would be incentives for cost control for both consumers and providers; freedom of choice for types of providers, settings, and delivery arrangements; reduced administrative costs through simplified bureaucratic controls and governance procedures; and payment policies connected to treatment effectiveness, to be determined by research on outcomes.

The nurses' plan would be implemented in steps, with priority given to pregnant women, infants, and children, the most cost-effective groups for improving the long-term health of the nation. Nurses would be gatekeepers, cost-saving providers, who would be positioned to encourage more appropriate care and a shift away from hospitalization and technology toward less costly providers in local health-care delivery settings. Accordingly, Medicare would include payments for nursing services to provide preventive services, primary care, and home care.

The nurses specifically included consumers in their plan. In a survey conducted through Hart Research Association, the NLN identified consumers' most pressing concerns. The study, whose results were published in a 1991 *NLN Public Policy Bulletin,* found that nurses were perceived more positively than other caregivers or caregiving institutions. Survey respondents were asked to rate groups and institutions on the extent to which they played a constructive role or attended to their own interests and were therefore part of the problem. Nurses were rated as playing a constructive role by 77 percent of the respondents, compared to physicians (42 percent), hospitals (43 percent), nursing homes (35 percent), hospital administrators (29 percent), the federal government (19 percent), and insurance companies (11 percent). Indeed, the survey demonstrated that the nurses' overall image was positive and their position was highly credible; thus, their plan for health-care reform should be well received. Furthermore, the survey also showed that many people would go to nurses for care instead of physicians and would support direct Medicare payments to nurses. As noted in chapter 9, nurse practitioners' fight to receive Medicare payments directly, regardless of specialty or geographic area of practice, was finally won in 1997.

Consumers were probably right in trusting nurses, because research on the quality of their care continued to show that they provided not only equivalent but *better* primary care than physicians. In a 1991 nationwide study by Jerry Avorn and colleagues, the potential of nurses is most clearly evident. Drawn from a stratified random sample, 501 internists and family or general practitioners were compared with 298 nurse practitioners in their responses to a case of a patient with abdominal pain. The participants were repeatedly asked by the researchers if there were any additional patient information needed before formulating a treatment plan. If they asked, additional standardized information was provided. The researchers found major "differences . . . in the diagnostic and therapeutic style of nurse practitioners when compared with physicians" (Avorn, Everitt, and Baker, 1991, p. 696). Twice as many physicians chose to initiate treatment *without* soliciting any additional patient information. The nurses much more frequently requested information on the patient's psychosocial circumstances, and especially on dietary factors.

The therapeutic interventions were also strikingly different: 63 percent of the physicians chose to write a prescription, but only 20 percent of the nurses did so, opting instead to recommend dietary changes or stress-reduction strategies, which were more appropriate for a patient with gastritis who also had high aspirin, caffeine, alcohol, and tobacco intake—facts that could only be known if the nurse or physician had chosen to ask for more information *before* starting therapy. According to the researchers, the nurses were far more likely to obtain the information needed "to make an intelligent treatment plan"; indeed, the nurse practitioners, who were reimbursed at a significantly lower level, nevertheless, performed the tasks of history taking and patient counseling more completely. Clearly, the gendered professional groups performed differently, presumably valuing different aspects of patient care.

A Fundamental Restructuring of the Health-Care "System"

Given the continued proof of advanced nurses' capabilities, Safriet (1992), as noted in chapter 9, called for a fundamental restructuring of the existing health-care "system," but questioned the accuracy of the term "system" since it connoted a considered structure involving organization and coordination, which obviously did not exist. The *quality* of American health care continued to be lower on a number of major health indices compared to that of other industrialized countries. There was also a continued high incidence of inappropriate or unnecessary care. The "system" was also characterized by overemphasis on medical services that stressed curing objectively defined illness and injuries and neglected the prevention of illness. The cost for this "system" of care had grown from 5.9 percent of the gross national product (GNP) in 1965 to 12.5 percent in 1990 or from $42 to $647 billion, mostly funded through public, not private, funds. Health-care costs are now 14 percent to 15 percent of the GNP.

Clearly, the regulation of licensing, accreditation, education, reimbursement, and activities of health-care providers needed thorough investigation. In the meantime, said Safriet, one small step could be taken immediately to improve access and quality at a lower cost, particularly for poor and rural people: "That step is simply to remove the unnecessary barriers to practice that certified nurse-midwives and nurse practitioners ... now face" (p. 421). By 1988, 63,000 RNs had received nurse practitioner training, but only 23,000 were in practice positions carrying the title. In 1990 there were 4,200 certified nurse midwives; in 1988 nurse midwives delivered 115,000 babies in hospitals, only 3.4 percent of all births.

As discussed in chapter 9, the quality of the care of APNs had been established in the review and analysis of studies published by the Office of Technology Assessment (1986); subsequent studies, considered later in this chapter, reinforced the earlier conclusions. To Safriet, proof of quality of care was crucial because the deployment of APNs depended on their safety and effectiveness, which had been repeatedly and severely questioned, primarily by physicians. Since the research had substantially disproved medical objections, it was very important to expand the use of APNs, particularly in rural and inner-city areas where physicians were less likely to practice. Nurses had already increased people's access to primary care in these areas and also in school-based clinics, long-term facilities and nursing homes, correctional institutions, industrial and community-health clinics, and free-standing birthing centers. In 1985 and 1988, the Institute of Medicine, part of the National Academy of Sciences, concluded that nurse practitioners and midwives were needed to increase the use of prenatal-care systems by lower-income women.

As a noted attorney and legal scholar, Safriet was particularly impressed that the nurses had accomplished such positive results, "despite the multiple legal and professional restrictions on their practices" (p. 433). Even though states required physicians' presence, they had usually refused to collaborate or to accept nurses' referrals. Furthermore, "a multitude of restrictive reimbursement schemes either refuse to pay them for their services or funnel their payment through physicians or hospitals and other institutions" (p. 433). When paid, these payment schemes usually "allow for only a portion of the fee that would be paid to a physician who provided exactly the same service with exactly the same quality outcome" (p. 433).

The cost-effectiveness of APNs, given the evidence by the 1990s, sustained the earlier findings discussed in previous chapters. But Dr. Claire M. Fagin, RN (1990), in a review of studies conducted between 1981 and 1990, admitted the complexity of the issue particularly given the inadequate or nonexistent data on the costs and efficiency of physicians' services. Furthermore, the wide variations in the legal and professional constraints by states and practice settings continued to make comparisons even more difficult. Defining discrete tasks by professional group, given the broad overlap of functions and control of these by physicians, also created problems. Nevertheless, Fagin largely reaffirmed the earlier findings and analyses made in the 1970s and 1980s: APNs were or potentially could be cost-effective alternatives to higher-priced physicians. These findings on cost-effectiveness also were confirmed in later studies. Since the research results were so repetitive for at least two decades, the failure to use APNs can only be traced to physician opposition and the medical monopoly.

The AMA Votes Again to Retain Its Monopoly: "Collaboration Equals Supervision"

Despite the positive research results on RN cost and care, a report and recommendations on independent nursing practice models by the AMA Board of Trustees were adopted by the AMA House of Delegates (American Medical Association, 1990c). In this report any nursing mode of care was considered to be independent if it impedes physician involvement in medical care within twenty-four hours of contact, admits patients to facilities or provides medical services without physician consultation, or assigns direct reimbursement for nursing service. Thus, as Safriet notes, "an 'independent' nursing practice is one in which the physician is replaced or supplanted as the paid 'gatekeeper' to health care" (Safriet, 1992, p. 455).

Collaborative practice between medicine and nursing was defined by the AMA as a "*moral* context" in which "autonomous" nursing practice "'*respects* and *supports* the autonomy of medical practice and vice versa'" (p. 455). This was contrasted with nursing models that adopt a "medical" model, "'*compete* for services . . . actively seek to increase the *hegemony* of the nursing profession, and *empower* nursing within the health care system. . . . Direct reimbursement is a major prerequisite for independent nurse practice'" (p. 455). To stop these competing models, the AMA board recommended and the House of Delegates resolved to insist on physicians' supervision as a qualification for nurses' reimbursement in state and federal legislation; to insist on physicians retaining their intermediary responsibility for direct patient care and to work for changes in federal and state legislation to ensure this; and to oppose any attempt at empowering non-physicians to become unsupervised primary "medical" caregivers and to be directly reimbursed for case-management activities (AMA, 1990b). A clearer restatement of a medical monopoly could not be made.

ANA Votes in Direct Opposition to the AMA

Summarily dismissing the AMA's report, the ANA board, after reviewing the report of their own Ad Hoc Committee on Credentialing in Advanced Practice, agreed with the committee's definitions of advanced specialty practice and with the requirement for graduate degrees, and further agreed that APNs are to be regulated by state boards of nursing (BONs) that have the *sole* authority to define and regulate advanced practice. These boards promulgate roles that include both diagnosing and prescribing privileges, "without reference to any requirements for physician collaboration, practice agreements, supervision, direction, protocols, or formularies" (*American Nurse,* 1993a, p. 22). State nurses' associations and affiliated specialty nursing associations were encouraged to develop and pursue strategies to achieve such definitions and regulatory systems, to promote educational opportunities for advanced nurse practice, to lobby for nondiscriminatory reimbursement requirements, and to support model legislative language and administrative rules based on the guidelines approved by the ANA board of directors.

Clearly, organized nursing and medicine were on a public collision course. Indeed, Winifred Carson of the ANA legal affairs department laid out in a series of four articles the legal barriers to practice, and specifically stated that "all too often nurses are restricted by legislation promoted by other health care professionals to protect their scopes of practice" (Carson, 1993a, p. 26). More precisely, she pointed to the use of terminology or regulations that "include language formalizing the physician-nurse relationships" (p. 26). However, the realities of practice, fortunately for patients, often bore little resemblance to statutes: "nurses are often treated as the primary care provider with little physician intervention, unless requested" (p. 26). Nevertheless, legislators continued to perceive nurses as needing supervision. The wide variations in state statutes created real problems in interstate reciprocity for APNs. Thirty-seven states authorized some form of advanced practice, but only two specified interstate reciprocity. Another major problem, as noted in the previous chapter, was the refusal of insurance carriers to reimburse independent nurse practitioners. Even though some states enacted laws to mandate that private insurers directly reimburse for nursing services, the laws varied widely and some insurers have continued to refuse reimbursement.

State laws were inconsistent in delineating the boundaries of medical and nursing practice, and some APNs were being charged with conducting "medical acts" and faced subsequent disciplinary action. Indeed, all nurses in some states were faced with new state laws that, for example, limited "invasive" procedures to the practice of medicine. In 1992 in Georgia, senate bill 159 would have prevented nurses from giving injections unless under *direct* supervision of a physician. The Georgia Nurses Association, unwavering in opposition to this invasion of their legal, autonomous practice, obtained a restraining order, and ultimately their position prevailed with the state supreme court. "The Medical Association of Georgia was the only party asking the [state] Supreme Court to preserve any part of the controversial legislation" (*American Nurse*, 1993b, p. 24). Despite the physicians' opposition, the law was found to be unconstitutional and the Supreme Court rejected lower court language mandating medically supervised nursing practice. To justify such monopolistic meddling, organized medicine must prove the health-care "system" they dominate is exceptional. Obviously, this is not the case.

The Consumer's Perspective on the Nation's Health-Care "System"

Physicians claim that their medical monopoly assures quality health care; if they are right, then the results should be readily apparent in the state of the nation's health. For a consumer perspective, presumably unbiased by either medicine or nursing, Consumers Union, noted from the 1930s onward for its objective analysis of everything from cars to insurance policies, presented a three-part series on health care in *Consumer Reports* (Consumers Union, 1992a, 1992b, 1992c). Though the editors failed to deal with nurses at all, focusing instead on physicians, hospitals, and drug and insurance companies, their exposé of the U.S. health-care system was startling. Of the $817 billion spent on health care in 1992, the editors claimed that at least $200 billion went for overpriced, useless, or even harmful treatments and a huge, unwieldy bureaucracy. Comparable countries spent half this amount, but their life expectancies and infant mortality rates were often much better than those in the United States. The price structure for medical care and the patterns of treatment and hospitalization in the United States were so inherently wasteful and inefficient that a total overhaul was needed. Trying to patch up the system with piecemeal reforms would not work because physicians and administrators would simply find spaces between the patches to use to their advantage.

Historically, the American "system" has allowed physicians to order any procedures they wanted and be paid whatever they think they should get. Similarly, hospitals have set their own costs and received whatever payments they could get. In contrast, Canada, Japan, and Western European countries have universal, standard payment schedules, directly negotiated with physicians and hospitals, and overall ceilings on national medical expenditures. Not one of these countries spends more than 10 percent of its gross national product on health care. The United States matched this percentage in 1985 and reached 14 percent in 1992. Ironically, Consumers Union seemed to assume that only physicians could provide care, entirely failing to consider nurses as a more cost-effective alternative. The sex-stratified system simply made invisible the largest group of health-care workers.

When Medicare, the government-sponsored program for the elderly, and Medicaid, the comparable program for the poor, were established by Congress in 1965, physicians were allowed to set their own charges in order to avoid allegations of "socialized medicine" by physicians and hospitals. With no effective constraints on costs, fees rapidly spiraled upward, particularly since hospitals were also allowed to build the cost of capital improvement into their rates. As Medicare began to set limits on physicians' fees and cut back on hospital budgets, through diagnostic related groups (DRGs), for example, physicians and hospitals charged privately insured patients more. With a "system" that virtually set no limits on what was done or charged, it was found in several studies that physicians often had only a vague idea of the costs of hospital tests and services. As new technologies, such as computerized tomography or magnetic resonance imaging, emerged, their use exploded even for patients who did not need such procedures; consequently, investment in technology has also been irrational and poorly planned.

According to *Consumer Reports* (Consumers Union, 1992a), ill and uninformed patients were unable to comparison shop, since physicians made almost all decisions that determined the costs of care. When nurses are excluded, true comparison shopping is not genuinely possible. To increase income, physicians might order more tests, schedule more appointments, provide less time to patients, and refer patients to facilities in which physicians have financial interests. In short, they profit from their own induced demand. Some even engage in actual fraud. According to the U.S. General Accounting Office, 10 percent to 12 percent of health-care costs are fraudulent, for example, in kickbacks some physicians receive for making referrals on phony diagnoses. More often, physicians create demand without knowing it. In areas with the greatest supply of physicians, people go to them more often, and in places that have more hospital beds, people are sent to them more frequently. Again, the possibility of using nurse practitioners in the community was not included in the discussion of physicians' income-making practices, which are only possible in an occupation that holds a total monopoly. Again, in this consumer-oriented analysis, monopolistic power was not specifically discussed and the sex-segregated system is assumed and left unexamined.

In a system of induced demand, a sizable amount of care is unnecessary, if not harmful. The Rand Corporation, a California research center, obtained consensus among recognized medical experts on a list of indications for certain procedures and then examined thousands of patients' records to see if the procedures were appropriate; "appropriateness" was simply defined as providing greater benefit than the risk involved in doing the procedure. Even with a substantial number of equivocal ratings, there was evidence of inappropriate treatment: for example, 17 percent of coronary angiograms, 14 percent of heart bypass operations, and 32 percent of operations to remove atherosclerotic plaque from the carotid artery were unnecessary. Using similar methodologies, various other studies have also found unnecessary procedures: for example, one study discovered that 27 percent of hysterectomies, 17 percent of surgeries for carpal tunnel syndrome, 16 percent of laminectomies, and 17 percent of tonsillectomies were unnecessary. Research on other procedures produced findings of 60 percent unnecessary preoperative laboratory screening, 50 percent unneeded cesarean sections, and 30 percent unnecessary upper gastrointestinal X-ray studies.

Consumers Union concluded that medical practice was conducted in a milieu of uncertainty and was affected by prevailing folklore in isolated medical referral networks. Thus, for example, the probability of tonsillectomies varied by towns: by age 15, 70 percent of patients in one Vermont community had had their tonsils removed, but only 10 percent of patients in a nearby town underwent this procedure. A number of research studies produced similar findings. Indeed, the only procedures that do not show regional and geographic variations are hospitalizations for heart attacks or strokes, for which there is only this option. Hospitalizations for other procedures have also been found to be unnecessary, ranging in some research from 15 percent to 30 percent.

With Medicare disincentives, the number of hospital days had dropped 22 percent, but there were still large regional variations. Nevertheless, in 1990, hospitals accounted for 38 percent of the national expenditures and earned a profit on $7 billion. Reductions in Medicare reimbursements had been offset by hospitals by increasing their outpatient, psychiatric, and rehabilitation services. Thus, patching one part of the system does not work. Indeed, hospitals had attracted more physicians by granting first-year guaranteed incomes or by giving subsidies for initial practice expenses. The average physician in 1990, according to Consumers Union, generated $513,000 in in-hospital revenue. Unleashing competition among hospitals during the 1980s actually *increased* costs as hospitals, for example, obtained more costly technology and created specialized units in order to compete for more patients.

Since the salaries of women workers, particularly nurses, are often inappropriately included in hospital room charges, it is impossible to analyze separately the cost to patients of these women's services. Hospitals are only possible if there are nurses; thus, nurses' views on the reduced number of hospital days for patients should have been included. Furthermore, care in the homes of released patients is given primarily by female family members and women health professionals. Cutting the number of hospital days does not mean that patients are capable of taking care of themselves when released. Someone must care for them at home. Yet the wives, mothers, grandmothers, friends, and community-health nurses, nursing aides, and home aides—mostly women— were excluded from a presumably consumer-oriented analysis. Furthermore, nurses, more than any other group, are most prepared by education and experience to critique the need for hospitalization and the appropriateness of physicians' interventions. When nurses are excluded, consumers lose the only group capable of daily surveillance of physicians. Consumers also lose the different health-care emphases of nurses, and reduce their authority to speak out on behalf of consumers.

Given the extreme medical monopoly in the United States, it is not surprising that American physicians earned 5.4 times more than the average worker, while for physicians in Germany the figure was 4.2; in Canada, 3.7; and in France, Japan, and Great Britain, 2.4. In the United States, the high proportion of specialists pushes income levels higher. Internists charged, in 1990, a fee of $110 for a comprehensive office visit that may take forty-five minutes, but charged a median fee of $126 for a ten-minute examination of the bowel with a sigmoidoscope. As new treatments are tried, the price is set high; after widespread usage, risk goes down, but the price does not. Primary-care and family physicians, general internists, and pediatricians had a median income between $93,000 and $100,000 in 1990, compared to $200,000 for surgeons and radiologists, and $500,000 for cardiovascular surgeons. Since specialization pays, only one-third of American physicians were in primary care, and in 1987 only a fourth of medical students entered primary care after their internships and residencies. While other countries maintain a 50–50 ratio, American specialists, despite insufficient cases, continue to run up higher bills for patients. Although, as noted in the previous chapter, the Physicians Payment Review Board developed the resource-based relative value scale in 1989, a standard, national fee schedule that increased the fees for evaluation and management in primary-care and reduced fees for specialized procedures, physicians could avoid these by increasing costs for privately insured patients or by "unbundling" services—charging, for example, not $1,200 for a hysterectomy, but $7,000 by billing separately for each component of the operation.

As discussed in chapter 9, several research studies demonstrate that nurses can give much of the primary care now provided by more costly physicians. Why then did Consumers Union exclude these possibilities for cost reduction by excluding competent women workers as alternatives to physicians? Particularly since research proved that nurses produced equal or better results than the physicians?

Not only physicians, but pharmaceutical companies also made profits on the ill, operating with a profit margin of 15 percent and producing a 25 percent average return to investors throughout the 1980s. Compared to other countries, costs of drugs and machinery are significantly higher in the United States. In 1992 an examination using magnetic resonance imaging cost $177 in Japan, compared to $1,000 in the United States. Indeed, of twenty-four industrialized nations, the United States spends more than two times more per capita than any other nation and a far greater proportion of the gross national product. Yet in 1992, the United States ranked twenty-first in infant mortality, seventeenth in male life expectancy, and sixteenth in female life expectancy (Consumers Union, 1992a). Compared to European countries, the United States ranked at or close to the bottom on the availability of quality primary care on a number of public-health indicators, and on public satisfaction with health care. Consumers Union concluded that the system was geared to services that produced the most money for physicians and hospitals, not the low-tech care that prevents ill health. Why then did Consumers Union not turn to the logical alternative, nurses? Certainly, women's wages in health care, in contrast to the inflated incomes of medical specialists, have been substandard; thus, the costs of nurse practitioners, even with equity increases, would be substantially lower.

According to *Consumer Reports,* to sustain the appearance of private medicine, the most bureaucratic system in the world had emerged, which required multiple forms from some 1,200 insurance companies and numerous government forms and review procedures; thus, American hospitals spent an average 20 percent of their budget on billing administration, compared to 9 percent in Canadian hospitals: "To run a health plan covering 25 million people, Canada employs fewer administrators than Massachusetts Blue Cross, which covers 2.7 million" (Consumers Union, 1992a, p. 448). Indeed, even the average private physician in the United States employed twice as many clerical workers than the average Canadian physician. According to the U.S. General Accounting Office, $70 billion annually would be saved if Americans adopted the single-payer Canadian system.

What solutions did Consumers Union suggest? A radically different system—different from the current patchwork mess. In the second part of the series (Consumers Union, 1992b), the editors considered HMOs as one possible alternative. In HMOs, which originated about forty years ago as alternatives to traditional, fragmented, fee-for-service medicine, salaried physicians provide prepaid care in group practices. Members or employers pay the same monthly fees regardless of whether people are sick or well; thus, there is a strong incentive to provide preventive services and to coordinate treatment, control hospital usage, and limit referrals to specialists. During the 1970s, the Nixon administration thwarted proposals for national health insurance by fostering HMOs, but a 1973 federal law allowed very different organizations from the earlier prepaid, mostly nonprofit group practice plans. By 1992 the 550 organizations created by hospitals, physicians, or entrepreneurs could be a loose collection of physicians who were practicing a variant of fee-for-service medicine. Many HMOs do little checking on physicians' qualifications and even less on the quality of work.

Choice of a primary-care physician, who sometimes coordinates contact with specialists and hospitals, is required in HMOs; thus, APNs are often eliminated as competitors in primary care. Some HMOs pay salaries and award bonuses if there is an annual profit. Others give capitation payments for the numbers of patients based on expected costs, but if these are above set levels, the physicians receive no additional monies; thus, there is no incentive to overtreat but there may be one to undertreat. Other HMOs pay according to fee schedules and penalize physicians if they exceed specified numbers of referrals and hospitalizations. As discussed later in this chapter, these and other restrictions imposed by HMOs have led to recent complaints by many physicians that they have lost control over their practices. As HMOs compete with the going rates in the wider marketplace, higher costs eventually enter the HMOs and negate the possibility of controlling health-care costs. This is exacerbated by little control of referrals to specialists external to the HMO, whose fees remain excessively high and are paid in large measure by the patients themselves.

Another serious problem is the lack of scientific measures for determining the quality of health care. Chart reviews show that total patients' visits obviously provide no appropriate outcome measures. In addition, it is clear that HMOs have not led the way to better preventive care since, for example, their immunization rates for children range only from 60 percent to 85 percent. Indeed, the quality of service could not be measured and was found to vary in the 46 largest HMOs studied by the Consumers Union. To keep costs lower, only 22 percent of the HMOs covered people who were not part of employer groups, and some of these groups were considered high risk and rejected. For example, one higher-rated HMO rejected any hospital employees, such as nurses, because of their exposure to drugs and technological hazards. There is a further problem of stability of service since a number of businessmen and physicians by the 1990s had sold out and merged with other HMOs and hospitals, or shut down completely.

From their own survey, Consumers Union concluded that in general the usage of medical services and hospitals and ambulatory care by HMO and privately insured patients was similar, except at HMOs located in clinics. The fastest growth in HMOs was of those in which physicians practiced for a fee-for-service in their own offices and where, despite group-based discounts, the pressure was toward uniformity in fees with physicians outside the HMOs. Finally the use of expensive, new technology did not seem to be less in the HMOs.

At the risk of being boringly repetitive, it must again be pointed out that Consumers Union's analysis of HMOs was focused entirely on physicians and that discussion of nurses' roles in such organizations or as alternatives to MDs was completely lacking. Yet public health, school, and industrial nurses have historically played a critical role in primary and preventive care—for example, in children's immunizations—in addition to many other practices and procedures. Again, the nurses were invisible even though they are currently the backbone of nonhospital clinics.

In a third article (Consumers Union, 1992c), other solutions were considered. The Canadian system, which was introduced thirty years ago as a single-payer provincial program, was under increasing attack from American special-interest groups that profit from the American non-system of health care. In fact, Canada does not practice "socialized medicine"; its program is one of social-health insurance like Social Security and Medicare. Canadian physicians do not work for a salary from the government, but are paid by patients, who have paid through payroll taxes for medical, hospital, long-term, and mental-health care, and for drugs, at least for those over sixty-five.

According to Consumers Union, the Canada Health Act is guided by five principles: universality, coverage for everyone; portability, benefits continue despite changes in employment or movement from one province to another; accessibility, all providers are available; comprehensiveness, coverage of all necessary treatment; and public administration, government-run and publicly accountable. Contrary to the charges of American critics, the Canadian system does not involve a terrible bureaucracy that tells physicians how to practice. Indeed, they practice in their own offices, but they may not charge whatever they want: their fees are negotiated by the provincial ministry of health and the medical associations. The result is that in 1992 the removal of a gall bladder in Ontario cost $348, compared to $945 across the border in Buffalo, New York. Even with lower fees, the average annual income of physicians ranged from $128,000 for general practitioners to $290,500 for cardiologists. Nevertheless, half of Canadian physicians were in general practice, compared to 13 percent of physicians in the United States.

Patients in Canada select their own physicians, whose bills are paid by the provincial insurance plans within two to four weeks of treatment. Patients go to general practitioners, seeing specialists usually by referral, which is probably still too frequent because general practitioners can increase the number of patients they see by referring difficult cases to specialists. Hospital beds have been reduced not because of the single-payer system, but because both Canadians and Americans overbuilt hospitals during the last few decades. In addition, deliberate government strategies to eliminate waste and duplication of services are possible because monies received by hospitals can be controlled through the annual national budgets, which make up 95 percent of each hospital's total funds; these can be used as the institution desires, although it may not run a deficit. The introduction and use of technology is also subject to control of overuse, inappropriate use, or duplication. Consumers Union argued that the waiting lists for care in Canada have been exaggerated by American critics and that Canadians get regular and emergency care as needed. In 1991 the British Columbia Royal Commission on Health Care found, after investigating all publicized cases of people claiming to be damaged by delays, that almost none were well founded. Waiting lists of eight hundred to nine hundred for heart surgery in British Columbia were alleged by American critics; however, about 66 percent of the patients were waiting not for the procedure but for one of three particular surgeons. However, by the end of the 1990s, after budget cuts, there was evidence of real delays in providing some services, particularly in some larger urban areas in Canada.

In contrast to conservative critics, Consumers Union asserted that Canadians are getting too much, not too little care. In a conference of provincial health ministers, a significant amount of ineffective or inappropriate care was reported, primarily because of the fee-for-service reimbursements to physicians; the problems caused by this system in America are similar. Indeed, Canada led the world in gall bladder surgeries and was second to the United States in heart-bypass surgeries. Although an American national insurance association charged that Canadian health-care costs were higher than in the United States, Consumers Union asserted that the costs were lower: $2,450 per American, but $1,800 per Canadian in 1989 and in 1990; 12.2 percent of the American gross national product, but only 9.5 percent of the Canadian, was expended on health care. About 25 percent to 35 percent of the difference in costs is due to hospital controls. In addition, the U.S. spent between 19 percent and 24 percent on administrative expenses, but Canada spent only between 8 percent and 11 percent. Unfortunately, Canadian physicians have used publicity releases to exaggerate negative circumstances in order to improve their negotiations with provincial governments. Consumers Union did, however, note the shortage of physicians in remote areas, a problem in the United States as well. There was also a trend toward greater numbers of specialists, in part influenced by the American precedent.

The most serious criticism of the Canadian health-care system is the tendency of provincial governments to be check writers rather than health managers, but this is changing with hospitals getting smaller increases and monies being distributed to other facilities. One- or two-day preoperative stays have been eliminated. The Canadian economy forced the federal government to decrease funding, but as Consumers Union concluded, the Canadians have at least answered affirmatively the question of whether everyone should be entitled to health care. Clearly, Canadians prefer their system: only one of 1,503 people testifying before the British Columbia Royal Commission on Health Care advocated the American way for paying for care. Observe, again, that Canadian nurses were completely eliminated from this analysis, making it impossible to consider the financial consequences of empowering the women by breaking the Canadian physicians' monopoly. Even with substantial incomes, physicians were still concerned with higher profits. As long as it remains a monopoly, organized medicine can still control nurses in a state-sponsored system if it excludes them from providing care at lower cost.

For comparison purposes, Consumers Union examined two states: Hawaii, which had coverage for nearly all residents, and Minnesota, which in some places had large HMO coverage. Hawaii spent 8 percent of its gross state budget on health care in 1989, while health care received 11 percent of the federal budget; nevertheless, there were indications that Hawaiians enjoyed better health than Americans as a whole. In addition, the Hawaii legislature established a state health insurance plan in 1989 to cover the unemployed and part-time workers who did not qualify for Medicaid; this left only 2 percent uninsured, compared with 14 percent on the mainland. Because two HMOs in Hawaii control a large share of the market, they were able to limit fee increases, paying only cost-of-living increases, and began to eliminate "unbundling," forcing one charge for an operation instead of allowing separate charges for incisions, removals, and suturing. Policies have been designed to favor outpatient and preventive care and to pay only the minimum rate for hospital rooms. Hawaiians did not overbuild hospitals; thus, they were 80 percent to 90 percent full. A health-planning agency controlled the duplication of expensive technology.

Still, Hawaiian hospitals were having difficulty keeping up with costs because of new technology and the failure of Medicare and Medicaid to pay adequately. To deal with inadequate coverage, patients with private insurers were charged more, and this cost shifting was passed to insurers, who in turn raised their premiums. Nearly universal coverage is not the same as universal coverage, since Medicaid patients are often refused by physicians and dentists, and employers pay higher copayments, again limiting access. Nevertheless, Consumers Union concluded that the clearest lesson was the *pernicious effects of cost shifting when public and private insurance try to coexist.* Again, nurses were not considered as low-cost alternatives to physicians. The only time in all three articles that Consumers Union referred to nurses was to note the "radical" wage inflation, presumably caused by nurses, who had recently won a 28 percent salary increase spread over three years.

In contrast to Hawaii, half the people in Minneapolis, Minnesota, were covered by HMOs in 1992; thus, "managed care" could be assessed. As a result of hard bargains for discounts, about half of the hospitals had collapsed, presumably eliminating unneeded hospital beds. In addition, inpatient services could be performed in outpatient settings, a result that was then transferred to the treatment of privately insured patients, causing a significant overall drop in hospitalization and in patient costs. However, with mergers, the fewer and stronger hospitals were able to force HMOs to accept less favorable packages. Thus, these organizations had increased their premiums by 18 percent in 1991, reflecting their inability to limit costs any better than private insurers. There is no planning agency to evaluate new procedures and no certificate-of-need law as in Hawaii to evaluate the need for new technology. According to the Consumers Union survey, the degree of satisfaction of Minnesota HMO participants was about the same as that of privately insured people.

Almost all HMOs did business only with large employers; therefore, this system had not been successful in expanding coverage to the 300,000 uninsured throughout Minnesota, and individuals who are already sick were rejected by both HMOs and private insurers. Even with recent state changes, 150,000 people are projected to remain essentially outside the system. Again, there was no analysis of the specific effects of the medical monopoly or the usefulness of nurses as alternative caregivers.

Another alternative considered by Consumers Union was the extension of Medicare for all Americans. From meeting with AMA officials, it was clear to Consumers Union that physicians, hospitals, and insurers envision only those changes that would *least* affect them—for example, limitations on fees or proposals for publicly set budgets to eliminate excess hospital capacity, or the right to choose who will be insured (Consumers Union, 1992c). Businesses want employee health insurance but want to pay less money for it. All these groups approve of "managed care," for example, in HMOs, because this would least disturb the current system. Such "managed care" does not deal with the uninsured or get rid of administrative waste or systemwide complexity. Ironically, despite the publicity received by *Nursing's Agenda for Health Care Reform*, published in 1991, the Consumers Union articles provided no evidence that their authors had read it, nor did they offer evidence of meetings with leaders of national nursing associations. In contrast, the nurses themselves had, as noted previously, conducted a consumer survey and related their proposal to consumers' thinking.

Consumers Union concluded that tinkering around the edges did not guarantee access or affordable care. To expand Medicaid and Medicare simply put the full burden on taxpayers and might continue the cost shifting as found in Hawaii; thus, a single-payer approach similar to the Canadian system was the best solution, but this prospect was rejected by physicians who were primarily concerned about fees, and by hospitals that wanted to become major medical centers, and by health insurance companies who feared they would go out of business. What the nurses wanted for themselves or for their clients was left unstated. Nevertheless, Consumers Union argued that the single-payer system was the best solution because it would eliminate private insurance costs and specific government programs and spread coverage and costs to everyone under a single, publicly financed insurance plan that would be strong enough to negotiate reasonable fees and the orderly and rational use of technology. Different managed-care techniques could be tried and compared to determine what worked, and under a single-payer system, cost shifting would stop.

Despite attacks from the medical industry, the proof is already available on cutting administrative costs: of the total money spent on health care in the United States, administering Medicare costs about 2.5 percent compared to costs of 4 percent to 12 percent for private insurers. Even with such savings, physicians must be stopped from adding on higher charges, gaps in coverage must be eliminated, and complex payment schedules have to be changed—these could best be done in a strong single-payer system. Would such a system break the medical monopoly and empower nurses to provide less expensive primary and preventive care in the community? Not unless consumers are provided information on these possibilities. Unfortunately, Consumers Union, noted for its objectivity on ratings of a wide range of services and products, did not provide such information in its analysis.

Ironically, the exclusion of nurses from the CU analysis occurred at roughly the same time that the results of a nationwide Gallup poll found that the vast majority (86 percent) of Americans were willing to receive everyday health-care services from nurses. Virginia Trotter Betts, then ANA president, said the survey proved widespread acceptance of nurses, except within the medical establishment, even though physicians had largely given up "family doctoring" over the last few decades. The AMA had strongly supported patients' choice of physicians, "yet it fights tooth and nail to maintain a monopoly on health services and limits choice of providers to medical doctors only" (Meehan, 1993b, p. 10). Nevertheless, it was clear from the national random sample of 1,000 adults that they would be willing to go to registered nurses with master's degrees for physical exams, prenatal care, immunizations, and treatment of common illnesses, such as colds and infections.

Congressional Proposals for Health-Care Reform

By 1992 more than two dozen congressional proposals for health-care reform had been put forward. None of these dealt directly with the sex-segregated marketplace; consequently, the use of nurses as alternatives to physicians was often missing. One group of proposals called for employers to in-sure their own employees or to contribute to government programs that included all Americans. Other proposals would have established a Canadian-style system or other forms of comprehensive government-sponsored pro-grams. Still others fostered the private sector, depending on insurance compa-nies. If current price structures remained intact, most of these would have required substantial sums of money—estimates ranged from $80 to $246 bil-lion—in the first years of operation.

Though necessary and appropriate goals, expanding health-care coverage to the uninsured millions and providing long-term care, may not *change* the system; these measures may simply expand it while leaving the hierarchical structure intact. Certainly, reducing the costs for pharmaceuticals and physi-cians' services would influence the availability of funds for other services; how-ever, without a recognition of the purposeful and intentional restrictions placed on women, who are the majority of health workers, and without a re-structuring of professional territories, the savings from lowered costs would do little to provide funds for the alternative caregivers who could genuinely refocus and redistribute services. Whether there would simply be more spend-ing at the beginning followed by subsequent savings was highly questionable if the entire "system" did not change. Indeed, in 1993, the League of Women Voters charged that a Bush administration advisory panel had flatly rejected calls for a systematic overhaul, suggesting only limited reforms and recom-mending that people "heal their lifestyles." Even a Senate task force, after months of meetings, proposed changes that would leave the current "system" basically intact. In addition, a group of congressional representatives, meeting weekly for more than six months, introduced no bill at all.

Some private-sector legislative proposals in the early 1990s even excluded pregnancy-related care and well-child care, areas usually important to women consumers and caregivers who value health promotion. The proposals often provided no long-term-care services, another area often related to the con-cerns of women clients and caregivers. Nor were outpatient prescription drugs or caps on personal out-of-pocket expenses for acute care addressed. Clearly, such proposals could hardly be considered reform. The National Leadership Coalition for Health Care Reform, in which nurses participated, produced one of the better universal employer-based plans, but though it offered wider cov-erage, even this proposal did not reconceptualize and restructure the entire "system."

In 1993 the ANA sponsored a national nursing summit on health-care reform. As a member of the National Leadership Coalition for Health Care Reform, the ANA focused its efforts on congressional hearings and public in-formation. Related to their work with the coalition, leaders from sixty-three major nursing organizations met in Chicago to achieve consensus on goals and strategies. Unity was a main theme. At the opening session Dr. Linda Aiken, RN, urged nurses to focus on legal, financial, and professional blockages to nursing practice: "The best single opportunity to make a lasting impact on nursing has to do with using the federal health initiative to remove the barriers to practice, particularly for advanced practice nurses" (cited in *American Nurse*, 1993e, p. 8).

Earlier, Dr. Lucille Joel (1992), then ANA president, had published a statement which acknowledged that managed care was the cornerstone of *Nursing's Agenda*, but surprisingly she then commented, "Quite as an afterthought, it is fair to ask 'Where is nursing in managed care?'" (p. 5). Existing regulations served as barriers to nurses' strategic positioning in managed care, and she had not observed any substantial nurse presence on HMO staffs. She warned that without plans, nurses would "be left to accommodate to what exists" and "possibly compromise the future of nursing" (p. 5). Although APNs could be accommodated, unlicensed assistive personnel would be used to fill regular RN positions. Although nurses had the necessary skills, "they lack experience and familiarity with the managed care setting. . . . The challenges are clear and time is of the essence. The nursing community should immediately reach consensus on the nature of the nurse's role in managed care" (p. 5). By 1993, 69 nursing and health-care organizations, representing one million registered nurses, had endorsed *Nursing's Agenda* (Gaffney, 1993).

The Clintons' Health-Care Reform: A Real Chance for Nursing

With the election of President Bill Clinton and the appointment of Hillary Rodham Clinton to head the President's Task Force on National Health Care Reform, there were rising expectations that nurses' vision of health care would finally be incorporated into national planning. In March 1993 nursing leaders met with Hillary Rodham Clinton, who supported *Nursing's Agenda* and agreed that access, quality, and cost must be reformed *simultaneously* and that anticompetitive barriers against APNs must be removed (Meehan, 1993a). Nurses were an untapped resource—not part of the problem, but part of the solution. Calling for a revitalized public-health system, the nurses noted the ongoing shortages of primary-care physicians and called for funding to support nurses as primary-care providers, removal of restrictive state laws that prevent nurses from working to their full potential within a wellness model of care, and funding to upgrade the competencies of over two million registered nurses, particularly necessary given the acute and complex care now required in hospitals. In May 1993, at a special ceremony honoring nurses, President Clinton recognized them as the backbone of the health-care system and a group that should do more in primary and preventive care to bring down medical costs.

The ANA gave testimony in mid-1993 to the Senate Finance Committee and called for the removal of all anticompetitive barriers. Managed competition in health-care reform requires that all competitors have the same opportunity to compete. Specifically, the nurses wanted removal of unnecessary nursing practice act restrictions and overregulation, unneeded limitations on prescriptive authority and hospital admitting privileges, and enactment of third-party reimbursement. Dr. Beverly L. Malone, RN, a member of the ANA board of directors, asserted that the nation could no longer afford "the inefficiencies of duplication or financial incentives that encourage technology at the expense of prevention" (*American Nurse*, 1993c, p. 36). The nurses took on directly the requirements for physician supervision, the use of insurance surcharges to increase malpractice premium coverage and create impediments to RN-MD collaboration, limitations on liability coverage for nurses without specific data, protocols and requirements for physician intervention into nurses' prescriptive autonomy, and the use of the Medical Practice Act to limit the scope of nursing practice that includes virtually every health-care action as a "delegated medical." Clearly, the nurses were *directly* confronting the medical monopoly. It was equally clear that the AMA was *directly* working to sustain the physicians' monopoly.

AMA Opposes APN Autonomy

At the interim meeting of its House of Delegates in December 1993, the AMA took a stand and released a report opposing the autonomy of APNs. Virginia Trotter Betts, ANA president, accused the AMA of using inaccuracy and innuendo to undermine the twenty-five-year track record of nurses' high quality, cost-effective primary care. More than 100,000 APNs, said Joan Meehan (1994), provided primary care, but had to navigate a patchwork of laws and regulations that hindered provision of service to a broader public. Alaska and Oregon allowed APNs to provide a full range of services, but other states, such as Illinois and Pennsylvania, still allowed little autonomy. To President Betts, "The issue is control, especially control of dollars. . . . The AMA wants physician supervision because then the physicians get the first dollar" (cited in Meehan, 1994, p. 3). Billing must still be submitted through a physician, who is reimbursed, and although the APN actually provided the care, she/he still gets only a salary. In 1992 the average net physician's income was $170,600 versus $43,500 for a nurse practitioner.

Although medicine had largely abandoned primary care, physicians "continue to object to anyone else picking up the pieces," said Betts (p. 3). At that time, there were 206,000 primary-care physicians, but it would take to the year 2040 to educate enough to meet the demand. President Clinton's Health Security Act removed barriers and allowed nurses to give "physical examinations, screenings, immunizations, well- and ill-baby care and treatment of acute and chronic illnesses" (p. 3). Hillary Rodham Clinton, in a speech to Georgia physicians, said bluntly that nurse practitioners' roles would be expanded. Meehan accurately accused the AMA of vigorously opposing all efforts to provide national health insurance and any autonomy for any other practitioners, including nurses. An AMA fund-raising brochure characterized non-physician providers as "flocks of daffy special interest groups" and "quacks." The gender implications are hardly disguised. Despite the widespread efforts of a bipartisan coalition concerned with health care, said Betts, "the AMA is still stuck in its status quo mentality, declaring open season on the nation's nurses—who are trying valiantly to meet the health care needs of the American public. Fortunately the AMA does not speak for all physicians . . . and we will continue to work closely with those physicians and other physician organizations who favor health care reform" (cited in Meehan, 1994, p. 3).

Nurses went public: "What's brewing is an in-your-face struggle between the female-dominated nursing profession and the male-dominated medical profession, and the battlefield is President Clinton's proposed health-care reform plan, which would expand the role of nurses" (Kleiman, 1994, p. B11). Nurses, said reporter Kleiman, had "finally earned the respect they deserve," improved their salaries, and some now wanted autonomy; specifically, they wanted to provide services without a physician's direct supervision. Some 100,000 APNs were already providing primary-health care, but the Clinton plan would increase their numbers and enable them to obtain direct reimbursement. Some ten physician associations supported the Clinton plan—for example, the American Academy of Family Physicians, American Academy of Pediatrics, American College of Obstetricians and Gynecologists, American College of Preventive Medicine, and the American Medical Women's Association (Associated Press, 1993)—but the AMA had ridiculed nurses in its brochure and questioned nurses' quality of care in its thirty-page 1993 report opposing autonomy for APNs. Indeed, Dr. James S. Todd, executive vice president of the AMA, said nurses did not have the same training as physicians and, therefore, the physicians must remain in charge of "teams." The AMA was objecting to nurses doing what many were already doing!

The media, increasingly aware of the struggle between nurses and physicians, expressed support for nurses, for example, in articles in *USA Today* entitled "Nurses Deserve a Bigger Role in Patient Care" (Jurgensen, 1993) and "Doctors and Nurses in Dispute Boundaries of Medical 'Domain'" (Keen and Wolf, 1993). Even the *Wall Street Journal* gave nurses favorable coverage in such articles as "Nurse Practitioners Fight Job Restrictions" (Petty, 1993).

Health-Maintenance Organizations: The Domino Effect

While the political struggles continued, HMOs steadily changed the structure of health-care delivery in the United States. In February 1993 a meeting of the Congress on Nursing Economics dealt with issues of managed competition, anticompetitive barriers, and price competition, all of which could lead to the crowding out of higher-priced providers and hospitals. Clearly, as hospitals lowered costs, the number of nurses would be reduced at some hospitals (O'Connor, Eckles, and Turner, 1993). In HMOs it was unlikely that nurses would be used to save on costs since physicians would be willing to give primary care in order to avoid their own displacement. Of seven major elements identified by the nurses at the congress analyzing the workforce in transition, two key points were, one, the removal of anticompetitive barriers for nurses in advanced practice, and, two, the evaluation and linkage between the cost of nursing service and patient outcomes.

The full implications of managed competition were, unfortunately, unclear for nursing because, as Peter I. Buerhaus (1994), professor and director of the Harvard Nursing Research Institute, said, "the role of nurses or how they will be affected by managed competition has not been seriously discussed in the health services literature" (p. 23). Four issues were critical: realizing opportunities for APNs, ensuring that the minimum package of benefits includes services provided by both RNs and APNs, ensuring nurses' clinical and economic interests, and making sure that the current turmoil does not distract from identifying the value of nursing services. Strong incentives for reduced costs should result in the expansion of nurses' clinical and managerial functions for which the public was ready: 66 percent of respondents in a 1993 Harvard national survey strongly or somewhat favored receiving their routine care from a well-trained nurse rather than a physician. But, said Buerhaus, nurses' "gains may come largely at the expense of physicians, . . . [whose] economic interests are likely to be increasingly threatened . . . [thus] nurses can expect some medical associations to withhold full support . . . unless legislators attach rules and regulations that restrict employment of APNs in prepaid health plans" (pp. 23–24). Physicians, said Buerhaus, would try to prevent independent, prepaid, primary-care arrangements for nurses; would favor restricting nurses from selectively contracting with health plans; would pressure legislators to restrict nursing ventures; would declare that independent nurse practitioners were conducting the illegal practice of medicine; and would limit the number of APNs an HMO could hire and further restrict state nurse practice acts.

Nurses could, said Buerhaus, expect "physician lobbying and distortions of their [nurses'] educational credentials and quality of care" (p. 24). Nursing would have to counter these charges with solid data and should anticipate congressional hearings. "In addition, the Federal Trade Commission's antitrust enforcement division should be consulted, or at least alerted to the possibility that incentives facing physicians may lead them to act in ways intended to keep APNs out of the market and thereby impede price competition" (p. 24). Here there is a clear summation of the ongoing efforts of medicine to sustain a lucrative monopoly.

Expecting the Clintons' national health-care reform to become a reality,

Buerhaus urged nurses to develop a consensus on what services or benefits must be included in a reform package. Nurses needed unanimity to avoid confusion since competition would be fierce and many nursing services would be claimed by others: "Nurses cannot blindly accept that those who control these organizations will be benevolent, public-minded, or unbiased brokers; the danger that these organizations become controlled by the very groups that health alliances oversee will be ever-present" (p. 25).

Expecting massive turmoil, Buerhaus nevertheless urged nurses to continue to focus on defining and demonstrating the value and cost-effectiveness of their care and the positive outcomes for their patients. He admitted that the short-term outlook would be difficult and fraught with disappointments and anxieties. Grossly inefficient or overbedded hospitals will "restrain growth in nurse wages, accelerate substitution of professional nurses by unlicensed and nonprofessional personnel, initiate layoffs or involuntary termination of RNs, and . . . take other steps to lower costs associated with providing nursing care" (p. 25). Nurses will be distracted from the hard work of defining the value of nursing, but it is this activity that would assure the long-term interests of nursing.

Defining the Value of Nursing

Nurses did try to publicize the extent and quality outcomes of the care they provided. The ANA continued to produce "Nursing Facts," short publications which in 1993, for example, noted that there were more than 100,000 advanced practice nurses who were prepared to provide 60 percent to 80 percent of the primary and preventive care traditionally done by physicians (ANA, 1993). There were roughly 30,000 nurse practitioners and about 150 NP programs, most conferring a master's degree. By 1993 at least 36 states required national certification by the ANA or a specialty nursing organization; in 35 states, APNs could prescribe medication. There were about 5,000 nurse midwives, who in 1990 delivered 148,728 or 3.6 percent of all U.S. births. About 40,000 clinical nurse specialists with master's or doctoral degrees were experts in specialized areas. They provided direct care, but also acted as clinical consultants. There were also 25,000 certified registered nurse anesthetists, who completed two to three years of additional education beyond their bachelor's degrees and administered more than 65 percent of all anesthetics given to patients. In 85 percent of rural hospitals, they were the sole providers of all anesthetics.

If APNs are accessible and cost-effective, and if they deliver quality care as proved by numerous studies, why were they not used to provide care to the more than 60 million uninsured and underinsured people? The answer? Again, unnecessary restrictions on scope of practice, which must be removed so that the health-care "system" can be restructured to focus on prevention and primary care rather than high-tech treatment and cure of disease. Despite the efforts of nurses to present their case to the public, the future of health-care reform seemed increasingly uncertain and unclear to many consumers, who instead listened to expensive television advertisements that rejected the Clinton health-care proposal.

By the end of 1993, as the debate intensified, the possibility of giving physicians broad immunity from antitrust laws was even considered by the Clinton administration in order to get passage of its health-reform proposal. Nurses and health-consumer groups opposed the proposed move, but physicians, such as Robert McAfee, then president-elect of the 294,000-member AMA, said, "It might make us feel a bit warmer toward the proposal. I'm not sure whether it will translate to support" (*Boston Globe*, 1993, p. A8E). Physicians from other medical organizations said it was a major concession and a "'significant loosening of the antitrust law'" (p. A8E). Consumers Union, among other groups, was not pleased since letting physicians collude and bargain a single fee was not consistent with cost control. Essentially, said one government official, the concession would create a loophole in antitrust laws large enough to drive a truck through.

A flood of campaign contributions and of special-interest money for lobbying bought access to decision makers in Washington for physicians, hospitals, insurance firms, and pharmaceutical interests, resulting in no major congressional action on health-care reform. The League of Women Voters agreed that the biggest culprits were medical and health industry PACs, special interest groups that had contributed tens of millions of dollars to shape or block a comprehensive health-care system.

By 1993 the AMA was reported in national newspaper articles to have swapped sides in the health-care fight. The AMA, with 300,000 members, was no longer trying to block sweeping changes, but was striving instead to shape and direct them. Publishing its own blueprint for revamping health care, the AMA accepted elements of "managed competition" after several meetings with Ira Magaziner, the top advisor to Hillary Rodham Clinton's health-care task force. Indeed, thousands of physicians descended on Washington on the AMA's first lobby day. This action was on top of the $2.9 million direct and $1.1 million indirect contributions to politicians in the 1992–1993 election cycle. Counting half the nation's physicians as members, the AMA had a budget of $6.5 million and a staff of nineteen lobbyists. It was this powerful group that had killed efforts to reform health care in previous decades. Ironically, the AMA complained in a formal letter about lack of access to the Clinton task force, which led to meetings and closer agreement on the principle of a "managed-competition" model that retained the patient's choice of a physician, did away with unnecessary regulatory requirements, and promoted liability reform. Nevertheless, the issues of cost controls and physicians' roles in the anticipated reform recommendations continued to be debated.

Whether the Clinton administration would have allowed a weakening of antitrust laws became less relevant when in October 1994 it was clear that health-care reform legislation, after a two-year struggle, was dead. Nevertheless, said Chris deVries and Marjorie Vanderbilt (1994), Congress had been educated by nurses and strong bipartisan support elicited for many nursing issues. Thousands of nurses had engaged in political activity, and by 1994, seventy-five separate nursing organizations had been brought together. N-STAT, the ANA grassroots network, had been created, and ANA-PAC (Political Action Committee) had raised $1.2 million to influence elections and Congress. Nevertheless, they had failed to achieve the health-care reform they had so strongly supported.

The Collapse of Federal Health-Care Reform: Millions Spent on Political Lobbying

What happened to health-care reform? Although powerful groups and institutions, such as organized medicine, the insurance industry, and business organizations, supported some provisions of the Clintons' proposal, "Unfortunately, they didn't support the same provisions. . . . All these groups had the will and the money . . . and they unleashed the biggest, most intense, most expensive lobbying campaign the country has ever seen . . . more than 650 individual groups spent over $100 million from January 1993 to March 1994 alone" (*American Nurse*, 1994c, p. 7). Funds went to elected officials as campaign contributions and to media advertising, and to huge phone and letter-writing campaigns. The ANA supported most of the reform package, but most of the other groups attacked at least some aspects of it. Raw political ambition to unseat Clinton led to charges of "socialized medicine." Eventually the public became confused and support waned. The nurses did not predict the sharp turn to the right in the subsequent elections in 1994.

Organized medicine was directly involved in the shift. In an important exposé, *The Serpent on the Staff*, journalists Howard Wolinsky and Tom Brune (1995) analyzed the unhealthy politics of the AMA, which in the last two decades had spent more than $100 million dollars to influence public policy. About a quarter of each member's dues of $420 went to finance lobbying, and this increased to one-third in 1994. The American Political Action Committee, the political funding arm of the AMA, raised another $34 million for political activities and since 1972 has ranked second out of more than 4,000 PACs in making direct contributions to candidates' campaign funds, donating much more than unions, educational associations, and even the National Rifle Association.

The AMA outspent all other health-related lobbies and contributed money to "nearly every representative and senator in the current Congress . . . to persuade doctors and scuttle major reform by persuading lawmakers to delay, dilute, or delete legislation it doesn't like. The AMA is banking that its investment in this Congress—a total of $11.4 million—will pay off" (Wolinsky and Brune, 1995, p. 69). This represented about $24,000 for each of the 464 members of Congress who took AMA money. Over $6.6 million had been invested in 241 Republicans and $4.6 million in 223 Democrats. Ironically, AMPAC's second largest investment, $248,108, was in Senator Robert Packwood: "It independently spent $227,808 in 1992 on television ads, polling, and other assistance to help Packwood, who was accused of sexually harassing several former female staff members" (p. 93). Forced to resign in disgrace, not only from the Senate Finance Committee but from the Senate, Packwood's support by organized medicine is a study in physicians' support of sexism.

Other health-related PACs, including the ANA-PAC, had increased their contributions. Unfortunately, research on the influence of special-interest groups in American politics from 1983 to 1998 by Ronald J. Hrebenar and Clive S. Thomas (publication pending) found that women's, victim's rights, and social issue groups were among the *least* influential in affecting legislation. Indeed, the medical lobby was still considered one of the top five by congressional staff. Clearly, organized medicine continued to be a formidable opponent for organized nursing and other reform groups. When the AMA reluctantly supported reform, it did so with so many provisions attached that it essentially limited the possibility of the passage of the Clintons' reforms. In December 1994 the AMA convention backed off from universal coverage. Annoyed at criticisms, the AMA "came up with a new formula for determining doctor compensation, making it lower by including the lower pay of physicians in training and those employed by the federal government" (Wolinsky and Brune, 1995, p. viii).

Whose interests does the AMA really represent, those of physicians or those of the public? The first time physicians' average yearly income exceeded $100,000 was in 1983; by 1989 it had risen to an average of $150,000; and in 1994 it was $186,600. Thus, noted Wolinsky and Brune, the AMA seemed to be looking after physicians' economic interests quite well. Whether the public's health was equally well served is open to question. According to Wolinsky and Brune, the 1990s saw the beginning of the sixth attempt by Americans in this century to reform the health-care system. And in all these efforts the AMA had opposed reform, losing only once—with Medicaid and Medicare. If we add the Sheppard-Towner Act, described in chapter 5, there were then at least seven reform battles. Despite nurses' losses in these battles, they did not give up efforts to put the public's health first. Nursing has had a formidable foe in the AMA, which represents the wealthiest profession and one that has spent more than $100 million to influence public policy in the last two decades. With the collapse of the battle for a nationwide health-care system, the AMA increased its lobbying in the states and continued to fortify its monopoly by restricting nurses and modifying any advances made in anticipation of a federal health-care system.

To John Robbins (1996), the medical monopoly is a game no one wins, yet the AMA's 1994 report on nurses' provision of primary care stated that it was unacceptable for nurses to function without the constant supervision of physicians. Lonnie Bristow, MD, AMA board chairman, claimed: "It's illogical and potentially dangerous to have this type of activity performed independently of the oversight and coordination of a physician" (Patterson, 1994; cited in Robbins, 1996, p. 199). The speaker of the AMA House of Delegates, Daniel Johnson, Jr., MD, warned that "some of the nurses are going to overstep their boundaries" (Patterson, 1994; cited in Robbins, 1996, p. 199), and another spokesperson said, "Nurses ought to go to medical school if they want to be doctors" (Wolinsky and Brune, 1995, p. 143; cited in Robbins, 1996, p. 199). Robbins was not impressed with these accusations or with those of another physician who in 1995 tried to explain the reasoning behind the AMA's position: "Sometimes a doctor needs an assistant at his side, someone who is not too full of herself to obediently perform menial tasks, and who is willing to follow orders. The role of a nurse is to fulfill that function" (Robbins, 1996, p. 199). To this, Robbins sarcastically responded, "I see" (p. 199). So do we see—an attitude unchanged since the turn of the century! So much for the AMA goal of "forging partnerships in healing."

Following a 1995 meeting of the American Nurses Association Constituent Assembly, consisting of presidents and executive directors of all fifty state nurses associations, Marva Wade, president of the New York State Nurses Association, reported that "the American Medical Association has set aside $6 million to try to regain supervisory control over nurses . . . [and] the ANA is lobbying against what I would describe as a tide of anti patient, anti quality care proposals" (Wade, 1996, p. 2).

Medicine Losing Control?

Ironically, organized medicine complained that they were losing control of the health-care "system." This was not a new complaint. Over the past forty years, several medical writers contended that physicians had lost authority. But had they? According to researcher J. Scott Osberg (1994), who examined longitudinal data on authority positions held by physicians, they had actually increased their faculty numbers in medical schools: up from 65.6 percent of all medical school faculty in 1970 to 72.8 percent in 1990. In professional associations, the AMA has always been headed by a physician and the ANA has always been headed by a nurse.

From 1930 to 1969, twenty-two (55 percent) of the forty presidents of the American Hospital Association were physicians, though none of the twenty presidents from 1970 to 1989 were medical men. Although the American Physical Therapy Association has never had a physician as president, its 1937 constitution clearly acknowledged its subordination to medicine, and until 1968 the association had an advisory board composed entirely of physicians. In 1973 the association voted to bypass the requirement for physician referral. In the American Public Health Association (APHA), thirty-two (80 percent) of forty presidents from 1930 to 1969 were physicians, but only nine (45 percent) of twenty from 1970 to 1989; however, 50 percent of the sixteen-member executive board in 1987 were physicians, for example, and all six of the officers were physicians.

In 1945 physicians accounted for 25 percent of hospital administrators; in the early 1950s, 32.5 percent; and by 1962 their numbers had dropped to 22.8 percent. From 1972 to 1982, there was a further decline of 75 percent. Probably the decline is a result of the shift of physicians to specializations. They are more likely now to head an array of departmental and research units within hospitals or head their own outpatient offices separate from hospitals. As Osberg said, other research was needed to show the extent to which physicians are "pulling the strings behind the scenes from powerful, but less conspicuous positions" (Osberg, 1994, p. 1574). Certainly, the success of their political lobbying was clear evidence that organized medicine was covertly, if not overtly, still very much in power. Indeed, they had sufficient power to produce a physician surplus at the public's expense.

The Physician Surplus and Lack of Integration of Nurses and Other Clinicians into a Comprehensive Model

In opposition to almost all other medical and governmental researchers in the 1980s and 1990s, Richard Cooper, MD (1995), concluded that the physician surplus would be trivial in the year 2000 and nonexistent by the year 2020. Nevertheless, even he admitted that medical models had not integrated the productivity of nurse practitioners, physician's assistants, optometrists, psychologists, and other clinicians. Alvin R. Tarlov (1995) agreed, but sharply questioned Cooper's assertion that the physician surplus would be trivial or nonexistent. Medical school admissions had doubled from 1965 to 1980, increased by 600 positions by 1993, and then remained flat. Residency positions exceeded the output of medical schools by 40 percent, and these were filled by foreign medical graduates, who numbered 7,000 in 1988 and have increased in number every year since. About 66 percent of these *stayed* in the United States after training, and about the same proportion became specialists, not general practitioners. In fact, Schroeder (1993) reported that less than 15 percent of medical students graduating in 1992 planned to become generalists. In New York City, where 17 percent of all physicians nationally are trained, the number of applicants for primary-care residencies had steadily declined—for example, in internal medicine from 49 percent in 1988 to 36 percent in 1992. MD education from 1945 to 1980 was *covertly* federally financed, but these costs had recently been partially shifted to student loans and to Medicare payments for residents in teaching hospitals. The increasing indebtedness of medical graduates leads them to choose the more highly paid specialties in order to reduce their debts quickly. This, in turn, contributes to the failure to change the generalist-specialist mix of MDs.

The 700,000 physicians projected by 2010 would be matched by an increase to 450,000 in non-physician clinicians. Unfortunately, "neither Cooper nor others have integrated all clinician groups into a comprehensive supply/ requirements model" (Tarlov, 1995, p. 1559). Indeed, Cooper said that the projected increase to 177,000 of APNs and PAs by 2010 was "double the number necessary to satisfy the current staffing needs in HMOs" (Cooper, 1995, p. 1541). The numbers of nurse anesthetists and nurse midwives would increase from 98,500 to 133,700 by 2010. Clearly, as Cooper noted, the degree to which patients used these non-physician clinicians would impact the demand for physicians' services. Tarlov concluded that the current models of physician supply and demand were inadequate because they did not account for the increased numbers of nurse and non-MD clinicians. If these were included, the MD surplus would certainly not be trivial or nonexistent.

In 1998, Cooper rectified the omission by publishing with his colleagues two articles in the *Journal of the American Medical Association* on the growth, scope, prescriptive authority, and independent practice of non-physicians (Cooper, Henderson, and Dietrich, 1998; Cooper, Laud, and Dietrich, 1998). Observing the blurring of lines between activities of physicians and non-MDs, Cooper and his colleagues noted that the number of NPs would equal that of family practice physicians by 2005. The authors recognize the growing acceptance by government agencies of direct reimbursement to NPs; the doubling of master's-level NP programs from 1992 to 1997; the quadrupling of nurse anesthetist programs; and the increased funding for these programs from $3 million in 1976 to $16 million in 1996. In the Cooper articles and the accompanying editorial by Grumbach and Coffman (1998), two strategies to deal with these trends are discussed: either physicians can learn to work with non-physicians or they fight for clinical turf and lobby against any further expansion. The latter strategy has been and still is dominant. For example, physicians are currently lobbying to prevent new federal rules eliminating MD supervision of nurse anesthetists. Cooper and his colleagues question whether or not there will be enough future jobs for the projected (by 2001) 7,250 NPs, 600 nurse midwives, 1,300 clinical nurse specialists, and more than 900 nurse anesthetists. And will they be willing to locate and practice in rural areas?

Nurses Anita J. Catlin and Maura McAuliffe (1999) published some nurse leaders' responses to the Cooper articles and the *JAMA* editorial. Nurse Ira A. Gunn reminded physicians that nurses have been anesthetists for more than a hundred years; they currently give 65 percent of all anesthetics nationally, are the sole providers of anesthetics in 75 percent of rural hospitals, and produce outcomes that are equal to or better than those of physicians. Although twenty-nine states do not require MD supervision, the AMA House of Delegates in December 1998 voted that administering anesthesia is the "practice of medicine" and decided to fight for clinical turf. Other nurse leaders dealt with research on acute-care specialists; discussed basing educational programs in rural areas; called for more research on such subjects as the effect of direct Medicare reimbursement; and stressed greater cooperation, for example, in joint course work for nursing and medical students. What is striking is the failure of nurses to deal directly with the AMA-led strategy of battling to retain or obtain more clinical turf.

Not What Percentage of Primary-Care Physicians, but Who Should Provide Primary Care

Not only did physicians fail to incorporate other clinicians into their models, and to admit openly their strategy of turf protection and extension; they also failed to deal adequately with the issue of the imbalance between primary and specialized care. Doug Bandow (1995), a senior fellow at the Cato Institute, asserted that the critical question is "not what percentage of doctors should provide primary care, but who should be allowed to provide primary care" (p. 89). Currently, there are over 2.5 million RNs, three times the number of physicians, and over 120,000 APNs, about half the number of physicians providing primary care. The number of nurses becoming APNs could easily reach 300,000 with only one or two years of training; however, they are blocked by the government-sustained physicians' monopoly. Because of the high cost of training medical personnel, "57 cents of every additional dollar in U.S. medical expenditures is eaten away by higher prices rather than added services . . . Physicians have [nevertheless] shown unyielding resistance to alternative professionals. . . . Working through state legislatures, physicians have won statutory protection from competition" (p. 89).

The Clintons' health-care reform proposal would have removed inappropriate barriers to practice—state laws that ban APNs from offering primary care—and would have approved insurance reimbursement for APNs' services. The AMA argued that these changes would "hurt patients, fragment the delivery of care, and even raise costs" (p. 90). The California Medical Association said it was dangerous to public health. Ironically, said Bandow, 86 percent of Americans would accept a nurse as a primary-care practitioner, according to a recent Gallup poll.

Advanced practice nurses could provide 60 percent to 80 percent of clinical services now monopolized by physicians and in process save between $6.4 billion and $8.8 billion annually, according to economist Len Nichols (1992). Lonnie Bristow, AMA official, admitted these facts but stressed that nurses were working under physicians' supervision; however, Bandow replied, this supervision was frequently loose and often unnecessary. Daniel Johnson, also of the AMA, emphasized the difference in years of education, but Bandow said, "No one is suggesting that nurses do anything but the tasks they are trained to do" (Bandow, 1995, p. 91), which the research shows they do as well or better than physicians.

If physicians were willing to give up some of their primary-care tasks to nurses who work independently, the nurses in turn would probably be less likely to balk at giving up some nursing tasks to LPNs, aides, and UAPs. However, if medicine does not loosen its monopoly, nurses' authority and control of the patient is simply eroded. They lose at both ends of the hierarchy. Bandow does not state this obvious fact. Instead, he stresses the $25 million that the Stanford University Hospital, for example, saved in five years by reducing RNs from 90 percent to 60 percent of the patient-care employees. Indeed, since 1987, American Practice Management (APM), a consulting firm, has assisted eighty other hospitals in saving $1 billion by using similar techniques. Unfortunately, Bandow said nothing about the impact of these changes on consumers as patients.

The Dizzying Speed of "Corporization": Who or What Represents Consumers?

Reducing the number of RNs does not reduce the need for sick people to receive quality nursing care. This was supposedly taken care of by hiring unlicensed nursing personnel. In January 1994 Dr. Ellen T. Fahy, editor of *Nursing and Health Care,* was very uneasy about the results of a survey in which nurses expressed concern about being fired and replaced with other types of workers. Although nurses had been aware of the privatization of health and hospital care at least since the 1980s, "the speed of increased corporization is dizzying. Further, it is combined with mergers and acquisitions of nonprofit hospitals" (Fahy, 1994, p. 3). Traditional hospitals were downsizing, merging, and acquiring community health agencies. In 1993 the two largest hospital chains, Columbia Healthcare Inc. and Hospital Corporation of America (HCA), agreed to merge and operate 190 hospitals in 26 states. Home-health-care agencies and intermediate and long-term care facilities were also being acquired. Had nursing leaders been involved in decisions about downsizing nursing staffs? Who was to train and supervise unlicensed personnel? What was nurses' involvement in mergers and acquisitions? And, finally, "Who or what is representing consumers?" (p. 8).

Though many hospitals in the United States were downsizing and reducing their RN staff, others were hiring APNs because of the decreased numbers of physicians practicing as generalists. Thus, in some major urban areas, APNs were extending their practices from primary to acute care. Dr. Mathy Mezey, Mary Dougherty, Patricia Wade, and Dr. Cynthia Mersmann (1994) reported on a survey of New York City hospitals and nursing schools to determine the current use of and projected demands for nurse practitioners, certified nurse midwives, and certified nurse anesthetists; the practice patterns in hospitals; and the enrollment and curriculum in advanced nurse practitioners' programs. Increasingly, they found hospitals were hiring APNs for positions in general medicine and pediatrics; thus, some of the 37,963 APNs in the United States were involved with inpatient acute care.

Using three questionnaires, Mezey and her colleagues found that only three of twenty-seven New York City hospitals returning the survey did *not* employ nurse practitioners, midwives, or anesthetists. The average numbers of APNs was 11 per hospital, and 74 percent of the hospitals expected to hire 311 additional advanced practitioners in 1994 and 282 in 1995. These local data support the national data from research by O'Neil, Leslie, Seifer, Kahn, and Bailiff (1993), which indicates increased contributions from APNs and a doubling of their numbers by 2000. However, sources of funding for current practitioners varied widely: using funds from existing or additional RN positions, vacant resident positions, or administrative positions. Additional personnel were to be funded from managed-care initiatives, new primary-care positions, and monies from the reduction in the number of residents.

The researchers also found that the nurses' hierarchies of authority were equally varied: "They reported to both nursing and medicine in 12 (44%) hospitals, to only nursing in 5 (19%) hospitals, and to only medicine in 3 (11%) hospitals" (Mezey et al., 1994, p. 15). Thus, nursing independence was *not* evident in the majority of hospitals. Of the 85 percent of the APNs employed by the hospital, only about 30 percent were hired by the nursing department and only 20 percent worked with three or more other APNs. Indeed, 83 percent of the APNs followed written protocols, 13 percent worked under standing orders, and about 88 percent had formal collaborative practice arrangements. Only 12 percent had hospital admitting privileges, and only 17 percent had discharge privileges; however, 87 percent had prescription privileges. Despite their *limited* autonomy, the demand for APNs would be high, and if the current trends continued, at least 40 percent would be caring for patients on acute-care units.

A Community-Based Model of Nurses as Primary Caregivers

According to Mary O. Mundinger (1995), dean of the Columbia University School of Nursing, despite the multiple problems faced by nursing as a result of the failure of broad federal health-care reform, there was still growing consciousness that the country had far too many physicians and states were expanding efforts to restrain costs, to collect data to support expenditures on the basis of outcomes and quality, and to empower APNs. Given these trends and in the absence of vigorous efforts by organized medicine to contain or decrease the numbers of physicians, "medicine and nursing are on a collision course for jobs" (p. 254).

Clearly, nursing must position itself for the twenty-first century. To do this, nurses must clearly enunciate their beliefs. The first belief is that APNs and primary-care physicians share a "large and identical body of knowledge about the detection and treatment of uncomplicated disease or illness . . . [and] are very similar in their abilities to provide high-quality, primary medical care" (p. 255). However, comparisons between primary-care RNs and MDs are usually based on disease-oriented care, not on health needs separate from the immediate medical problems. Thus, the second belief: physicians and APNs are not indistinguishable. Physicians have a deeper knowledge of disease detection and treatment. Nurses are able to do health-risk assessments based on individual, environmental, and family factors; they stress health promotion and disease prevention strategies, provide counseling and health education, and have the knowledge to create care regimens using community resources. Given these differences, would patients receive better care from MD-APN partnerships? Or, as Mundinger put it, an "even more wrenching and unasked question is, should we be encouraging large numbers of MDs to adopt primary care careers at all?" (p. 255). Probably the country needs "about half the number of MDs we are now producing, with all, or nearly all, practicing in the specialties, and with APNs as their partners in primary care" (p. 255).

If there is to be a regulatory expansion of nurses' authority, the gap between expanding practice and lagging criteria for high-quality training must be bridged. In 1992, 130 institutions offered nurse-practitioner programs, but by 1994 this number had increased to 152. The numbers of tracks within these institutions had increased from 173 to 364 (Harper and Johnson, 1995), but existing state and professional oversight was, said Mundinger, "minimal." Without rigorous educational standards, it was pointless to discuss the development of teams and the attribution of authority over services.

Mundinger's faculty shifted its program to accept students with baccalaureate degrees in non-nursing fields with "academic backgrounds indistinguishable from the medical, dental and public health students" (p. 256), thus erasing age and educational differences and enabling nursing students to enter multidisciplinary courses and research on an equal footing. A clinical preceptor program (Columbia Advanced Practice Nurse Associates—CAPNA) was begun with faculty located in 100 different agencies in which new partnerships were formed. A doctoral program was started to train clinical experts in health-services research. In 1994 the Center for Advanced Practice, an ambulatory site staffed by faculty-nurse practitioners with full hospital admitting privileges, was founded. These included direct admissions, writing "medical" orders, managing patients, making rounds, ordering tests and medications, requesting medical and surgical consultations, and discharging patients. Prescriptive authority was limited to a collaborative agreement with a physician, initiated by the nurse, who also advised the MD of a patient's admission so that the physician could see the patient within twenty-four hours. Pediatric patients were jointly admitted.

Obviously, medical supervisory control, not simply collaboration, still prevailed in this model. Indeed, Mundinger stressed, "This is not a project to show that nurses can be doctors. Just the opposite, it is a project to elucidate how seamless advanced nursing care—across sites and in its most comprehensive configuration—can be a valued addition to care delivered by physicians. We also believe we will begin to demonstrate how nurses use resources differently, including hospitalization or extended community resources, to solve the same health problems physicians solve" (p. 257). It was already clear that pediatric nurse practitioners hospitalized children for different reasons than physicians did. The nurses used the hospitals when the home was inadequate, but did not hospitalize if they judged the mother capable of handling the child at home; thus, their final reasons were not simply medical, but family- and community-based.

Ideally, managed care should value health and healthy lifestyles since it caps the amount of money it will pay for care: "Prevention pays. Health promotion pays" (p. 258). As Mundinger said, "Not only is solo medical practice a thing of the past, but physician-only practices are equally outmoded" (p. 258). The support for nurses in creating ambulatory clinics in areas where there were insufficient physicians came from those physicians who were aware there was a shortage of primary-care physicians, knew that most physicians at Columbia-Presbyterian Medical Center were specialists, recognized that hospital occupancy rates left beds unfilled that APNs could fill with patients from the community, and realized that MDs as specialists could have a larger number of referrals from nurses. The nurses created the Center for Advanced Practice model in the framework of a well-designed, randomized control trial with adequate funding to assess quality and comprehensiveness of care and timing and utilization of other resources, and patient satisfaction and outcomes. The research also was funded to create a model for replacement of medical residents in hospitals.

The success of Mundinger's CAPNA program is evident in the recent coverage given to it by the media (*American Nurse*, 1998b). This program is seen as a significant prototype for a new branch of primary care, and an example of "broken barriers" for nurse practitioners' practices. Insurance companies are backing the center, and although some physicians claim that the nurses "might miss diagnoses or overlook symptoms" (p. 17), Mundinger asserted that nurses "don't miss things" (p. 17). Indeed, they spent twenty-five minutes with each patient while physicians spent seventeen minutes.

By the end of the decade, Mundinger's assertion was supported by research she conducted with several colleagues over a year's period (Mundinger, Kane, Lenz, Totten, Tsai, Cleary, Friedewald, Siu, and Shelanski, 2000). For the 1,316 patients who were randomly assigned to NPs or physicians for primary care, there were comparable rates in number of patients seen per hour, patient outcome, numbers of referrals to specialists, number of hospitalizations, cost levels, and degree of patients' satisfaction. In an editorial that appeared in the same issue of *JAMA* as Mundinger et al., Harold C. Sox, Jr., MD (2000), criticized the study because it was conducted only in the satellite clinics of the Columbia-Presbyterian Medical Center system, the patients were predominantly Hispanic, and the study, he claimed, was only six months long. (This was an error: it was actually conducted over a one-year period, with the exception of one element of the study.) Mundinger responded that every researcher wants more data, subjects, and time, but "the fact remains that this study showed that NPs were generally indistinguishable from physicians in regard to primary care practice" (*American Journal of Nursing*, 2000a). Unfortunately, in the absence of a national health-care system, it is uncertain whether this new model will be widely adopted.

Medicine's Milestone Year?

Unlike nurses, many physicians were happy with the demise of the Clintons' health-care reform, hardly questioning whether this was best for consumers. Indeed, "Medicine's Milestone Year" was applauded in the AMA's *American Medical News:* "At no time in recent history has medicine's voice been heard so clearly and forcefully, and on such a broad array of topics" (American Medical Association, 1995, p. 1). In the 1995 battle over Medicare, the impact of medicine had been "dramatic," and the AMA had provided House Speaker Newt Gingrich a detailed proposal to change the Medicare program. This was followed by intensive lobbying by the AMA that led to congressional support for major aspects of their proposal. President Clinton vetoed the Republican proposal, forcing the AMA to redouble its efforts to obtain antitrust reform, a key element in their program, aimed at excluding medicine from antimonopolistic regulations by the Federal Trade Commission.

As organized medicine was experiencing a milestone year with the newly elected Republican Congress, the National Women's Health Network was damning the congressional legislative proposals—for example, those dealing with welfare reform—as a direct attack on children and women (Kasper, 1995). The push toward managed care was also questioned: for example, in the Health-Care Reform Act of 1994, pregnant women were restricted to twenty-four hours or less for childbirth in hospitals, regardless of the opinions of the women, their families, or their caregivers. Profit-driven HMOs were already implementing such changes, forcing feminist groups to attack the twenty-four-hour restriction. The feminist action, said Ellen R. Shaffer (1995), was only the first push in a longer struggle against health-care corporations that had already "concentrated economic power in a handful of companies in some areas of the country" (p. 4). Kaiser was the only nonprofit corporation of the ten largest HMOs, which now accounted for over half the 50 million privately insured enrollees in managed care. It was the proactive efforts by feminist groups that influenced the Clinton administration in 1997 to convince Congress to mandate longer hospital stays for childbirth.

Women's health groups, including providers, had called for universal coverage and cost containment, and agreed that HMOs had the potential for delivering preventive and primary care, particularly if nurses' independent practice was extended. However, Shaffer concluded that there was little evidence that managed care had led to substantially lower costs; indeed, they often excluded classes of sick people and shifted costs to individuals. For-profit HMOs were primarily responsible to their stockholders: "At the end of 1994, these plans were sitting on an excess of $9.5 billion, and the *Wall Street Journal* reported that they were having trouble finding enough places to invest so large a sum. (This amount would subsidize health insurance for 3.2 million Americans for a year.)" (p. 4).

Since women and children use health care more frequently than men, and low-income women and children are the majority of Medicaid beneficiaries, they are most affected by the shift to HMOs. If these limit office visits to between 7.5 and 20 minutes and speed up nurses' work, women, whom research has already found to receive less attention from physicians than men, would again be more negatively affected. If choice of providers is limited, women may not be able to choose reproductive services offered, for example, by Planned Parenthood. Indeed, women's health centers are often excluded by large HMOs that may dominate entire geographic areas. Women need control over health-care decisions that affect them and the right to choose health professionals who respect women—without having to go out of their HMOs. What women needed was real quality improvement programs, not arbitrary limits and bureaucratic hassles. Instead, "Cost-cutting hospitals have shrunk staff so seriously that nurses led a march on Washington in March, 1995, warning that patient care has deteriorated significantly" (p. 4).

Census Bureau figures showed that in 1992 and 1993 48 percent of the chronically poor were children (Associated Press, 1996a). The average poverty threshold for a family of four in 1993 was $14,763. In an average month, single-parent families, generally headed by women, were much more likely to be poor, nearly 38 percent, compared to families headed by couples (7.7 percent); and 17.2 percent versus 1.6 percent were continuously poor for the whole of 1992 and 1993. Indeed, the proportion of children without health insurance was growing: 10 million children under eighteen were uninsured in 1994, according to the government General Accounting Office; this represented 14.2 percent of the total, up from 12.4 percent in 1992 (Knight Ridder News Service, 1996). In 1980, 74 percent of U.S. workers had insurance fully paid by their employers, but by 1993, that number had dropped to 21 percent. Indeed, the number of insured children had been dropping every year since 1987. The 1990 expansion of Medicaid insurance did not help the third of uninsured children who came from ineligible families. Welfare reforms in 1996 would certainly not help improve the situation of female-headed families, given the lower earning power of women coupled with dead-end jobs that included few or minimal health-care benefits. Indeed, the Foundation for Women's Health, in collaboration with the American College of Women's Health Physicians, concluded that women's health care is fragmented and inadequate (K. Phillips, 1999). Statewide surveys support this assertion. For example, a survey of eleven HMOs in Arizona found serious gaps in health care for midlife women, who lacked proper preventive care for osteoporosis and heart disease and did not routinely receive lifesaving screenings such as bone-density scans and cholesterol tests (West, 1999). Clearly, the piecemeal shift to managed care and profit-making institutions was not helping a substantial proportion of children, women, and families.

Evaluating HMOs: Only Four Rated as Excellent

By mid-1996, 53.3 million people had been shunted into HMOs, and another 50 million were shifted by 2000. Ironically, there was no central source of information about and no authoritative ranking of HMOs. Indeed, according to Ellyn Spragins (1996), "The industry can't even agree on a definition of quality" (p. 56). Of the existing 593 HMOs in 1996, the Foundation for Accountability (a nonprofit health-care information group) surveyed 75 of the largest in order to assess their quality; 43 of them, covering 24 million people, responded. Some, such as United Health Care, operating more than 40 HMO plans covering 14 million people, would not participate because, as they asserted, measures of quality were not yet clear. This, despite the fact that the National Committee for Quality Assurance, a group that accredits HMOs, had developed a database on 50 different characteristics used to evaluate HMOs for accreditation. Only 37 percent of the 222 plans reviewed as of June 1996 won full accreditation; 39 percent, partial; 11 percent, provisional; and 12 percent were denied.

In 1989 several corporations, including Xerox and General Electric, developed HEDIS, the Health Plan Employer Data and Information Set, in order to compare the quality of HMOs. Surprisingly, most HMOs could not say how healthy or unhealthy their members are; only one plan merited the highest rating in this category. Furthermore, only the top-rated HMOs bothered to analyze the outcomes of their health care treatment. Prevention and screening, the quality of maternity care, the degree of consumer satisfaction, and numbers of complaints were also considered in the survey. *Only four of the forty-three plans surveyed were given an overall rating of excellent.*

"This Isn't Managed Care: It's a Move to Create a Physician-Controlled Monopoly"

The shift to HMOs and profit-making institutions had severe effects on nursing. For example, the Rochester Community Individual Practice Association (RCIPA), a prominent HMO that had cornered more than 70 percent of the managed-care market in Rochester, New York, announced it would not reimburse for extended patient visits with NPs because, it stated, "The *physician* should be the focus of the individual patient's care. . . . A nurse practitioner may be utilized to assist in the provision of that care, but *at no time* should the nurse practitioner be considered the primary caregiver" (New York State Nurses Association, 1994e, p. 3). Indeed, she or he should be "appropriately supervised" by physicians. Nursing official Karen Ballard asserted that limiting reimbursements for nurse practitioners essentially limited access to alternative services, saying: "This isn't managed care. It's a move to create a physician-controlled monopoly" (cited in *NYSNA Report,* 1994e, p. 3). More precisely, it was another move to *sustain* physicians' monopoly. Nurses contacted the attorney general's Antitrust Bureau about this issue and also about the state law requiring collaboration, not supervision. Ballard claimed that "Anything more than collaboration would be a duplication of services and increase health care costs" (cited in *NYSNA Report,* 1994e, p. 3). RCIPA officers refused to delay implementation of their policy, but agreed to form a working committee and to monitor the effect on patient care. Thus, a delaying tactic was coupled with asking the fox to monitor the chickens! The RCIPA continued to ignore the efforts of nurses and the New York State Nurses Association to resolve the conflict. Thus, by the fall of 1995, the state attorney general's office had forwarded the nurses' complaint for review to the Federal Trade Commission (New York State Nurses Association, 1995f).

Given the conservative shift to the Republican-controlled Congress and the collapse of the Clintons' health-care reform plan, nurses were forced into taking the lead in opposing the Republican-sponsored proposals to restrict and reduce costs of Medicare ($270 billion) and Medicaid ($182 billion) in seven years. These cuts would accelerate the cost-reduction efforts already underway in hospitals and agencies; the first and biggest cuts would be in patient-care services and staffing, lowering levels of quality, and accelerating job losses for RNs.

"Incredibly, the American Medical Association (AMA) supports these draconian proposals. It endorsed the House version after the House leadership offered several concessions, including smaller reductions in Medicare fees to physicians, a cap on malpractice awards for noneconomic damages and removal of many antitrust restrictions on anticompetitive behavior by physicians" (New York State Nurses Association, 1995f, p. 1). ANA President Betts charged that the "AMA [has] put blatant self-interest above the medical professional ethic of 'do no harm'" (Vanderbilt and Keepnews, 1995, p. 1). Shifting to block grants to states would jeopardize federal mandates and standards; the incentives built in for special populations, including children; remove hard-won protections for the elderly in nursing homes; and exclude provisions for APNs. The ANA opposed these changes and was thus once again in opposition to the AMA.

Merger Mania, Downsizing, and Skill Mix: Frightening Trends That Must Be Challenged

The mergers of health-care organizations rapidly and substantially increased their power. For example, in Minneapolis, Northwestern Hospital merged with Abbott Hospital, and then it joined with other hospital and physicians' groups to form a large conglomerate called Life Span. This merged with another jumbo system and was called Health Span, which was in the process of merging with yet another large HMO. The same pattern, reported Joni Ketter (1994c) was obvious in Rhode Island, Florida, Texas, Massachusetts, and other states across the nation. Indeed, a 1993 survey reported in *Hospitals* magazine showed that more than two-thirds of hospitals had entered into mergers with other institutions, mostly other hospitals. Consolidation or closure of units directly impacted nurses' jobs, and their job descriptions, benefits, workloads, cross-training, and collective bargaining contracts.

Nurses were asking how this had happened. According to Ketter, "Many hospitals are using health care reform as an excuse for their plans to restructure" (Ketter, 1994d, p. 22). The ANA had funded research on the impact of RN workforce changes on the safety and quality of care in hospitals and to determine the linkages between organization and delivery of nursing care and patient outcomes. The U.S. Department of Health and Human Services was also conducting a study of a number of "redesigned" facilities in several geographic areas to determine the impact on nurses, quality of patient care, safety, and cost savings. Working with the Institute of Medicine in a study funded by Congress, the ANA was researching the levels of quality of care as these related to nurse staffing levels and mix, educational levels, and other variables.

In the meantime, unlicensed assistive personnel were rapidly taking over some nursing functions and nurse administrators were again, as in the 1960s, facing a different staffing mix as hospitals reduced beds and changed the nurse-patient ratio from 1:6 to 1:8. Called by dozens of different names—aides, nursing assistants, patient-care techs, OR techs, maternity techs, patient aides, attendants—these people had "literally hundreds of different job descriptions, and their numbers were growing. According to a 1991 study, 80% of hospital RNs and 98% of long-term care RNs surveyed were working with unlicensed assistive personnel, and the Bureau of Labor Statistics predicted that by the year 2000, nursing-assistant positions will increase by 33% and home-health aides by 80%" (New York State Nurses Association, 1994c, p. 1). However, some nurse administrators were talking optimistically about RNs directing and managing assistants and were actually complaining about nurses as primary caregivers who did not know how to delegate and supervise. Other nurses were concerned about loss of close relationships with patients and the renewed emphasis on tasks or functions as demanded in the 1920s and periodically, in different guises, in subsequent decades.

At the same time, research showed that a "higher proportion of RNs in the staff mix is linked to fewer patient deaths, fewer complications, shorter lengths of stay, and increased patient satisfaction. In a 1993 study of 281 hospitals reported by *Modern Healthcare,* those facilities that reduced their staffing by 7.75% or more were *400 times* more likely to see an increase in patient illness and mortality" (New York State Nurses Association, 1994d, p. 10). Nevertheless, RNs were still losing out in hospitals, although their numbers were expected to increase in new community settings, where an additional 766,000 would be needed by 2005, according to the Bureau of Labor Statistics. In the meantime, RNs were increasingly unclear about the growing numbers of unlicensed assistants and were calling the state associations to determine what their supervisory and legal responsibilities were. Unfortunately there were no clear answers (New York State Nurses Association, 1993d, p. 3).

If an increased number of nurses external to hospitals were needed in the future, the trend was for an increase in UAPs in home care in for-profit agencies to cut costs. Thus, caregivers in some geographical areas did not have any nursing credentials (RN) in public health. Even baby- and school-health programs were being administered—for example, in Florida—by unlicensed, inadequately trained, and unqualified individuals, many of whom were not even high school graduates: "It's not a public health program but a bunch of fragmented pieces done on the cheap," said one Florida nurse (Ketter, 1994a, p. 18). In home-health care, according to this nurse, "Wounds are becoming severely infected or dressing changes are not done appropriately" (p. 18), because nurses' caseloads have increased tremendously and the assistive personnel cannot be properly supervised.

Colorado—one of three states, along with Florida and Minnesota, used as pilot sites to investigate school nurses' training of paraprofessionals—was finding that there was no consensus on the proper role, training, or credentialing of such assistive personnel. In New York, the state Department of Health was nevertheless planning to eliminate nursing titles, remove the educational requirements for supervising community-health nurses, and drop the title of director of patient services. Community-health nurses could then work with a supervising nurse with no training or experience in public health and no field staff to assist in making decisions about case management. Nurses' testimony before the state Hospital Review and Planning Council Code Committee was rejected along with the nurses' alternative proposal. The Department of Health planned "to proceed with 'reform' that will further dismantle the only health care system that brings any primary care . . . to a needy, vulnerable patient population" (New York State Nurses Association, 1993b, p. 3). Ironically, in the same issue of the *NYSNA Report,* the expanded role for nurse practitioners and removal of barriers is espoused as a solution to the shortage of primary-care physicians. A further irony is obvious in the trend to demote nurses: "The facility where I've been working is downsizing its professional nursing staff and refilling these positions with LPNs. I've lost my RN position but, since I have an LPN license, I've been offered a job as an LPN. Should I take the job? I can't afford not to work" (New York State Nurses Association, 1993d, p. 3). The response? The RN might be "unofficially" expected to continue RN responsibilities, but the employer could, at the same time, initiate disciplinary action if the nurse placed her RN license on inactive status. On the other hand, if she faced a situation that demanded action beyond the scope of the LPN, the state could hold her to the highest standard of her training as an RN, but she could still be subject to disciplinary actions. In short, this nurse and many others found themselves in ridiculous double binds.

The Latest Version of "Do the Best with What You've Got"

According to nurse administrator Eloise Balasco (1995), managed care was used to redesign work by assuming that nursing was simply doing tasks that could be rank-ordered. Only those requiring high-level skills would be done by RNs, who would supervise non-nurses performing low-level tasks; thus, a "new" skill mix was introduced. This presumably justified fewer RNs. But, said Balasco, a continuous trusting relationship was often made possible through the performance of "routine" tasks, during which the nurse assesses the patient's conditions and decides on the most effective ways to promote healing. Human caring cannot be measured from a distance as simply a set of tasks. Expert clinical judgments cannot be rank-ordered by a set of tasks. These cannot replace "care that respects the integrity of the human person and contributes to the restoration and promotion of health in the community" (p. 5).

Is the "new" skill mix just a return to team nursing, in which a registered nurse directs a group of caregivers and coordinates their care? Nurse Theresa M. Stephany said, "I've nursed through Team/Functional Nursing, Primary Nursing, Modified Primary Nursing, several versions of 'do the best you can with what you've got', and now Case Management, so I *know* better! The change in skill mix to fewer RNs and more LVNs [licensed vocational nurses] and aides is a frightening trend that *must* be challenged" (Stephany, 1992, p. 4). This was not a return to team nursing of the 1970s, another recycled idea; rather, "Skill mix changes are *entirely* driven by cost" (p. 4). There are no benefits to patients or nurses, but only to hospitals that will profit off nurses' backs without regard for patient safety.

What was vastly different in the 1990s was the acuity of patients' illnesses and the more technical duties now routinely expected of nurses:

Comical though it must sound today, in the '70s nurses did not routinely carry stethoscopes, much less use them for anything except blood pressures. . . . We were neither educated nor expected to listen to breath, heart, or bowel sounds. Physicians started and managed IVs; central lines did not exist; nurses did not draw blood. . . . Only the head nurse spoke to the doctors; hyperal was done in the ICU; we gave IM Demerol every four hours PRN for terminal cancer pain; MDs pushed what rudimentary chemo existed; and, even in our worst nightmares, we could not have imagined AIDS. (p. 4)

When team nursing was popular, said Stephany, nurses still wore caps, white hose and shoes, and white uniform dresses. Now nurses wear scrubs and athletic shoes and own the finest stethoscopes for good reasons. "To say that the proposed changes in skill mix are nothing more than a return to Team Nursing is simplistic, misleading and downright *dangerous*. We must not let anyone tell us that it's okay to have fewer RNs today" (p. 4). Stephany called for more seasoned, mature nurses to speak out against this "latest euphemistic outrage." In sharp contrast, Patricia Keen agreed that skill mix was driven by costs, but claimed that now RNs did not need to draw blood or give baths; instead they could plan care, delegate to non-RNs, and get away from task-oriented nursing (Keen, 1992).

"We've Given Up on Quality": The Struggle to Provide Safe Care amid All the Restructuring and Cost-Cutting

The debate on skill mix and staffing ratios led many nursing analysts to claim that restructuring plans were still not including the impact on patient outcomes and were often dangerous to patient safety. Instead, hospital labor costs were the main focus; nursing constituted 20 to 30 percent of total hospital expenditures and half the labor costs. At the 1994 ANA convention, the House of Delegates chose to focus on a plan to link cost, quality, and staff mix with patient outcomes and conduct research on how nurses affected these. A California delegate said the all-RN staff had gone to a 60–40 mix and more cuts were to come: "We've given up on quality. We're hoping for safe" (Ketter, *American Nurse*, 1994e, p. 26). Unlicensed assistants were now replacing rather than assisting. For example, in Washington, OR scrub nurses were being replaced with scrub technicians. At University of Illinois Hospital, more than 100 RN positions had been filled with UAPs, and the hospital had refused to enter collective bargaining over the change. At the University of Chicago Hospital, the reduction of RNs from 90 percent to 70 percent of the total nursing care staff had reached an impasse as the hospital asserted the management's right to determine the number of nurses and the mix of staff. At both hospitals, nurses were raising union and other issues with the appropriate arbitrators. Ironically, nurses were being asked to train the UAPs to take over their jobs and to delegate nursing tasks to them.

By late 1994 organized nursing groups testified before the Institute of Medicine's Committee on the Adequacy of Nurse Staffing that nurses were very concerned with the trend to slash nursing budgets and replace nurses with UAPs at the same time that patients were now being admitted to hospitals only when acutely ill (*American Nurse,* 1994d). Ironically, fewer nurses were now expected to provide for a greater number of sicker patients. Indeed, in a 1988 study, Flood and Diers (cited in *American Nurse,* 1994d, p. 14) compared patients on a well-staffed unit to those on an inadequately staffed unit and found that the length of stay was shorter in the units with an adequate number of RNs. The researchers estimated that "the extra hospital costs incurred by a greater length of stay for patients on the understaffed unit cost the hospital more than $37,000 for a three-month period" (*American Nurse,* 1994d, p. 14). Additional data provided evidence for increased costs for training unlicensed personnel and training RN staff to oversee work, and increased overtime costs of RNs to finish work left undone because of insufficient numbers of RNs or the incompetence of UAPs. Unfortunately, the American Organization of Nurse Executives disagreed with other nursing organizations on restructuring, asserting that the data on nurses' impact on the quality of care were limited. The representatives of the American Hospital Association and the nursing home industry agreed. Nevertheless, in a recent study conducted by researchers at the University of Iowa College of Nursing, inpatient care units with higher numbers of RNs were found to have lower rates of medication errors, patient falls, and other negative patient outcomes (*American Nurse,* 1998c). Clearly, using unlicensed assistive personnel in preference to registered nurses has severe health-care consequences for patients.

Increasingly concerned about RN layoffs, failure to fill vacant positions, and reliance on unlicensed personnel, the ANA stressed these issues with the President's Task Force on National Health Care Reform and with Donna Shalala, secretary of the Department of Health and Human Services (HHS), calling for a transition plan with interim quality protection to safeguard patient care and for the retraining and redeployment of nurses into preventive and primary care. Although hospital executives continued to receive high salaries and bonuses, women nurses were an easy target for cost-cutting, despite the fact that labor as a percentage of total hospital expense "actually declined between 1985 and 1992, while capital costs soared and excessive tests and procedures became more widespread. RNs made up an average 22 percent of hospital staff in 1991–92, essentially unchanged from the 21 percent of 1985, even as patients as a whole grew 'sicker' and hospital services became increasingly intense" (Scott, 1993, p. 3).

Hospitals had increased spending on costly new buildings and equipment at a rate that was almost double that of other industries, according to a report from the Department of Health and Human Services. At the same time, Tampa General Hospital, to use one example, fired 213 employees, which led to the dismantling of care for indigent mothers and their newborns, and then later to the rehiring of 19 of those who had been laid off and to advertisements for nurses to fill vacant positions. In one survey, hospital chief executive officers said that nursing care was the single most important factor contributing to overall hospital quality and patient satisfaction. In another study, a short-staffed hospital unit actually drove up costs because of the costs of extra patient days caused by complications. Obviously, decreasing the use of inappropriate, ineffective, or unnecessary tests and procedures would be more cost-effective than cutting labor; nevertheless, Ketter (*American Nurse*, 1994h), reported a continuation in the replacement of RNs, who were, however, fighting the trend. More than three hundred RNs in Michigan finally went on strike over the reduction of RNs and increase of UAPs on the oncology unit. Preceding the strike, the negotiating team for the nurses, who were represented by the Michigan Nurses' Association, advocated that current staffing patterns be maintained, but hospital management rejected the proposal, failed to make a counterproposal, and presented its final offer to the local media: a three-month cooling-off period. The nurses went on strike to prevent the erosion of care in the community, which generally supported the nurses; indeed, some people joined the nurses on the picket line and held a rally outside the hospital. In response, the hospitals ran ads for replacements, hiring mostly LPNs.

Nurses at the University of Chicago Hospital did not have the strike option, because their contract called for arbitration when impasses occurred. The Illinois Nurses' Association reported that the hospital would not agree to minimum staffing ratios or limits on RN replacement or assistive-worker jobs. The nurses would not budge on these issues. In New York, informational picketing on unsafe staffing, RN substitution, and substandard quality of care was underway. The nurses in New York were in a tough fight over home-health care, continuing a grueling year-long struggle with the state Department of Health that was, as noted previously, in the process of eliminating key public health nursing positions and lowering the educational qualifications required for home-health caregivers (New York State Nurses Association, 1994a). The Department of Health, ostensibly changing regulations to conform to federal guidelines, had actually lowered educational standards *selectively,* eroded high nursing standards, and become impatient with the numerous letters from nurses. In the end, NYSNA won retention of nursing titles, such as "Public Health Nurse," but lost the level of educational preparation previously required for these positions (i.e., BS in Nursing degree).

By the end of 1994, nursing practice was being challenged on still another front: the use of emergency medical technicians (EMTs), who could, with more training, provide primary care (in addition to their ambulance duties) to patients outside of hospitals. Trained to provide basic life support, an ambulance company in Syracuse, New York, for example wanted to move into the home-health-care business for financial reasons. Nurses, who had originally trained the emergency personnel, were now to be replaced by them. Ambulance companies had made similar proposals in other areas of New York State and in other states (New York State Nurses Association, 1994i).

Indeed, hospital aides were now doing tracheal suctioning, post-op gastrostomy tube feeding, and giving medications and immunizations. NYSNA reported on two teacher aides who, after brief instruction from a school nurse, "performed daily catheterizations on a child with severe cerebral palsy. The procedure required one aide to hold the student's legs while another inserted the tubing. After about a week, the mother noticed a problem with the child's leg. It was found to be broken" (New York State Nurses Association, 1994j). As more children with special needs were mainstreamed into regular classes, teachers and their aides were calling the New York State Education Department about practicing nursing illegally. However, the special education services unit of the State Education Department was proposing an amendment to the current Nurse Practice Act, allowing teachers and their aides to provide nursing care to special needs children. Obviously this was opposed by nurses, who forced the unit to form a work group to draft guidelines. The more fundamental problem was that school nurses were still practicing under the outdated restrictions specific to school nurses delineated in the 1913 Nurse Practice Act and had not been allowed to expand their functions in school settings.

With these struggles occurring in all fifty states, the ANA produced in 1994 a consumer brochure, "Every Patient Deserves a Nurse," that underscored the direct impact of registered nurses on reducing patient mortality, readmission rates, and length of hospitalizations. In the same year, the ANA met with the secretary of labor in Washington, D.C., to find out whether a plan of action was being developed to assist a dislocated nursing workforce to demand re-training services. The ANA certainly supported retraining efforts for RNs, but the strategies of cross-training, restructuring, and the use of multiskilled workers, which had been implemented in manufacturing industries where tasks were routine, were not appropriate when applied to hospitals where the "product" to be processed was a sick individual, not an inanimate object. Downward substitution strategies were dangerous for such high-performance workplaces (Ketter, 1994b).

"We Got What We Wanted at the Worst Possible Time"

Barbara Stevens Barnum, RN (1994) asserted that the reality of nursing practice was resource constrictions, overwhelming demands for more service from fewer professionals, and increasing technological demands. Yet Barnum thought that nursing for once was on top of the change in health care, even though brutal economic restraint, dislocation of professionals, and limitations in patient care were part of the revolution: "The brave new world of ideal patient care some nurses envisioned a few decades ago simply never happened" (p. 401). Nevertheless, nurses now headed new entrepreneurial health-care ventures or were independent practitioners, or worked as partners with other providers, creating private psychotherapy firms, independent rehabilitation facilities, nursing-management consulting firms, forensic nursing businesses, and partnerships in independent, managed-care organizations. Much of this growth *outside* of the usual institutions was due to the rise of nurse practitioners. Nurses, said Barnum, had actually, for the first time, beaten the system by going out of it. The nurses were getting paid for providing independent services, whether or not they had real or titular physician partners.

However, Barnum admitted that traditional institutions still represented the major domain of practice and never before had as many "well educated, masters-and doctorally-prepared nurses been out of work . . . never have the nurses . . . been so overstressed and overburdened in their day-to-day roles" (pp. 401–402). Ironically, said Barnum, this was partially caused by nurses' success in making respectable salaries; now they were forced to supervise less-costly technicians and aides. "We got what we wanted at the worst possible time, becoming a powerful player when it might have been easier to fade into the woodwork" (p. 402). Now nurse leaders had to play hardball in the corporate world and deal with restructured nursing practice, in which all tasks are placed into new job constellations based on skill levels. Skill-mix reassessment is key to determining which tasks are complex or repetitive, which require judgment and analysis.

According to Barnum, nursing practice patterns and ideologies occurred in cycles determined by scarcity of resources, but always varying on patient versus task orientation and ratio of nurses per patient. If the total quantity of resources is plentiful, a goal-driven model of comprehensive care prevails, but when they are scarce, the resource-driven model dominates with care determined by the quantity, for example, of nurses' time. There is, however, a level at which a critical lack of resources presents an overt hazard. Historically, private-duty nursing was resource-rich, but when World Wars I and II intervened, nursing at home became a scarce commodity. Nurses were directed away from private patients to hospitals, where, to maximize nurses' time, functional tasks could be organized on a factory model and also redistributed to subordinates.

As World War II ended, resources increased and team nursing developed with a return to a patient orientation, but also focused on functions directed by team leaders. Primary-care nursing was an attempt to return to the one-to-one orientation, but now, given the drive for cost containment, the shift is again to functional nursing, but in a more complex form. Indeed, "no wave of care delivery returns in exactly the same form" (p. 405). The new factor in a return to task analysis is the added element of patient outcomes based on planned recovery expectations derived from the imposition of diagnostic related groups (DRGs). Hiring cheaper, less educated workers requires someone to hold together the elements of restructured practice; thus, the introduction of the case manager, who assesses the outcomes of diverse activities and mediates cross-professional goals. Now, in a restructured matrix, the head nurse is responsible to the case managers.

Higher Profits the Primary Consideration?

Was Barnum's analysis of resource scarcity and nursing models correct? If correct, hospital profits should have plummeted as resources shrank. This was not the case: Hospital profits soared, with hospitals posting some of the highest profit margins of the last two decades; acute-care hospital aggregate profits for 1992, for example, were $11.9 billion, *up nearly 19 percent* from 1991 (*American Nurse*, 1994a). While nurses were experiencing scarcity of resources, most hospitals were not. According to data produced by the American Hospital Association (AHA), the profit margins had reached double-digit increases for four years in a row. Only 24 percent of hospitals had negative profit margins, down from 28 percent in 1987. Women nurses and other women workers made an easy target, despite the fact that "labor as a percent of total hospital expense actually declined between 1985 and 1992" (p. 30). Even though patients were "sicker," nurses made up an average 22 percent of hospital staff in 1991–1992, relatively unchanged from 21 percent in 1985. Downsizing, cuts in nursing jobs, and use of UAPs were evidently producing not cost savings but higher profits, which, as ANA president Virginia Trotter Betts said, should *not* be the primary consideration in restructuring the health-care "system" (*American Nurse*, 1994a). Indeed, a 1994 ANA white paper asserted that restructuring had produced not simply a new cycle of nursing care but a *fragmentation* of care, serious understaffing, and overworked RNs and other caregivers. Obviously, the industrial factory model was not working well with very ill human beings in need of intensive services. Nonetheless, by 2000, more than half of the nation's HMOs were reporting profit losses, and some were forced to claim bankruptcy. To maintain their solvency, most HMOs were dropping Medicare patients and increasing their rates. Not good news for the consumer.

Manipulating the Presentation of MD Income

Had changes in health-care services also negatively affected physicians? According to Robert Reno (1996), physicians see the meteoric rise of HMOs and power of insurance companies as the major culprits for physicians' loss of control, autonomy, and reduced incomes. "Only 43 percent of doctors participated in managed care as recently as 1986, and the rest said they would sooner eat worms than join. Now 83 percent participate" (p. AA5). Indeed, the media reported that for the first time in the fourteen years that the AMA has been keeping such records, physicians' incomes dropped (*New York Times* News Service, 1995). The median earnings reportedly dropped 3.8 percent from $156,000 in 1993 to $150,000 in 1994, although they had risen 9.9 percent in 1992–1993. However, as noted previously, at its annual meeting in mid-1994 the AMA had changed the way it calculated physicians' median income when it decided to include the income of young physicians in training and of those employed by the federal government. Obviously this produced a lower overall median income. The AMA secretary-treasurer alleged that press reports had previously left out the footnotes about which physicians were included or excluded from the calculations; however, "Health consumer groups called the change 'unabashed deception'" (New York State Nurses Association, 1994g, p. 6). Given the previous increase from $164,300 in 1990 to $177,400 in 1992 (Wolinsky and Brune, 1995), the new way of reporting data was, even if partially accurate, hardly an indication of scarce resources for the medical practitioners, who, nevertheless, continued to work to restrict nurses, causing a confusing mix of state laws.

The Continuing Hodgepodge of Restrictions on Nurses

Researchers at SUNY Buffalo, led by Patricia Burns, had by 1995 produced data that showed the national geographic distribution of nurse practitioners and defined the barriers whose removal would stimulate providers to relocate in areas where they are most needed (New York State Nurses Association, 1995c). The heaviest concentration of NPs was on the East and West Coasts (California, 5,770, and New York, 3,062), but some western states had fewer than 100. Only 5.5 percent worked in rural areas, compared to 85 percent in metropolitan areas. Ironically, the ANA reported in 1994 that APNs who lived in these metropolitan areas but provided care outside them were experiencing difficulty in being directly reimbursed through Medicare, even though the law provided for such compensation. The ANA had to assure nurses that they did not have to *live* in a more rural area in order to receive direct payment for *work* in those areas!

The ten states that imposed the fewest restrictions on APN practice were Alaska, Arizona, Iowa, Montana, New Hampshire, New Mexico, North Dakota, Oregon, Washington, and West Virginia. The ten most restrictive states were Alabama, Arkansas, Hawaii, Illinois, Louisiana, Maine, Massachusetts, Michigan, Ohio, and Wisconsin. The most restrictive—Hawaii and Illinois—did not even recognize NPs as a group. And only five states—Alaska, Arizona, Montana, New Mexico, and Wyoming—granted full prescriptive authority with no additional directives or written protocols (*American Nurse*, 1995).

Restrictiveness was rated in nine categories: legal recognition, standards of practice, prescriptive authority, educational requirements, certification examination requirements, continuing education requirements, temporary practice, grandfather clause exempting NPs from new regulations, and private insurance reimbursement. Burns and her colleagues concluded that the current legislative situation limited the influence nurses could have on the nation's health (New York State Nurses Association, 1995c). Nurse practitioners were not accepting this state of affairs, and in February 1994 they formally created the National Nurse Practitioner Coalition, an umbrella organization bringing together separate specialty groups in order to achieve greater visibility and a single unified voice.

Still More Research Proves Advanced Practice Nurses' Cost-Effectiveness and Competence

Research continued to produce the same positive results on APNs' competence as in earlier decades. The cost-effectiveness of nurse practitioners in long-term-care facilities in new HMOs was again researched, this time by Jeffrey Burl, Alice Bonner, and Maithili Rao (1994). In the late 1980s they compared the efforts of a physician practicing alone in providing care to residents of long-term-care facilities to those of a nurse practitioner who consulted and worked with an MD when needed. The patients cared for by the NP-MD team had fewer emergency-room visits and hospitalizations. There were also significant increases in patient, family, and staff satisfaction. Later, in 1992, three more NPs were added to the staffs to care for three hundred residents in seven area nursing homes. The researchers then compared the results for patients under the care of the NP-MD team to those with physician-only care. There were statistically significant lower costs for the NP-MD patients, even though they were on average older than those covered only by MDs. In addition, among the patients of the NP-MD team, hospital admissions were 25 percent fewer, hospital stays were significantly shorter, and emergency-room visits and specialty visits were significantly fewer. The costs were $2,500 lower per patient; the average hospital costs were 30 percent lower, emergency room costs 16 percent lower, and ambulatory-care costs 10 percent lower. Overall, the average cost for a nursing-home patient cared for by the NP-MD team was 42 percent lower than for patients cared for by physicians alone. The quality of care was better, reflecting a more comprehensive approach. The savings exceeded the cost of salaries for the NPs. Subsequently, more NPs have been added to care for the patients in this HMO, proving that cost-effectiveness and quality care are not mutually exclusive.

Lower Death Rates with Empowered Nurses

In the absence of educated and experienced RNs, people may not only visit emergency rooms more frequently and stay longer in hospitals, they may also be more likely to die. To save money at the expense of quality of care is obviously no saving at all. Dr. Linda Aiken, RN, and colleagues found in their study of 244 hospitals across the United States that the number of deaths among Medicare patients was lower by 5 percent in the 39 magnet hospitals in which nurses had reorganized nursing and empowered nurses (*American Nurse*, 1994b). These hospitals were compared to 195 hospitals that were similar in all respects except for the organization and delivery of nursing. Patients were more likely to survive at hospitals that give nurses' professional autonomy, control over practice setting, more egalitarian relations with physicians, and the right to routinely exercise their own professional judgment. Thus, the issue of empowering nurses is very fundamental, involving even the mortality of patients. Other research focused on the reduction of house staff workload by using trauma nurse practitioners, whose quality of care and cost-effectiveness were again established (Spisso, O'Callaghan, McKennan, and Holcroft, 1990). Still other research proved APNs' effectiveness in ICUs (Schulz, Liptak, and Fioravanti, 1994).

The trend in positive research results continued even among patients with HIV infection. Aiken and her colleagues (Aiken, Lake, Semaan, Lehman, O'Hare, Cole, Dunbar, and Frank, 1993) compared the outcomes of care provided by a physician and care provided by a nurse practitioner. Despite the fact that the nurses' patients were *three times* more likely to report that their health was fair or poor, they functioned at comparable levels and used no more health-care services than the patients cared for by physicians alone. The nurses' patients also reported 45 percent fewer problems with their care. Clearly, nurses could successfully care for severely, chronically ill patients.

Performing Medically Coded Functions without MD Supervision

The depth of the severity was matched by the breadth of conditions covered by nurses from a variety of different specialties. Dr. Hurdis M. Griffith, RN, and Dr. Karen R. Robinson, RN, (1993) surveyed a random sample of nurses from nine specialties to identify the procedures they used that were part of the Current Procedural Terminology, universally used by physicians to file claims for payment. Following up on an earlier questionnaire completed by 4,869 RNs (Griffith and Fonteyn, 1989), who indicated they used a number of physicians' codes with little MD supervision, Griffith and Robinson asked randomly selected nurses by specialty whether and how often they performed the coded functions and how often they were directly supervised by a physician. This well-constructed study indicated that nurses in all specialty groups performed at least 493 coded functions; critical-care nurses performed the largest number of functions. Again, as in the 1989 study, respondents reported *very little* direct physician supervision. Clearly, registered nurses were performing independently a significant number of medically coded functions. To what degree physicians or hospitals were charging for the functions actually performed by nurses remained to be researched.

A National Disgrace: Widespread Cutbacks Continue to Degrade Patient Care and Safety

Given these findings, we could logically expect that legislators would be clamoring to extend the roles of nurses for primary care and hire more, not fewer, nurses. This was *not* the case. In all the states across the nation, nurses had to campaign against initiatives to waive licensure requirements for RNs and other licensed health-care professionals; protect the title "nurse" from being used by technicians; eliminate exemptions that allowed unlicensed individuals to practice as nurses in all related institutions, for example, in mental health and mental retardation; lobby for adequate reimbursement levels and RN staffing in agencies, facilities, and private practices; and work to secure funding to retrain acute care nurses for primary care and stop RN cutbacks.

By 1995, after the U.S. Congress had debated and abandoned comprehensive health-care reform, the "restructuring" by corporate managers was aimed at cutting costs, not necessarily broadening access to care or improving the quality of care. Instead of going after waste and changing misplaced priorities, hospitals instead altered staffing policies, particularly those pertaining to the mostly female RNs, who historically had delivered 90 percent of hospital services and were now considered too "expensive." An ANA national survey showed that RN cutbacks were widespread. Some 200,000 RNs nationwide reported on conditions in their hospitals: 68.4 percent reported that RNs in their facilities had been cut back; 44.7 percent reported the increased use of UAPs; of those reporting cutbacks, 78.6 percent said these had degraded patient care, and 64 percent indicated patient safety had been negatively affected (New York State Nurses Association, 1995a).

Thus nurses faced a crisis in RN understaffing that directly affected their patients. After intense nurses' lobbying in New York, for example, four state assembly committees (Social Services, Labor, Health, and Higher Education) held a joint hearing to investigate the impact on patients of RN cutbacks (New York State Nurses Association, 1995d). At one hospital, a woman visited her father after heart bypass surgery, only to find him lying in a pool of blood. She contacted the nurse, who had forty patients to care for and who said the father could not be a priority when compared to other patients. In another facility, many RNs were on duty three hours beyond their eight-hour days, and one RN, with only one medical technician and one aide, was caring for thirty-five patients. The nurses were refusing to sign non-RN notes. Such anecdotal evidence was supported by statistics: RNs, who once provided 90 percent of hospital care, now constituted only 65 percent to 75 percent of patient-care staff. These reductions were occurring despite a steady rise in patient acuity, reliably estimated in research to have increased about 20 percent over the previous ten years, accompanied by a 14 percent decline in admissions and a 12 percent decrease in hospital stays. Most hospital administrators, although asked, chose not to testify before the state assembly committees. Many RNs were afraid to testify because they feared retaliation for whistle-blowing. Nevertheless, those who testified demanded retraining and placement of RNs, assurances that the state Nurse Practice Act would be controlled by the nursing division of the State Education Department, not by non-nursing departments or agencies, and that there would be protection for nurses who speak out about unsafe conditions.

Regardless of such efforts by New York nurses, hospital administrators at Mt. Vernon announced it would fire 32 of 270 RNs and replace them with 6 LPNs and 24 aides. The nurses organized a rally at the town hall, but the hospital said cuts in Medicaid had forced their actions (New York State Nurse Association, 1995e). Indeed, proposed national Medicare cuts of $200 billion could, said Ursula Himali (1995), spur further RN layoffs. The funding cuts would reduce nursing education and hit not only the elderly but the entire healthcare "system," particularly the quality and safety of care, stretching RNs to their limit.

On March 31, 1995, twenty-five thousand nurses, frustrated and angry over RN layoffs and substitutions of aides, marched in Washington, D.C., sponsored by many national nurses' organizations. They and the women and men who joined them deplored the emphasis on cuts, not care, and compared these with the 1994 data that proved that CEOs at the top privately owned HMOs received between $2.8 million and $15.5 million in salary and stock options, among the highest in any industry (New York State Nurses Association, 1995b).

Supreme Court Ruling Threatens Nurses' Organizing and Bargaining Rights

The attack on nurses and nursing was not limited to legislative bodies, hospitals, and organized medicine; it extended to the judicial arena as well. On May 23, 1994, in a 5 to 4 decision, the U.S. Supreme Court ruled that nurses who direct the work of others may be considered supervisors and thus they are not protected by the National Labor Relations Act (NLRA), which assures non-management employees the right to bargain collectively and to not be fired for "whistle-blowing" or complaining against management. The case, National Labor Relations Board v. Health Care and Retirement Corp. of America, involved three LPNs at an Ohio nursing home who had some limited supervisory responsibilities and openly expressed concerns about working conditions and were subsequently discharged. They filed charges of unfair labor practices with the National Labor Relations Board (NLRB), which ruled they were not supervisors so they should be reinstated in their positions (Ketter, 1994f). The Sixth Circuit Court of Appeals refused to reinforce the NLRB order. Subsequently, the Supreme Court ruled against the nurses; however, Justice Ruth Bader Ginsburg in her dissent said there was a difference between employers whose level of control places them in management and highly skilled employees who perform limited supervisory roles in relation to their skilled work.

Expressing grave concern, nurses such as Catherine Cornu-Quinn (1994) feared that the decision would lead to a loss of job security and a decline in health standards. Delegating, directing, and functioning with some autonomy are acts that are simply part of professional credentials; thus, to deny nurses the protection given to other workers is to deny the professionalism that aims at setting reliable, objective standards: "If every manager is free to decide professional standards for his/her health care institution, the profession as a whole has no way to protect the rights of its members to decide their own standards of practice. If any person who may use independent judgment to assign a task to others cannot be protected under the National Labor Relations Act, fair organized labor practices will not be intelligently implemented" (Cornu-Quinn, 1994, p. 28). Nurses must stop management from intimidating and coercing nurses into unsuitable practices.

Another nurse protested: "The Supreme Court must have been misled to believe that an ordinary charge nurse has the same power as a Director of Nursing. Even a nurse manager is rarely regarded as 'management' in terms of budgetary regulations, staffing levels, and disciplinary actions involving the hospital staff and doctors" (Agboola, 1994, p. 14).

The ANA quickly created a task force to develop and lobby for legislation that would amend the NLRA. In the meantime, hospitals immediately began using the new ruling against nurses. For example, negotiations over contracts were stalled because hospitals could not identify any nurses eligible for collective bargaining since they claimed that even assistant head and charge nurses were supervisors and thus *in*eligible: "They even claim that RNs who occasionally *fill in* as charge nurses are supervisors" (New York State Nurses Association, 1994g, p. 1). At one New York hospital, administrators labeled "almost every member of the negotiating team a supervisor" (p. 1). Yet these nurses did not hire or fire, promote or demote, or discipline employees, or handle budgets.

Since this development came at the same time as severe cost-cutting, nurses were very concerned. Said Virginia Trotter Betts, ANA president: "Now is not the time to tell the front-line caregivers in U.S. hospitals that they can be fired for complaining about management decisions that are detrimental to patient care" (Ketter, 1994f, p. 13). As Carolyn McCullough, director of NYSNA's collective bargaining program, said, the decision would be used to shrink the size of the bargaining unit, but "We have struggled long and hard for our right to representation. We are *not* going to give it up. Not now. Not ever" (McCullough, 1994, p. 1).

Organized nursing was ready to take legal action against employers who used the Supreme Court decision to obstruct and undermine nurses. Collective-bargaining units and state associations had already moved to influence state and national legislators to affirm the importance of labor law protection for employees who direct assistive personnel and exercise independent professional judgment. The RN license gives nurses the right to speak on behalf of patients and to question the actions and judgments of physicians, administrators, or insurance companies. But the license "cannot protect the nurse when she tells management the unit is understaffed, or that the patient is not ready to be discharged, or that conditions on the third floor are unsafe. The risk of being disciplined or fired for standing up for patients undermines the nurse's role as patient advocate" (New York State Nurses Association, 1994f, p. 7). Collective bargaining safeguards this advocacy because the contracts produced protect nurses against being dismissed without "just cause." Cornu-Quinn concluded that the Supreme Court decision was influenced by the majority of Republican appointees, who reached a politically biased decision in favor of management. In her view, the court was not immune to the big business special-interest groups that were gaining control of the health-care industry (Cornu-Quinn, 1994).

It became increasingly clear that management was using the ruling against nurses. For example, in Bozeman, Montana, one hospital's board of directors decided to terminate the contract between the hospital and the Montana Nurses' Association. In Maine, three employers filed petitions with the NLRB to exclude from bargaining most, and in some hospital units *all*, nursing positions from the all-RN units, claiming these positions were "supervisory" and thus that the nurses were not eligible to be represented by the Maine State Nurses' Association. In Washington, D.C., one week after the Supreme Court decision, another hospital that had agreed to include almost all RN positions sought to withdraw from this agreement and reopen a hearing to take evidence on excluding charge nurses and, indeed, any nurse who worked in this capacity, even if for only 10 percent of her shift. Since staff nurses rotated charge-nurse duties, about 25 percent of the nurses would be considered supervisors and therefore excluded from bargaining and thus from union protection. In Anchorage, Alaska, Providence Hospital claimed that almost half a unit was made up of supervisory employees, including charge nurses and even team leaders. The Alaskan nurses joined the ANA in presenting an oral argument before the NLRB, as did many other supporting union and labor groups (Ketter, 1994g). The Alaska Nurses' Association won the decision before the NLRB regional director, but the employer appealed.

After several years of concerted efforts, the ANA finally forced the NLRB to issue a decision stating that registered nurses, including charge nurses, are not statutory supervisors and are indeed protected by federal labor laws. Thus, they have the right to organize for collective bargaining and for other activities, such as speaking out as a group regarding job conditions or management decisions that compromise the safety and quality of patient care. Therefore, patient advocacy and nursing judgment were inherent in the professional role (Ketter, 1996a). However, Providence Hospital in Alaska still refused to bargain, even following the NLRB decision, and engaged in further stalling tactics, despite the nurses' 305–193 vote for collective bargaining representation by the Alaska

Nurses Association (Ketter, 1996b). Even with the support of forty-five physicians for the nurses' position and the NLRB ruling, it was not until 1999 that a federal mediator created a contract agreeable to both sides (Nawar, 1999).

"Let the Market Provide and the Buyer Beware!"

Clearly, nursing was beleaguered from many directions. As ANA president Virginia Trotter Betts said at the June 1995 meeting of the ANA House of Delegates, indescribable high hopes and expectations for health-care reform had been dashed and replaced with enormous concern for nursing. The nation moved from a "progressive social agenda for all to a philosophy of 'let the market provide' and 'the buyer beware.' Since we met last year, the nation has missed its best chance in 50 years to provide health care for all, and with that loss, nursing is now pitted in what I would call a fight for our profession" (Betts, 1995, p. 5).

Generalist nursing practice was being eroded, continued Betts, by UAPs, who were replacing RNs; by hospital associations that were striving to obtain institutional licensure and, thus, damage nurse practice acts and weaken the control of nurses over nursing; and by state governments and even foundations through their efforts to reduce professional licensure to the lowest common denominator. Advanced and specialty practice nursing was also facing vast challenges and potential closure of opportunities by state-level discrimination against nurses as a specific class of providers; by legislative efforts to diminish nurses' prescriptive authority, hospital privileges, and professional corporate practices; and by the efforts of the AMA and its state medical associations to substitute collaborative practice models with supervised clinical practice.

Organized nursing, said Betts, had had a "year like no other—from the pinnacle of expectation of expanded opportunities to provide care for all to the depths of anxiety about the future of health care, its quality and the maintenance of the role of the nurse as a unique, essential health care provider" (p. 5). Nevertheless, to stay firmly committed to universal access, "even if we alone do so, is a powerful statement of the core values of nursing. . . . To demand quality of care in all institutions and to call attention to quality failures, even if we are speaking alone, is courageous and reflects our commitment to our patients. . . . To pursue the data that link professional nursing care to patient outcomes and link staffing patterns to that care" (p. 5) will continue to create a record of credibility.

Foundations: Helping or Hindering Nurses?

Despite the failure of federal health-care reform, debate continued, particularly on changing regulations governing nursing. In Oregon, "recent proposed legislation (defeated through the efforts of the Oregon Nurses' Association) would have greatly restricted the authority of nurses and the nursing board over patient care activity. In Maine, a proposal has been submitted to the governor, after almost two years of dialogue . . . that would totally restructure the state's current health professions licensure system" (Whittaker and Minich, 1995, p. 1).

Although some initiatives were honestly motivated by concerns for consumers, others were more interested in "removing government interference in an effort to cut costs through substitution of unlicensed personnel for RNs" (p. 1). The origin of these initiatives include the various foundations that were engaged in analyzing the health-care system. One such foundation was the Pew Charitable Trusts, which set up the Pew Health Professions Commission. The commission initially included two nurses, Dr. Rheba deTornyay and Dr. Sheila A. Ryan, who proposed a change toward a model focused on health-promotion and community-based care. The failure of federal reform led the commission to concentrate on state initiatives on workforce reform in Alabama, California, and Missouri and on regulatory systems in Virginia, Washington, Maine, and Colorado. Gary Filerman, PhD, hired as director of the commission's Washington, D.C. office, told the July 1995 conference of the National Council of State Boards of Nursing that there was no profession other than nursing that was defined by another profession, in this case medicine. Admitting that this situation was not in the public interest, he used it not to advocate greater nursing independence, but to argue for the creation of a "superboard" of nursing and medical and other professionals combined with lay members. The obvious consequence would be an increase in medical monopolistic control.

In November 1995 *Critical Challenges: Revitalizing the Health Professions for the Twenty-First Century,* the third report of the Pew Health Professions Commission, was disseminated. This report was widely reported by the media, particularly the recommendation to shut down 20 percent of the 141 medical schools and 10 percent to 20 percent of the 1,470 nursing programs during the next decade. As many as half the nation's 5,000 hospitals were expected to close as a result of the shift to managed care, which, it was estimated, would cover 80 percent to 90 percent of the insured population in the next few years. The panel recommended that the 141 medical colleges admit 20 percent to 25 percent fewer students by 2005, thus lowering the size of entering classes from 17,500 to 13,000 or 14,000, not through reductions of students but by complete closure of schools. The numbers of training positions for residents and interns would be reduced, particularly since a quarter of these were currently filled by foreign-trained physicians, whose visa process should be tightened in the future to ensure their return to their native countries (Pew Health Professions Commission, 1995).

Predictably, the AMA disagreed with the report, saying it would dismantle the best system of medical education in the world. Nevertheless, by 1993 specialists outnumbered generalists among the 600,000 physicians by a 2-to-1 ratio and the imbalance was growing. Fifteen thousand new physicians graduated each year from medical schools, and Medicare and private health insurance subsidized graduate medical education through the rates paid for patient care, particularly at the 400 major teaching hospitals.

The ANA challenged the Pew report recommendation to close 10 percent to 20 percent of nursing schools, primarily associate degree and diploma programs. Nurse-attorney David Keepnews asserted: "The fact is that even as RN positions appear to be drying up . . . the unmet health-care needs of the American people . . . are growing . . . access to care for underserved and uninsured populations continues to suffer . . . the goal of providing care [to them] . . . simply does not appear to fit into the priorities of a 'market-based' system" (Keepnews, 1996, p. 3).

In January 1996, the Institute of Medicine's Committee on the Adequacy of Nursing Staffing called for adjusting the current mix of nursing personnel, twenty-four-hour RN coverage in nursing homes, and expanded hospital use of advanced practice nurses. The ANA responded that the report and recommendations fell short because the committee members did not grasp the urgency of the problems (*American Nurse*, 1996).

While various non-nursing groups came up with recommendations, nurses were involved with the immediate problem of protecting patient safety by developing quality safety indicators to guide the collection, tracking, and measurement of data. After defining seven indicators, the ANA moved to fund a demonstration project (Canavan, 1996a). Eventually, national data would provide "report cards" on hospitals so consumers could assess their safety in relation to nursing staff and care. Given the research data on RNs reducing mortality rates, such information could be literally related to life or death.

Concern for Patient Safety Increases as More RNs Lose Jobs

Though Mezey and her coauthors (1994) found that the majority of New York City hospitals were adding APNs to their staffs, the New York City municipal health system announced plans in mid-1996 to eliminate 1,600 jobs, including 1,156 RNs, and another 8,000 positions during 1997. In addition, public hospitals would be leased or sold to private corporations. "The most recent job cuts, which account for one-sixth of the RN staff, come on top of a severance program that 16 months ago coaxed 300 RNs out the door. Another 500 or so positions have also been lost through attrition" (New York State Nurses Association, 1996f, p. 1). The New York State Nurses Association (NYSNA) was "unilaterally opposed" to selling public health facilities "to private hospitals that have no statutory commitment to serving the poor" (p. 1). NYSNA joined others in a lawsuit against the city (headed by Republican Mayor Giuliani) for slashing the legally required funds "by $117 million in just two years to half the level it was in 1994" (p. 5). In June hundreds of nurses also protested in front of the city hospitals, nursing homes, and treatment centers. Ironically, the City Health and Hospitals Corporation had on the same day honored thirty nurses for their excellence and commitment while giving seven of them termination notices! (New York State Nurses Association, 1996g).

With increasing numbers of nurses losing their jobs, concern for patient safety was understandable. Thus, in 1996, the ANA drafted the legislation which led to H. R. 3355, the Patient Safety Act. The legislation included protection for nurses who disclosed unsafe patient care practices and required public disclosure of patient quality care indicators, including RN-patient ratios, and review of plans for mergers, closures, or acquisitions (Franklin, 1996). The public was becoming more aware of the problems, as is clear from an ANA-sponsored survey conducted by Princeton Survey Research Associates, which found that 67 percent of adults are worried about the use of unlicensed personnel to provide traditional nursing care. About 86 percent of the respondents wanted to know the hospital survival rates for patients treated for major illnesses, 84 percent wanted to know the number of patients who contract new infections during their hospital stays, and 87 percent wanted satisfaction ratings from recently treated patients. (New York State Nurses Association, 1996i). These data were used by the ANA to develop the legislative model that led to the Patient Safety Act noted above.

Union-Busting and Direct Confrontation Continue

Despite strong political and organizing efforts in opposition, the trend toward eliminating nurses and rejecting their right to organized bargaining continued. Union-busting was breaking out in many states. In New York State, for example, after an eight-month battle with Olean General Hospital, nurses finally won their right to representation by their state association, after a ruling by the NLRB (New York State Nurses Association, 1996h). But hospitals continued to eliminate RN positions and rely more on UAPs. According to one report, "Many nurses see bits and pieces of their practice being handed over to unlicensed assistive personnel (UAPs)" (New York State Nurses Association, 1996b, p. 5). Ironically, in New York State, UAPs could not be legally challenged for illegally practicing nursing because the state education department could take action only against *licensed* professionals. In the meantime, dozens of job descriptions for unlicensed hospital workers "clearly violated the nurse's scope of practice and represented a real threat to patients" (New York State Nurses Association, 1996e, p. 1). NYSNA officer Karen Ballard said that hiring unlicensed workers "would turn out to be more, not less, costly . . . and would hasten the historical cycle of oversupply and undersupply in the RN workforce" (New York State Nurses Association, 1996a, p. 8). It was only unionized nurses with strong contracts and supportive nursing administrations who were not telling horror stories. Indeed, the Institute of Medicine (IOM) noted that there was a lack of uniformity in training and testing UAPs, whose rapidly expanding responsibilities included functions they could not perform safely and reliably (New York State Nurses Association, 1996c). In the absence of an external licensing process, only hospitals were left to set and maintain training standards for UAPs. As the IOM report asserted, the shifts in how hospitals do business were causing notable disruptions among nursing staffs. Ironically, the efforts to save money were happening at the same time that a few hospitals, such as Mount Sinai in Toronto, were laying off LPNs and using only RNs *without incurring higher costs* than comparable Canadian hospitals that had replaced RNs with lower-paid workers. Nevertheless, in Ontario, 5,000 RNs had lost their jobs and 15,000 more were also expected to do so (New York State Nurses Association, 1997).

Peculiarly, the IOM report found a 15.7 percent increase from 1988 to 1994 in the number of RNs employed in the United States (New York State Nurses Association, 1996c). This trend was clearly being offset in the late 1990s. Certainly, the experience of nurses at Mt. Sinai Medical Center in New York reflects this later trend. In 1996 this hospital considered replacing up to 40 percent of the RN staff with UAPs (New York State Nurses Association, 1996d). The nurses placed ads in seven newspapers, including the *New York Times,* explaining the dangers to patients. The response was overwhelmingly in favor of the 1,600 RNs, who also staged a hospital-wide work-to-rule that excluded "pitching in" and overtime. After elective surgeries were canceled and the costs to the hospital became clear, the hospital agreed to a contract that limited RN replacements.

In July 1996, nurses at Columbia-Presbyterian Hospital in New York called a one-day strike to oppose management's right to replace any and all RNs with UAPs (New York State Nurses Association, 1996k). The hospital responded by refusing to allow most RNs to return to work for three days. Management also wanted to eliminate flextime and to increase "floating" nurses outside their clinical areas without adequate orientation; thus, for example, dialysis nurses could be "floated" to recovery rooms, and from there to cardiac care or oncology without regard to clinical competencies. On these and other issues, the hospital refused to negotiate; instead, it threatened a lawsuit against NYSNA, the bargaining agent, and hired a national strike-busting agency to supply new nurses who would cross the picket lines. At other institutions RNs were also demonstrating publicly against replacing nurses with UAPs. Job descriptions, for example, at Albany Medical Center, New York, clearly violated nurses' scope of practice and represented a real threat to patients (New York State Nurses Association, 1996e). After going to the media, NYSNA forced the medical center to stop UAPs from performing several functions: "insertion of nasogastric tubes and urinary catheters, changing of sterile dressings, care of tracheostomies, and performing arterial punctures" (p. 1).

These confrontations were only a few of many over several years. Indeed,

NYSNA had fought since 1990 for legislation to stop UAPs from working illegally in New York. Finally in 1996, both houses in the New York state legislature passed legislation that gave the state authority to pursue sanctions against persons who practice nursing illegally (New York State Nurses Association, 1996l). Still, in an unexpected move, Republican governor George Pataki vetoed the bill in October 1996, claiming the bill's provisions were counter to the "well-established policies" of his administration (New York State Nurses Association, 1996m).

Downsizing, Speed-Up, Cost-Saving: Dangerous for Patients and Nurses

Obviously, nurses had good reason to be distressed about the increased use of UAPs. Indeed, the *American Journal of Nursing* released a survey in June 1996 of some 5,000 nurses from all geographic areas that found almost nine out of ten nurses polled expressed serious concerns that cost-saving practices were diminishing the safety and quality of patient care. As Sara Foer and Anita Bauman (1996) noted, more than two-thirds of the RNs had seen an increase in the number of patients assigned to them, and three-quarters said patient acuity had increased. More than half observed a marked decrease in length of stay and an increase in the number of unexpected readmissions. More than 60 percent reported reductions in the numbers of RN staff. Dr. Judith Shindul-Rothschild, RN, who conducted the survey, said all the factors led to a "speed-up" trend, with nurses "expected to work harder and faster with fewer resources, providing care for greater numbers of sicker patients in the same amount of time" (Foer and Bauman, 1996, p. 19). Almost 75 percent of the nurses reported "less time to teach patients and families, comfort and talk to patients, document nursing care and consult with the health care team" (p. 19). Patient complaints had increased, said more than 50 percent of those polled, and patient complications, medication errors, nosocomial infections, skin breakdown, and injuries to patients had also increased, according to two out of five nurses. The most damning finding was that 37 percent "would not recommend that a family member receive care in their hospitals" (p. 19). Almost 15 percent rated the quality of care as poor or very poor, and only 10 percent as excellent.

Consumers, as well as nurses, are very concerned about the effects of downsizing and cost-saving strategies. A recent Harris Poll commissioned by Sigma Theta Tau International and Nurseweek Publishing Inc. (1999) revealed that more than half of the approximately one thousand Americans polled believe that the quality of health care is seriously affected by the worsening shortage of skilled registered nurses. In addition, 92 percent of the public responding said they trust health-care information provided by nurses as much as physicians. Indeed, a recent Gallup Organization survey of 1,028 adults has found, for the second year in a row, that Americans believe that the nursing profession has the highest standards of honesty and ethics of all professions surveyed. Physicians ranked third, after veterinarians (*American Journal of Nursing*, 2001).

Hospital downsizing and nursing "speed-up" are dangerous not only to patients, but to nurses as well. A study by the Minnesota Nurses Association found a positive relationship between hospital downsizing and the incidence of workplace injury and illnesses among RNs (Canavan, 1996c). Analysis of employers' documents, required by the federal Occupational Safety and Health Act (OSHA), by nurse Elizabeth Shogren proved there was a 61.8 percent increase in RN injuries (from 569 to 921) between 1990 and 1992. Adding in the 1994 data, the increase was 65.2 percent. During the same four-year period, the total number of RN positions fell 10.22 percent. At the same time, the nurses were providing 20 percent more hours of direct RN care. The ANA used the research data in testimony before the National Institute for Occupational Safety and Health, which subsequently placed the issue on the agenda to guide subsequent research (Wilburn, 1996). However, the research may be too little, too late. States with the largest decrease in employed RNs are those with the highest managed-care infiltrations and those with the largest numbers of for-profit hospitals—both rapidly expanding trends (Williams, 1996). Countering these trends was the unification of nurses with other groups in the Consumer Coalition for Quality Health Care, backing legislation to ensure patient safety, which would at the least make public the number of RNs providing direct care, the number of unlicensed workers providing direct care, the average number of patients per registered nurse, patient mortality rates, incidence of adverse patient-care incidents, and methods used to determine and adjust staffing levels and patients' needs (Ketter, 1996c).

Profit-Making Managed Care and the Erosion of Nursing Principles

At the core of nurses' and patients' concerns was the "disconnect" between the original concept and the current practice of managed care: "To advocate a system that runs more cost-effectively by emphasizing primary and preventive services, eliminating waste and providing a true continuity of care is not the same as accepting a system that emphasizes cost savings (and profit-making) at the expense of needed services and care" (Keepnews and Stanley, 1996, p. 5). The nursing principles enunciated before the 1994 collapse of comprehensive federal health reform espoused the original concept, not the current practice, which many nurses could not defend. Indeed, as Dr. Mary Ann Thompson, RN, said, "It is not clear to me who the managed care nurse *IS* serving: is it the company, the patient or both? How does the managed care nurse ethically integrate the professional standard of patient advocacy with the employer's primary goal of cost containment?" (Thompson, 1996, p. 5).

Ironically, a similar problem confronted sensitive physicians, but from a position of relative power. For example, Dr. Linda Peeno (1998) switched to medical administration in 1987, but after functioning as a HMO executive, she left the industry in frustration. Beginning with enthusiasm and convinced she could balance economics and quality care, Peeno found "the pressure was always there to deny as much care as possible to cut costs—even if that meant pushing physicians toward some practices that endangered patients" (Peeno, 1998, pp. 150–151). She continued: "I'd begun to feel we were part of some psychology experiment designed to see how quickly we would abandon our humanity" (p. 151). Unlike nurses, she was removed from patients, "distanced from their pain and anxiety" no longer looking them in the eye, hearing their complaints, and examining them for a myriad of subtleties. Dr. Peeno was accused of expecting the company to pay for the "creative comforts" of some of her patients: "I hate what I have come to be. I am sick of being the good company doctor" (p. 152). At least one man and maybe other patients could have died as a result of her denials of payment for treatments; however, she did not know how many there were since "Managed-care plans don't track the outcomes of their denials" (p. 152).

The AMA "Seal of Approval" as MD Incomes Rise

Instead of dealing directly with managed-care systems that had lost the principles espoused by conscientious nurses and physicians, the AMA announced in 1997 that it would create a seal of approval for physicians who met certain quality standards (Associated Press, 1997a). Supposedly an antidote to consumers' worries about physicians cutting corners to reduce costs, the AMA plan could hardly deal with quality, because, unlike nurses, they had little data on how to define, let alone measure, quality outcomes, particularly for the elderly and the chronically ill. The data collected on physicians would not go to consumers, but would be *sold* to interested health plans! Nor would the public even get to see whether a physician tried and failed to get accredited. Nor would standards of measuring clinical performance, patient care, and satisfaction be in place for several years. Nor were there any plans to withhold accreditation from physicians based on poor performance or results. The AMA standards were minimal: they involved, for example, meeting perfunctory standards such as state and specialist certification and adhering to specified office procedures, not achieving actual clinical performance and patient outcomes. Obviously, consumers would not have access to a history of malpractice litigation, disciplinary action by state regulators, drug violations, charges of sexual harassment or other sexist treatment of women, or violations against children. The move to accreditation would simply provide the organization with more monopolistic power, to obtain even more control over their own constituency and provide another facade for consumers based on the latter's continuing ignorance.

The power of the medical monopoly was more than evident in physicians' continued rise in income, which, despite managed care, reached $200,000 a year on average in 1996 (*Salt Lake Tribune*, 1998). This represented an increase of about 10 percent from 1994 and of 50 percent from 1987, covering the period of rapid expansion of HMOs and for-profit hospitals. These results were obtained from random telephone interviews with 4,000 physicians nationwide. Some physicians were complaining of working longer hours for less money under managed care and "being crushed" under the proliferation of HMO rules and regulations. Indeed, by the end of the 1990s, the AMA voted to endorse the creation of a national union, Physicians for Responsible Negotiations (PRN), for those MDs employed by HMOs to give the profession more leverage with managed-care organizations (Associated Press, 1999). Furthermore, a large portion of the AMA's $18 million lobbying budget was to be set aside to pressure Congress to change antitrust laws that currently bar self-employed physicians from joining a union. Of the 684,000 physicians in the nation, only about 110,000 are currently not self-employed and thus eligible for union membership (*The American Nurse*, 1999). The status of 96,000 residents as employees or students was already an issue before the NLRB, which ruled recently that doctors-in-training at Boston Medical Center are employees, who have the same rights as other workers. This has reversed a twenty-three-year-old ruling that claimed interns and residents were students.

Despite their complaints and actions, physicians, unlike nurses, were not suffering the loss of employment and income, the "speed-up" with more and sicker patients over an eight-hour period of constant contact, and the struggle with hospital administrators over patient safety and working conditions. Indeed, a number of physicians were selling their practices for lump sums to physician practice management companies, new organizations that now "manage" between 5 percent and 10 percent of the nation's physicians and in 1997 constituted a $13.5 billion industry, up from $6.4 billion in 1995 (Chandler, 1997). Physicians pay an annual fee to these companies for providing office support, handling administrative details, maintaining computer equipment, and offering cut-rate office and medical supplies. In addition to initial cash payments and annual incomes, physicians also often get company stock and productivity incentives, making their status as employees somewhat ambiguous, particularly since share prices of these companies rose substantially from 1995 to 1997.

Not only were many physicians doing quite well with managed care, 1,025 medical schools and centers were to receive over a five-year period hundreds of millions of dollars *not* to train physicians in order to reduce the number of people entering medicine, thus eliminating their growing surplus (Goldstein,

1997). Previously, medicine had underwritten residency-training programs, some $7 billion a year paid for by the taxpayers. Indeed, every residency produced an average subsidy of $100,000 a year. Obviously, physicians had worked to blunt any negative effects of managed care and downsizing on physicians' education.

Nursing Schools: Fewer Training Sites and Less Money

As managed care and downsized hospitals were driving health care beyond the hospital, nursing was suffering the problem of finding training sites, particularly for advanced practice nurses. Federal estimates suggested 100,000 primary-care providers were needed; thus, more advanced nurses should be trained. However, from a survey by Lewin-VHI, Inc. (American Association of Colleges of Nursing, 1997), it was clear that the nursing schools were already at full capacity and some had cut admissions because of the limited training sites available and the insufficient number of faculty. Medical students, who were urged to consider primary care, were now going to sites they would have avoided in the past, but ones that had commonly been part of nurses' training for decades. Many HMOs no longer hired nurse practitioners presumably because of productivity concerns, claiming the NPs spent too much time with patients. Many preceptors no longer took on nurse practitioners because of these productivity concerns, and some companies would not allow preceptor arrangements at all. The move to employ UAPs reduced the number of RNs and, thus, reduced the number of students allowed per shift since appropriate RN/student ratios could not be guaranteed. As Dan Mezibov of the AACN said, "[O]f all the roadblocks cited by deans, one of the largest remains financial ... practitioners have refused to take students ... because of reimbursement issues" (AACN, 1997, March, p. 4). Many agencies and practitioners were now requiring monetary payment for student placements, rather than the more traditional remitted-tuition system of payment. Nursing organizations were lobbying Congress to redirect Medicare dollars from hospital diploma schools to support training for advanced practice nurses, who were seeing more opportunities, but still facing varying reimbursement laws and negative lobbying by physician organizations that left the nurses "struggling to operate at a level of autonomy for which they've been prepared" (Canavan, 1996d, p. 24). The most negative effect is to become "managed care puppets," seeing patients every ten or fifteen minutes, practicing a medical model and losing the nursing focus. In 1993, 40 percent of the firms provided Medigap coverage, but by 1997, this had dropped to 31 percent. Only 5 percent of companies with more than a thousand workers gave free care to retirees under the age of sixty-five and just 12 percent to those sixty-five and over (Lewis, 1998).

A Patchwork "System": Errors, Waste, Abuse, and Fraud

In the meantime, the health-care "system" continued to be a patchwork mess. In 1995 a survey by Louis Harris and Associates found that 55 percent of the respondents (1,081 Americans) had not heard of managed-care plans and did not understand the term, and about 33 percent were unfamiliar with HMOs (Associated Press, 1996b). This was in spite of the fact that more than half of all Americans with health-care coverage were now in HMOs. Stephen Isaacs, author of the study, also found that respondents in HMOs complained of more unmet medical needs, even though they saw physicians more. Of those not in HMOs, 37 percent had unmet medical needs because they could not afford the cost. This compared to 26 percent in HMOs.

Even with Medicare, health care was costly. People sixty-five and older spend 19 percent of their income (almost $1 of every $5) on health care, *excluding* home-care and nursing-home-care costs. In a study sponsored by the American Association of Retired Persons (Findlay, 1998), HMO enrollees paid a third less than those in traditional, fee-for-service Medicare. But even the HMO seniors were not protected, as previously predicted, since they spent an average of $1,775 every year, compared to $2,454 for non-HMO seniors. The poor (income up to $7,755 for individuals) paid 35 percent of their annual incomes on health care; the near poor (up to $9,693), 23 percent; the middle income (up to $31,020), 17 percent, and upper income, 10 percent. Unreimbursed drug costs were a major drain on Medicare recipients, leading President Clinton to urge coverage of prescription drugs; Republicans created a task force to study the problem, while Democrats tried to force a vote on the issue. According to the AARP, 39 million Medicare-qualifying Americans do not have prescription plans, and about a quarter of these spend more than $500 a month for drugs. In the meantime, Medicare benefits are being tightened, causing severe funding problems for nursing homes; about 10 percent are claiming bankruptcy in 2000. Clearly, the elderly poor were hardest hit from all directions, and staffing shortages exacerbated the problems. At the same time, more companies were terminating the health coverage of their retirees or requiring them to pay a larger share of the costs. A survey by William M. Mercer, Inc., of nearly 4,000 firms with 500 or more employees showed a steady decline in health benefits.

In 1997 a Senate investigation reported a staggering loss of $24 billion in Medicare claims because of errors, waste, abuse, and fraud (McLeod, 1998b). The audit found rapid increases in illegal billing, especially in home health care; however, $4.1 billion involved hospital bills and $5.9 billion involved *physicians'* bills. By 1998 a well-intentioned effort by the federal Health Care Financing Administration (HCFA) to get rid of fraud and abuse had threatened thousands of elderly homebound patients. HCFA now requires home-health-care agencies to put up surety bonds of 15 percent of their annual Medicare business, but the 8,000 owners of independent businesses cannot find underwriters to take on the risk because the government can recover *all* past overpayments, which would result in unlimited liability for insurers (Knight Ridder News Service, 1998). The American Hospital Association (AHA) accused the Justice Department of unfair treatment and harassment and lobbied to exempt hospitals from major parts of the False Claims Act, particularly the 1986 amendments, and to raise the standard of proof, making it more difficult for the government to win judgments. The U.S. inspector general's office in 1997 recovered between $500 million and $600 million from health-care fraud. Consumer groups wanted no change in the existing laws. Why, they asked, should there be a special exemption for the health-care industry? By the end of the decade, the General Accounting Office said Medicare officials had overlooked their own rules and procedures and had negotiated deals to settle the debts of three of the largest Medicare overpayment cases of the past decade. Providers had been overpaid $332.4 million by Medicare, but the cases were settled for only $120 million, or 36 cents on each dollar.

Ironically, the Public Citizen Health Research Group in 1997 claimed that illegal "patient dumping" (rejecting Medicare patients and/or restricting services to them) by hospitals and home-care agencies had reached alarming proportions, particularly of patients requiring intensive and costly home-health care. The abandonment of patients has been reported from many states and involves a variety of conditions, such as multiple sclerosis, diabetes, rheumatoid arthritis, osteoporosis, and colon cancer (Associated Press, 1997b; McLeod, 1998a). HMOs are also under federal scrutiny for fraudulent practices. Columbia/HCA, the nation's largest for-profit hospital chain, has been accused of overcharging Medicare, Medicaid, and other government health programs. By 1997 key executives were indicted and charged with overbilling of at least $1.8 million. In 1998 further indictments were added (Associated Press, 1998). Recent analysis of Medicare data shows that more than 730,000 elderly and disabled Medicare beneficiaries have been dropped by their HMOs, who have quit Medicare or reduced coverage areas. Indeed, it was projected that by January 2000, 325,000 more Medicare enrollees in twenty-nine states would be dropped by their HMO providers and forced to seek alternative coverage (Gannett News Service, 1999).

The failure of the Clintons' health-care reform plan has imposed piecemeal and insufficient reform on both the government and consumers. By 1997 Republicans were accusing Clinton of surreptitious efforts to reform health care step by step. The Republicans were aligned with a campaign to block federal standards for health-care quality, led by the Health Insurance Association of America and the National Federal of Independent Business, part of the lobby against the Clinton plan earlier in the decade (*Salt Lake Tribune*, 1997). Now they wanted to avoid regulations and audits that might cut into profits.

The Clinton advisory committee recommended a bill of rights for patients—legislation that would guarantee a choice of health plans, access to specialists, coverage of necessary drugs, information on physicians' experience, the right to appeal clinical and payment decisions, prohibition of gag clauses that prevent discussing *all* care options, protection of the privacy of health data, and freedom for patients to sue health plans. Though several Patient's Bill of Rights proposals and bills had been introduced in Congress over the past years by both Republicans and Democrats, none had been accepted by both the Senate and the House. The ANA and APHA supported a *full* Patient's Bill of Rights, reflected in S.R. 1890 and H.R. 3605, unlike the Republican leadership's watered-down bills, H.R. 4250 and S.R. 2330 (Helmlinger, 1998). Indeed, as ANA president Beverly Malone stated: "The proposals offered by Republican leaders are not credible alternatives. . . . The ANA will be steadfast in its support for genuine, comprehensive reform" (Reed, 1998, p. 17).

By 1997, many states had passed new managed-care reform laws or were trying to extend insurance coverage to low-income children. Obviously, something had to be done. More than 45 million Americans lacked health insurance—even more than in 1992 when health care was considered in crisis. In 1998 Republicans came up with a weak reform bill that would have done little to mend the fractured "system" itself (Gannett News Service, 1998). In 1999 a Republican bill that passed the Senate (S.R. 1344) fell short of many consumer protections. President Clinton promised to veto the bill because it was weak, unenforceable, and an empty promise that applied to only those 48 million Americans who have employer-based self-funded health insurance. The Democratic version would have applied to all 161 million Americans in private insurance managed-care plans (American Public Health Association, 1999). In the meantime, the Health Care Financing Administration issued six fundamental standards that hospitals must meet to participate in Medicare/Medicaid programs. These, at least, provide a minimum set of rights for hospital patients.

At the end of 1997, Massachusetts nurses and physicians, in a reenactment of the Boston Tea Party, joined together in boarding a ship in Boston harbor and dumping the cargo overboard (American Public Health Association, 1998a). The crates contained the annual reports of the major for-profit health-care firms in the United States. Members of the Ad Hoc Committee to Defend Health Care pitched overboard crates labeled Corporate Greed, Bonuses for Denying Care, and No Care for the Uninsured. The protest was timed to coincide with the publication of "For Our Patients, Not for Profits: A Call to Action" in the December 3, 1997, issue of the *Journal of the American Medical Association.* Signed by 2,300 Massachusetts nurses and physicians, and subsequently endorsed by 700 more, it protested "being prodded by threats and bribes to abdicate allegiance to patients, and to shun the sickest, who may be unprofitable . . . [while] the ranks of the uninsured continue to grow . . . [and]

public hospitals and clinics shrink and public health programs erode" (American Public Health Association, 1998a, p. 7).

International Health Rankings Down: Medically Caused Injuries and Deaths Up

There was good reason for concern. American per capita health expenses ranked third highest in the world, but the other rankings *dropped* in almost *every* health category in the 1990s. In 1986 there were twelve nations with lower infant death rates than the United States; now there are twenty-eight. The maternal death rate ranking slipped from fifteenth to sixteenth, women's life expectancy from ninth to fifteenth, and men's from nineteenth to twenty-second. Adding to these grim statistics is the lack of quality control in American hospitals which results in at least 1 million injuries and 120,000 deaths each year. Dr. David Lawrence, CEO of Kaiser Permanente, estimates that the numbers are actually much higher—up to 500,000 deaths each year (reported on C-Span, "Town Hall Meeting on America's Health Care System, 1999," December 11). Seldom are the results of "suboptimal" treatments (to use the medical profession's term) reported. At one major teaching center, the Medical College of Pennsylvania Hospital (MCPH), records show that hundreds of patients have been seriously injured in the last decade, and at least 66 died after medical mistakes. Of 598 incidents reported in the last decade, *none* of the physicians involved were disciplined and often patients and their families were not told that the injuries were caused by medical errors (Gerlin, 1999a). The only reason the records became public is that bankruptcy proceedings forced the new owner to file a detailed report. According to Harvard professor Lucian Leape's research (Leape, Brennan, Laird, Lawthers, Localio, Barnes, Hebert, Newhouse, Weiler, and Hiatt, 1991), the estimated 120,000 annual deaths caused by hospital injuries in the United States is *three times* the 43,000 that die in car crashes each year. In New York State, Leape and his colleagues found that one of every 200 patients admitted to a hospital during 1991 died because of a hospital error.

The medical monopoly has succeeded in making such statistics confidential even under state statutes. Internal audits of physician performance, reviews of physician success and failure rates, and morbidity and mortality rates cannot be used in some malpractice trials! The carefully guarded "honor system" of "self-policing" is not working. Clearly, the medical culture is seriously flawed. Even some medical professors, such as Robert Brook of the University of California, admit that the system is out of control.

The *Philadelphia Inquirer,* after learning of the mistakes at the MCPH, sought similar information from thirty-four other large hospitals, but only twenty-five responded, and *none* would provide any insurance information (Gerlin, 1999a). The cover-up was obvious in a 1991 *JAMA* article which reported that 54 percent of medical residents discussed their mistakes with attending MDs, but only 24 percent of these told patients or families about the errors (Gerlin, 1999b). Consumers cannot easily obtain internal reviews of physicians' competence because these are "privileged" and unavailable to patients or the public.

At the present time, there is no comprehensive effort to minimize errors; this will not happen until physicians admit that self-policing is not working and that their monopoly over nurses is self-defeating. Although the Joint Commission on Accreditation of Healthcare Organizations visits and surveys the 5,000 participating hospitals every three years, the hospitals are not required to open their incident files or inform the visiting committee of medical errors. Indeed, since 1995, the commission has received fewer than 500 error reports from the 5,000 hospitals (Gerlin, 1999c).

There is no central system to track medical errors, which are costing the nation about $9 billion a year, according to a November 1999 report issued by the Institute of Medicine, an arm of the National Academy of Sciences. The IOM's recommendations include mandatory reporting of serious errors and creation of the new National Patient Safety Center. Although the IOM report called for a National Patient Safety Center, there is little recognition in the report that empowered nurses, as noted earlier in this chapter, actually *reduce* mortality rates in their hospitals. Following the publication of the report, President Clinton immediately ordered federal agencies to take actions to reduce medical errors, ranging from preventing pharmacists from dispensing the wrong drugs to encouraging hospitals to investigate errors. Any health insurance plan covering federal employees would be required to have plans to reduce medical errors by the year 2001. This would affect more than 300 private plans and 9 million people. In addition, Senator Edward Kennedy has introduced a bill to carry out the IOM's recommendations. Although AMA representatives claim there is no evidence that mandatory reporting reduces errors, some states have such laws; for example, in New York State, since 1985 mandatory information has been required on *all* heart bypass patients, and the death rate for this type of surgery has dropped 30 percent since 1989.

Clearly incremental reform had not created a systemwide solution, and health care was less, not more accessible, and less, not more safe. Rhoda H. Karpatkin (1999), president of the Consumers Union, said that although Consumers Union's original 1992 proposal of a single-payer system had not been adopted, there were still other options: Medicare could be expanded or states could create reform models to expand coverage for all. Or the Federal Employees Benefits Program could be opened to all who wanted to join. At the same time, the individual health insurance market could be overhauled and target subsidies provided to make premiums more affordable. According to Karpatkin, the current reforms had only created health-care insecurity as coverage costs, reimbursements, medical staffs, and HMOs kept changing. Consumers still needed a health-care system that ensured quality care regardless of age, income, job, or health conditions; a system that was run efficiently without excessive administrative costs and paperwork; a system that is accountable, with fair and speedy resolution of complaints; a system that provides freedom of choice of providers and fair-share financing based on savings from cost-containment so that the sickest and poorest do not pay a disproportionate share of their earnings for health care. Karpatkin concluded that "fixing a dysfunctional system is a tough job, but our elected representatives must not be let off the hook" (p. 7).

They were clearly off the hook for the uninsured, who were, by the beginning of the twenty-first century, still more likely to be female, young (18–24), less educated, foreign-born, of Hispanic origin, or working part-time. By 1999 the public was more concerned about the lack of health insurance than at any time since 1992. In a bipartisan poll, about 7 out of 10 Americans said that they would pay higher taxes to ensure health insurance for everyone. According to the U.S. Census Bureau, one million more people lacked health insurance in 1998 than did in 1997—seven million more than in 1993 when President Clinton proposed a national health-care system. About 29 percent of the respondents of the bipartisan poll said they had been uninsured at some time in the last three years, and 43 percent said they knew of others who were uninsured during that period. Few of the uninsured were "deadbeats"; 85 percent were in low-wage jobs in small businesses. Almost half of poor, full-time workers were uninsured in 1998. Many of these were women, retrained to go off welfare, who had entered the workforce. Indeed, in 1998, the number of women with no health insurance rose by 947,000, bringing the total to 21.3 million, while the number of uninsured men declined by 116,000 to 23 million. The number of uninsured children also rose: 11.1 million under age 18 were uninsured in 1998, up 330,000 from 1997. In poor families, one out of every four children, or 3.4 million, were uninsured.

At the same time, total health-care spending rose 5.6 percent in 1998, compared to 4.7 percent in 1997, the biggest increase since the 8.7 percent jump in 1993. Government spending dropped 4.1 percent. In 1998 health care cost $4,094 per person, for a national total of $1.1 trillion. In 1998 prescription drugs rose 15.4 percent to $90.6 billion. Employers were seeing insurance premium increases as much as 10 percent for large companies and 15 percent for smaller ones. These costs impact the nearly two out of three workers who buy health insurance on the job. Premiums are outstripping the average annual salary raise of 3.8 percent and the general inflation rate of 2.8 percent. HMOs are also caught up in higher costs; half of the nation's 576 HMOs lost money in 1998, and the total loss for all HMOs was $490 million. With nearly 85 percent of working Americans enrolled in such plans, they and their employers would, by 2000, find that their plans were not providing the expected cost reductions. However, in 1999, many HMO profits increased because they raised their rates and left unprofitable markets, leaving thousands of patients unprotected.

Some physicians are now refusing to accept reimbursement from HMOs or Medicare or insurance companies, saying that repayments to them are minimal and often delayed for months. Thus, patients must pay for some physicians' services in cash and then submit their own bills to the agencies for reimbursement, accepting whatever is paid to them. Obviously, a two-tier health-care system will develop if this trend continues. Another strategy used by physicians is to file class-action suits, as the AMA did in New York against the United Healthcare Corporation for reducing payments to MDs by using invalid data to determine rates and then forcing patients to pay the difference. In February 2000, in Georgia, the AMA sued Aetna, Inc., for failing to pay physicians promptly. These actions simply do nothing to change the fundamental problems. Obviously, the health-care "system" is a chaotic mess. Nothing has taken the place of the Clintons' proposal for a universal health-care solution, and the market solution is disastrous. Markets control costs and answer to shareholders, not to patients. Indeed, in early 2001, the IOM issued a second report of 320 pages that essentially states that America's health-care system is broken. The report calls for a vast improvement in the way that physicians, nurses, and other professionals communicate with each other, and a great need for training them for teamwork.

A Health-Care System Simply Does Not Exist

Although politicians and the public heard reports and complaints from physicians and consumers, they seldom heard those of nurses. The poor international health rankings of the United States and the large numbers of medically caused deaths and injuries are not helped by the minimal training levels of unlicensed assistive personnel, who in 41 percent of hospitals had less than 40 hours of training; in 58 percent they had 41 to 120 hours; in less than 1 percent did they have 201 to 280 hours; and none had more than 281 hours. Julia Rossi, RN, asked, "What kind of administrator would say that cutting back on registered nurses better meets the needs of patients? I'll tell you the kind: The Administrator who hasn't a clue of what patient care is all about. Someone who breaks nursing care into little tasks and says, 'Anybody can be trained to do that!'" (Rossi, 1997, p. 1).

As Rossi noted, an article in the February 20, 1997, issue of *Hospitals and Health Networks* reported on the AHA series of thirty-one focus groups of consumers and their consensus was that a health-care "system" simply does not exist. Blocking access to care and reducing quality of care while increasing profits does not constitute a "system." The only positive experience reported were with skilled nurses. Speaking of her own experience, Rossi said:

> I not only treat the problems at hand, but I also guard against the problems lurking around the corner. I will watch for early signs of a blood reaction, of

infection, of overwhelming grief and loss. Yes, I may empty a urine container, but I have also suspected hepatitis because I looked at that urine, matched it with other signs and symptoms and alerted the physician that the patient needed to have liver enzymes checked. . . . I have watched people suffer in ways I cannot describe and I, myself, have suffered ways I cannot share. . . . I've cried for the patients and, more recently, I've cried over the distressingly poor care I've witnessed. (p. 2)

A nurse anesthetist, Kelly DeFeo (1997), shared Rossi's observations. To her the only thing now certain in health care was that money talks and hospitals want the cheapest bottom line. This was amply clear when her husband recently had surgery on his hip. DeFeo warned: "[N]o one should go into the hospital without a guardian person to watch over them. I work at the hospital where he had surgery, but he still was not safe" (p. 1). Managed care had created a health-care machine focused on costs, not care. The pharmacy was late with critical antibiotics because of a new cheaper and slower service. There were only three RNs for twenty-one surgical patients, which translated into no more than one hour for each patient during eight hours. Bleeding at the surgical site, requiring four units of blood, could have been avoided had the nurses had time for a proper evaluation. Bedsores developed, again because of insufficient time to turn the patient frequently. DeFeo said corporate downsizing may sound good, but losing one nurse on a unit can make a serious difference in care. While visiting her husband, DeFeo answered phones for other patients. She could not stand by when the elderly man next door could not reach his phone. She cut up food and opened drinks, because when she walked past patients' rooms, she heard them call out for help. Again she advised everyone to not go to a hospital without a guardian person. In the meantime, hospital CEOs get big bonuses for cutting costs, which they achieve by eliminating nurses, social workers, and pastoral care. DeFeo concludes, "I know that this system should not be allowed to continue" (p. 3).

Currently, DeFeo is fighting to gain hospital privileges at McKay-Dee Hospital in Ogden, Utah, to practice as a certified registered nurse anesthetist (CRNA) so that she can provide services to children needing anesthesia services at the hospital's school-based clinic. Though DeFeo is credentialed to work at other area hospitals with no direct supervision required, McKay-Dee medical anesthesiologists have refused her practicing privileges because she is "not known" to them and their policy requires direct supervision, which is not possible at the school clinic. DeFeo blames this refusal on "a cadre of anesthesiologists who feel threatened by the skills of certified registered nurse anesthetists. . . . They won't let me come on board, yet none of them have volunteered" (Kapos, 1998, p. B1). She claims, "The medical profession has been at odds over the growing number of nurse practitioners providing care that has typically come from doctors" (p. B1). Unfortunately, it is the children at the school-based clinic who are suffering from the restrictions placed on DeFeo's practice.

Despite these damning critiques, closures, downsizing, and mergers continue. In 1996 the Bureau of Labor Statistics projected an average annual increase in RN jobs of only 1.4 percent from 1994 through 2005. Hospital nurses were expected to decline from 63.8 percent of all employed RNs in the United States to 57.4 percent. There would be a 127 percent increase in RN home-health jobs, or an average annual increase of 11.6 percent. This represents a change from 5.95 percent of all RN jobs to 10.8 percent (American Nurses Association, 1997). A similar rise is occurring in nursing home positions. The 1996 National Sample Survey of Registered Nurses found a *very* rapid shift: in 1992, 66.5 percent (1,232,717) of RNs were employed in hospitals, but by 1996 only 60 percent (1,270,870) out of the 2,115,815 employed RNs in the nation were working in hospitals. *In only four years, there had been a 6 percent drop* (Keepnews, 1998).

Nurses Working on Community-Based Care

To cope with this movement from hospitals to nursing homes, the Kellogg Foundation—which had since the early 1930s consistently provided support for nursing (Lynaugh, 1995) and strongly influenced the development of the profession—focused in the 1990s on community-based, affordable health care and on grassroots reforms, as it had in the 1930s. Accordingly, with the Community Partnership Initiative, seven institutions in Georgia, Hawaii, Massachusetts, Michigan, Texas, and West Virginia were funded to increase the number of primary-care practitioners committed to community-based health care. Stressing multidisciplinary team work, the reforms are also oriented toward giving nurses a direct role in health-care delivery.

Under the federal Health Services Act, public-supported grants have been made to a variety of programs, for example, the Pennsylvania-based Resources for Human Development, an agency devoted to serving disadvantaged people in Philadelphia, where a primary health-care center in an urban housing project is staffed and managed by nurse practitioners, receiving direct third-party payment and contracting for physicians' services (McCarty, 1992). According to nurse Donna Torrisi, the center's director, the nurses plan to do as much in the community as in the center itself.

Nursing centers that originated in the 1970s (see chapter 9) were usually associated with university nursing programs, and these have continued into the 1990s. For example, under Dean Linda K. Amos, the University of Utah College of Nursing faculty established a family health-care center in Salt Lake City in 1985. In 1994 the center advertised nurse midwives as "specialists in the normal" and claimed that "10,000 Babies Can't Be Wrong!"; it provides care for women where they would feel "confident and secure," and "tender, compassionate care" for their most precious assets, their children.

Family nurse practitioners treat the total health of the whole family and promise "comfortable, convenient" scheduling coordinated for all its members, who are seen at the same time. Nurse therapists are available as personal confidants, dealing with sensitive issues with *no* taboo subjects (College of Nursing, University of Utah, 1995). Indeed, the *Salt Lake Tribune* reported on the facility as part of a national trend to control costs. Amos emphasizes that care is offered with no more than a fifteen-minute wait (Siegal, 1994). Uncomplicated vaginal deliveries, said center director Marcia Scoville, cost $1,000— compared to $2,500 to $4,000 for a hospital delivery, depending on whether a nurse midwife or a physician is involved. In addition to deliveries, the center provides pre- and postnatal care; immunizations and other pediatric care; physical examinations and a wide variety of lab tests; treatment for common illnesses; birth control services; and education for weight-control, stopping smoking, stress-reduction, nutrition, and exercise counseling, as well as for depression, abuse, addiction, and other problems. These services are available on a sliding fee scale and are covered by most insurance plans.

How have physicians responded? "Amos said some doctors are skeptical of a health-care facility run entirely by nurses, but 'it's mostly just grumbling'" (Siegal, 1994, p. B1). Obstetrician Richard Chapa said that the new physicians were grumbling because they wanted more business. Nevertheless, the university nurses have extended into rural areas as well, for example, in Wendover, Utah, a small town of 6,500 beyond the Bonneville Salt Flats and the Great Salt Lake. There on the Utah-Nevada border, four nurse practitioners began the newest clinic, which now draws forty to sixty patients a day (Baggaley and Klein, 1995). The nurses deal with all kinds of problems, from delivering a premature, twenty-week-old baby, to caring for patients in cardiac arrest and even one with a gunshot wound to the head. A physician is available for consultation and is at the clinic one day each week.

Another program, Health of the Public (HOP), has sought to construct a new model of health care that emphasizes community-based professional collaboration. Angela McBride, dean of the Indiana University School of Nursing, says that, despite the presence of the largest nursing school in the country, her institution is still dominated by a hospital-based, disease-treatment approach. The HOP program, led by nurses, is changing this. Funded by the Pew Charitable Trusts and by the Robert Wood Johnson Foundation in collaboration with the Rockefeller Foundation, the HOP program is designed to redirect academic health centers toward strategies to address major systemwide deficiencies and involves more than thirty-three academic health centers in the United States and Canada. McBride said she sees more understanding of the importance of community-based health care from other professionals, and, she adds, "I also see the style of collaboration changing. . . . The old model had the physician as captain of the team. Now, the community is the center of attention and the disciplines are responding together to its needs rather than acting from their own mandates" (Health of the Public, 1995, p. 1).

Certainly, the old model must change to incorporate the approximately 34,000 PAs and 66,000 NPs that were available by 1998. Unfortunately, turf protection, espoused by the AMA, does not bode well for the needed changes in health care. Nevertheless, in 1999, the number of graduating nurse practitioners rose by 15.8 percent from the previous year. In fall 1998, more than half (60.8 percent) of master's degree students in nursing schools were in NP tracks, compared to 40.2 percent in 1994. Of 358 institutions, 312 (87 percent) offered master's degree NP programs. To incorporate these highly educated nurses requires a drastic change in the medical monopoly.

Are "Tears and Rage" Sufficient? Political Action Needed

Probably the most important move nurses can make to attack the sick system of health care and break the medical monopoly pertains to direct political action. There are now seventy-one nurses serving as state legislators. Marilyn Goldwater, RN, said that she has done more for nursing in her fourteen years in the Maryland state legislature than she could have done in direct nursing practice (Canavan, 1996b). One of her major accomplishments was legislation in 1978 to reimburse advanced practice nurses without physician supervision or referral. Joan Barry, RN, winner of a legislative seat in Missouri, is focused on the negative changes in hospitals and on job security of nurses.

Anything nurses, and especially advanced practice nurses, can do to raise their visibility to the public and lay out the dimensions of their unnecessary subordination, is critical. The media still almost completely ignore nurses, making them invisible (Mann, 1998). The late Nancy Woodhull's 1997 study on "Nursing and the Media" (cited in Mann, 1998, p. 38) examined health care and nursing coverage in seven newspapers, four general-interest magazines, one business magazine, and five health industry publications. Health coverage constituted 10 percent of all articles. But in 142 articles published in news magazines, nurses were mentioned only *three* times. The health-care industry publications used nurses as references only 1 percent of the time.

Given these data, what can nurses do to be heard? Unfortunately, too many feel "Tears and Rage" over "The Nursing Crisis in America," as the title of Jane Schweitzer's book expressed it (1997). Expressing the anger and grief over the radical upheaval in health care and the transition to concern for profits, not patients, Schweitzer diagnosed a countrywide "morale crisis" among nurses, who are "miserable" and at times "desperate." Unfortunately, having a "gripe-fest" and attacking other nurses and nursing organizations, rather than taking on administrators and the medical monopoly are, as in the past, insufficient and inadequate. Indeed, Schweitzer's worthy recommendation that individuals change to enhance their self-esteem cannot succeed unless the sick "system" of health care is *directly* attacked. Being "angry as hell" and uniting to express their anger certainly would make nurses more visible, but their analysis and action must target systemwide changes. These cannot be achieved without greater autonomy, and this cannot be obtained without cracking the medical monopoly. It really is time to use "tears and rage" to get the autonomy needed to become visible and to use that visibility in direct political action on behalf of people to prevent illness, sustain health, and provide the kind of compassionate and competent care for the sick that nurses want to give. These goals cannot be achieved if nurses' every action depends on prior approval of physicians. Nor can decent care be given in for-profit "factories" that predetermine the value of nurses according to the costs of their care without recognition of nursing values and principles. It is time to transmute tears and rage into constructive action.

Nursing and the Medical Monopoly in the Twenty-First Century

We have laid out some of the historical roots of the current conflicts between organized nursing and medicine. Obviously, much more research in the earlier periods is necessary. Equally obvious is the need for nursing to confront the medical monopoly directly. If nurses can do this successfully, they can reorient the fragmented and disease-oriented system toward community-based preventive health care and provide the primary-care services needed to sustain health for *all* the people. This cannot be achieved with the monopolistic perspective of medicine precisely because of the limitations in the medical view of health.

We have seen a number of models developing in specific locations across the nation, even as organized medicine works to place greater restraints and influence more constrictive legislation in all the states. The medical monopoly is still largely intact, and the twenty-first century will continue to see interprofessional conflicts between the still largely gendered professional groups. The extent to which nurses can achieve greater autonomy is still highly dependent on the extent to which women maintain a liberated sense of self and continue to seek equality. If, as in some previous decades, the gender matrix of sex roles becomes more conservative, nurses, still predominantly female, will find it extremely difficult to sustain, let alone increase, their independence from predominantly male physicians. Only time will tell whether the women healers of the past will live in their sisters of the future.

The twenty-first century will bring major changes in health care. The Human Genome Project promises to map all human genes, providing a very different approach to diagnosis and treatment. The continued advance in computerized technology has already heavily impacted all aspects of health care and will continue to substantially alter the work of health-care providers.

Coupled with these changes, the invention of lasers, as well as other new procedures in surgery, and other technological processes to see into the human body will have far-reaching consequences. However, none of these changes reduces the need for compassionate and intelligent care of sick human beings. And none reduces the demand for the prevention and primary care that nurses can provide.

Given these and many other expected changes in the twenty-first century, can we afford to lumber along with an outmoded, gender-derived "system" that fosters a predominantly male-dominated profession at the expense of the full usage of nurses and the members of other female-dominated professions? We think not. The overlap of functions is too great; the antiquated system of order giving too time-consuming and bureaucratic in its consequences; the intrusive control too confining to allow immediate and needed caregiving activities; the control of nationwide health care too limited to those with money and too often denied to those without adequate funds to pay for care. We can no longer afford the medical monopoly. It is too costly for patients and too restrictive of the full expression of the predominantly female nurses' intelligence and capabilities.

This fact is particularly obvious when it is applied to the international scene. It is a truism that we live in a global village. And it is a fact that the United States is a critical resource in the world. Although this could and will probably change in the next century, the proliferation of the American model of health care to other countries of the world, more particularly the developing ones, does not bode well for the world's rapidly growing population. Indeed, what American nurses' model of care demands—autonomy, an emphasis on compassionate care and on community-based prevention and primary care—is what the world's poorest people require. And this is a model that cannot be achieved if the medical monopoly is transported to other countries. No one denies the valuable achievements in research from the basic sciences that have been applied to medical care. But these must be placed in a more holistic context—one that honors the work of women healers and nurses in their communities. Such honor cannot be extended to women who are subordinated to men, or to nurses, male or female, who are restricted in the full expression of their intellects and capacities to provide the kind of care they know is needed.

We have come full circle in this volume to repeat once again: The medical monopoly is a gender-based relic from previous decades and centuries. It is no longer appropriate to carry it into the twenty-first century. It is time for nurses and other health professionals to be heard and for organized medicine to realize that excessive medical control is no longer appropriate. Both professions need to think globally and create a new vision for the twenty-first century and the new millennium.

REFERENCES

AARP. (1998, September). Finding health insurance. *AARP Bulletin, 39* (8), 6.

Abdullah, F. (1972). Evolution of nursing as a profession. *International Nursing Review, 19* (3), 219–235.

Abel-Smith, B. (1960). *A history of the nursing profession.* London: Heinemann.

Aber, C. S., and Hawkins, J. W. (1992, Winter). Portrayal of nurses in advertisements in medical and nursing journals. *Image: Journal of Nursing Scholarship, 24* (4), 289–293.

Achterberg, J. (1991). *Woman as healer.* Boston: Shambhala.

Adams, E. K. (1921). *Women professional workers.* New York: Macmillan.

Adamson, T. E. (1971). Critical issues in the use of physician associates and assistants. *American Journal of Public Health, 61* (9), 1765–1779.

Agboola, A. (1994, October/November). To the editor: NYSNA must challenge court ruling. *NYSNA Report, 25* (9), 14.

Aiken, L. H. (Ed.) (1982). *Nursing in the 1980s.* Philadelphia: J. B. Lippincott Co.

Aiken, L. H., E. T. Lake, S. Semaan, H. P. Lehman, P. A. O'Hare, C. S. Cole, D. Dunbar, and I. Frank. (1993, Fall). Nurse practitioner managed care for persons with HIV infection. *Image: Journal of Nursing Scholarship, 25* (3), 172–177

Alfano, G. I., K. Kowalski, L. R. Levin, and G. B. McFadden (1976, Fall). Prerequisite for nurse-physician collaboration: Nursing autonomy. *Nursing Administration Quarterly, 1,* 45–63.

Allen, D. (1986). Nursing and oppression: "The family" in nursing texts. *Feminist Teacher, 2* (1), 14–20.

Allport, F. (1909). The graduate nurse versus the patient of moderate means. *Chicago Medical Report, 31,* 404.

American Association of Colleges of Nursing. (1997, March). As schools produce for primary care, training sites grow slim. *AACN Issue Bulletin,* 1–4.

———. (1998, May/June). Advanced practice multi-state recognition. *Syllabus, 24* (3), 2, 6.

American Journal of Nursing. (1908, February). Progress and reaction [Editorial comment]. *8* (5), 333–336.

———. (1910). The medical attitude [Editorial comment]. *10,* 1000–1001.

———. (1970, April). AMA unveils surprise plans to convert RN into medic. *70* (4), 691, 724, 727.

———. (1978, August). Nurse practitioners fight move to restrict their practice. *78* (8), 1285, 1308, 1310.

———. (1981, April). Nurse practitioner privileges attacked in Oregon. *81* (4), 653.

———. (1998, February). ANA lobbying team named in top 100. *98* (2), 16.

———. (2000a, March). Study shows NP care is comparable to physician care. *100* (3), 21.

———. (2000b, November). Nursing organizations unite. *100* (11), 23.

———. (2001, February). NewsCaps. *101* (2), 20.

American Medical Association. (1972, May 29). Extending the scope of nursing practice: A report of the secretary's committee to study extended roles for nurses. *Journal of the American Medical Association, 220* (9), 1231–1236.

———. (1985). Resolution: To combat legislation authorizing medical acts by unlicensed individuals. Chicago: American Medical Association.

———. (1990a, June 24–28). Board of trustees, independent nursing practice models. *Proceedings of the American Medical Association,* 192.

———. (1990b). *Proceedings of the House of Delegates.* 139th annual meeting, June 24–28. Board of Trustees #LL. *Independent nursing practice models. Proceedings of the American Medical Association,* 141–152.

———. (1995, December 18). Medicine's milestone year. *American Medical News,* 1.

American Medical Association, Committee on Nursing. (1970, September 14). Medicine and nursing in the 1970s: A position statement. *Journal of the American Medical Association* 213 (11), 1881–1883.

American Medical Association, Council on Health Manpower and Council on Medical Education. (1972, June). A report on education and utilization of allied health manpower. Adopted by the AMA House of Delegates, June 1972.

American Medical News. (1970, February 9). AMA urges major new role for nurses.

American Nurse. (1988, July/August). Nursing opposes RCTs: AMA proposal short-sighted, says ANA. *20* (7), 2.

———. (1993a, February). ANA Board acts on advanced practice issues. *25* (2), 22.

———. (1993b, February). Georgia RNs fight law. *25* (2), 24.

———. (1993c, June). ANA asks Congress to end medical monopoly of health care system. *25* (6), 36.

———. (1993d, July/August). Final rule published on DEA numbers for mid-level practitioners. 25 (7), 22.

———. (1993e, October). National nursing summit unites organizations and targets key issues for health care reform. *25* (9), 8.

———. (1994a, September). Hospital profits soar. *26* (8), 30.

———. (1994b, September). Study: Nursing tied to lower mortality rates. *26* (8).

———. (1994c, October/November). Whatever happened to health care reform? *26* (9), 7.

———. (1994d, November/December). ANA and SNAs testify on risks of decreasing skill mix. *26* (10), 11, 14.

———. (1995, January/February). Study finds NPs still face barriers. *27* (1), 7.

———. (1996, March). IOM issues nurse staffing report. *28* (2), 8, 23.

———. (1998a, September/October). ANA continues talks with NCSBN on interstate compact. *30* (5), 3.

———. (1998b, September/October). *U.S. News and World Report* covers NPs. *30* (5), 17.

———. (1998c, September/October). Surprise! More nurses, better outcomes. *30* (5), 7.

———. (1999, July/August). Docs vote for unionization. *31* (4), 6.

American Nurses' Association. (1980). *Nursing: A social policy statement.* Kansas City, Mo.: ANA.

———. (1991). *Nursing's agenda for health care reform.* Kansas City, Mo.: ANA.

———. (1993). *Nursing facts.* Washington, D.C.: ANA.

———. (1997, May). Skills for the 21st century: Preparing for the emerging workplace. *Nursing Trends and Issues, 2* (5), 1–8.

American Nurses' Association and American Medical Association. (1964, February 13–15). *Proceedings of First National Conference for Professional Nurses and Physicians.*

Williamsburg, Va.: American Nurses' Association and American Medical Association.

American Public Health Association. (1998a, January). Massachusetts health professionals protest practices of profit-oriented care systems. *The Nation's Health, 28* (1), 7.

———. (1998b, July). Study reveals excellent results of births attended by midwives. *The Nation's Health, 28* (6), 12.

———. (1999, August). Republican bill passes, falls short of APHA-backed patient protections. *The Nation's Health, 29* (7), 1, 7.

Andreoli, K. G., and E. A. Stead. (1967, July). Training physician's assistants at Duke. *American Journal of Nursing, 67,* 1442–1443,

Ashley, J. A. (1976). *Hospitals, paternalism, and the role of the nurse.* New York: Teachers College Press.

———. (1980, April). Power in structured misogyny: Implications for the politics of care. *Advances in Nursing Science, 2,* 3–22.

Associated Press. (1993, December 16). Doctors' groups support Clinton health care plan. *Syracuse Herald-Journal,* A4.

———. (1996a, August 20). Half of U.S. poor are kids. *Salt Lake Tribune,* A1, A4.

———. (1996b, November 12). Survey blasts health-insurance industry. *Salt Lake Tribune,* B12.

———. (1997a, November 19). Doctors to get AMA seal; Critics call it a bum deal. *Salt Lake Tribune,* A3.

———. (1997b, December 21). 2 Utah hospitals dispute 'patient dumping' charges. *Salt Lake Tribune,* B8.

———. (1998, February 14). Columbia/HCA: More charges coming. *Salt Lake Tribune,* B9.

———. (1999, June 24). Doctors launch volley at HMOs. *Salt Lake Tribune,* F1, F2.

Aungier, G. J. (1840). *The history and antiquities of Syon Monastery.* London: J. B. Nichols and Son.

Aveling, J. H. (1872). *English midwives: Their history and prospects.* Reprint 1967. London: Hugh K. Elliott Ltd.

Avorn, J., and S. Soumerai (1983). Improving drug-therapy decisions through educational outreach: A randomized controlled trial of academically based "detailing." *New England Journal of Medicine, 308,* 1457–1463.

Avorn, J., D. E. Everitt, and M. W. Baker (1991). The neglected medical history and therapeutic choices for abdominal pain: A nationwide study of 799 physicians and nurses. *Archives of Internal Medicine, 151,* 694–697.

Baggaley, S., and J. Klein. (1995, Spring). Wendover Clinic: An oasis in the desert. *Excellence, 14,* 4–7.

Balasco, E. M. (1995, July/August). Nursing is not just rank-ordered tasks. *American Nurse, 27* (5), 5.

Baly, M. (1986). *Florence Nightingale and the nursing legacy.* Dover, N.H.: Croom Helm.

Bandow, D. (1995, Fall). M. D. monopoly. *Policy Review,* no. 74, 89–91.

Bapna, J. (1989). Education on the concept of essential drugs and rationalized drug use. *Clinical Pharmacology and Therapeutics, 45* (3), 217–219.

Barnum, B. S. (1994, October). Realities in nursing practice: A strategic view. *Nursing and Health Care, 15* (8), 400–405.

Bates, B. (1970). Doctor and nurse: Changing roles and relations. *New England Journal of Medicine, 283* (3), 129–134.

Bates, B. (1972, Spring). Changing roles of physicians and nurses. *Washington State Journal of Nursing, 44* (2), 3–9.

Batey, M. V., and J. M. Holland. (1983, Summer). Impact of structured autonomy accorded through state regulatory policies on nurses' prescribing practices. *Image: Journal of Nursing Scholarship, 15* (3), 84–89.

———. (1985). Prescribing practices among nurse practitioners in adult and family health. *American Journal of Public Health, 75* (3), 258–261.

Bayne-Smith, M. (1996). *Race, gender and health.* Thousand Oaks, Calif.: Sage.

Beard, R. O. (1913, December 13). The trained nurse of the future. *Journal of the American Medical Association, 61* (24), 2149–2152.

Beers, M., J. Avorn, S. Soumerai, D. Everitt, D. Sherman, and S. Salem. (1988). Psychoactive medication use in intermediate-care facility residents. *Journal of the American Medical Association, 260,* 3016–3020.

Bell, K. E., and J. I. Mills (1989). Certified nurse-midwife effectiveness in the health maintenance organization obstetric team. *Obstetrics and Gynecology, 74* (1), 112–116.

Bergeson, P. S., and D. Winchell. (1977, August). A survey of Arizona physicians' attitudes regarding pediatric nurse practitioners. *Clinical Pediatrics, 16* (8), 678–681.

Bergman, A. B. (1971, May). Physician's assistants belong in the nursing profession. *American Journal of Nursing, 71* (5), 975.

Betts, V. T. (1995, July/August). A fight for our profession. *American Nurse, 27* (5), 5.

Bezjak, J. E. (1987). Physician-perceived incentives for association with nurse practitioners. *Nurse Practitioner, 12* (3), 67–74.

Bianchi, E., and R. Reuther. (1976). *From machismo to mutuality: Woman-man liberation.* New York: Paulist Press.

Bigbee, J. L., S. Lundin, J. Corbett, and J. Collins. (1984, February). Prescriptive authority for nurse practitioners: A comparative study of professional attitudes. *American Journal of Public Health, 74* (2), 162–163.

Billings, F. (1924, March 23). Remarks. *Journal of the American Medical Association, 82,* 967.

Blake, S. J. (1886). Medical women: A thesis and a history. London: Hamilton, Adams and Co.

Bok, S. (1979). *Lying: Moral choice in public and private life.* New York: Vintage Books.

Boston Globe. (1993). Clinton dangles antitrust immunity for doctors. *Syracuse Herald-Journal,* November 1, A8E.

Boston Medical and Surgical Journal. (1889, October 24). Editorial. The reciprocal relations of the nurse and the physician. *121* (17), 417–418.

———. (1903, July 2). Editorial. Preliminary training of nurses. *149* (1), 23.

———. (1903, July 30). Editorial. Nursing as a profession. *149* (1), 133.

Breay, M. (1897, June 19). Nursing in the Victorian Era. *Nursing Record and Hospital World,* 493–502.

Brent, K. A. (April, 1949). Are nurses getting too much education? *Hospital Management, 67,* 68–70.

British Medical Journal. (1897, June 19). The nursing of the sick under Queen Victoria, *1,* 1644–1648.

Brook, R., K. Williams, and A. Avery. (1976). Quality assurance today and tomorrow: Forecast for the future. *Annals of Internal Medicine, 85,* 809–817.

Brooke, E. (1993). *Women healers through history: Portraits of herbalists, physicians, and midwives.* London: The Women's Press Ltd.

Brown, L. (1948). *Nursing for the future.* New York: Russell Sage Foundation.

Brown, S. A., and D. E. Grimes (1992). A meta-analysis of the process of care, clinical outcomes, and cost-effectiveness of nurses in primary care roles: Nurse practitioners and certified nurse-midwives. Washington, D.C.: American Nurses' Association.

Brumgardt, J. R. (Ed.). (1980). *Civil War nurse: The diary and letters of Hannah Ropes.* Knoxville: University of Tennessee Press.

Buerhaus, P. I. (1994, January). Managed competition and critical issues facing nurses. *Nursing and Health Care, 15* (1), 22–26.

Bullough, B. (1975). Barriers to the nurse practitioner movement: Problems of women in a woman's field. *International Journal of Health Services, 5* (2), 225–233.

———. (1976, September). Influences on role expansion. *American Journal of Nursing, 76* (9), 1476–1481.

———. (1986). The state nurse practice acts. In *Nurses, nurse practitioners: The evolution of primary care,* ed. M. D. Mezey and D. O. McGivern, 350–367. Boston: Little, Brown and Co.

Bullough, V. L. (1983, Fall). Nurses and women physicians: The case of Ida May Wilson. *Bulletin, American Association for the History of Nursing,* (3), 4.

———. (1985, Winter). Elizabeth Kenny. *Bulletin, American Association for the History of Nursing,* (7), 4.

Bullough, V. L., and B. Bullough. (1978). *The care of the sick: The emergence of modern nursing.* New York: Prodist.

———. (1984). *History, trends, and politics of nursing.* Norwalk, Conn.: Appleton-Century-Crofts.

Burl, J. B., A. Bonner, and M. Rao. (1994, December). Demonstration of the cost-effectiveness of a nurse practitioner/physician team in long-term care facilities. *HMO Practice, 8* (4), 157–161.

Butler, P. E. (1978, August). Self-assertion key to new roles. *Association of Operating Room Nurses Journal, 28* (2), 215–218.

Butter, I. H. (1989, March/April). Women's participation in health-care delivery: Recent changes and prospects. *Health Values, 13* (2), 40–44.

Butter, I., E. Carpenter, B. Kay, and R. Simmons. (1985). *Sex and status: Hierarchies in the health work force.* APHA Public Health Policy Series. Ann Arbor: University of Michigan, School of Public Health.

Buys, D. (1977). Nurse-practitioners—are they a threat to doctors? *Modern Medicine, 45* (8), 50–54.

Cabot, R. (1901, November 21). Suggestions for the improvement of training schools for nurses. *Boston Medical and Surgical Journal, 960,* 21, 567–569.

Campbell, J. (1981). Misogyny and homicide of women. *Advances in Nursing Science, 3* (2), 67–85.

Campbell, M. A. (1974). *Why should a girl go into medicine?* Old Westbury, N.Y.: The Feminist Press.

Canavan, K. (1996a, March). ANA asserts attacks on practice threaten patient safety. *American Nurse, 28* (2), 1, 9.

———. (1996b, April/May). Nurse ranks grow in legislative bodies nationwide. *American Nurse, 28* (3), 13.

———. (1996c, October). Minnesota study supports link between hospital downsizing and workplace injury/illness. *American Nurse, 28* (7), 15.

———. (1996d, October). Specialty fields practice differences spawned by managed care. *American Nurse, 28* (7), 24.

———. (1996e, October). Nursing addresses troubling trends in managed care. *American Nurse, 28* (7), 1, 9.

Canham, J. (1982, September 29). Time to speak our minds. *Nursing Mirror, 155* (13), 50–51.

Caraher, M. T. (1988, April). The importance of third-party reimbursement for NPs. *Nurse Practitioner, 13* (4), 50, 52, 54.

Cargill, V. A. (1986/87, Winter). Nurses as colleagues, not servants: A win-win proposition for everyone. *Health Matrix, 4* (4), 33–35.

Carson, W. (1993a, January). Nurses and professional boundaries: Legal barriers to practice. *American Nurse, 25* (1), 26.

———. (1993b, February). Nursing and professional boundaries: Legal barriers to practice. *American Nurse, 25* (2), 24.

———. (1993c, June). Gains and challenges in prescriptive authority. *American Nurse, 25* (6), 19–20.

Cassetta, R. A. (1993, June). Opening doors for advanced practice opportunities. *American Nurse, 25* (6), 18–19.

Catlin, A. J., and M. McAuliffe. (1999, Second Quarter). Proliferation of non-physician providers as reported in the *Journal of the American Medical Association* (*JAMA*), 1998. *Image: Journal of Nursing Scholarship, 31* (2), 175–177.

Celentano, D. D. (1982). The optimum utilization and appropriate responsibilities of allied health professionals. *Social Science and Medicine, 16* (6), 687–698.

Chaffee, K., C. Kingstedt, J. Reiss, B. Baron, K. Brady, E. Lee, H. P. Kyung, I. Stuart, and B. Bullough. (1974). *A study of the doctor-nurse game.* Unpublished manuscript.

Chandler, M. (1997, December 30). Doctors giving up practices, headaches. *Salt Lake Tribune,* D11. (Reprinted from the *Miami Herald.*)

Chaney, J. A., and P. Folk. (1993). A profession in caricature: Changing attitudes toward nursing in the *American Medical News,* 1960–1989, *Nursing History Review, 1,* 181–202.

Chapman, C. M. (1977, November/December). Image of the nurse. *International Nursing Review, 24* (6), 164–167, 170.

Chaucer, G. (1957). The merchants tale. In *The complete works of Geoffrey Chaucer,* ed. F. N. Robinson, 1133. Boston: Houghton Mifflin Co.

Chinn, P. L., and Wheeler, C. E. (1985). Feminism and nursing. *Nursing Outlook, 33* (2), 74–77.

Clark, A. (1919). *Working life of women in the seventeenth century.* London: George Routledge and Sons.

Cohen, N. W., and L. J. Estner (1983). *The silent knife: Cesarean prevention and vaginal birth after cesarean.* South Hadley, Mass.: Bergin and Garvey Publishers.

Cohn, S. (1984). Prescriptive authority for nurses. *Medical and Health Care, 12,* 72–73.

Cohn, S. D. (1989). Professional liability insurance and nurse-midwifery practice. In *Medical professional liability and the delivery of obstetrical care,* ed. V. P. Rostow and R. J. Bulger, 104–112. Washington, D.C.: National Academy Press.

College of Nursing, University of Utah. (1995). *Birthcare/Healthcare.* Clinic brochure.

Congressional Budget Office. (1979). *Physician extenders: Their current and future role in medical care delivery* (Background Paper #1005-A). Washington, D.C.: Government Printing Office.

Conley, F. (1991, June 2). Associated Press. *San Francisco Chronicle.*

Connell, M.-T. (1983, October). Feminine consciousness and the nature of nursing practice: A historical perspective. *Topics in Clinical Nursing, 5* (3), 1–10.

Connelly, S. V., P. A. Connelly. (1979). Physicians' patient referrals to a nurse practitioner in a primary care medical clinic. *American Journal of Public Health* 69 (1), 73–75.

Consumers Union. (1992a, July). Health care in crisis, part 1: Health care dollars. *Consumer Reports, 57* (7), 435–443.

———. (1992b, August). Health care in crisis, part 2: Are HMOs the answer? *Consumer Reports, 57* (8), 519–523.

———. (1992c, September). Health care in crisis, part 3: The search for solutions. *Consumer Reports, 57* (9), 579–592.

Cooper, R. A. (1995, November). Perspectives on the physician workforce to the year 2020. *Journal of the American Medical Association, 274* (19), 1534–1543.

Cooper, R. A., T. Henderson, and C. L. Dietrich (1998). Roles of nonphysician clinicians as autonomous providers of patient care. *Journal of the American Medical Association, 280* (9), 795–802.

Cooper, R. A., P. Laud, and C. L. Dietrich. (1998). Current and projected workforce of nonphysician clinicians. *Journal of the American Medical Association, 280* (9), 788–794.

Cope, Z. (1958). *Florence Nightingale and the doctors.* London: Museum Press.

Corea, G. (1985). *The hidden malpractice: How American medicine mistreats women.* New York: Harper and Row.

Cornu-Quinn, C. (1994, July/August). Supreme Court decision penalizes independent judgment. *American Nurse, 26* (7), 5, 28.

Cowan, B. (1977). *Women's health care.* Ann Arbor, Mich.: Anshen.

Culpepper, M. M., and P. G. Adams. (1988, July). Nursing in the Civil War. *American Journal of Nursing, 88* (7), 981–984.

Dachelet, C. Z. (1978, Winter). Nursing's bid for increased status. *Nursing Forum, 17* (1), 18–45.

Daly, M. (1968). *The church and the second sex.* 1st ed. New York: Harper and Row.

Daly, M. (1978). *Gyn/ecology: The metaethics of radical feminism.* Boston: Beacon Press.

Daniels, D. (1976). *Lillian D. Wald: The progressive woman and feminism.* Unpublished doctoral dissertation, City University of New York.

Dannett, S. G. L. (Ed.). (1959). *Noble women of the North.* New York: Thomas Yoseloff.

D'Antonio, P.O. (1993). The legacy of domesticity: Nursing in early nineteenth-century America. *Nursing History Review, 1,* 229–246.

Darbyshire, P. (1987, January 28). The burden of history. *Nursing Times, 83* (4), 32–34.

Davies, C. (1976, July). Experience of dependency and control in work: The case of nurses. *Journal of Advanced Nursing, 1* (4), 273–282.

Davies, C. (Ed.). (1980). *Rewriting nursing history.* Totowa, N.J.: Croom Helm.

Davis, L. (1971, March). Physician's assistant: A threat or a challenge? *Association of Operating Room Nurses Journal, 13* (3), 53–54.

Davis, S. W., D. L. Best, G. Marion, and G. H. Wall. (1984, August). Sex stereotypes in the self- and ideal descriptions of physician's assistant students. *Journal of Medical Education, 59* (8), 678–680.

De Angelis, C. D. (2000, February). Women in academic medicine: New insights, same sad news. *New England Journal of Medicine, 342* (6), 426–427.

DeFeo, K. (1997, April 30). You'd better bring your own nurse. Salt Lake City, Utah: *Citizens,* West edition, 1, 3.

DeFleur, M. (1964). Occupational roles as portrayed on television. *Public Opinion Quarterly, 25,* 54–74.

Denny, F. P. (1903, June 11). The need of an institution for the education of nurses independent of the hospitals. *Boston Medical and Surgical Journal, 148* (25).

———. (1910, May 5). The need of instruction and experience in nursing as part of medical education. *Boston Medical and Surgical Journal, 162* (18), 596–598.

de Normandie, R. L. (n.d., c. 1927). Standards of prenatal care. U.S. Children's Bureau *Bulletin,* no. 157, 17.

de Tornyay, R. (1971, May). Expanding the nurse's role does not make her a physician's assistant. *American Journal of Nursing, 71* (5), 974, 976.

deVries, C., and M. Vanderbilt (1994, November/December). Nurses gain ground during reform debate. *American Nurse, 26* (10), 2–3.

Diers, D. (1992). Diagnosis-related groups and the measurement of nursing. In *Charting nursing's future: Agenda for the 1990s,* ed. L. Aiken and C. Fagin, 139–156. Philadelphia: J. B. Lippincott Co.

Diers, D., and S. Molde. (1979). Some conceptual and methodological issues in nurse practitioner research. *Research in Nursing and Health, 2,* 73–84.

Dobrzynski, J. H. (1995, September 21). Women say they still face bias on the job. New York Times News Service. *Syracuse Herald-Journal,* D3.

Dock, L. L. (1890). *Text-book of materia medica for nurses.* 1st ed. (8th ed., 1926). New York: G. P. Putnam.

———. (1903). Hospital organization. *National Hospital Record, 6,* 10–14.

———. (1903, March). Hospital organization. *American Journal of Nursing, 3,* 413–421.

———. (1906, June 16). Our foreign letter: From the United States. *British Journal of Nursing, 36,* 486–487.

———. (1907, August). Some urgent social claims. *American Journal of Nursing, 7,* 895–905.

———. (1909a, February 28). Letter to Dr. Baldy, New York Public Library, Wald Mss.

———. (1909b, May). The relation of the nursing profession to the woman movement. *Nurses' Journal of the Pacific Coast, 5,* 197–201.

———. (1929, August). Nurses' debt to the feminist movement. *Equal Rights,* 221.

———. (1949). The relationship of training schools to hospitals. In *Nursing of the sick, 1893,* ed. I. Hampton, 83. New York: McGraw-Hill.

Dock, L. L. (Ed.). (1900). *Short papers on nursing subjects.* New York: M. Louise Longeway Publisher.

Dock, S. E. (1917, February). The relation of the nurse to the doctor and the doctor to the nurse. *American Journal of Nursing, 17,* 394–396.

Doering, L. (1992). Power and knowledge in nursing: A feminist poststructuralist view. *Advances in Nursing Science, 14* (4), 24–33.

Dolan, A. K. (1980, Winter). Antitrust law and physician dominance of other health practitioners. *Journal of Health Politics, Policy and Law, 4* (4), 675–691.

Dolan, J. A. (1958). *Goodnow's history of nursing.* 10th ed. (11th ed., 1963). Philadelphia: W. B. Saunders Co.

———. (1973). *Nursing in society: A historical perspective.* 13th ed. (14th ed., 1978). Philadelphia: W. B. Saunders Co.

Dolan, J. A. (Ed.). (1968). *History of nursing.* 12th ed. Philadelphia: W. B. Saunders Co.

Donnelly, G., A. Mengel, and E. King. (1975, November). The anatomy of a conflict. *Supervisor Nurse, 6* (11), 28–33, 36–38.

Donnison, J. (1977). *Midwives and medical men.* London: Heinemann.

Dorland, W. A. (1908). The sphere of the trained nurse. Address given at the Philadelphia School of Nursing, May 27, 1908.

Doyal, L. (1995). *What makes women sick: Gender and the political economy of health.* New Brunswick, N.J.: Rutgers University Press.

Doyle, A. (1929, July). Nursing by religious in the United States, part I, 1809–1840. *American Journal of Nursing, 29* (7), 775–785.

Dusky, L. (1997). *Still unequal: The shameful truth about women and justice in America.* New York: Crown.

Duttera, M. J., and W. R. Harlan. (1978, February). Evaluation of physicians assistants in rural primary care. *Archives of Internal Medicine, 138* (2), 224–228.

Edmunds, M. W. (1978, Spring). Evaluation of nurse practitioner effectiveness: An overview of the literature. *Evaluation and the Health Professions, 1* (1), 69–82.

———. (1979, November/December). Conflict. *Nurse Practitioner, 4* (6), 42, 47–48.

———. (1981). Nurse practitioner—physician competition. *Nurse Practitioner, 6* (2), 47, 49–51, 53–54.

———. (1991, May). Lack of evidence could exclude NPs from reimbursement-reform legislation. *Nurse Practitioner, 16* (5), 8.

Ehrenreich, B., and D. English. (1972). *Witches, midwives, and nurses: A history of women healers.* Old Westbury, N.Y.: The Feminist Press.

———. (1973). *Complaints and disorders: The sexual politics of sickness.* Old Westbury, N.Y.: The Feminist Press.

Elliott, M. D. (1978, August). Assertion opens options for OR nurses. *Association of Operating Room Nurses Journal, 28* (2), 219–226.

Emerson, J. H. (1892, July 9). Phases of nursing. *New York Medical Journal, 56.*

Etheridge, P. (1991). A nursing HMO: Carondelet St. Mary's experience. *Nursing Management, 22* (7), 22–27.

Etzioni, A. (1969). *The semi-professions and their organization: Teachers, nurses, social workers.* New York: Collier Macmillan.

———. (1980). *A sociological reader on complex organizations.* 3rd ed. New York: Holt, Rinehart and Winston.

Everett, S. (1974). Florence Nightingale. *British Historical Illustration, 1* (5), 12–25.

Everitt, D. E., J. Avorn, and M. W. Baker. (1987, October). The use of medication by physicians, nurse practitioners and older patients. Special issue. *The Gerontologist, 27,* 34a.

Ewen, J. (1981). *Canadian nurse in China.* Canada: McClelland and Stewart.

Fagin, C. M. (1983, March). Concepts for the future. Competition and substitution. *Journal of Psychiatric Nursing and Mental Health Services, 21* (3), 36–40.

———. (1990). Cost-effectiveness of nursing care revisited: 1981–1990. *American Journal of Nursing, 90* (10), 16–18.

Fagin, C., and H. Lehman. (1971, Spring). Professional nursing: The problems of women in a microcosm. *Journal of the New York State Nurses Association, 2,* 8–12.

Fahy, E. T. (1994, January). Attention, attention must be paid! *Nursing and Health Care, 15* (1), 3, 8.

Faludi, S. (1991). *Backlash: The undeclared war against American women.* New York: Crown.

Fee, E. (1983). *Women and health: The politics of sex in medicine.* Farmingdale, N.Y.: Baywood.

Feinman, C. (1992). *The criminalization of a woman's body.* Binghamton, N.Y.: The Haworth Press.

Feldman, M. J., M. Ventura, and F. Crosby. (1987, September-October). Studies of nurse practitioner effectiveness. *Nursing Research, 36* (5), 303–308.

Fennell, K. (1991, June). Prescriptive authority for nurse-midwives. *Nursing Clinics of North America, 26* (2), 511, 515.

Ferguson, E. D. (1901a, April). The evolution of the trained nurse, part 1. *American Journal of Nursing, 1* (7), 463–468.

———. (1901b, May). The evolution of the trained nurse, part 2. *American Journal of Nursing, 1* (8), 535–538, 620–626.

Ferguson, M. (1979, November). Reflections on teaching a history of nursing—2. Occasional Papers. *Nursing Times, 75* (30), 121.

Ferry, M., P. Lamy, and L. Becker. (1985, September). Physicians' knowledge of prescribing for the elderly: A study of primary care physicians in Pennsylvania. *Journal of the American Geriatrics Society, 33* (9), 616–625.

Findlay, S. (1998, March 5). Study: Care costs seniors dearly. *USA Today,* 3A.

Fine, R. (1969, March/April). Nurse-doctor relationships. *Washington State Journal of Nursing, 41,* 12–13.

Fiorino, D. (1980). *An historical study of the National Association of Pediatric Nurse Associates/Practitioners (NAPNAP), 1973–1978.* Thesis, Wright State University, Dayton, Ohio.

Fisher, S. (1986). *In the patient's best interest.* New Brunswick, N.J.: Rutgers University Press.

Flexner, E. (1970). *Century of struggle: The women's rights movement in the United States.* Cambridge: The Belknap Press of Harvard University Press.

Flores, F. (1957). The nurse: Handmaiden or partner? *Boston Medical Quarterly, 8* (2), 52–55.

Foer, S., and H. Bauman. (1996, July/August). RNs voice critical concerns about patient care. *American Nurse, 28* (5), 19.

Fondiller, S. H. (1995, January/February). "Loretta C. Ford: A modern olympian—She lit a torch." *Nursing and Health Care: Perspectives on Community, 16* (1), 6–11.

Ford, L. C. (1995, March). Nurse practitioners: Myths and misconceptions. *Journal of the New York State Nurses Association, 26* (1), 12–13.

Ford, L. C., and H. K. Silver. (1967, September). The expanded role of the nurse in child care. *Nursing Outlook, 15,* 43–45.

Fox-Grage, W. (1996). States study scope of practice and reimbursement. *Issues: A Newsletter of the National Council of State Boards of Nursing, 17* (2), 1, 4–5.

Frankfort, E. (1972). *Vaginal politics.* New York: Quadrangle.

Franklin, K. R. (1996, November/December). Patient Safety Act progresses in 1996. *American Nurse, 28* (8), 17.

Freeman, R. B. (1971, May). Practice as protest. *American Journal of Nursing, 71* (5), 918–921.

Freund, C. M., and G. A. Overstreet. (1981, March/April). The economic potential of nurse practitioners. *Nurse Practitioner, 6* (2), 28–32.

Friedan, B. (1963). *The feminine mystique.* New York: Dell Publishing Co.

Friedson, E. (1970). *Profession of medicine.* New York: Dodd, Mead and Co.

Froh, R. (1988, September/October). An interview with AMA's James Sammons: Responding to critics of the RCT proposal. *Nursing Economics, 6* (5), 221–230.

Gabel, J. B. (1978, Winter). Medical education in the 1890s: An Ohio woman's memories. *Ohio History, 87* (1), 53–66.

Gaffney, T. (1993, April). Preparing nursing for the 21st century. *American Nurse, 25* (4), 2.

Gage, M. J. (1893). *Woman, church and state. A historical account of the status of women through the Christian ages.* Chicago: Charles H. Kerr and Co.

Gairdner, J. (Ed.). (1900–1901). The Paston letters. London.

Galewitz, P. (1999, August 18). Just what the doctor would have ordered. Associated Press. *Salt Lake Tribune,* C5.

Gamarnikow, E. (1978). Sexual division of labour: The case of nursing. In *Feminism and materialism: Women and modes of production,* ed. A. Kuhn and A. Wolpe, 96–123. Boston: Routledge and Kegan Paul.

Gannett News Service. (1998, July 16). GOP unveils managed-care reform plan. *Salt Lake Tribune,* A3.

———. (1999, August 5). HMOs' break with Medicare forces 730,000 to find new coverage. *Salt Lake Tribune,* A8.

Gardner, M. S. (1916). *Public health nursing.* New York: Macmillan.

Garrard, J., R. L. Kane, D. M. Radosevich, C. L. Skay, S. Arnold, L. Kepferle, S. McDermott, and J. L. Buchanan. (1990, March). Impact of geriatric nurse practitioners on nursing-home residents' functional status, satisfaction, and discharge outcome. *Medical Care, 28* (3), 271–283.

Géraud, H. (Ed.). (1843). *Chronique latine de Guillaume de Nangis.* Vol. 2. Paris: Société de l'Histoire de France.

Gerlin, A. (1999a, September 19). Cause of death: Medical mistake. Knight Ridder. *Syracuse Herald American,* D1, D7–8.

———. (1999b, September 21). Few survivors learn of fatal errors. Knight Ridder. *Syracuse Post-Standard,* A6.

————. (1999c, September 22). Hospitals loath to report fatal errors. Knight Ridder. *Syracuse Post-Standard,* A11.

Gibson, K. W. (1977). If you've ever thought about being a nurse-practitioner: 'One nurse said we weren't fit to work in a hospital.' *R.N., 40* (5), 38–40.

Gies, J. (1993, June). Oregon NPs gain hospital privileges. *American Nurse, 25* (6), 26.

Giles, H., and J. E. Williams. (1979). Medical students' descriptions of self and ideal physician. *Social Science in Medicine,* 13A, 813–815.

Godfrey, M. A. (1978). Job satisfaction—or should that be dissatisfaction? *Nursing '78, 8* (4), 89–102.

Goldmark, J., and the Committee for the Study of Nursing Education. (1923). *Nursing and nursing education in the United States.* New York: Macmillan.

Goldstein, A. (1997, August 24). How to cure the doctor glut: $$$$$$. *Salt Lake Tribune,* A-1, A-19. (Reprinted from the *Washington Post.*)

Goldstein, H., and M. A. Horowitz. (1978). *Utilization of health personnel: A five hospital study.* Germantown, Md.: Aspen Systems Corp.

Goodnow, M. (1916). *Outlines of nursing history.* 1st ed. (2nd ed., 1919; 3rd ed., 1923; 4th ed., 1928; 5th ed., 1933; 6th ed., 1938; 7th ed., 1942; 8th ed., 1949; 9th ed., 1953). Philadelphia: W. B. Saunders Co.

Goodrich, A. W. (1950, October). To explain happiness. *American Journal of Nursing, 50* (10), 598.

Gordon, L. (1986). What's new in women's history. In *Feminist studies/critical studies,* ed. T. DeLauretis, 20–30. Bloomington: Indiana University Press.

Gould, G. M. (1889, June). Graduation speech. *Bulletin of the Johns Hopkins Hospital, 10* (99), 103–105.

Grace, Sr. (1898, January 8). Practical aspects of a nurse's life. *Hospital,* 127.

Green, M. (1989, Winter). Women's medical practice and health care in medieval Europe. *Signs: Journal of Women in Culture and Society, 14* (21), 434–473.

Greenbaum, L. S. (1980, May). Nurses and doctors in conflict: Piety and medicine in the Paris Hôtel-Dieu on the eve of the French Revolution. *Clio Medica, 13* (3/4), 247–267.

Greer, G. (1971). *The female eunuch.* New York: McGraw-Hill.

Griffith, H. M., and M. Fonteyn, M. (1989). Let's set the payment record straight. *American Journal of Nursing, 89,* 1051–1058.

Griffith, H. M., and K. R. Robinson. (1993, Fall). Current procedural terminology (CPT) coded services provided by nurse specialists. *Image: Journal of Nursing Scholarship, 25* (3), 178–186.

Grissum, M., and C. Spengler. (1976). *Womanpower and health care.* Boston: Little, Brown and Co.

Gross, W., and E. Crovitz. (1975). A comparison of medical students' attitudes towards women and women medical students. *Journal of Medical Education, 50,* 392–394.

Grumbach, K., and J. Coffman. (1998). Physicians and nonphysician clinicians: Complements or competitors. *Journal of the American Medical Association, 280* (9), 825–826.

Guy, M. E. (1986, January/February). Interdisciplinary conflict and organizational complexity. *Hospital and Health Services Administration, 31* (1), 111–114.

Guy's Hospital Reports. (1871). Ed. Fagge and Durham. Vol. 16, 3rd series, 541–555.

Hagell, E. I. (1989). Nursing knowledge, women's knowledge: A sociological perspective. *Journal of Advanced Nursing, 14,* 226–233.

Halloran, E. (1986/87, Winter). Nurse and physician relationships in acute care hospitals. *Health Matrix, 4* (4), 35–36.

Hampton, I. (1889, December). Speech given at the opening of the Nurses' Home. *Bulletin of the Johns Hopkins Hospital, 1,* 6–8.

Hampton, I. (Ed.). (1949). *Nursing of the sick, 1893.* New York: McGraw-Hill.

Harkless, G. E. (1989, August). Prescriptive authority: Debunking common assumptions. *Nurse Practitioner, 14* (8), 57–61.

Harper, D.C., and J. Johnson. (1995). Preliminary data. National Organization of Nurse Practitioner Faculties National Nurse Practitioner Database Initiative. (Supported by the Kellogg Foundation.)

Harris, J. D. (1922). *The Royal Devon and Exeter Hospital.* Exeter, England: Eland Bros.

Hawker, R. (1987). For the good of the patient? In *Nursing history: The state of the art,* ed. C. Maggs, 143–152. Wolfeboro, N.H.: Croom Helm.

Hawkings-Ambler, G. A. (1897, July 31). The etiquette of nursing. *Hospital,* 163.

Hawkins, J. W., and C. S. Aber. (1988). The content of advertisements in medical journals: Distorting the image of women. *Women and Health, 14* (2), 43–59.

Health Planning Report. (1981, June 17). AMA: Cut federal funds for advanced nurse training. 8–9.

Health of the Public. (1995, Spring). HOP nurses focus on collaboration. *Challenge: Academe and the Health of the Public, 4* (2), 1–6.

Helmlinger, C. (1998, September). Washington Watch: Act now to get key bill passed. *American Journal of Nursing, 98* (9), 16.

Henry, S. (1992, Summer). Exclusive *Revolution* interview with Susan Faludi. *Revolution, 2* (2), 39–45, 134.

Herzog, E. L. (1976). The underutilization of nurse practitioners in ambulatory care. *Nurse Practitioner, 2* (1), 26–29.

Hiestand, D. L. (1966). Research into manpower for health services. (Part 2) *Milbank Memorial Fund Quarterly, 44* 148.

Himali, U. (1995, July/August). Medicare cuts could spur further RN layoffs. *American Nurse, 27* (5), 13.

Hofling, C. K., E. Brotzman, S. Dalrymple, N. Graves, and C. M. Pierce. (1966). An experimental study in nurse-physician relationships. *Journal of Nervous and Mental Disorders, 143* (2), 171–180.

Holcombe, L. (1973). *Victorian ladies at work.* Hamden, Conn.: Archon Books, Shoestring Press.

Holmes, G. (1907, December). The doctor as the nurse knows him. *American Journal of Nursing, 8,* 181–182.

Holt, L. E. (1923). American pediatrics, a retrospect and a forecast. *Transactions,* American Pediatric Association.

Hospital. (1913, March 8). Review of Nutting and Dock, *History of Nursing,* Vol. III and IV.

Howell, M. (1977). Can we be feminist physicians? Mirages, dilemmas and traps. *Journal of Health Politics, Policy, and Law, 2,* 168–172.

Huey, F. L. (1988, November). How nurses would change U.S. health care. *American Journal of Nursing, 88* (11), 1482–1493.

Hughes, M. J. (1943). *Woman healers in medieval life and literature.* New York: Books for Libraries Press.

———. (1968). *Women healers in medieval life and literature.* New York: Books for Libraries Press.

Hurd, H. M. (1910, June). Florence Nightingale—A force in medicine. *Johns Hopkins Alumnae Magazine, 9,* 68–81.

Hurd-Mead, K. C. (1938). *A history of women in medicine from the earliest times to the beginning of the nineteenth century.* Haddam, Conn.: Haddam Press.

Hutchinson, W. (1905, December). The origins of medicine. *American Journal of Nursing, 5,* 148–157.

Illich, I. (1976). *Medical nemesis: The expropriation of health.* New York: Pantheon Books.

Ingles, T. (1976, Spring). The physicians' view of the evolving nursing profession: 1873–1913. *Nursing Forum, 15* (2), 123–164.

Inlander, C. B., L. S. Levin, and E. Weiner. (1988). *Medicine on trial.* New York: Prentice Hall.

Institute of Medicine. (1988). Brown, S. S. (Ed.). *Prenatal care: Reaching mothers, reaching infants.* Washington, D.C.: National Academy Press.

Jacobson, A. C. (1972, July). 1915—A medical view of women's lib. *Medical Times, 100* (7), 71–72.

Jacox, A. (1982). Role structuring in hospital nursing. In *Nursing in the 1980s,* ed. L. H. Aiken, 75–99. Philadelphia: J. B. Lippincott Co.

James, J. W. (Ed.). (1985). *A Lavinia Dock reader.* New York: Garland Publishing.

Jameson, A. B. (1856). *The communion of labour.* London: Longman.

Jensen, D. M. (1943). *A history of nursing.* 1st. ed. (2nd ed., 1950; 3rd ed., 1955; 4th ed., 1959; 5th ed., 1965). St. Louis: C. V. Mosby Co.

Joel, L. (1992, January). Uncharted waters of managed care. *American Nurse, 24* (1), 5.

Journal of the American Medical Association. (1901, October 12). The trained nurse and her position [Minor comments]. *37,* 982.

———. (1906). Nurses' schools and illegal practice of medicine [Minor comments]. *47* (22), 1835.

———. (1924, October). The scope of the public health nurse [Current comment]. *83* (17), 1339–1340.

———. (1927, May 21). Minutes of the seventy-eighth annual session of the A.M.A. *88,* 1642–1643.

Jurgensen, K. (Ed.). (1993, December 10). Nurses deserve a bigger role in patient care. *USA Today,* 10A.

Kahn, L., and P. Wirth. (1978). Perceptions and expectations of physician supervisors. *Nurse Practitioner, 3* (1), 27–31.

Kaiser, A. D. (1948, January). The public health nurse, the physician's ally. *Pediatrics, 1* (1), 23–27.

Kalisch, B. J., and P. A. Kalisch. (1977, January). An analysis of the sources of physician-nurse conflict. *Journal of Nursing Administration, 7* (1), 51–57.

———. (1983). An analysis of the impact of authorship on the image of the nurse presented in novels. *Research in Nursing and Health, 6,* 17–24.

———. (1984a). The Dionne Quintuplets legacy: Establishing the "good doctor and his loyal nurse" image in American culture. *Nursing and Health Care, 5* (5), 242–250.

———. (1984b). Sex-role stereotyping of nurses and physicians on prime-time television: A dichotomy of occupational portrayals. *Sex Roles, 10* (7/8), 533–553.

Kalisch, P. A., and B. J. Kalisch. (1978). *The advance of American nursing.* Boston: Little, Brown and Company.

Kampen, N. B. (1988). Before Florence Nightingale: A prehistory of nursing in painting and sculpture. In *Images of nurses: Perspectives from history, art, and literature,* ed. A. H. Jones, 6–39. Philadelphia: University of Pennsylvania Press.

Kane, R., J. Garrard, B. Skay, D. Radosevich, J. Buchanan, S. McDermott, S. Arnold, and L. Kepferle. (1989). Effects of a geriatric nurse practitioner on the process and outcome of nursing home care. *American Journal of Public Health, 79* (9), 1271–1277.

Kansas Nurse. (1972, August). Legal implications relative to orders from physician's assistants. *47* (1).

Kapos, K. (1998, July 2). Helping kids to stop hurting. *Salt Lake Tribune,* B1, B3.

Karpatkin, R. H. (1999, August). Americans need fair share health care. *Consumer Reports, 64* (8), 7.

Karpf, A. (1988a). Doctoring the media: The reporting of health and medicine. London: Routledge.

———. (1988b, May 18). Broken images. *Nursing Times, 84* (20), 16–17.

Kasper, A. S. (1995, July/August). Target . . . women and children: Welfare in the wrong direction. National Women's Health Network *Network News,* 1, 5.

Kearnes, D. (1992). A productivity tool to evaluate NP practice: Monitoring clinical time spent in reimbursable, patient-related activities. *Nurse Practitioner, 17* (6), 55–67.

Keddy, B., K. Acker, D. Hemeon, D. MacDonald, A. MacIntyre, T. Smith, and B. Vokey. (1987, December). Nurses' work world: Scientific or "womanly ministering"? *Resources for Feminist Research, 16* (4), 37–39.

Keddy, B., M. J. Gillis, P. Jacobs, H. Burton, and M. Rogers. (1986). The doctor-nurse relationship: An historical perspective. *Journal of Advanced Nursing, 11* (6), 745–753.

Keen, J., and R. Wolf. (1993, December 8). Doctors and nurses dispute boundaries of medical "domain." *USA Today,* 12A.

Keen, P. (1992, November/December). Letters to the editor: Changing the skill mix. *American Nurse, 24* (10), 5.

Keepnews, D. (1993, September). HCFA clarifies Medicare payment for advanced nursing services. *American Nurse, 25* (9), 18.

———. (1996, January/February). ANA challenges Pew Health Professions' findings. *American Nurse, 28* (1), 3.

———. (1998, May/June). The National Sample Survey of RNs: What does it tell us? *American Nurse, 30* (3), 10.

Keepnews, D., and Stanley, S. (1996, October). Managed care and nursing principles. *American Nurse, 28* (7), 5.

Keller, N. S. (1973, April). The nurse's role: Is it expanding or shrinking? *Nursing Outlook, 21* (4), 236–240.

Kelly, L. Y. (1979, February). How to start a counterculture. *Nursing Outlook, 27* (2), 149.

Kett, J. (1968). *The formation of the American medical profession: The role of institutions, 1780–1860.* New Haven, Conn.: Yale University Press.

Ketter, J. (1994a, June). Use of UAP on the rise in public health. *American Nurse, 26* (6), 18, 20.

———. (1994b, June). ANA, Department of Labor discuss workplace issues. *American Nurse, 26* (6), 1, 3.

———. (1994c, July/August). When 1 + 1 = 1: How 'merger mania' is impacting nurses across America. *American Nurse, 26* (7), 22.

———. (1994d, July/August). RNs and restructuring: An overview. *American Nurse, 26* (7), 22.

———. (1994e, July/August). Restructuring spurs debate on staffing ratios skill mix. *American Nurse, 26* (7), 26.

———. (1994f, July/August). Ruling questions NLRA protection for nurses. *American Nurse, 26* (7), 10, 13.

———. (1994g, October). Employers use Supreme Court decision against RNs; ANA devises legal, legislative strategies. *American Nurse, 26* (9), 1, 7.

———. (1994h, October). RNs strike back against unfair staffing and jeopardized patient care. *American Nurse, 26* (9), 10, 11.

———. (1996a, March). Nurses score victory in NLRB decision. *American Nurse, 28* (2), 1, 6.

———. (1996b, April/May). Providence refuses to bargain. *American Nurse, 28* (3), 6–7.

———. (1996c, July/August). Consumer Coalition for Quality Health Care launches aggressive campaign. *American Nurse, 28* (5), 8.

Kinlein, M. L. (1977). *Independent nursing with clients.* Philadelphia: J. B. Lippincott, Co.

Kjervik, D. K., and I. M. Martinson. (1979). *Women in stress.* New York: Appleton-Century-Crofts.

———. (1986). *Women in health and illness.* Philadelphia: W. B. Saunders.

Kleiman, C. (1994, February 23). Registered nurses take on AMA over range-of-care issue. *Syracuse Herald-Journal,* B11. (From *Chicago Tribune.*)

Kletke, P. R., W. D. Marder, and A. B. Silberger. (1990, March). The growing proportion of female physicians: Implications for U.S. physician supply. *American Journal of Public Health, 80* (3), 300–304.

Knight Ridder News Service. (1996, August 17). Kids without medical insurance: Unhealthy trend. *Salt Lake Tribune,* A1, A7.

———. (1998, February 21). Medicare-fraud rules put home-health care at risk. *Salt Lake Tribune,* A8.

Kölbing, E., and Day, M. (Eds.) (1932). *The siege of Jerusalem.* Early English Text Society, original series, no. 188. London: Oxford University Press.

Kollock, C. W. (1904, July 30). Nurses' training schools. Letter to the editor. *New York Medical Journal and Philadelphia Medical Journal,* 235.

Kraman, C. (1989). Women religious in health care: The early years. In *Pioneer healers: The history of women religious in American health care,* ed. U. Stepsis and D. Liptak, 15–38. New York: Crossroad.

Krantzler, N.J. (1986). Media images of physicians and nurses in the United States. *Social Science and Medicine, 22* (9), 933–952.

Kritek, P. B. (1991). Editorial. *Nursing Forum, 26* (4), 3–4.

LaBar, C. (1986, January). Filling in the blanks on prescription writing. *American Journal of Nursing, 86* (1), 30–33.

Lagemann, E. C. (Ed.). (1983). *Nursing history: New perspectives, new possibilities.* New York: Teachers College Press.

Lake, E. (1992). Medicare prospective payment and the changing health care environment. In *Charting nursing's future: Agenda for the 1990s,* ed. L. Aiken and C. Fagin, 121–138. Philadelphia: J. B. Lippincott Co.

Lambertsen, E. C. (1969, January). Knowing roles aids doctor-nurse accord. *Modern Hospital, 112* (1), 75–77.

Lancet. (1880, December 11). Editorial. 946–947.

———. (1881, June 4). Editorial. Trained nurses for the sick poor. 923.

Lanese, R. R. (1961). *Authoritarianism in nurses: Hospital-significant attitudes and nursing performance.* Columbus, Ohio: Systems Research Group, Engineering Experiment Station.

Lang, N. M. (1983, September). Nurse-managed centers: Will they thrive? *American Journal of Nursing, 83* (9), 1290–1293.

Lapius, S. K. [pseud.]. (1983, March). Physicians and midlevel practitioners: Can the conflict be resolved? *Postgraduate Medicine, 73* (3), 94–95.

LaPlante, L. J., and F. V. O'Bannon. (1987, April). NP prescribing recommendations. *Nurse Practitioner, 12* (4), 52–53, 57–58.

Larsen, R. L. (1904, July 30). Letter to the editor. Nurses' training schools. *New York Medical Journal and Philadelphia Medical Journal,* 235.

Laslett, B., S. Kohlstedt, H. Longino, and E. Hammonds, E., eds. (1996). *Gender and scientific authority.* Chicago and London: University of Chicago Press.

Lawrence, R. S., G. H. DeFriese, S. M. Putnam, C. G. Pickard, A. B. Cyr, and S. W. Whiteside (1977). Physician receptivity to nurse practitioners: A study of the correlates of the delegation of clinical responsibility. *Medical Care, 15* (4), 298–310.

Lawry, R. P. (1986/87, Winter). Nurses and physicians: An ethical prospective. *Health Matrix, 4* (4), 36–37.

Leape, L. L., T. A. Brennan, N. Laird, A. G. Lawthers, A. R. Localio, B. A. Barnes, L. Hebert, J. P. Newhouse, P. C. Weiler, and H. Hiatt. (1991, February). The nature of adverse events in hospitalized patients. Results of the Harvard Medical Practice Study, II. *New England Journal of Medicine, 324* (6), 377–384.

Leavell, H. R. (1955, January). The public health physician learns from the public health nurse. *Nursing Outlook, 3* (1), 15.

Leonard, R. C. (1966). The impact of social trends on the professionalization of patient care. In *A sociological framework for patient care,* ed. J. Folta and E. Deck, 71–82. New York: John Wiley and Sons.

Leopoldt, H. (1977, February 3). Responsibility and the doctor/nurse relationship. *Nursing Mirror, 144* (5), 59–61.

LeRoy, L. (1982). The cost effectiveness of nurse practitioners. In *Nursing in the 1980s,* ed. L. H. Aiken, 295–314. Philadelphia: J. B. Lippincott Co.

Letourneau, C. U. (1969, August). Authority in the hospital. *Hospital Management, 108* (2), 36–37.

Levine, J. I., S. T. Orr, D. W. Sheatsley, J. A. Lohr, and B. M. Brodie. (1978). The nurse practitioner: Role, physician utilization, patient acceptance. *Nursing Research, 27* (4), 245–253.

Levy, B., F. Wilkinson, and W. Marine. (1971). Reducing neonatal mortality with nurse midwives. *American Journal of Obstetrics and Gynecology, 109,* 50–57.

Levy, J. (1981, May). Physicians lack economic incentive to get along with hospital nurses. *Modern Health Care, 11* (5), 47.

Lewenson, S. B. (1993). *Taking charge: Nursing, suffrage, and feminism in America, 1873–1920.* New York: Garland Publishing.

Lewin, E. (1985). *Women, health and healing.* London: Tavistock.

Lewis, C. E., and T. K. Cheyovich. (1976, April). Who is a nurse practitioner? Processes of care and patients' and physicians' perceptions. *Medical Care, 14* (4), 365–371.

Lewis, C. E., and B. Resnick. (1967). Nurse clinics and progressive ambulatory patient care. *New England Journal of Medicine, 277,* 1236.

Lewis, J. A., and J. Bernstein. (1996). *Women's health: A relational perspective across the life cycle.* Boston: Jones and Bartlett.

Lewis, R. (1998, March). Retiree medical coverage fading away. *AARP Bulletin, 39* (3), 4.

Lipman, M. (1972, May). Challenging physicians' orders. *R.N., 35* (5), 54–55, 84–86.

Little, M. (1978). Physicians' attitudes toward employment of nurse practitioners. *Nurse Practitioner, 3* (4), 27–30.

Lopate, C. (1968). *Women in medicine.* Baltimore: Johns Hopkins University Press.

Lorber, J. (1984). *Women physicians: Career, status, and power.* New York: Tavistock Publications.

Lovell, M. C. (1980). *An historical study of the development of the medical profession as a business: Impact on nursing and society, 1896–1979.* Unpublished master's thesis, Wright State University, Dayton, Ohio.

———. (1982). Daddy's little girl: The lethal effects of paternalism in nursing. In *Socialization, sexism, and stereotyping: Women's issues in nursing,* ed. J. Muff, 210–220). St. Louis: C. V. Mosby Company.

Ludlam, G. P. (1906, April 28). The organization and control of training schools. *New York Medical Journal, 73* (16), 850–853.

———. (1908, February). The reaction in training school methods. *National Hospital Record, 11,* 4.

Lynaugh, J. (1995, June). Nursing and the W. K. Kellogg Foundation. *Nursing and Health Care, 16* (4), 174–183.

Maggs, C. (Ed.). (1987). *Nursing history: The state of the art.* Wolfeboro, N.H.: Croom Helm.

Mahoney, D. F. (1988, March). An economic analysis of the nurse practitioner role. *Nurse Practitioner, 13* (3), 44–45, 48–50, 52.

———. (1992). Nurse practitioners as prescribers: Past research trends and future study needs. *Nurse Practitioner, 17* (1), 44–51.

———. (1994, Spring). Appropriateness of geriatric prescribing decisions made by nurse practitioners and physicians. *Image: Journal of Nursing Scholarship, 26* (1), 41–46.

Mankiewicz, F., and J. Swerdlow. (1977–1978). Sex roles in TV: Co-opted liberation. *Television Quarterly, 14* (4), 5–17.

Mann, J. (1998, First Quarter). A lot of care, but little credit. *Reflections, 24* (1), 38–39. (Reprinted from the *Washington Post,* 1997.)

Manning, A. (1998, February 23). Operating with sexism. *USA Today,* 1D–2D.

Marieskind, H. I. (1980). *Women in the health delivery system: Patients, providers, and programs.* St. Louis: C. V. Mosby.

Martin, P. D., and S. A. Hutchinson. (1997, January). Negotiating symbolic space: Strategies to increase NP status and value. *Nurse Practitioner, 22* (1), 89–102.

Mauksch, H. O. (1957, January). Nursing dilemmas in the organization of patient care. *Nursing Outlook, 5* (1), 31–33.

———. (1963, March). Becoming a nurse: A selective view. *Medicine and Society.* Special issue of *The Hands of the American Academy of Political and Social Science, 346,* 88–98.

May, F. (1784). *Unterricht für Krankenwärter.* Mannheim.

McCarty, P. (1992, March). NPs will operate health care center. *American Nurse, 24* (3), 28.

McConville, B. (1983, March). Only when I laugh. *Nursing Times, 79* (12), 11–12.

McCullough, C. (1994, June). Supreme Court decision muddies RN collective bargaining rights. *NYSNA Report, 25* (5), 1.

McElmurry, B. J., N. F. Norr, and R. S. Parker. (1993). *Women's health and development: A global challenge.* Sudbury, Mass.: Jones and Bartlett Publishers.

McGrath, J. (1990). The cost-effectiveness of nurse practitioners. *Nurse Practitioner, 15* (7), 41–42.

McGuire, M. A. (1980, March). Nurse-physician interactions: Silence isn't golden. *Supervisor Nurse, 11* (3), 36–39.

McLeod, D. (1998, May). Patient "dumping" on the rise. *AARP Bulletin, 39* (5), 8–9.

———. (1998, June). Medicare anti-fraud drive hits a snag. *AARP Bulletin, 39* (6), 8–9.

Mechanic, D. (1978). *Medical sociology.* New York: Free Press.

Mechanic, D., and L. H. Aiken. (1982, September). A cooperative agenda for medicine and nursing. *New England Journal of Medicine, 307* (12), 747–750.

Medical Times and Gazette. (1852, January 10). no. 80, new series, p. 40.

———. (1860, August 16). Editors. The imbroglio at Guy's. p. 463.

Meehan, J. (1993, April). Hillary Clinton seeks nursing's input on reform. *American Nurse, 25* (4), 1–2.

———. (1993, October). Consumers willing to see a nurse for routine "doctoring." *American Nurse, 25* (9), 10.

———. (1994, January). ANA expresses disappointment over AMA opposition to APN autonomy. *American Nurse, 26* (1), 1, 3.

Mellett, H. (1986, March/April). Nurse practitioners in New York State: A case study in institutional licensure? *Nursing Outlook, 34* (2), 56–57.

Melosh, B. (1983). Doctors, patients, and "Big Nurse": Work and gender in the postwar hospital. In *Nursing history: New perspectives, new possibilities,* ed. E. C. Lagemann, 157–179. New York: Teachers College Press.

Mendelsohn, R. S. (1982). *Malepractice: How doctors manipulate women.* Chicago: Contemporary Books.

Mercer, M. (1992, January). DEA rule still pending. *American Nurse, 24* (1), 8.

———. (1992, October). DEA reconsiders regulations on prescriptive authority. *American Nurse, 24* (9), 13.

Mezey, M., M. Dougherty, P. Wade, and C. Mersmann. (1994, December). Nurse practitioners, certified nurse midwives, and nurse anesthetists: Changing care in acute care hospitals in New York City. *Journal of the New York State Nurses Association, 25* (4), 13–17.

Mill, H. T. (1851, July). Enfranchisement of women. *Westminster Review, 60,* 150–161.

Mill, J. S. (1869). *The subjection of women.* Bungay, Suffolk, England: Richard Clay, Ltd.

Minkowski, W. L. (1992, February). Women healers of the middle ages: Selected aspects of their history. *American Journal of Public Health, 82* (2), 288–295.

———. (1994). Physician motives in banning medieval traditional healers. *Women and Health, 21* (1), 83–96.

Minor, A. F. (1989). The cost of maternity care and childbirth in the United States, 1989. *Health Insurance Administration of America.*

Mitchell, C. A. (1975, November). Professional nursing practice and the hospital milieu. *Journal of the New York State Nurses Association, 6* (3), 14–16.

Mitchell, J.R.A. (1984, January 21). Is nursing any business of doctors? A simple guide to the "nursing process." *British Medical Journal, 288,* 216–219.

Mittelstadt, P. (1992a, January). New Medicare fee schedule will affect many nurses. *American Nurse, 24* (1), 2.

———. (1992b, January). Bill would increase reimbursement for advanced practice nurses. *American Nurse, 24* (1), 3.

———. (1992c, June). ANA successful in change of HCFA CNS definition. *American Nurse, 24* (6), 2.

———. (1992d, October). DOT rule reflects ANA stance on advanced practice nurses. *American Nurse, 24* (9), 24.

———. (1993, February). ANA advocates APNs for primary care. *American Nurse, 25* (2), 18.

Monteiro, L. A. (1987, March/April). Insights from the past. *Nursing Outlook, 35* (2), 65–69.

Moore, J. (1988). *A zeal for responsibility: The struggle for professional nursing in Victorian England, 1868–1883.* Athens: University of Georgia Press.

Morantz, R. M. (1977, June). Making women modern: Middle class women and health reform in 19th century America. *Journal of Social History, 10,* 490–507.

Morgan, A. P., and J. M. McCann. (1983, Summer). Nurse-physician relationships: The ongoing conflict. *Nursing Administration Quarterly, 7* (4), 1–7.

Morris, M. (1909). Editorial statement. *Southern California Practitioner, 22,* 180.

Moss, R. W. (1993, November/December). Privileging essential to APN autonomy. *American Nurse, 25* (10), 7, 21.

Muff, J. (Ed.). (1982). *Socialization, sexism, and stereotyping: Women's issues in nursing.* St. Louis: C. V. Mosby.

Muller, T. G. (1959, May). Let's talk it over. *Nursing World, 133,* 28–29.

Mundinger, M. O. (1995, September/October). Advanced practice nursing is the answer. . . . What is the question? *Nursing and Health Care, 16* (5), 254–259.

Mundinger, M. O., R. L. Kane, E. R. Lenz, A. M. Totten, W. Y. Tsai, P. D. Cleary, W. T. Friedewald, A. L. Siu, and M. L. Shelanski, M. L. (2000, January). Primary care outcomes in patients treated by nurse practitioners or physicians: A randomized trial. *Journal of the American Medical Association, 283* (1), 59–68.

Munroe, D., J. Pohl, H. H. Gardner, and R. E. Bell. (1982). Prescribing patterns of nurse practitioners. *American Journal of Nursing, 82* (10), 1538–1540.

National League for Nursing. (1991, March). *NLN Public Policy Bulletin.* New York: National League for Nursing.

National League of Women Voters. (n.d.). *Memorandum* of the Child Welfare Committee, United States Children's Bureau Files.

Nawar, M. (1999, May/June). Providence nurses win contract after long, hard-fought battle. *American Nurse, 31* (4), 6.

Nelson, K. R. (1964, February 13–15). Changing patterns of practice—Nursing and medical. In *Proceedings of First National Conference for Professional Nurses and Physicians,* ed. American Nurses Association and American Medical Association, 22–31. Williamsburg, Va.: American Nurses Association and American Medical Association.

New England Journal of Medicine. (1929, April). A committee on relationships of nurses and physicians. Editorials. *200* (15), 786.

———. (1931a, January). The doctor and the bedside nurse. Editorials. *204* (3), 115, 122.

———. (1931b, February). The doctor and his patient's nurse. Editorials. *204* (8), 394–395.

———. (1931c, March). Miscellany: Maternity cases and nursing care. Editorials. *204* (11), 571–572.

———. (1931d, May). Doctors as nursing school teachers. Editorials. *204* (20), 1074–1075.

———. (1931e, May). Excerpts from Bulletin of the Committee on the Grading of Training Schools for Nurses. Editorials. *204* (19), 980, 993.

———. (1948, July 1). Medicolegal Abstract. Hospitals—Dismissal of nurse at request of physician. *239* (1), 31.

New York State Nurses Association. (1989, May). Editorial. *NYSNA Report, 20* (4), 1.

———. (1992, July). Persistence on DEA numbers pays off. *NYSNA Report, 23* (6), 3.

———. (1993a, April). Mandatory third party reimbursement for RNs will foster patient access to primary care. *NYSNA Report, 25* (3), 8.

———. (1993b, September). NYSNA fights to maintain quality public health care. *NYSNA Report, 24* (8), 3.

———. (1993c, September). News Briefs. *NYSNA Report, 24* (8), 10.

———. (1993d, December). Ask the experts: RNs working as LPNs. *NYSNA Report, 24* (10), 3.

———. (1994a, January/February). Tough fight over home health care saves nursing positions, but not qualifications. *NYSNA Report, 25* (1), 1.

———. (1994b, May). The reimbursement maze. *NYSNA Report, 25* (4), 9.

———. (1994c, May). RNs troubled by use of unlicensed assistive personnel. *NYSNA Report, 25* (4), 1, 10.

———. (1994d, May). RNs and UAPs. *NYSNA Report, 25* (4), 10.

———. (1994e, July). Nurse practitioners under fire in Rochester. *NYSNA Report, 25* (6), 3.

———. (1994f, July). Why the Court's decision is bad news for patients. *NYSNA Report, 25* (6), 7.

———. (1994g, August). News briefs. *NYSNA Report, 25* (7), 6.

———. (1994h, August). Is every RN a supervisor? Nurses work under shadow of Supreme Court ruling. *NYSNA Report, 25* (7), 1, 5.

———. (1994i, October/November). Nurses oppose EMT push to provide primary care. *NYSNA Report, 25* (9), 10.

———. (1994j, October/November). NYSNA fights to ensure safe health care in schools. *NYSNA Report, 25* (9), 11.

———. (1994k, October/November).Whatever happened to health care reform? *NYSNA Report, 25* (9), 7.

———. (1995a, January/February). Concern for patients spurs nurses to action. *NYSNA Report, 26* (1), 1.

———. (1995b, April/May). Nurses march on Washington to protest use of unlicensed workers. *NYSNA Report, 26* (3/4), 1.

———. (1995c, June). News briefs. Nurse practitioners face barriers in many states. *NYSNA Report, 26* (5), 7.

———. (1995d, June). NYS Assembly holds hearing on crisis in RN understaffing. *NYSNA Report, 26* (5), 1.

———. (1995e, June). Mt. Vernon tries to justify replacement of RNs with unlicensed personnel. *NYSNA Report, 26* (5), 11.

———. (1995f, October/November). FTC to review nurses' complaint against RCIPA. *NYSNA Report, 26* (9), 5.

———. (1996a, January). Brooklyn forum targets RN staffing problems. *NYSNA Report, 27* (1), 8.

———. (1996b, February). The coming shakeup in professional regulation. *NYSNA Report, 27* (2), 5.

———. (1996c, February). Nurse staffing report calls for more research. *NYSNA Report, 27,* 2, 3.

———. (1996d, March). Campaign against replacements shocks Mt. Sinai. *NYSNA Report, 27* (3), 13.

———. (1996e, April). NYSNA blows whistle on improper use of technicians. *NYSNA Report, 27* (4), 1.

———. (1996f, May). Will New York City abandon care for the poor? *NYSNA Report, 27* (5), 1, 5.

———. (1996g, June). Nurse educators confront a changing healthcare system. *NYSNA Report, 27* (6), 1, 10.

———. (1996h, June). Nurses protest cuts to NYC public health system. *NYSNA Report, 27* (6), 13.

———. (1996i, June). NYSNA wins final labor board battle with Olean General. *NYSNA Report, 27* (6), 6.

———. (1996j, June). News briefs: Americans worried about cost cutting. *NYSNA Report, 27* (6), 7.

———. (1996k, July/August). Nurses strike at Columbia-Presbyterian. *NYSNA Report, 27* (7), 13.

———. (1996l, July/August). Nurses win sanctions against illegal practice. *NYSNA Report, 27* (7), 8.

———. (1996m, December). NYSNA resolves to fight illegal practice. *NYSNA Report, 27* (10), 1, 13.

———. (1997, February). News briefs: Hospital finds RNs are cost effective. *NYSNA Report, 28* (2), 10.

New York Times News Service. (1995, November 19). Doctors' salaries shrink as managed-care grows. *Syracuse Herald-American,* H1.

Newton, L. H. (1981, June). In defense of the traditional nurse. *Nursing Outlook, 29* (6), 348–354.

Nichols, L. (1992). Estimating costs of underusing advanced practice nurses. *Nursing Economics, 10* (5), 343–351.

Nightingale, F. (1859). *Notes on nursing: What it is and what it is not.* In Nightingale Collection. London: London School of Economics.

———. (1867). *Suggestions on the subject of providing, training and organising nurses, for the sick poor in workhouse infirmaries.* Letter to the President of the Poor Law Board. In Nightingale Collection. London: London School of Economics.

———. (1874). *Suggestions for improving the nursing service of hospitals and the method of training nurses for the sick poor.* In Nightingale Collection. London: London School of Economics.

———. (1893). Sick nursing and health nursing. In *Nursing of the sick, 1893,* ed. I. Hampton, 24. New York: McGraw-Hill.

———. (1928). Cassandra. In *"The cause": A short history of the women's movement in Great Britain,* ed. R. Strachey, 395–418. London: G. Bell and Sons, Ltd.

Nuckolls, K. B. (1974, October). Who decides what the nurse can do? *Nursing Outlook, 22* (10), 626–631.

Nursing Outlook. (1981, September). Responses to "Traditional Nurse." *29* (9), 500–503.

Nutting, M. A. (1913, July). Letter to the editor. *American Journal of Nursing, 13* (660), 743–744.

Nutting, M. A., and L. L. Dock. (1907; 1912). *A history of nursing.* 4 vols. (Vols. 1 and 2, 1907; Vols. 3 and 4, 1912). New York: G. P. Putnam's Sons.

O'Brien, P. (1987, January/February). All a woman's life can bring: The domestic roots of nursing in Philadelphia, 1830–1885. *Nursing Research, 36* (1), 12–17.

O'Connor, K., E. Eckles, and G. Turner. (1993, May). CNE discusses nurses' role in managed competition. *American Nurse, 25* (5), 42.

Office of Technology Assessment. (1986). *Nurse practitioners, physicians' assistants, and certified nurse-midwives: A policy analysis.* (Case Study 37, OTA-HCS-37). Washington, D.C.: Government Printing Office.

Oliver, D. R., R. D. Carter, and J. E. Conboy. (1984, December). Practice characteristics of male and female physician assistants. *American Journal of Public Health, 74* (12), 1398–1400.

O'Neil, E. H., J. Leslie, S. Seifer, J. Kahn, and P. Bailiff. (1993). *Nurse practitioners: Doubling the graduates by the year 2000.* Pew Health Professions Commission. Philadelphia: Pew Charitable Trusts.

Osberg, J. S. (1994, October). Changes in positions of authority held by U.S. physicians: A fresh look at existing data. *American Journal of Public Health, 84* (10), 1573–1575.

Osler, Sir W. (1913, July). Commencement address. *Johns Hopkins Alumnae Magazine, 12,* pp. 72–81.

———. (1932). *Aequanimitas.* Philadelphia: P. Blakiston's Son and Co., Inc.

Otis, E. (1883, November). The trained nurse, a criticism. *Boston Medical and Surgical Journal, 109* (18), 429–430.

Packard, J. H. (1876, November). On the training of nurses for the sick. Speech delivered before the American Social Science Association. *Boston Medical and Surgical Journal, 95* (20), 573–575.

Park, J. (1979, November). Negotiating ambiguity: An aspect of the nurse-doctor relationship. *New Zealand Nursing Journal, 72* (11), 14–16, 36.

Patterson, E. (1994, June). Nursing our medical system back to health. *Delicious,* 10–11.

Pearson, L. J. (1986, November). NPs write prescriptions regardless of enabling legislation. *Nurse Practitioner, 11* (11), 6–7.

———. (1992, January). 1991–92 update: How each state stands on legislative issues affecting advanced nursing practice. *Nurse Practitioner, 17* (1), 14, 16–23.

———. (1996, January). Annual update of how each state stands on legislative issues affecting advanced nursing practice. *Nurse Practitioner, 21* (1), 10, 12ff.

———. (1997, January). Annual update of how each state stands on legislative issues affecting advanced nursing practice. *Nurse Practitioner, 22* (1), 18–86.

Peeno, L. (1998, March 9). A voice for Elizabeth. *U.S. News and World Report.* (Reprinted in *Reader's Digest,* August 1998, 149–153.)

Petty, A. (1993, September 3). Nurse practitioners fight job restrictions. *Wall Street Journal,* sec. B1.

Pew Health Professions Commission. (1995, November). *Critical challenges: Revitalizing the health professions for the twenty-first century.* The Third Report. Washington, D.C.: American Hospital Publishing.

Phillips, J. R. (1979, November). Health care provider relationships: A matter of reciprocity. *Nursing Outlook, 27* (11), 738–741.

Phillips, K. (1999, July/August). Weaving women's health together: A report on the Foundation for Women's Health and the American College of Women's Health Physicians. National Women's Health Network *Network News, 24* (4), 3, 6.

Physician Associate Program. (1972, January). State University of New York at Stony Brook, Health Science Center, School of Allied Health Professions.

Physicians Payment Review Commission. (1991). *Annual report to Congress.* Washington, D.C.: U.S. Congress, House Committee on Ways and Means, Subcommittee on Health.

Piggott, B. M. (1971, June). Disarray in the house of nursing. *Association of Operating Room Nurses Journal, 13,* 56–64.

Pirquet, C. (1927, September). Should the nurse take part in the scientific work of the medical profession? *American Journal of Nursing, 27* (9), 757–758.

Potter, T. (1910, May 14). The nursing problem. *New York Medical Journal, 91,* 995–999.

Power, E. (1921). Women practitioners of medicine in the Middle Ages. *Proceedings of the Royal Society of Medicine.*

Pratt, H. (1965, August). The doctor's view of the changing nurse-physician relationship. *Journal of Medical Education, 40* (8), 767–771.

Preston, A. (1863). *Nursing the sick and the training of nurses.* Philadelphia: King and Baird.

Pulliam, L. (1991). Client satisfaction with a nurse-managed clinic. *Journal of Community Health Nursing, 8* (2), 97–112.

Punnett, L. (1976, July/August). Women-controlled medicine—theory and practice in 19th century Boston. *Women and Health, 1* (4), 3–11.

Raisler, J. (1974). A better nurse-doctor relationship. *Nursing '74, 4,* 21–23.

Ray, W., C. Federspiel, and W. Schaffner. (1980). A study of antipsychotic drug use in nursing homes: Epidemiologic evidence suggesting misuse. *American Journal of Public Health, 70,* 485–491.

Record, J. C., and M. R. Greenlick. (1976). New health professionals and the physician role: An hypothesis from Kaiser experience. *Journal of Nurse-Midwifery, 21* (3), 6–12.

Record, J. C., M. McCally, S. O. Schweitzer, R. M. Blomquist, and B. D. Berger. (1980, Fall). New health professions after a decade and a half: Delegation, productivity, and costs in primary care. *Journal of Health Politics, Policy and Law, 5* (3), 470–497.

Reed, S. (1998, November). Washington Watch. Legislation stalls in Congress. *American Journal of Nursing, 98* (11), 17.

Reiser, S. (1978). *Medicine and the reign of technology.* New York: Cambridge University Press.

Reno, R. (1996, September 8). Health costs still insane, but docs aren't culprits. *Salt Lake Tribune,* AA4–AA5. (From *NewsDay.*)

Report of the Graduate Medical Education National Advisory Committee. (1981). *Nonphysician provider panel.* Vol. 6 (DHHS Publication No. HRA 81–656). Washington, D.C.: Government Printing Office.

Reverby, S. M. (1979). The search for the hospital yardstick: Nursing and the rationalization of hospital work. In *Health care in America: Essays in social history,* ed. S. Reverby and D. Rosner, 206–225. Philadelphia: Temple University Press.

———. (1987). *Ordered to care: The dilemma of American nursing, 1850–1945.* Cambridge: Cambridge University Press.

Rial, W. Y. (1982, April). Who's in charge? *Pennsylvania Medicine, 85* (4), 22, 24.

Richard, Le P. (1868). *La Conquête de Jerusalem.* Published by C. Hippeau (365). Paris: A. Aubry.

Robbins, J. (1996). *Reclaiming our health.* Tiburon, Calif.: H. J. Kramer.

Roberts, H. (1992). *Women's health matters.* New York: Routledge.

Roberts, J. I., and Group, T. M. (1995). *Feminism and nursing: An historical perspective on power, status, and political activism in the nursing profession.* Westport, Conn.: Praeger, Greenwood Publishing Group.

———. *Gender and the nurse-physician game: The impact of changing interrelationships on autonomy and range of practice in health care.* Publication pending.

———. *Men in nursing: Historical perspectives on prejudice and privilege.* Publication pending.

———. *Nurses as caregivers at work and at home: The impact of triple duty, inadequate support, and changing gender expectations on their families and the nursing profession.* Publication pending.

———. *Sexism and nursing: Historical perspectives on the struggle to overcome educational and economic inequities.* Publication pending.

Roberts, M. M. (1932, December). Fusing the triple viewpoints on nursing—Doctors', nurses', and hospital executives'. *Bulletin of the American College of Surgeons, 16,* 32–37.

Robertson, J. D. (1929, February 14). Home and public health nurses and their training. *Journal of the American Medical Association, 74* (7), 481–483.

Robinson, F. N. (Ed.). (1957). *The complete works of Geoffrey Chaucer.* Boston: Houghton Mifflin Co.

Rogers, M. (1972). Nursing: To be or not to be? *Nursing Outlook, 20* (1), 42–46.

Rooks, J. P., N. L. Weatherby, E. K. Ernst, S. Stapleton, D. Rosen, and A. Rosenfeld. (1989, December). The National Birth Center Study: Outcomes of care in birth centers. *New England Journal of Medicine, 321* (26), 1804–1811.

Rosenaur, J., D. Stanford, W. Morgan, and B. Curtin. (1984, January). Prescribing behaviors of primary care nurse practitioners. *American Journal of Public Health, 74* (1), 10–13.

Rosenberg, C. (1984, October). Nurse/physician relations: A perspective from medicine. *Bulletin of the New York Academy of Medicine, 60* (8), 807–810.

Ross, G. (1939, April). Is the health officer fulfilling his responsibility in relation to the nursing program? *American Journal of Public Health, 29* (4), 305–310.

Rossi, J. (1997, April 30). Nursing profession is undervalued. Salt Lake City, Utah: *Citizens,* West edition, 1–2.

Rothberg, J. S. (1973). Nurse and physician's assistant: Issues and relationships. *Nursing Outlook, 21* (3), 154–158.

Rothman, S. M. (1978). *Woman's proper place: A history of changing ideals and practices, 1870 to the present.* New York: Basic Books, Inc.

Rude, H. E. (1922, July 7). Letter, Director, Division of Hygiene, Children's Bureau, to the Hon. Morris Sheppard, Files of the United States Children's Bureau, National Archives, Washington, D.C.

Russell, H. (1854, October 9). The Crimea. *Times* (London), *21* (867), 6–9.

———. (1854, October 12). The Crimea. *Times* (London), *21* (870), 6–9.

———. (1854, October 13). The Crimea. *Times* (London), *21* (871), 6–9.

Ruzek, S. B. (1978). *The women's health movement: Feminist alternatives to medical control.* New York: Praeger Publishers.

Ruzek, S. B., V. Oleson, and A. E. Clarke. (Eds.) (1997). *Women's health: Complexities and differences.* Columbus: Ohio State University Press.

Sackett, D. L., W. O. Spitzer, M. Gent, and , R. Roberts. (1974). The Burlington randomized trial of the nurse practitioner: Health outcomes of patients. *Annals of Internal Medicine, 80,* 137–142.

Safriet, B. J. (1992, Summer). Health-care dollars and regulatory sense: The role of advanced practice nursing. *Yale Journal on Regulation, 9* (2), 417–488.

St. John's House Sisterhood (1874). Statement of the Lady Superior addressed to the Right Honourable, the Lord Hatherley. Privileged communication for Governors of King's College Hospital only.

Salt Lake Tribune. (1997, November 17). Health reform risks. Editorial. A8.

———. (1998, April 23). Doctors' income rises, despite managed care, B6.

Samuel, M. (1906, April 28). What nurses should be taught. *New York Medical Journal, 83* (16), 853–854.

Sandelowski, M. (1980). *Women, health and choice.* St. Louis: C. V. Mosby.

Saunders, L. (1954, September). The changing role of nurses. *American Journal of Nursing, 54* (9), 1094–1098.

Schechter, D. S. (1954, April). Changes in relationships. *Nursing Outlook, 2* (4), 192–193.

Schill, F. (1904, October). Should the medical profession encourage the state registration of nurses? *American Journal of Nursing, 5,* 33–35.

Schoen, E. J., R. J. Erickson, G. Barr, and H. Allen. (1973). The role of pediatric nurse practitioners as viewed by California pediatricians. *California Medicine, 118* (1), 62–68.

Schroeder, S. A. (1993, Winter). The U.S. physician supply: Generalism in retreat. *Bulletin of the New York Academy of Medicine, 70* (3), 103–117.

Schulman, S. (1958). Basic functional roles in nursing: Mother surrogate and healer. In *Patients, physicians, and illness,* ed. E. G. Jaco, 528–537. Glencoe, Ill.: The Free Press.

Schulz, J., G. S. Liptak, and J. Fioravanti. (1994). Nurse practitioners' effectiveness in NICU. *Nursing Management, 25* (10), 50–53.

Schweitzer, J. (1997). *Tears and rage: The nursing crisis in America.* Fair Oaks, Calif.: Adams Blake Publishing.

Scott, K. (1993, June). RN layoffs of growing concern to ANA. *American Nurse, 25* (6), 3, 14.

Seaman, B. (1972). *Free and female.* New York: Coward.

Segal, J., J. Thompson, and R. Floyd. (1979). Drug utilization and prescribing patterns in a skilled nursing facility: The need for a rational approach to therapeutics. *Journal of the American Geriatrics Society, 27* (3), 117–122.

Select Committee of Lords on Metropolitan Hospitals. (1890). *Report: Parliamentary papers, 16* (555), Third International Congress of Nurses, 803.

Sermchief v. Gonzales (1983). 600SW 2nd 683.

Shaffer, E. R. (1995, July/August). Managed care: Your money or your life. National Women's Health Network *Network News, 1,* 4–5.

Sheps, C. G., and M. E. Bachar (1964, September). Nursing and medicine: Emerging patterns of practice. *American Journal of Nursing, 64* (9), 107–109.

Shetland, M. L. (1971, October). An approach to role expansion—The elaborate network. *American Journal of Public Health, 61* (10), 1959–1964.

Shryock, R. H. (1959). *The history of nursing: An interpretation of the social and medical factors involved.* Philadelphia: W. B. Saunders Co.

Siegel, L. (1994, April 17, Sunday). Nurses—not doctors—to run new child, family health clinic. *Salt Lake Tribune,* B-1, B-3.

Sigma Theta Tau International and Nurseweek Publishing. (1999, July 7). Press Release—Harris Poll. From Sigma Theta Tau Web site: http://www.nursingsociety.org.

Silver, H., and J. Hecker (1970). The pediatric nurse practitioner and the child health associate: New types of health professionals. *Journal of Medical Education, 45,* 171–176.

Sims, J. M. (1889). *The story of my life.* New York: Appleton.

Skoblar, S. M., and L. J. Amster. (1977, September). Doctors write an unsolicited Rx for nursing education. *RN, 40,* 40.

Sloane, P., and D. Lekan-Rutledge. (1988). Drug prescribing by telephone: A potential cause of polypharmacy in nursing homes. *American Geriatrics Society, 36* (6), 574–575.

Smeal, E. (1998). Emergency special message. *The Feminist Majority.* Washington, D.C., 1–4.

Smith, L. (1987, July 29). Doctors rule, OK? *Nursing Times, 83* (30), 49–51.

Smoyak, S. A. (1987, January 28). Redefining roles. *Nursing Times, 83* (4), 35–37.

Smoyak, S. A. (1971, June). "A marriage between physicians and nurses." Thanks—but no thanks. *Association of Operating Room Nurses Journal, 13* (6), 53.

———. (1977). Problems in interprofessional relations. *Bulletin of the New York Academy of Medicine, 53* (1), 51–59.

South, J. F. (1857). *Facts relating to hospital nurses.* London: Richardson.

Sox, H. C., Jr. (1979, September). Quality of patient care by nurse practitioners and physician's assistants: A ten-year perspective. *Annals of Internal Medicine, 91* (3), 459–468.

———. (2000, January). Independent primary care practice by nurse practitioners. *Journal of the American Medical Association, 283* (1), 106–108.

Speakman, E. H. (1902). Womanliness in nursing. *American Journal of Nursing, 3,* 182.

Spisso, J., C. O'Callaghan, M. McKennan, and H. J. Holcroft. (1990). Improved quality of care and reduction of house staff workload using trauma nurse practitioners. *Journal of Trauma, 30* (6), 660–665.

Spitzer, W. O., D. L. Sackett, J. C. Sibley, R. Roberts, M. Gent, D. Kergin, B. Hackett, and A. Olynich. (1974). The Burlington randomized trial of the nurse practitioner. *New England Journal of Medicine, 290,* 251–256.

Spragins, E. (1996, June 24). Does your HMO stack up? *Newsweek,* 56–61.

Stanley, I. (1983, September, 21). Where do we stand with doctors? *Nursing Times, 79* (38), 46–48.

Starr, P. (1982). *The social transformation of American medicine.* New York: Basic Books.

Steele, Dr. (1871). The nursing arrangements in Guy's Hospital. In *Guy's Hospital Reports,* ed. Fagge and Durham. Vol. 16, 3rd series, 541–555.

Stein, L. (1967, June). The doctor-nurse game. *Archives of General Psychiatry, 16,* 699–703.

Stephany, T. M. (1992, May). Skill mix change may be a trap. *American Nurse* 24 (5), 4.

Stepsis, U., and D. Liptak. (Eds.) (1989). *Pioneer healers: The history of women religious in American health care.* New York: Crossroad.

Stevens, B. J. (1984, October). Nurse/physician relations: A perspective from nursing. *Bulletin of the New York Academy of Medicine, 60* (8), 799–806.

Stillman, W. O. (1910, January 15). A successful experiment in educating efficient nurses for persons of moderate income. *New York Medical Journal, 91,* 110–112.

Styles, M., and M. Gottdank. (1976, December). Nursing's vulnerability. *American Journal of Nursing, 76* (12), 1978–1980.

Sullivan, E. M. (1992, May). Nurse practitioners reimbursement. *Nursing and Health Care, 13* (5), 236–241.

Tarlov, A. R. (1995, November). Estimating physician workforce requirements. *Journal of the American Medical Association, 274* (19), 1558–1560.

Thayer, W. S. (1919, December). Nursing and the art of medicine. *American Journal of Nursing, 20,* 187–192.

Thompson, M. A. (1996, October). Letter to the editor. *American Nurse, 28* (7), 5.

Thompson, W. G. (1906, April 28). The over-trained nurse. *New York Medical Journal, 83* (11), 851.

Thornton, L. (1983, June 29). Giving in to the stereotype. *Nursing Times, 79* (26), 11–12.

Times (London) (1884, October 3). 9.

Titus, S. (1952, September). Economic facts of life for nurses. *American Journal of Nursing, 52* (9), 1109–1110.

Todd, A. D. (1989). *Intimate adversaries: Cultural conflict between doctors and women patients.* Philadelphia: University of Pennsylvania Press.

Torrence, G. (1917). The trained nurse. *Boston Medical and Surgical Journal, 176,* 573.

Trall, R. (1850). Allopathic midwifery. *Water Cure Journal, 9,* 121.

U. S. Commission on Civil Rights. (1979). *Window dressing on the set.* Washington, D.C.: Government Printing Office.

Vanderbilt, M. W. (1992, January). Bills would benefit advanced practice RNs. *American Nurse, 24* (1), 7.

———. (1993, May). Medicaid bill introduced for nurse reimbursement. *American Nurse, 25* (5), 11.

———. (1994, July/August). Senate committee votes yes on amendment providing Medicare reimbursement to RNs. *American Nurse, 26* (7), 2.

Vanderbilt, M. W., and D. Keepnews. (1995, November/December). Nurses denounce proposed cuts, changes in Medicare, Medicaid. *American Nurse, 27* (10), 1, 3.

Vanderbilt, M. W., and S. Reed. (1996, April/May). ANA posts big wins in contentious/ challenging 104th Congress. *American Nurse, 28* (3), 10–11.

Van Ness, E. (1927, March). Teamwork from the doctors. *American Journal of Nursing, 27* (3), 167–170.

Versluysen, M. C. (1980). Old wives' tales? Women healers in English history. In *Rewriting nursing history,* ed. C. Davies, 175–199. Totowa, N.J.: Croom Helm.

Vintras, L. (1894, April 14). The ethics of nursing. *Hospital,* xxiii–xxx.

Wade, M. (1996, January). From the president. *NYSNA Report, 27* (1), 2.

Wald, L. (1912a). *New aspects of an old profession.* Speech, Wellesley College. New York Public Library, Wald Mss.

———. (1912b, October). Lecture, Board of Health, New York Public Library, Wald Mss.

———. (1930, March 10). Letter to Agnes Leach, New York Public Library, Wald Mss.

Walsh, L. V. (1988, April). Alternative health care delivery systems—nursing opportunity or threat? *Nurse Practitioner, 13* (4), 56, 61, 64.

Walsh, M. R. (1977). *Doctors wanted: No women need apply—Sexual barriers in the medical profession, 1835–1975.* New Haven, Conn.: Yale University Press.

Warrington, J. (1839). *The nurses guide: Containing a series of instructions to females who wish to engage in the important business of nursing mother and child in the lying-in chamber.* Philadelphia: Thomas, Cowperthwaite.

Wear, D. (Ed.). (1996). *Women in medical education: An anthology of experience.* Albany: State University of New York Press.

West, M. (1999, December 8). Women face care gap, report says. *Arizona Republic,* B1, B6.

White, R. (1978). *Social change and the development of the nursing profession.* London: Henry Kimpton Publishers.

Whittaker, S., and L. Minich. (1995, October). Pew efforts seek to change how health professions are regulated. *American Nurse, 27* (7), 1, 14.

Wilburn, S. (1996, October). MNA study captures national attention. *American Nurse, 28* (7), 15.

Wile, I. S. (1924, February). The relation of the public health nurse to the practicing physician: The viewpoint of the physician. *American Journal of Public Health, 14* (2), 106–111.

Williams, J. (1996, April/May). Labor groups strive to protect workers in growing managed care era. *American Nurse, 28* (3), 23.

Williams, J. E., and D. L. Best. (1982). *Measuring sex stereotypes: A thirty-nation study.* Beverly Hills, Calif.: Sage Publications.

Williams, K. (1980). From Sarah Gamp to Florence Nightingale: A critical study of hospital nursing systems from 1840 to 1897. In *Rewriting nursing history,* ed. C. Davies, 41–75. Totowa, N.J.: Croom Helm.

Wolfe, S. M. (1997). Editorial. *Worst pills/best pills news.* Washington, D.C.: Public Citizen.

Wolinsky, H., and T. Brune. (1995). *The serpent on the staff: The unhealthy politics of the American Medical Association.* New York: Tarcher/Putnam.

Woodham-Smith, C. (1950). *Florence Nightingale.* London: Constable.

Worcester, A. (1887, August 25). The training of nurses in private practice. *Boston Medical and Surgical Journal, 117* (9), 193–194.

Wright, E. (1975, December). Family nurse clinicians: Physicians' perspective. *Nursing Outlook, 23* (12), 771–773.

Yankauer, A., J. P. Connelly, and J. J. Feldman (1970, March). Pediatric practice in the United States—With special attention to utilization of allied health worker services. *Pediatrics, 45* (3), Suppl: 521–554.

Yankauer, A., and J. Sullivan. (1982). The new health professionals: Three examples. *Annual Review of Public Health, 3,* 249–276.

Zaslove, M. O., J. T. Ungerleider, and M. Fuller. (1968, October). The importance of the psychiatric nurse: Views of physicians, patients, and nurses. *American Journal of Psychiatry, 125* (4), 74–78.

INDEX

THETIS M. GROUP is Professor Emerita at Syracuse University, where she was Dean of the College of Nursing for ten years. She is also adjunct faculty member at the University of Utah College of Nursing. She is co-author of *Feminism and Nursing* and has published numerous articles in professional nursing journals.

JOAN I. ROBERTS, social psychologist, is Professor Emerita at Syracuse University. A pioneer in Women's Studies in higher education, she is co-author of *Feminism and Nursing* and author of numerous books and articles on gender issues and racial and sex discrimination.